Human Tumor Cells *in Vitro*

Human Tumor Cells *in Vitro*

EDITED BY JØRGEN FOGH

Donald S. Walker Laboratory
Sloan–Kettering Institute for Cancer Research
Rye, New York

SPRINGER SCIENCE+BUSINESS MEDIA, LLC

Library of Congress Cataloging in Publication Data

Fogh, Jørgen.
Human tumor cells in vitro.

Includes bibliographies and index.
1. Cancer cells. 2. Pathology, Experimental. 3. Human cell culture.
I. Title. [DNLM: 1. Cell transformation, Neoplastic. QZ206 F655h]
RC268.F63 616.9'92'0028 74-26959

ISBN 978-1-4757-1649-8 ISBN 978-1-4757-1647-4 (eBook)
DOI 10.1007/978-1-4757-1647-4

Originally published by Plenum Press, New York in 1975
Softcover reprint of the hardcover 1st edition 1975

Contributors

Michael A. Bean Memorial Sloan–Kettering Cancer Center, New York, New York.

June L. Biedler Memorial Sloan–Kettering Cancer Center, New York, New York.

Relda M. Cailleau Department of Medicine, M. D. Anderson Hospital and Tumor Institute, University of Texas at Houston, Houston, Texas.

Leon Dmochowski Department of Virology, The University of Texas, M. D. Anderson Hospital and Tumor Institute at Houston, Texas Medical Center, Houston, Texas.

Audrey Fjelde Roswell Park Memorial Institute, Buffalo, New York.

Jørgen Fogh Walker Laboratory, Sloan–Kettering Institute for Cancer Research, Rye, New York.

Steven I. Hajdu Memorial Sloan–Kettering Cancer Center, New York, New York.

Teddy Holmström Department of Pathology, University of Helsinki, Helsinki, Finland.

Etienne Y. Lasfargues Institute for Medical Research, Camden, New Jersey.

Albert Leibovitz Scott and White Clinic, Temple, Texas.

Joseph Leighton Cancer Bioassay Laboratory, Department of Pathology, The Medical College of Pennsylvania, Philadelphia, Pennsylvania.

George E. Moore Surgical Oncology, Denver General Hospital, and University of Colorado Medical Center, Denver, Colorado.

Jan Pontén Division of Cell Biology, The Wallenberg Laboratory, University of Uppsala, Uppsala, Sweden.

Arnis Richters University of Southern California, School of Medicine, Department of Pathology, Los Angeles, California.

F. KINGSLEY SANDERS Walker Laboratory, Sloan–Kettering Institute for Cancer Research, Rye, New York.

GABRIEL SEMAN Department of Virology, The University of Texas, M. D. Anderson Hospital and Tumor Institute at Houston, Texas Medical Center, Houston, Texas.

RUSSELL P. SHERWIN University of Southern California, School of Medicine, Department of Pathology, Los Angeles, California.

JOHN A. SYKES Research Department, Southern California Cancer Center, California Hospital Medical Center, Los Angeles, California.

RUY TCHAO Cancer Bioassay Laboratory, Department of Pathology, The Medical College of Pennsylvania, Philadelphia, Pennsylvania.

GERMAIN TREMPE Memorial Sloan–Kettering Cancer Center, New York, New York.

EM. WOLFF Laboratoire d'Embryologie Experimentale, Collège de France, Nogent S/Marne, France.

ET. WOLFF Laboratoire d'Embryologie Experimentale, Collège de France, Nogent S/Marne, France.

Preface

The study of cultured human tumor cells is a most obvious approach in experimental human cancer research. For many techniques in virology, immunology, biochemistry, and biophysics, for example, large amounts of cells may be required and such quantities are usually provided only when the cultures develop into established cell lines; when this happens, thorough characterization also becomes possible. The development of cell lines, therefore, is of prime importance. Recent major advances in research with animal cell systems seem to be a prologue for present and future efforts directed toward work with human tumor cells in culture. Conceivably, the most significant results in cancer research may develop from work with such cells, and so the time seemed right to define the present state of our knowledge. This is the first book dedicated exclusively to the subject: human tumor cells *in vitro.* Although some of the fundamental aspects in the cultivation of human tumor cells, and the extent to which they represent human cancer *in vivo* are still unclear, I asked a number of the leading investigators in this area of research to collect and evaluate previous and present contributions, and to offer their thoughts on the questions to which answers are not yet available.

Many of the chapters are concerned with techniques of cultivation. Cultures from some types of tumors have grown well; in many cases they have given rise to established cell lines. Other types have shown less encouraging results, and there are still tumors which are not represented as cell lines. Although many tumor cell lines have become available, considering the numerous attempts, success has usually been the exception.

Some of the problems faced daily in the tissue culture laboratory may seem trivial. For example, are the cells we observe in early cultures actually the tumor cells, or are they derived from other cells of the tumor tissue? Contamination with extraneous cells is known to occur in work with established cell lines. Unfortunately, there is evidence that many investigations have been carried out without proper attention to such problems. This book contains information about new and old methods for monitoring and evaluation of the cultured cells as to malignancy and confirmation of origin. Other chapters are oriented more toward explorative research approaches employing human tumor cells, for example, search for causative viruses.

If future trends in cancer research will be toward further exploration of human tumor cell systems as model systems for human cancer, and toward greater attention to cell characterization, the efforts that have gone into this book will not have been needless. I am grateful to all the contributors and to the staff of Plenum Publishing, Inc. A special thanks to Shirley DeVore and Gwendolyn Holmes for their work in attending to the many details of the book and to the preparation of the list of published cell lines established from human tumors.

Rye, New York Jørgen Fogh

Contents

2 Development of Media for Isolation and Cultivation of Human Cancer Cells

ALBERT LEIBOVITZ

3 New Approaches to the Cultivation of Human Breast Carcinomas

ETIENNE Y. LASFARGUES

4 Old and New Problems in Human Tumor Cell Cultivation

RELDA M. CAILLEAU

5 New Human Tumor Cell Lines

JØRGEN FOGH AND GERMAIN TREMPE

6 Human Brain Tumor Cells in Matrix Culture

TEDDY HOLMSTRÖM

7 Neoplastic Human Glia Cells in Culture

JAN PONTÉN

8 Current Research with Organ Cultures of Human Tumors

ET. WOLFF AND EM. WOLFF

9 Metabolic Gradients in Tissue Culture Studies of Human Cancer Cells

JOSEPH LEIGHTON AND RUY TCHAO

10 Human Lung Cancer in Tissue Culture

RUSSELL P. SHERWIN AND ARNIS RICHTERS

11 Cell Lines from Humans with Hematopoietic Malignancies

GEORGE E. MOORE

12 Cytological Characterization of Human Tumor Cells from Monolayer Cultures

MICHAEL A. BEAN AND STEVEN I. HAJDU

13 Chromosome Abnormalities in Human Tumor Cells in Culture

JUNE L. BIEDLER

14 Ultrastructural Characteristics of Human Tumor Cells *in Vitro*

GABRIEL SEMAN AND LEON DMOCHOWSKI

15 The Strategy of a Search for Viral Involvement in Human Cancer

F. KINGSLEY SANDERS

16 Helper Activity for the Defective Friend Leukemia Virus in Human Malignant Cell Cultures

AUDREY FJELDE

Separation of Tumor Cells from Fibroblasts 1

JOHN A. SYKES

1. Introduction

It is well known that clinical and experimental microbiology made little progress until 1881, when Robert Koch described his method of preparing cultures on solid media. The use of solid media permitted rapid separation of different types of bacteria, and thus allowed the selected organisms to be grown out into pure cultures for further study. The art of tissue culture is somewhat akin to microbiology before the year 1881. It is very difficult to obtain "pure" cultures of selected cell types from most organs and tissues of man and animals. In studies of human tumors, this problem is particularly exasperating; the desired cell is the tumor cell, but the cell usually obtained is the fibroblast from the connective tissue elements associated with the tumor. The technique most widely used to obtain cultures of cells from organs and tissues of mammals utilizes controlled enzyme activity to break down the tissue fragment into a suspension of single cells or small groups of cells. The technique has proved effective for many tissues, particularly those derived from embryos or from organs without much fibrous stroma; however, adult tissues and those with abundant fibrous stroma provide a challenge and a stumbling block for the tissue culturist, who as it were wants the wheat, not the chaff and weeds. The methodology to be described, when tailored to the

JOHN A. SYKES Research Department, Southern California Cancer Center, California Hospital Medical Center, Los Angeles, California system being studied, has usually proved effective in separating a high proportion of tumor cells from the "contaminating" fibroblasts.

2. *Methodology of Others*

The literature on centrifugal methods for the separation of different types of blood cells is voluminous and is well documented by Abeloff *et al.* (1970) and by Böyum (1968). Methods for the separation of different cell types are few and in most cases particular to the problems of specific scientific studies (Ali and Fletcher, 1971; Giorgi, 1971; Johnson *et al.*, 1970; Leeman *et al.*, 1971; Schindler *et al.*, 1970). Separation of tumor cells from normal cells was attempted by Mateyko and Kopac (1963), who tested more than 200 substances and showed that although "isopycnotic" solutions could be prepared that were suitable for the centrifugation of cells of different types, none was ideal. Preservation of cellular morphology, staining, and viability were generally rather poor. All tissue culturists are familiar with the scraping technique for the physical removal of colonies of the cell type desired from a mixed culture and the lack of success in obtaining the desired result—growth of a "clean" cell type. The introduction of Ficoll (Holter and Møller, 1958) as a suitable material for aqueous density gradients made possible successful cell separations by centrifugation such as those for mast cells by Uvnäs and Thon (1959) and by Johnson and Moran (1966), who compared use of Ficoll solutions with other methods. They considered Ficoll preferable to other substances, such as sucrose, for isolation of rat peritonal mast cells as osmotic damage was negligible. Walder and Lumseth (1963) used Ficoll gradients in their studies of rabbit gastric mucosal cells. More recently, the problem of preparing pure cell populations from solid human tumors was studied by Boone *et al.* (1968). They used a continuous Ficoll gradient with an A-1X zonal centrifuge rotor and a book of computer-prepared charts relating sedimentation position, velocity, and time for the particular cells being studied. The cost and complexity of their system led us (Sykes *et al.*, 1970*b*) to seek a simpler and cheaper method. Our technique is described in the following pages.

3. *Experimental Studies—Materials and Methods*

3.1. *Cells*

The preliminary studies were made with epithelioid cells from established lines derived from human tumors and with fibroblasts from early passage cultures originating from biopsies of human breast tumors. The following established cell lines of human origin were used: BT-20 (Lasfargues and Ozzello (1958), derived from a human breast carcinoma (obtained from Dr. L. Ozzello, Institute de Pathologie, Hospital Cantonal University, Lausanne, Switzerland; CMP (Rounds, 1970), from an adenocarcinoma of the bowel (obtained from Dr. D. Rounds, Pasadena Foundation for Medical Research, Pasadena, Calif.); HeLa (Gey *et al.*, 1952), from a carcinoma of the cervix (obtained from Dr. E. P. Byatt, University of California, Los Angeles, Calif.); and ME-180 (Sykes *et al.*, 1970*a*), from a metastatic carcinoma of the cervix in our own laboratory.

Fibroblasts were grown and maintained in Eagle's minimal essential medium (MEM) supplemented with 30% heat-inactivated fetal calf serum (CM). The tumor cell lines were grown and maintained in MEM supplemented with 10% heat-inactivated fetal calf serum. The antibiotics streptomycin and neomycin were added to all culture media, the former at 0.1 g/liter, the latter at 0.25 g/liter.

Cells were detached from the surface of the culture vessels with trypsin–versene solution (0.25% trypsin, 0.01% versene in phosphate-buffered saline at pH 8.0).

3.2. Density Gradients

Following unsuccessful experiments with sucrose and with various other substances, density gradients were constructed with solutions of Ficoll, a synthetic sucrose polymer of average molecular weight 400,000 (Pharmacia Fine Chemicals, Piscataway, New Jersey).

Various concentrations of Ficoll were prepared with MEM as solvent, and the osmotic effect of these solutions was tested on different cell lines. No detectable differences were noted in the cell diameters of any of the cell lines before or after exposure to these Ficoll solutions.

3.3. Ficoll Solutions

A stock solution of Ficoll was prepared by dissolving 100 g of the polymer in 100 ml of MEM at pH 7.0 heated to 60°C in a water bath. The fine white powder was stirred into the warm MEM until it formed a homogeneous mixture; the container was covered with aluminum foil and left at 60°C until the solution had become water clear. It was then removed from the water bath and allowed to cool to ambient temperature (23°C). Three or more random dilutions were prepared from this stock solution using MEM as

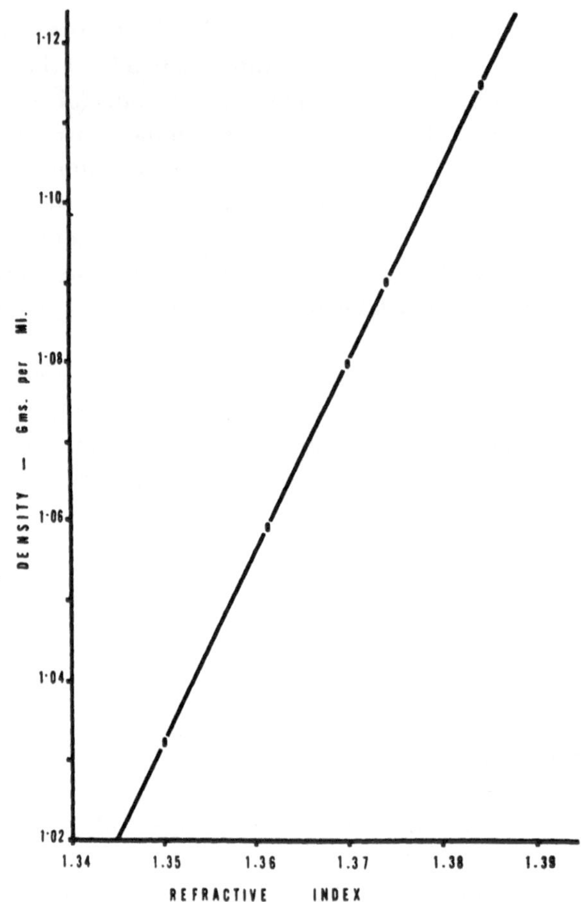

FIG. 1. Relationship of density to refractive index for solutions of Ficoll in MEM at 23°C.

diluent. The refractive index of each dilution was measured at 23°C (room temperature) using a Zeiss Abbé refractometer, and the density of each of these solutions was determined by weighing 50 ml in a specific gravity bottle. Refractive index was then plotted against density (Fig. 1). This graph was used thereafter to determine the refractive index of the Ficoll solutions having the desired densities. Stock solution was diluted with MEM to obtain the desired refractive index, which therefore gave a solution of the desired density. Ficoll solutions with densities ranging from 1.025 to 1.100 g/ml in steps of 0.005 g/ml were prepared, and samples of these solutions were taken at random for a density check by weighing. Absolute correlation with the plot was obtained, therefore, until a given batch of Ficoll was finished; densities were calculated by determining the refractive index and using the plot.

As the purpose of the studies was to obtain cell cultures of a single cell type from a population of cell types, it was necessary to observe strict asepsis in all procedures. Ficoll solutions in phosphate-buffered saline sterilized by autoclaving were found inhibitory to the growth of some cells. Therefore, all solutions were sterilized by filtration through 0.22-μm membrane filters (Millipore Filter Corp., Bedford, Mass., Nalge Sybron Corp., Rochester, N.Y.). To facilitate filtration, the solutions were warmed to 60°C to lower their viscosity and simplify the filtration.

For cells obtained from surgical specimens and in current experimental studies, the Ficoll solutions have been made with Ca^{2+}– free MEM. It has been found desirable to prepare duplicate density series of Ficoll, one containing phenol red as indicator, the other not; the gradient then is built by alternating densities of colored and uncolored solutions. This facilitates collection of material from the interface zones of the discontinuous gradients.

3.4. Preparation of Gradients

Linear gradients were prepared using Ficoll solutions having densities of 1.025 and 1.100 g/ml with an apparatus modified from that described by Britten and Roberts (1960).

Discontinuous or step gradients were prepared by sequential addition of appropriate volumes of the chosen solutions (Table 1), beginning with the most dense. These solutions were pipetted into sterile 4- by 1.3-cm cellulose nitrate centrifuge tubes. The tubes were sterilized with ultraviolet light by overnight exposure with tops facing upward 20 cm below a G.E. 18-inch germicidal lamp. These tubes fit the buckets of the Beckman Spinco SW-40

TABLE 1

Discontinuous Gradient Structure

Volume (ml)	Density[a] (g/ml)	Refractive index[a]
0.5	1.025	1.3490
0.5	1.050	1.3590
1.0	1.055	1.3612
1.0	1.060	1.3635
1.0	1.065	1.3652
0.5	1.085	1.3736

[a]Measured at 23°C.

and SW-50 rotors. Occasionally, tubes were sterilized by soaking in 75% ethanol for 10 min followed by rinsing with sterile distilled water and then sterile MEM. The tubes were shaken free of almost all traces of liquid before building of the gradients.

Before addition of Ficoll solutions, 12 drops of light mineral oil (viscosity 80–90) was placed in each tube to insure smooth layering of the solutions, to protect the centrifuge by preventing evaporation under the vacuum during centrifugation, and to help preserve the sterility of the tube contents.

3.5. Centrifugation

All density gradient centrifugations were done in a Beckman Spinco L2-HV preparative ultracentrifuge using the SW-50 rotor at an ambient temperature of 23°C. Gradients were centrifuged at an average RCF of 8161 g (10,000 rpm). Linear gradients were centrifuged for 60 min and discontinuous gradients for 10 min under the above conditions unless otherwise specified.

3.6. Fraction Collection

Opalescent bands seen after centrifugation of continuous gradients and the interface zones of the discontinuous gradients were collected by bottom puncture, with the apparatus previously described (Sykes *et al.*, 1964) and

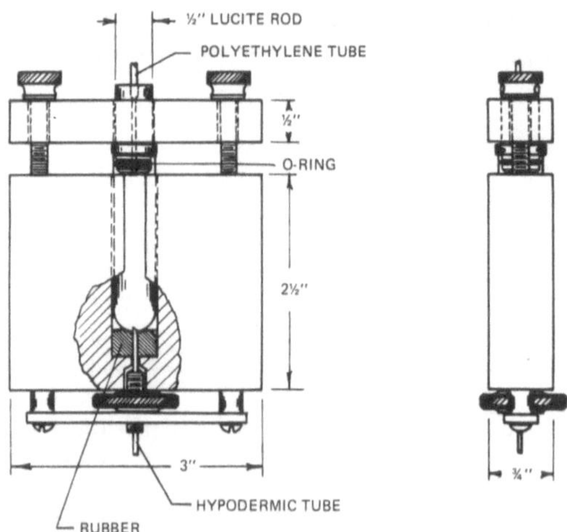

FIG. 2. Mechanical drawing of the apparatus used for collecting fractions by bottom puncture.

illustrated in Fig. 2. Before insertion of the centrifuge tube, the needle and rubber pad were flushed with 95% ethanol and blown dry with Freon.

Fractions from both linear and discontinuous gradients which were to be cultured were collected directly into 5–10 ml of culture medium. Cultures were made from these fractions in glass T-30 culture flasks (Bellco Glass Inc., Vineland, N.J.) or in plastic T-30 flasks (Falcon Plastics, Los Angeles, Calif.). Cultures were fed and maintained with MEM enriched with 30% fetal calf serum (heat inactivated). Fractions that were to be used for counting and measuring of cells were collected into 1–2 ml of the same culture medium.

3.7. Density Determinations

For linear gradients, the density of the Ficoll above and below the opalescent bands was determined by measurement of the refractive index of 2 drops of solution, and after taking the arithmetic mean of the two refractive indices, reference to the density–refractive index plot gave the density for the centre of the band. For discontinuous gradients, measurements indicated that bands of cells collected only at the interface zones between adjacent densities.

3.8. Cell Counts and Cell Diameters

Cells were counted in a bright-line hemocytometer chamber using low-magnification phase contrast optics, and diameters were measured using a focusing eyepiece equipped with a suitable micrometer disc. Using this combination with a 40× objective permitted measurements of cell diameters with an accuracy of ± 3 μm.

The weighted mean cell diameter was calculated by application of the formula $\sum_0^n A_iB_i/\sum_0^n A_i$ to the results obtained from counting and measuring the cells in a particular sample; A_i represents the number of cells of a specific diameter B_i.

3.9. Virus Studies

The following viruses were used with ME-180 cells as substrate: vaccinia, poliovirus I (Mahoney), and echovirus (type 1); in addition, a culture of ME-180, carrying influenza A_0-WSN in its thirteenth passage, was used. Cultures were infected with an amount of virus sufficient to produce a gross cytopathogenic effect within 7 days, but insufficient to visibly affect the cultures at 2 days. (No virus titrations were made for these preliminary studies.) Identical uninfected cultures served as controls. Infected and uninfected cells were removed (with trypsin–versene) from the flasks 48 h after infection with a particular virus. Exposure of the cells to the enzyme mixture was limited to 10 min at 37°C. Cell suspensions were than diluted with Ca^{2+}-free MEM, and the cells were sedimented by centrifugation at 900 g for 15 min at a temperature of 5°C. The cells were resuspended in a volume of fresh Ca^{2+}-free MEM and counted before centrifugation as before. the cell pellets were resuspended in Ficoll solution of density 1.025 g/ml, and the volumes were adjusted to give equal numbers of cells per unit volume from the infected and uninfected cell cultures. The resuspended cells in volumes of 0.5 ml were layered onto discontinuous gradients which included an additional step of 1.075 g/ml. The opalescent zones at the density interface areas following centrifugation at an RCF of 8151 g for 10 min at 23°C were aseptically collected by bottom puncture of the tubes into 2-ml volumes of CM. The cells from each zone were counted and measured before the addition of 8 ml CM to each sample tube and the transfer of the material to T-30 culture flasks. Cultures from the different zones were examined daily for evidence of cytopathic changes and discarded at 10 days if no changes had been observed.

3.10 Evaluation of Cultures

Cultures were washed with Hank's BSS, stained with Wright's stain, and examined by bright-field microscopy to determine the cell types grown from a particular zone.

4. Results

To determine the buoyant densities of the fibroblasts and of the epithelial cells, centrifugation experiments patterned after those described by Boone *et al.* (1968) were made. Fibroblasts derived from cultures of more than 20 human breast tumors were examined and found to have an average maximum buoyant density of 1.049 g/ml under the conditions described. The epithelial cells examined were found to have an average maximum buoyant density of 1.067 g/ml. When the opalescent zones from continuous Ficoll gradients which had been overlaid with mixtures of fibroblasts and epithelial cells were examined after centrifugation at 8161 g for 60 min, it was found that mixtures of the cell types were present in each band. Centrifugation of replicate tubes for an additional 30 min failed to produce either separation of the two cell types or movement of the bands of cells. These findings suggested that either the technique (linear Ficoll gradients) was at fault or the tubes used (4 by 1.3 cm) were too short to obtain separation of epithelial cells from fibroblasts. It was evident, therefore, that some other technique would be needed if the desired separation of cell types was to be obtained with the tubes and rotors available.

In disc gel electrophoresis, the behavior of macromolecules crossing a density interface suggested that a "sieving" effect on the different molecular sizes was occurring because of the sudden discontinuities in density. It was theorized that if such a system could be used with centrifugal force rather than an electromotive force then the desired separation to cell types might result. Preliminary studies with discontinuous Ficoll gradients using densites of 1.0125, 1.055, and 1.085 g/ml overlaid with mixtures of fibroblasts and epithelial cells gave encouraging results. Discontinuous gradients having more density steps were next investigated and appeared to give complete separation of some of the epithelial cells from the fibroblasts as judged from cultures of the material collected from the interfaces. The results were reproducible except when large numbers of cells were overlaid on the gradient.

The method was refined by investigation of different density combinations and cell numbers, leading to the adoption of a standard discontinuous gradient structured as indicated in Table 1. It was found that when mixtures of fibroblasts and epithelial cells not exceeding 3×10^6 total cells were centrifuged on gradients of this type for 10 min at 8161 g only epithelial cells (determined by culture) were recovered from the material at the 1.065–1085 g/ml interface zone. The appearance of a gradient of this type before loading is shown in Fig. 3a. Cultures made from the density junctions or interfaces of such a gradient used to separate fibroblasts from ME-180 cells demonstrated that the two upper junctions (1.025–1.050 and 1.050–1.055 g/ml) consisted of fibroblasts with relatively few ME-180 cells (Fig. 3b); cultures from the next two junctions or interfaces (1.055–1.060 and 1.060–1.065 g/ml) showed an increase in the number of ME-180 cells relative to the number of fibroblasts which was greater at the 1.060–1.065 g/ml interface (Fig. 3c). Cultures from the 1.065–1.085 g/ml interface yielded only ME-180 cells (Fig. 3d). When more than 3×10^6 cells were used for the overlay, fibroblasts were occasionally found in the cultures from the 1.065–1.085 g/ml interface.

These studies were repeated using cells from different fibroblast cultures and other epithelial cell lines, with the same result—cultures of only epithelial cells were obtained from the lowest interface. To determine how

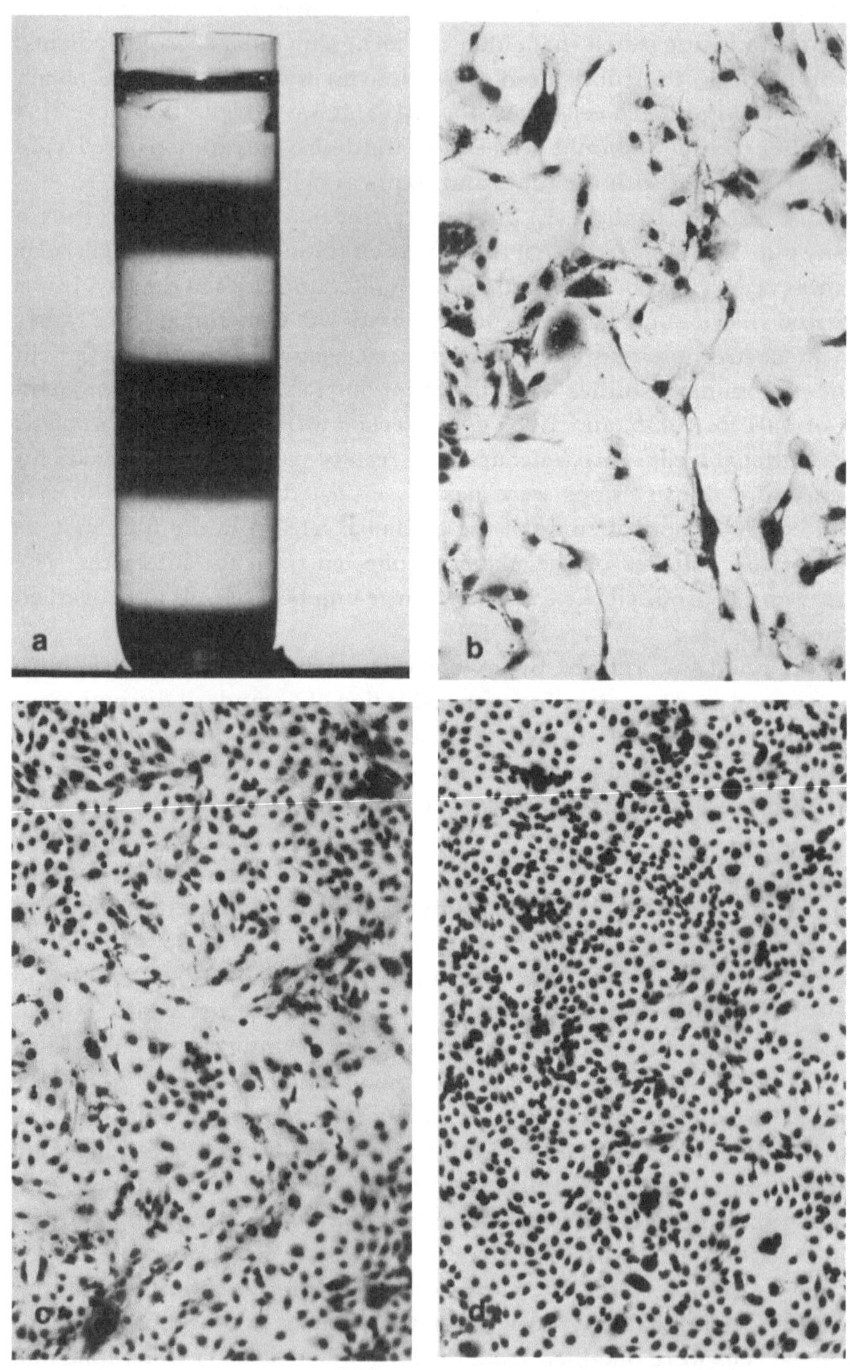
a
b
c
d

the experimental results using 3×10^6 cells compared to theoretical considerations, calculations were made to determine the number of epithelial cells that might form a monolayer on an interface in a tube with diameter of 1.3 cm. Assuming a cell diameter of 16–20 μm, a monolayer would be obtained with 60×10^4 cells. As the gradients used had four interfaces at which fibroblasts could be held back, it was theorized that $2–3 \times 10^6$ cells could be centrifuged on the standard gradient without overloading and break-through of fibroblasts to the 1.065–1.085 g/ml interface. Thus theory and practice were in agreement. Repeated experiments with different fibroblasts and epithelial cells and with different proportions of one to the other were carried out using 2–3 times the theoretical maximum number of cells ($2–3 \times 10^6$), and all gave satisfactory separation of epithelial cells from fibroblasts at the 1.065–1.085 g/ml interface. As a routine procedure and in an attempt to make the method more "foolproof," a maximum loading of 3×10^6 cells per tube was adopted.

In experiments to determine the minimum of cells that could be loaded on a standard discontinuous gradient and still permit recovery of epithelial cells at the lowest interface, various numbers of ME-180 were used. ME-180 cells have a plating efficiency of about 50% (Sykes *et al.*, 1970*a*), and positive cultures could be obtained from the lowest interface when as few as 900 cells were layered on the gradient.

As a result of the experimental studies described above, this technique was applied to surgical biopsy specimens from different types of tumors, particularly breast tumors. Two major problems have been encountered with tumor material: difficulty in obtaining a single cell suspension and the presence of fatty material which appears to coat some cells, usually the tumor cells, and to prevent (by flotation) their migration to the proper interface. Studies so far carried out with lipase treatment of the cell suspensions have been unsuccessful. The method has been shown to be applicable to some breast tumors when the fat content is minimal. Cells derived from a fibroadenoma of the breast in a 25-year-old female gave a satisfactory single cell suspension when the tissue was digested with trypsin–versene rather than trypsin alone, and cultures from the upper

FIG. 3. (a) Appearance of a standard discontinuous Ficoll gradient before centrifugation. The appearance does not change during centrifugation. (b) Typical appearance of a culture taken from the 1.025–1.050 or 1.050–1.055 g/ml zone of a discontinuous Ficoll gradient which had been loaded with a mixture of fibroblasts and ME-180 cells. The preponderant cells in these cultures are fibroblasts. Wright's stain. Magnification × 60. (c) Appearance of cultures taken from the same gradient as in (b), but at the 1.055–1.060 or 1.060–1.065 g/ml zone. Relatively few fibroblasts can be found in cultures from these zones. Wright's stain. Magnification × 60. (d) Appearance of cultures taken from the same gradient as in (b), but at the 1.065–1.085 g/ml zone. Only tumor cells (ME-180) can be found in these cultures. Wright's stain. Magnification × 60.

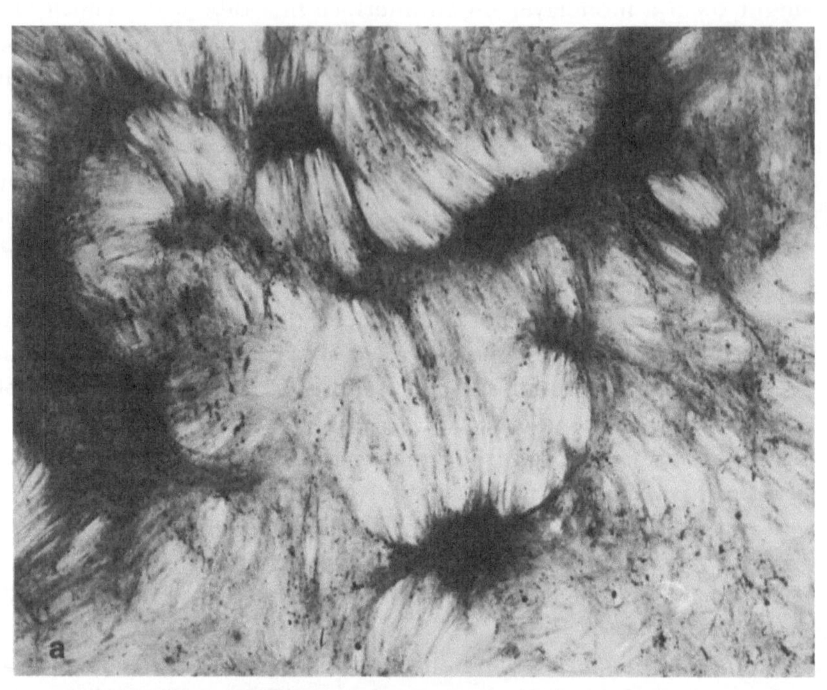
a

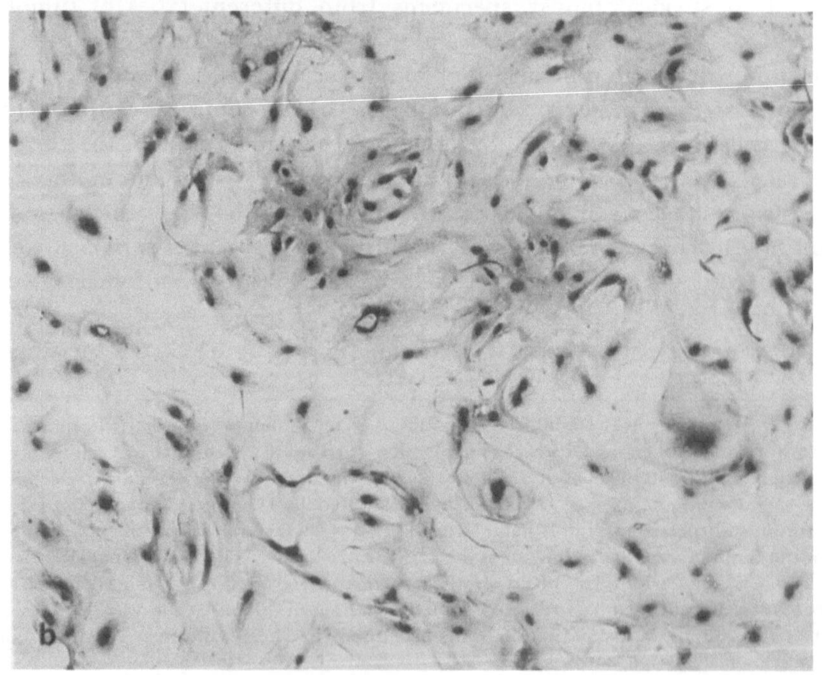
b

TABLE 2

Centrifugal Force and Cell Recovery[a]

Relative centrifugal force	Zone	Number ($\times 10^6$) cells recovered	Weighted mean cell diameter (μm)
	A	2.660	20.588
	B	0.954	18.108
8000*g*	C	1.820	17.105
	D	1.681	16.958
	E	3.870	16.499
	A	2.40	20.249
	B	1.03	19.440
16,000*g*	C	1.45	17.363
	D	1.46	17.756
	E	3.42	16.632
	A	1.80	21.231
	B	1.18	18.113
32,000*g*	C	1.27	17.269
	D	2.84	17.369
	E	3.22	16.717

[a]Tubes were loaded with 12×10^6 cells of ME-180 in 0.5 ml.

zones of the gradient are shown in Fig. 4a, with many fibroblasts, present, and from the 1.065–1.085 g/ml interface in Fig. 4b, where only epithelioid cells were isolated.

In an attempt to further improve the method, some of the parameters which might be thought to influence the cell separation, such as time of centrifugation and centrifugal force (RCF), were investigated. Using the standard gradient and different epithelial cells, centrifugal forces of 8000, 16,000, and 32,000*g* for 10 min at 23°C were used. In these experiments, a higher than normal cell load of 12×10^6 cells per gradient was used. Following centrifugation, the cells from each interface were collected, counted, and measured. It was found that no matter which epithelial cell line was used, the size distribution of cells within each zone varied little for that cell line even with twofold and fourfold increases in RCF, as shown by a comparison of the weighted mean cell diameters by zone for ME-180 cells (Table 2). In similar studies in which the RCF was kept constant, but the time

FIG. 4. (a) Appearance of cultures taken from the top two zones (1.025–1.050 and 1.050–1.055 g/ml) of a discontinuous Ficoll gradient overlaid with cells obtained from a human fibroadenoma. The few tumor cells present are overgrown by fibroblasts. Wright's stain. Magnification × 72. (b) Appearance of cultures taken from the same gradient as in (a) but at the 1.065–1.085 g/ml zone. Only epithelioid cells are found in these cultures. Wright's stain. Magnification × 72.

TABLE 3

Centrifugation Time and Cell Recovery[a]

Density (g/ml)	Interface	Number (× 10^4) cells recovered after		
		10 min	20 min	30 min
1.025				
	A	32.6	27.3	27.3
1.050				
	B	8.4	6.6	6.0
1.055				
	C	26.0	45.0	40.0
1.060				
	D	88.0	74.4	91.0
1.065				
	E	149.0	147.0	147.0
1.085				

[a]Tubes were loaded with 5 × 10^6 cells of ME-180 in 0.5 ml.

of centrifugation was varied (10, 20, and 30 min), cell counts from the zones (Table 3) showed a degree of uniformity similar to that obtained when the RCF was varied. That the technique was reproducible was demonstrated by recentrifugation of the cells from a specific zone on a fresh, identical discontinuous gradient—the cells banded only at the interface from which they had been taken.

Experiments were then carried out to determine the behavior of cells from a specific interface of a standard discontinuous gradient when centrifuged on a continuous Ficoll gradient (1.025–1.085 g/ml). ME-180 cells were centrifuged on a discontinuous gradient, the cells from each zone (except the topmost) were collected, and the number of cells and their diameters were determined for each zone. Cells from the upper zones showed a wide range of diameters compared to the cells from the lower zones and to those from the bottom zone (Fig. 5), which were almost exclusively of the modal diameter previously determined for ME-180 (Sykes *et al.*, 1970*b*). The cells from each zone were then centrifuged on continuous gradients, and the gradients were sampled in 10-drop aliquots obtained by bottom puncture (Sykes *et al.*, 1964). The cells in each aliquot were counted and the average density of each aliquot was determined before plotting the percentage (of the input) against density (Fig. 6). It can be seen that the cells from a specific interface showed a considerable spread in buoyant density and that on the basis of the results from the linear gradients these cells should have banded (in the discontinuous gradient) at a lower interface than

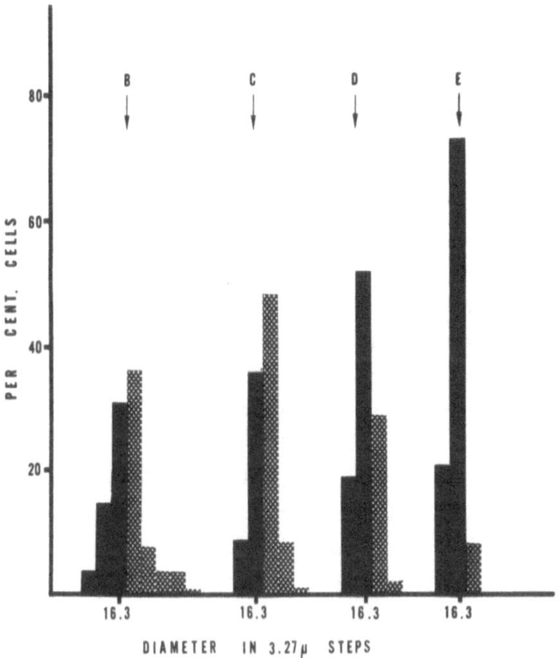

FIG. 5. Results of a typical centrifugation experiment with tumor cells (ME-180) on a standard discontinuous Ficoll gradient showing size distribution of cells by zone. Solid areas represent cells with the modal or less than modal diameters.

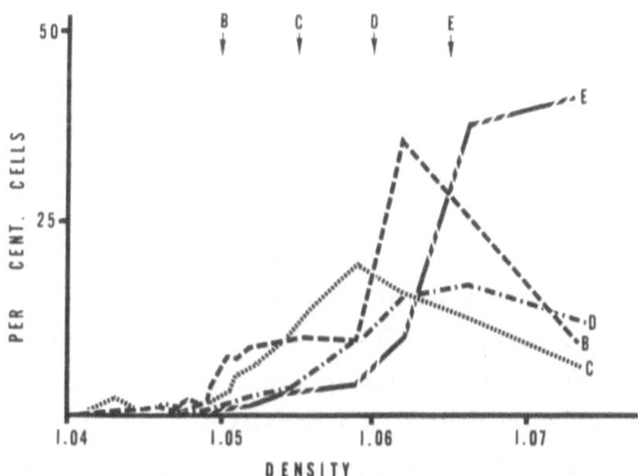

FIG. 6. Density distribution of cells from the discontinuous gradient zones shown in Fig. 5 after being recentrifuged on linear Ficoll gradients (1.025 to 1.085 g/ml). Letters and arrows indicate the starting densities of the zones from which the cells were taken.

the one from which they were taken. The converse of this experiment was also found to be true: cells from a narrow zone of a linear gradient when centrifuged on a discontinuous gradient banded one step higher than indicated by their buoyant density on the linear gradient.

As a result of these findings, it was theorized that part of the "sieving" effect might be due to a distortion of the cells at the interface causing an artificial lessening of density which prevented them from moving through the interface to the next zone. Plastic density marker beads (Sondell Scientific Instruments, Inc., Palo Alto, Calif.) of approximately 1 mm diameter centrifuged on both linear and discontinuous gradients, under the same conditions used in the cell separation studies, always located at the correct density in either continuous or discontinuous Ficoll gradients. As these marker beads were of rigid plastic, further studies were undertaken using silicone oil of density 1.068 g/ml (No. 550 kindly provided by Dow Corning Corp., Midland, Mich.). One drop of the oil was sonicated for 60 sec at an output intensity of 50 watts with the standard tip in 10 ml Ficoll of density 1.020 g/ml using a model No. W1850 sonifier cell disruptor (Heat Systems Co., Melville, Long Island, N.Y.). Phase contrast microscopy of the resulting emulsion showed oil droplets with minimum and maximum diameters of 3 μm and 30 μm. The majority of the droplets had diameters of 3–10 μm. Aliquots of this emulsion centrifuged for 60 min on continuous Ficoll gradients of density 1.040–1.085 g/ml showed a faint diffuse opalescent band near the top of the gradient (mean density 1.0498 g/ml) composed of droplets with an average diameter of 1.3 μm, and a dense opalescent zone where the bulk of the oil droplets were tightly banded at a density of 1.070–1.077 g/ml. The diameter of the oil droplets in this lower band varied from 3 to 18 μm, with most of the droplets measuring 5 μm. The same material centrifuged on a discontinuous gradient banded at the 1.065–1.070 g/ml interface, thus mimicking in a remarkable way the behavior of the tumor cells. Attempts to carry these studies one step further by centrifuging "microcapsules" of silicone oil No. 550 or polybutene–mineral oil coacervated with different amounts of gelatin (courtesy Dr. K. Assar, N.C.R. Capsule Products Division, Dayton, Ohio) were unsuccessful. Gelatin has a density of 1.27 g/ml, and the maximum useful density of the Ficoll solutions being used was 1.15 g/ml because of the viscosity problem (Ficoll solution at a density of 1.060 g/ml has a viscosity of 11.84 centipoises and at a density of 1.065 g/ml a viscosity of 14.27 centipoises).

As the use of discontinuous density gradients of Ficoll solutions had been demonstrated to yield reproducible results in the separation of epithelial cells from fibroblasts, it was felt that the same technique might prove helpful in separating virus-infected cells from uninfected cells. It was thought that virus-infected cells, because of the additional nucleic acid, might have a greater buoyant density than uninfected cells. The standard discontinuous gradient (Table 1) was therefore modified by insertion of an additional zone of density 1.075 g/ml.

Vaccinia virus was used with cultures of CMP and ME-180 cells. Poliovirus and echovirus were used with cultures of ME-180, and the same cell line carrying influenza virus A_0-WSN in passage 13 was also studied.

In the vaccinia virus experiments, cell percentages in each zone of the total recovered cells were calculated and compared with the percentages recovered from the same zones of infected cell cultures of the same age. In this study with vaccinia virus, as well as in the comparable experiments with poliovirus, echovirus, and the A_0-WSN-carrying line of ME-180, the results were contrary to expectations. The cells collected from each of the interface zones were counted and measured (Fig. 7) and used for culturing in T-30 plastic flasks (Falcon Plastics). The cultures were maintained with MEM enriched with 10% fetal calf serum (heat inactivated). Cultures were examined daily for cytopathogenic changes and discarded after 10 days, except those cultures carrying influenza virus A_0-WSN, which were

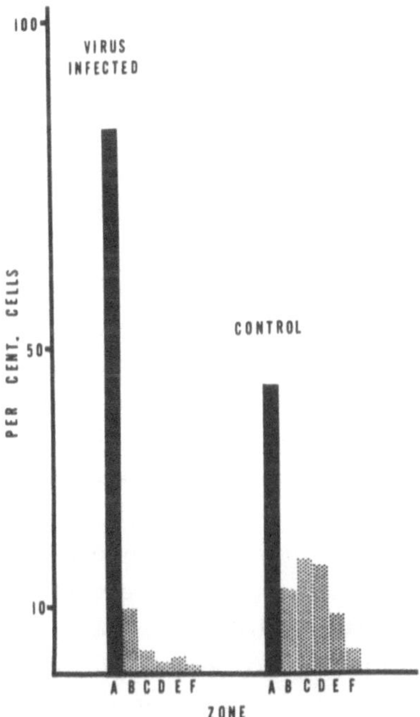

FIG. 7. Total cells per zone for discontinuous density gradients (as in Table 1 with addition of a 1.075 g/ml band) overlaid with poliovirus 1 (Mahoney) infected and uninfected ME-180 cells after centrifugation at 8161*g* for 10 min. The solid bars emphasize the difference in cell numbers in the upper zone between infected and uninfected samples.

discarded after 21 days. The A_0-WSN infected cultures were tested for hemadsorption activity at 8 and 21 days.

In these preliminary virus studies, cultures from the upper zones showed massive cytopathic changes 4 days after culture, but cultures from the lowest zone were apparently normal at the time of discard. In one instance, a culture from the lowest zone in the vaccinia series was subcultured to maintain the cells and cultures remained free of gross cytopathic changes for 6 wk. Hemadsorption studies on the A_0-WSN carrier culture series gave positive results from the upper zones at 8 and at 21 days, but cultures from the lowest zone were hemadsorption negative at the time of discard.

5. *Discussion*

The very detailed studies of Böyum (1968) on methods and parameters encountered in separating leukocytes from bone marrow and from blood indicated some of the complexities in the separation of cells of different types. The problems associated with the separation of hematopoietic cells from one another are analogous to but different from those encountered with solid tissues and tumors. These problems were discussed by Boone *et al.* (1968) and restated by Sykes *et al.* (1970*b*). A close study of the methodology of Boone *et al.* (1968) and of our own preliminary investigations suggested that two problems required solutions, the separation of different cell types from cultures and the mixture of cells which composed tissues and tumors. To provide controlled populations of cells for the experimental studies demanded cells grown in tissue culture, and the most variable cells, the fibroblasts, were obtained from cultures derived from human breast tumors. The more stable cell types, tumor cells, on which our prime interest was centered, were selected from cell lines derived from solid tumors of human origin and readily available in our laboratory.

The linear gradients of different solutions such as sucrose, cesium chloride, sodium citrate, sodium tartrate, bovine albumin, and dextran which were used initially with cells from solid tumors had proved disappointing. The report by Boone *et al.* (1968) provided a stimulus for further studies using Ficoll. The studies by Walder and Lumseth (1963) with this substance directed our attention to the use of discontinuous gradients. The preliminary studies using three different densities of Ficoll solutions, although promising, made it evident that more than three densities, as used by others (Boone *et al.*, 1968; Britten and Roberts, 1960; Johnson and Moran, 1966; Uvnäs and Thon, 1959; Walder and Lumseth, 1963), would be necessary. It seemed also that as low an RCF as possible should be used in order to avoid the necessity of an ultracentrifuge. Although Pretlow and Boone (1968) had described a technique using low-speed centrifugation and linear Ficoll gradients for separation of latex microspheres with different modal diameters, in our hands their technique was ineffective when used with cells. Their method was tested with various combinations of fibroblasts and ME-180 cells, but failed to bring about the desired separation. Higher centrifugal forces and discontinuous gradients were therefore tested in an attempt to overcome some of the factors which appeared to affect the satisfactory separation of mammalian cell types—notably size, density, and stickiness.

As our methodology was refined and led to a reproducible technique, attempts were made to identify some of the factors responsible for, or influencing, the successful separation of cell types on discontinuous Ficoll. It is of interest that when the RCF was kept constant and the time of centrifugation was varied or the RCF was varied and the time of centrifugation was kept constant, little significant difference could be detected, and the pattern of interface banding remained unchanged for the cell lines studied. A puzzling feature of the method was evident when cells from each interface of a discontinuous gradient were separately centrifuged on linear gradients and failed to band at the position of their interface density. When buoyant densities were plotted against percent cells, the densities displayed a spread (Fig. 6). Cells that banded at a particular interface because of their buoyant density in a linear gradient should have banded at a lower interface in a discontinuous gradient. For a small proportion of the cells at a given interface, the converse was also true. When the experimental procedure was reversed and cells taken from a linear Ficoll gradient at any specific density were centrifuged on a discontinuous Ficoll gradient, they were found to band at an interface of lower density than expected from their position on the linear gradient. This appeared to be something of a paradox. When opposed by the drag of the viscous fluid, the centrifugal force (8161*g*) acting on the cells was more than enough to move them to their point of equilibrium in a fraction of the experimental time (10 min). However, this force was insufficient to move the cells through a density interface to their position of density equilibrium. Obviously, other factors than RCF and cell density were involved in the successful separation of cell types. In an effort to explain this paradox, it was theorized that some cells might flatten more easily than others; that is, the plasma membrane might for some reason be more plastic. If this assumption were correct, then it provided a reasonable explanation for the observed differences in behavior of cells on continuous and discontinuous gradients. The more rigid the plasma membrane the further down the discontinuous gradient it would travel. There was no means of visualizing the cells during centrifugation; therefore cells being subjected to different osmotic pressures were measured to determine what changes in volume were induced by different concentrations of salt. It was felt that changes in diameter of cells under osmotic stress might be considered to be a reflection of changes in cell shape under centrifugation, although other factors such as cell membrane permeability would be active in the experimental case, but not during centrifugation in isoosmotic Ficoll solutions. It is interesting that under these conditions tumor cells showed markedly less distortion than did fibroblasts (Fig. 8). Other data which supported the hypothesis, but did not prove it, were the difference in behavior on continuous and discontinuous Ficoll gradients of silicone oil droplets of density and size range comparable to those of cells, whereas solid plastic marker beads behaved correctly in both situations. Also, it was found that glutaraldehyde-fixed cells behaved in a similar fashion to the marker

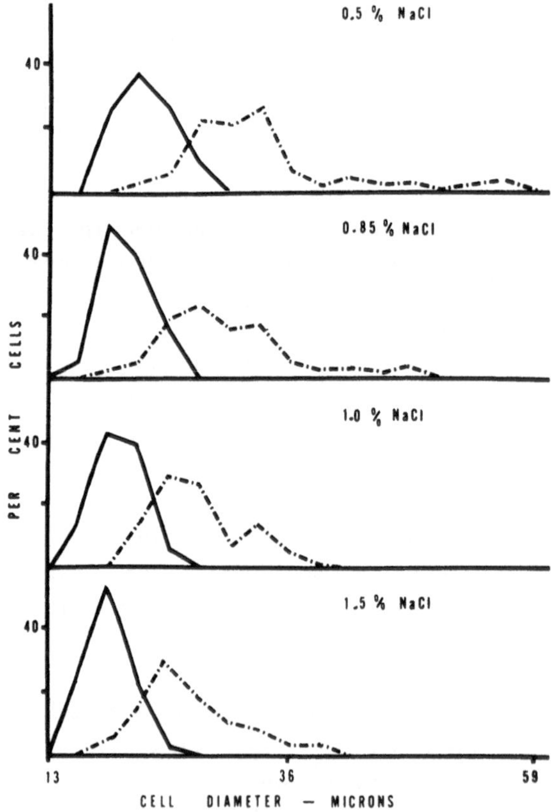

FIG. 8. Percentages of cells having a given diameter after exposure to solutions of sodium chloride with different tonicities. Solid lines represent the findings with tumor cells, broken lines the findings with fibroblasts.

beads. It is unfortunate that so far we have not found an analogous system to Ficoll with higher usable densities in which our theories could be tested using the microcapsules supplies to us by N.C.R. If the above theory is correct, then it would help to explain the results of the preliminary studies using virus-infected cells. In these studies, the virus-infected cells did not vary grossly in morphology from their uninfected neighbors. However, with cell–virus systems studied, the behavior of the virus-infected cells on discontinuous Ficoll gradients was quite different from that of the uninfected cells (Fig. 7). This observed difference could be explained if the theory of cell plasma membrane plasticity as it relates to position in a discontinuous gradient is accepted. It is reasonable to expect that biochemical and biophysical changes occur in the plasma membrane of a cell invaded by a virus and that an indication of this change could be a "softening" of the membrane, leading to an apparent decrease of buoyant density on a discontinuous gradient.

The preliminary studies using virus-infected cells suggested that the discontinuous Ficoll gradient described brought about the separation of infected from uninfected cells. Whether similar results will be obtained with other cell–virus systems remains to be demonstrated. It seems evident that whether or not complete separation is obtained of infected from uninfected cells a high degree of concentration of virus-infected cells could be expected. The described technique has been shown to be a useful tool for the separation of tumor cell from fibroblasts, both from cultured cell mixtures and from cells obtained from some tumors.

6. *Summary*

Use of discontinuous density gradients constructed with solutions of Ficoll in Ca^{2+}-free MEM having densities varying from 1.025–1.085 g/ml and centrifuged at 8000*g* for 10 min at 23°C has permitted separation of epithelial (tumor) cells from fibroblasts. The technique has been successfully applied both to cells grown in tissue culture and to cells derived by use of enzymes from some human tumors. Preliminary studies with cells from cultures infected with different viruses suggest that the technique may make possible the separation of virus-infected and uninfected cells. The paradoxical nature of the technique *vis à vis* continuous Ficoll gradients has not been categorically explained, but the theoretical explanation appears to fit the experimental data so far obtained.

7. *References*

Abeloff, M. D., Mangi, R. J., Pretlow, T. G., and Mardiney, M. R., 1970, Isolation of leukemic blasts from peripheral blood by density gradient centrifugation, *J. Lab. Clin. Med.* **75:**703–710.

Ali, S. N., and Fletcher, K. A., 1971, Zonal centrifugation as a technique for the separation of malania-infected erythrocytes, *Trans. R. Soc. Trop. Med. Hyg.* **65:**4–5.

Boone, C. W., Harell, G. S., and Bone, H. E., 1968, The resolution of mixtures of viable mammalian cells into homogeneous fractions by zonal centrifugation, *J. Cell Biol.* **36:**369–378.

Böyum, A., 1968, Separation of leucocytes from blood and bone marrow, *Scand. J. Clin. Lab. Invest.* **21:**9–29.

Britten, R. J., and Roberts, R. B., 1960, High resolution density gradient sedimentation analysis, *Science* **131:**32–33.

Gey, G. O., Coffman, W. D., and Kubicek, M. T., 1952, Tissue culture studies of the proliferative capacity of cervical carcinoma and normal epithelium, *Cancer Res.* **12:**264.

Giorgi, P. P., 1971, Preparation of neurons and glial cells from rat brain by zonal centrifugation, *Exp. Cell Res.* **68:**273–282.

Holter, M., and Møller, K. M., 1958, A substance for aqueous density gradients, *Exp. Cell Res.* **15:**631–632.

Johnson, A. R., and Moran, M. C., 1966, Comparison of several methods for isolation of rat peritoneal mast cells, *Proc. Soc. Exp. Biol. Med.* **123:**886–889.

Johnson, L., Morrow, J., Kasten, F. H., and Dizerega, G., 1970, Isolation of viable neurons from embryonic spinal ganglia by centrifugation through albumin gradients, *Exp. Cell Res.* **63:**189–192.

Lasfargues, E. Y., and Ozzello, L., 1958, Cultivation of human breast carcinomas, *J. Natl. Cancer Inst.* **21:**1131–1147.

Leemann, U., Weiss, S., and Schmutz, E., 1971, A centrifugation technique for cytochemical preeparations, *J. Histochem. Cytochem.* **19:**758–760.

Mateyko, G. M., and Kopac, M. J., 1963, Cytophysical studies on living normal and neoplastic cells, *Ann. N.Y. Acad. Sci.* **105:**183–286.

Pretlow, T. G., II, and Boone, C. W., 1968, Centrifugation of mammalian cells on gradients: A new rotor, *Science* **161:**911–913.

Rounds, D. E., 1970, A growth-modifying factor from cell lines of human malignant origin, *Cancer Res.* **30:**2847–2851.

Schindler, R., Ramseier, L., Schaer, J. C., and Grieder, A., 1970, Studies on the division cycle of mammalian cells. 3. Preparation of synchronously dividing cells by isotonic sucrose gradient centrifugation, *Exp. Cell Res.* **59:**90–96.

Sykes, J. A., Grey, C. E., Scanlon, M., Young, L., and Dmochowski, L., 1964, Density gradient centrifugation studies of the Bittner virus, *Texas Rep. Biol. Med.* **22:**609–627.

Sykes, J. A., Whitescarver, J., Jernstrom, P., Nolan, J. F., and Byatt, P., 1970*a*, Some properties of a new epithelial cell line of human origin, *J. Natl. Cancer Inst.* **45:**107–122.

Sykes, J. A., Whitescarver, J., Briggs, L., and Anson, J. H., 1970*b*, Separation of tumor cells from fibroblasts with use of discontinuous density gradients, *J. Natl. Cancer Inst.* **44:**855–864.

Uvnäs, B., and Thon, I. L., 1959, Isolation of "biologically intact" mask cells, *Exp. Cell Res.* **18:**512–520.

Walder, A. I., and Lumseth, J. B., 1963, A technic for separation of the cells of the gastric mucosa, *Proc. Soc. Exp. Biol. Med.* **112:**494–496.

Development of Media for Isolation and Cultivation of Human Cancer Cells 2

ALBERT LEIBOVITZ

1. Introduction

The advances in our knowledge of the growth, nutrition, and metabolic requirements of established tissue cell cultures (Rothblat and Cristofalo, 1972) have not solved the problems of developing permanent cell cultures from human solid tumor tissues. There has been little progress in our knowledge of the mechanisms by which cancer cells can become adapted to survive *in vitro.*

Most permanent cell cultures were established from human tumor tissues after many fruitless efforts (Gey *et al.*, 1952; Cailleau, 1960). Although short-term cultures can be established (Southam and Goettler, 1953; Southam, 1954; Cobb *et al.*, 1961; Walker *et al.*, 1965; Foley and Aftonomos, 1965; Lazarus *et al.*, 1966; Feller *et al.*, 1972), most of these die within a few weeks, some survive for several months, but few develop into permanent cell lines (Ioachim, 1970).

Most of our present knowledge of the human cancer cell *in vitro* is based on the poorly differentiated cell. When Gey *et al.* (1952) isolated the first permanent cell culture (HeLa) from a human epidermoid carcinoma of the cervix, they established an epithelial-like cell that grew quite rapidly and as a monolayer directly on glass surfaces. During the next decade, similar

ALBERT LEIBOVITZ Scott and White Clinic, Temple, Texas

long-term cultures were established from human solid tumors originating in various sites (Eagle, 1955*b*; Frisch *et al.*, 1955; Berman and Stulberg, 1956; Baron and Rabson, 1957; Cailleau, 1960; Reed and Gey, 1962). Some human tumors that were successfully transplanted into conditioned animals (Toolan, 1953, 1954, 1957) were also sources of tissue culture cell lines (Fjelde, 1955; Moore *et al.*, 1955; Yohn *et al.*, 1962). During the same period, cell lines were also being established from normal tissues (Chang, 1954; Jordan, 1956; Ginsberg, 1957; Henle and Deinhardt, 1957; Føgh and Lund, 1957; Syverton and McLaren, 1957).

All of the above cell cultures were similar in their rapid growth (generation time from about 18 to 24 h), approximately triploid chromosome stemlines, infinite life, and lack of contact inhibition and were characteristic of poorly differentiated or "dedifferentiated" cell lines. This "sameness" of cell lines originating from a variety of human tumor tissues and "normal" tissues indicated that they were poor models of oncogenesis *in vivo* (Eagle and Foley, 1958; Hsu and Kellog, 1960).

Although relatively few in number, permanent cell lines have been established from human solid tumors that differ significantly from the above cell lines in growth requirements, chromosome stemlines, and metabolic byproducts. Gey (1954–1955) isolated a second cell line (ElCu) from a tumor of the cervix which grew very slowly and was maintained with great difficulty. Lasfargues and Ozzello (1958) established the first permanent cell culture from a human breast tumor; in order to proliferate, this cell line required the complex mucopolysaccharides found in human umbilical cord extract.

Auersperg (1964) cultivated six permanent cell cultures from three human cervical carcinomas that had hypodiploid (43–45 chromosomes) karyograms.

Pattillo and Gey (1968) established the first functioning cell line of a hormone-synthesizing trophoblastic cell. Their cell line originated from the 304th serial passage in hamsters (Hertz, 1959) of a human choriocarcinoma. Kohler *et al.* (1971) obtained similar material from Hertz after the 387th passage in hamsters and also established a hormone-synthesizing cell line.

This chapter is an attempt to take a fresh look at the formulation of media that may enable the reasonably consistent establishment of long-term cultures of human cancer cells from solid tumors. No medium available today has been singled out as the medium of choice for cultivating newly isolated cancer cells, although the more complex ones are usually preferred (Feller *et al.*, 1972). Even though our present means of isolating cancer cells from solid tumor tissues may be highly traumatic, enough cells survive to obtain outgrowth from most specimens (Foley and Aftonomos, 1965; Lazarus *et al.*, 1966).

The reason for the failure of most of these cells to survive *in vitro* may be that only the stem cells have this capability (Patuleia and Friend, 1967; Pierce and Johnson, 1971) or that essential nutrients are missing, or both.

An approach to this problem is to theorize how cancer cells may proliferate *in vivo*. It is logical to assume that cancer cells are derived from normal cells that have been injured *in vivo*, whether by oncogenic viruses, chemical carcinogens, X-irradiation, environment, or something else (Foulds, 1954). Initially, they may differ little from their normal counterparts (Weinhouse, 1972), but they may be giving off strong proteases (Santesson, 1935). As the cancer cells become established, they are loosely adherent to the stromal cells (Cameron and Chambers, 1937; Coman, 1942; Royle, 1946; Lasfargues and Ozzello, 1958) and are embedded in a stroma rich in glycoproteins (Ozzello and Speer, 1958; Ozzello *et al.*, 1960). They may use the stromal fibroblasts as a channel for spread (Leighton, 1957*b*; Wolff, 1956*a*, *b*) and as a source of nutrients (Foley, 1973). As the cell becomes more anaplastic, its isoenzyme patterns change (Weinhouse, 1972), its chromosome stemline may start to deviate significantly from the normal, and it eventually becomes a self-sustaining cell that can readily metastasize. This highly simplified version of *in vivo* growth of cancer cells is presented in order to stress that cancer cells may require the nutrients furnished by the stromal cells to become established.

Santesson (1935) studied the relationship of malignancy to the interaction of cancer cells and fibroblasts. He cocultured mouse mammary tumors with mouse embryo heart and noted that the most anaplastic tumors were the most invasive, whereas the benign tumors were surrounded by a capsule of connective tissue which appeared to wall off their further growth. It has been shown that malignant cells may use the fibroblasts as channels for invasion of normal tissue (Leighton *et al.*, 1957; Wolff, 1956*a,b*). In some of the permanent cell cultures noted above, especially those from normal tissues (Henle and Deinhardt, 1957), only fibroblast-like cells were seen for the first few passages. On subsequent passages, clones of epithelial-like cells would appear which subsequently overgrew the fibroblasts. The fibroblasts may have functioned as a feeder layer until the neoplastic cells had proliferated sufficiently to be self-sustaining (Puck and Marcus, 1955; Puck *et al.*, 1956; Aaronson *et al.*, 1970).

The complex carbohydrates may be significant in the development of a medium for human solid tumor cells. These compounds include the glycoproteins, the glycolipids, and the glycosaminoglycans (mucopolysaccharides) and are recognized to be vital constituents at the cellular level of life. Extensive reviews have been written in this field, which are summarized by Kraemer (1972). The stromal matrix of human tumors is rich in complex carbohydrates (Ozzello and Speer, 1958; Ozzello *et al.*, 1960; Williams *et al.*,

1966; Sumegi *et al.*, 1954; Sumegi and Rajka, 1972). It is unknown whether these compounds are given off by the tumor cells or the stromal cells or both. Recent indirect evidence by Foley (1973), indicates that adult fibroblasts in culture emit complex carbohydrates, especially hyaluronic acid, into the surrounding medium. Lasfargues and Ozzello (1958) found that they needed the mucopolysaccharide-rich umbilical cord extract in their medium to propagate their human breast tumor line. Glycoproteins, such as collagen, have proven to be of value in the culturing of fastidious cells (Ehrmann and Gey, 1956; McLimans *et al.*, 1966).

The invasion of tumor tissue by lymphocytes and/or macrophages may be significant in establishing cancer cells *in vitro*. It is known that antilymphocyte and antithymus sera may enhance tumor growth *in vivo* (Anigstein *et al.*, 1965, 1966; Allison and Law, 1968; Gaugas *et al.*, 1969; Traub, 1972). *In vitro* studies by Sinkovics *et al.* (1972) indicate that cocultivation of sensitized or nonsensitized lymphocytes with neoplastic cells may be detrimental to the latter. If the lymphocytes are sensitized to the neoplastic cells *in vivo*, they will exert their cytotoxic effect *in vitro* immediately. If the lymphocytes are not sensitized, they will become sensitized after a few days of coculture and then exert a cytotoxic effect. Not all cancer cells are sensitive; those emerging are resistant to the cytotoxic effect of the lymphocytes, and the supernatant fluid of such cell cultures will also inhibit lymphocyte cytotoxicity.

Hibbs *et al.* (1972), working with a mouse model, hypothesize that activated macrophages play a role in the normal immunological surveillance of the host. They presume that when cells become "altered" *in vivo*, the activated macrophages exert a selective destructive effect on cells with abnormal growth characteristics by a nonimmunological mechanism. They showed this phenomenon *in vitro* by coculturing activated macrophages and cancer cells. The activated macrophages had no obvious effect when cocultured with "normal" cells.

2. *Isolation of Cancer Cells from Human Solid Tumors*

Three methods have been in common use for the preparation of freshly isolated tissues for cell cultures: (1) chopping with scissors or knives, (2) careful dissection to obtain desired tissue fragments, and (3) treatment of the tissues with enzymes or chelating agents to disperse the cells (Parker, 1961). When normal tissues are treated by any of the above techniques, most of the cells are badly traumatized or destroyed (Anderson, 1953; Kaltenbach, 1954; Laws and Strickland, 1956), and key enzyme systems cannot be detected (Laws and Strickland, 1956; Kalant and Young, 1957; Lata and

Reinerston, 1957; Zimmerman *et al.*, 1960) or are markedly reduced (Burlington, 1959). Usually less than 0.02% cells survive (McLimans *et al.*, 1966), and these must adapt to growth media that are devoid of many of the growth-regulating factors found *in vivo* (Morgan, 1958; Levintow and Eagle, 1961; Zaroff *et al.*, 1961; Pious *et al.*, 1963). The system is therefore highly selective for the type of cell that can survive and proliferate. The isolated of cancer cells from solid tumors is further compromised, as many of these cells were already dead or dying *in vivo* (Vaage, 1968; Wespic, 1970; Leibovitz *et al.*, 1973*a, b*).

2.1. Tissue Fragments or Minces

Optimal outgrowth of cellular elements occurs when the fragment is firmly attached to a solid surface. Many techniques have been devised to accomplish this.

2.1.1. Plasma Clots

Harrison (1907) used clotted frog lymph in his classical studies on the developing nerve fiber. Burrows (1910) popularized the use of chicken plasma clots. Since then, this method has been used in combination with a variety of methods to obtain optimal cell outgrowth. Carrel (1923) developed special flasks for this purpose, and Gey (1933) developed the roller tube technique, which permitted the cells to be grown on the wall of the tube in a thin coagulum of plasma. Leighton (1954) found plasma clots helpful in enabling cells to grow on his cellulose sponge matrices. Plasma clots were difficult to use because actively growing tissues frequently digested the fibrin. This necessitated frequent repairs with fresh coagulum and often entailed the loss of the culture (Parker, 1961). The development of better media and cell lines that grew readily on glass surfaces turned most investigators away from the plasma clot methods. Fibrinogen clot cultures (Ebeling, 1921) and reconstituted rat-tail collagen (Ehrmann and Gey, 1956) have proved useful, but these substrates are also subject to lysis (Whitescarver *et al.*, 1968).

2.1.2. Perforated Cellophane

Evans and Earle (1947) advocated perforated cellophane as a support in growing tissue fragments in fluid media. The cells often preferred to grow on the cellophane rather than the glass surface of the vessel. Better growth was usually attained when the tissues were placed under the cellophane rather than over it. Lazarus *et al.* (1966) could not obtain a consistent outgrowth of cells in replicate cultures, but this method has proved useful for the isolation of cancer cells from solid tumor tissues (Sinkovics *et al.*, 1971).

2.1.3. Tantalum or Stainless Steel Grids

The "grid" technique was first advocated by Trowell (1953, 1959) and improved on by Jensen and Castellano (1960) and Jensen *et al.* (1964). Tantalum or stainless steel mesh platforms, 2 by 2 cm and 3 mm high, processed to remove toxic products and sterilized in dry heat, are placed in small petri dishes. Discs of open-mesh paper (tea-bag paper), 12 mm in diameter, are processed to remove toxic products, dry heat sterilized, and placed on the metal mesh platform. Tissue fragments placed on the paper readily adhere to this surface and do not wash away when the medium is added. This is both a short-term organ culture and a potential cell culture. Cells may migrate from the tissue fragment and proliferate as colonies on the petri dish floor. Jensen *et al.* (1964) were able to maintain tumor cells collected in this manner up to 90 days. Lazarus *et al.* (1966), although successful with some explants, were not able to get consistent outgrowth in replicate cultures from human solid tumors on such grids. They believe that cells do not migrate from human tissue explants as readily as they do from rodent tissue. Feller *et al.* (1972) adhered 1- to 2-mm^3 tissue fragments from breast tumors to 1-cm^2 tantalum mesh and incubated these with the tumor tissue on the underside of the mesh in contact with the glass. They found that epithelial cells migrated from the tissue fragments, especially from intraductal carcinomas, and grew as monolayers in the areas adjacent to the tumor. However, the maximum time they could maintain these was 4 months.

2.1.4. Agar Cultures

It was noted that cells transformed by polyoma virus would form colonies in soft agar whereas their normal counterparts failed (Sanders and Burford, 1964; Macpherson and Montagnier, 1964). Macpherson and Montagnier (1964) noted that malignant cells such as HeLa, HEp-2, and the L strain of mouse fibroblasts would also form colonies in soft agar. To determine whether this would be a useful technique in the isolation of malignant cells from human neoplasms, McAllister and Reed (1968) incorporated minces and trypsin-dispersed cells from solid tumors in 0.33% agar and overlaid this mixture on a 0.5% agar bed. Minces were obtained from 29 tumors; cell migration occurred with 27 of the minces and colony formation was evident in 14 cultures. Trypsin-dispersed cells were obtained from 17 solid tumors; nine of these showed colony formation. The efficiency of colony formation was low, ranging from one to 133 colonies per 10^6 cells inoculated. Bone marrow specimens were obtained from 14 children with various types of acute leukemia; none of these cultures developed colonies. Five specimens of normal human embryonic tissues failed to form colonies, but four of seven tissue specimens obtained from patients with hyperplastic disease with no evidence of neoplasia did form colonies. Attempts to heterotransplant colonies obtained from five of the tumor tissues to adolescent hamsters failed.

Patuleia and Friend (1967) used an agar "pearl" technique. They suspended 10^4–10^5 cells in 0.45% agar and placed 0.5 ml on the floor of a flask. After setting, a "pearl," 20 mm in diameter, was formed. Growth medium was added and medium changes were made once per week. About 21 days were required to produce visible colonies. The efficiency of colony formation was low, which, they speculate, might have been because of false viability results obtained with the trypan blue exclusion test (DeLuca, 1965) and/or because only the stem cells present in the inoculum could proliferate indefinitely; the other cells may have been in an advanced state of maturity and thus have had limited growth capacity (see Pierce and Johnson, 1971).

Costachel *et al.* (1969) devised a modification of the suspension culture technique using agar. When they dispersed hamster sarcoma cells over solid agar (2.7%), the cells remained in suspension and formed growing islands of cells. This negated the need for stirring or the use of chelating agents for suspension cultures. This laboratory is investigating this method for the isolation of cancer cells from human solid tumor minces and for growing dispersed cells obtained by mechanical or enzymatic means. Theoretically, the stromal cells will not be able to proliferate, as they do not have a solid footing (Rubin, 1965–1966), but may still act as a feeder layer for the cancer cells which may be able to grow in suspension (Lasfargues *et al.*, 1972).

2.1.5. Feeder Layers

Bichel (1938) cocultivated mouse leukemia leukocytes with stromal cells to establish a continuous culture; Debruyn *et al.* (1949) similarly established mouse lymphosarcoma cultures. Beynish-Melnick *et al.* (1963) determined that spontaneous lymphoblastoid transformation in bone marrow cultures obtained from leukemic and nonleukemic children was enchanced by the fibroblasts present acting as feeder cultures. X-Irradiated fibroblasts (Puck and Marcus, 1955; Puck *et al.*, 1956) are good feeder layers for enabling growth of single cells, although the fibroblasts are unable to multiply, they continue to metabolize actively and thereby furnish essential nutrients. However, their use for the isolation of malignant cells from tumor tissues is limited as these feeder layers start to degenerate in 7–10 days. Aaronson *et al.* (1970) eliminated the need to irradiate fibroblast feeder layers by using diploid strains of human adult foreskin fibroblasts that were relatively late in their *in vitro* lifetime expectancy (e.g., 20th–30th passage). These fibroblasts did not form a dense monolayer, and developing colonies of cancer cells could be readily detected by microscopic and macroscopic techniques. They obtained colony proliferation in eight of 18 tumor tissues, three of four normal embryonic tissues, and none of 15 normal adult tissues. The authors state that this method may be useful in the isolation of malignant cells from specimens containing large numbers of stromal cells as up to 10^5 normal stromal cells can be inoculated on a monolayer without attaining colonies.

Lasfargues and Moore (1971) were able to maintain long-term mixed cultures of mouse mammary epithelial cells and their fibroblast stroma by the judicious use of collagenase. In this laboratory, we are investigating variations in this technique to maintain malignant cells in coculture with their fibroblast stromal cells (see Section 3).

Lasfargues *et al.* (1972) cocultivated human breast malignant cells with a human lymphoblastic cell line, NC-37, in suspension cultures. NC-37 cells grow rapidly in suspension cultures, are free of any obvious virus infection, and because of their small size are readily differentiated from the breast cancer cells. The larger cancer cells appeared to feed on the small NC-37 cells and proliferated about twice as fast as usual.

2.1.6. *Microcultures*

The concentration of cells in a given volume of medium may significantly affect their capability to proliferate (Lockhart and Eagle, 1959; Eagle, 1958–1959; Eagle and Piez, 1962; Ham, 1963; Waymouth, 1967). As relatively few of the malignant cells isolated from tumor tissues may have the capacity to proliferate (Patuleia and Friend, 1967), microcultures may be of value. Lazarus *et al.* (1966) investigated a number of techniques in attempting to devise a method that would yield consistent outgrowth of replicate cultures of tumor tissues. They determined that coverslip microculture is the most reliable. Four to eight fragments of tissue less than 1 mm^3 in size were placed on a drop of medium in the center of a 35- by 10-cm Falcon plastic petri dish. A 22-mm^2 coverslip was placed firmly over the minces and 1 ml of medium was added to the dish. These were not disturbed for 3–5 days, and then the medium was changed twice weekly. Outgrowths were usually attained in 1–2 wk. Of 1369 cultures attempted from 95 specimens, growth was obtained in 1201 (88%) from 90 specimens; these included 61 out of 63 tumor tissues and 29 out of 32 normal tissues. About 14 replicate cultures were attempted from each specimen; in 75% of their cultures, growth was attained in all replicates. Many of the outgrowths reached confluency and could be passed. However, the authors do not state whether any effort was made to establish permanent cell lines or whether any other studies were done with these isolates except for chemotherapeutic screens.

The microculture multiwell plastic dishes originally devised by Rightsel *et al.* (1956) did not give consistent outgrowths of replicate cultures in the above study (Lazarus *et al.*, 1966), but proved to be of value in the isolation of human breast tumor cell cultures. Bassin *et al.* (1972) transferred clones of epithelial-like cells found in collagenase-dispersed cultures of breast tumors to such microculture dishes. Although they consider the establishment only four cell lines from about 100 specimens to be fortuitous, they have succeeded in developing more human breast tumor cell lines directly from tumor tissues than all previously recorded successes combined. Further investigation of this method appears warranted.

2.2. Spillout Techniques

Cameron and Chambers (1937), while working with explants of breast tumors, noted that tumor cells spilled or migrated away from the explants in the form of "hollow nodules." Coman (1942) and Royle (1946) noted the relatively loose arrangement of the tumor cells in their fibrous stroma. Lasfargues and Ozzello (1958), utilizing this information, developed the "spillout" technique. They anchored the tissue specimen with a pair of forceps and then carefully cut thin slices. When the thin slices were further cut, a dense population of cells, almost entirely epithelial, flowed from the minces. Unfortunately, the growth media available were not adequate for the establishment of permanent cell lines and only one line was established. Recently, Lasfargues (see Chapter 3) has devised a new medium which may enhance long-term cell cultures. Leibovitz *et al.* (1973*a*, *b*) applied the spillout technique to all human solid tumor tissues. This method was expanded to include the spinner spillout and the trypsin–versene spillout techniques. These methods are summarized in Section 2.5.

2.3. Ascites and Pleural Fluids

Pomerat *et al.* (1950) devised the simplest means of isolating cancer cells from such body fluids as ascites or pleural fluid. They recommend that the fluid stand for several hours, permitting the cancer cells to settle to the bottom of the collection bottle. The sediment is harvested with a pipette and then concentrated by centrifugation. They warn that greenish ascites fluids indicate bile contamination and recommend thorough washing of such sediments to remove this toxic contaminant.

Ascites fluids and pleural fluids are often badly contaminated by whole blood. In the course of standing for several hours, clotting is quite possible. Such fluids should be heparinized (about 1 unit/ml) to prevent cancer cell loss in the ensuing clots. Separation of red blood cells from tissue cells is readily attained by the albumin flotation methods (Ferrebee and Geiman, 1946; Fawcett *et al.*, 1950; Fawcett and Vallee, 1952; Parker, 1961). The cell mixture is concentrated into about 2–5 ml of the supernate, overlaid on 10 ml of bovine albumin with a specific gravity of about 1.067 (Calbiochem, Miles Laboratory) in a 40-ml centrifuge tube, and centrifuged at about 2000–2500 rpm for 20–25 min. The red cells are concentrated in the bottom of the centrifuge tube, and the desired cells form a "buffy coat" at the albumin–supernate interface. This is removed to a fresh centrifuge tube, which is then filled to the top with a basic salt solution or saline. Following centrifugation at about 1000 rpm for 5 min, the cell yield will be concentrated in the bottom of the tube. This method is also useful for the separation of viable from nonviable cells in processed tumor tissues (Wespic, 1970).

2.4. *Enzymes*

Rous and Jones (1916) introduced the use of trypsin to disperse cells from tissue cultures for subcultures. Moscona (1952) noted better dispersion of embryonic rudiment cells when calcium and magnesium were omitted from the buffered saline.

Rinaldini (1958, 1959) studied the effect of trypsin, pancreatin, elastase, and papain and determined that crude trypsin preparations carry tissue digestion to the cell-free stage only because they also contain other enzymes as impurities; crystalline trypsin left a viscous mucin-like residue that was dissolved by crude trypsin preparations, pancreatin, and elastase.

Collagenase was introduced for the dispersion of cells from organs rich in connective tissue (Lasfargues, 1957; Hinz and Syverton, 1959). This enzyme is not inhibited by serum (Lasfargues and Moore, 1971), whereas trypsin, pancreatin, and elastase are. Pronase, an actinomycette protease, is recommended by a number of investigators for the dispersion of cells from tissues (Wilson and Lau, 1963; Gwatkin and Thomsen, 1964; Houba, 1967). Wilson and Lau (1963) noted that this enzyme would separate the cells from chicken pectoral muscle, whereas trypsin and versene failed to do so. Similarly to trypsin, the enzyme is inactivated by serum (Gwatkin and Thomsen, 1964).

Enzyme dispersion of tumor tissues invariably disperses stromal cells, which are released in probably much greater numbers than the cancer cells. Most neoplastic cells have difficulty adapting to their new environment, and

FIG. 1. A "cancer cell" clone developing in a culture of an endometrial adenocarcinoma (accession No. SW-409) which was on collagenase medium for 1 month. Note the "cancer cells" starting to invade the fibroblast stromal cells.

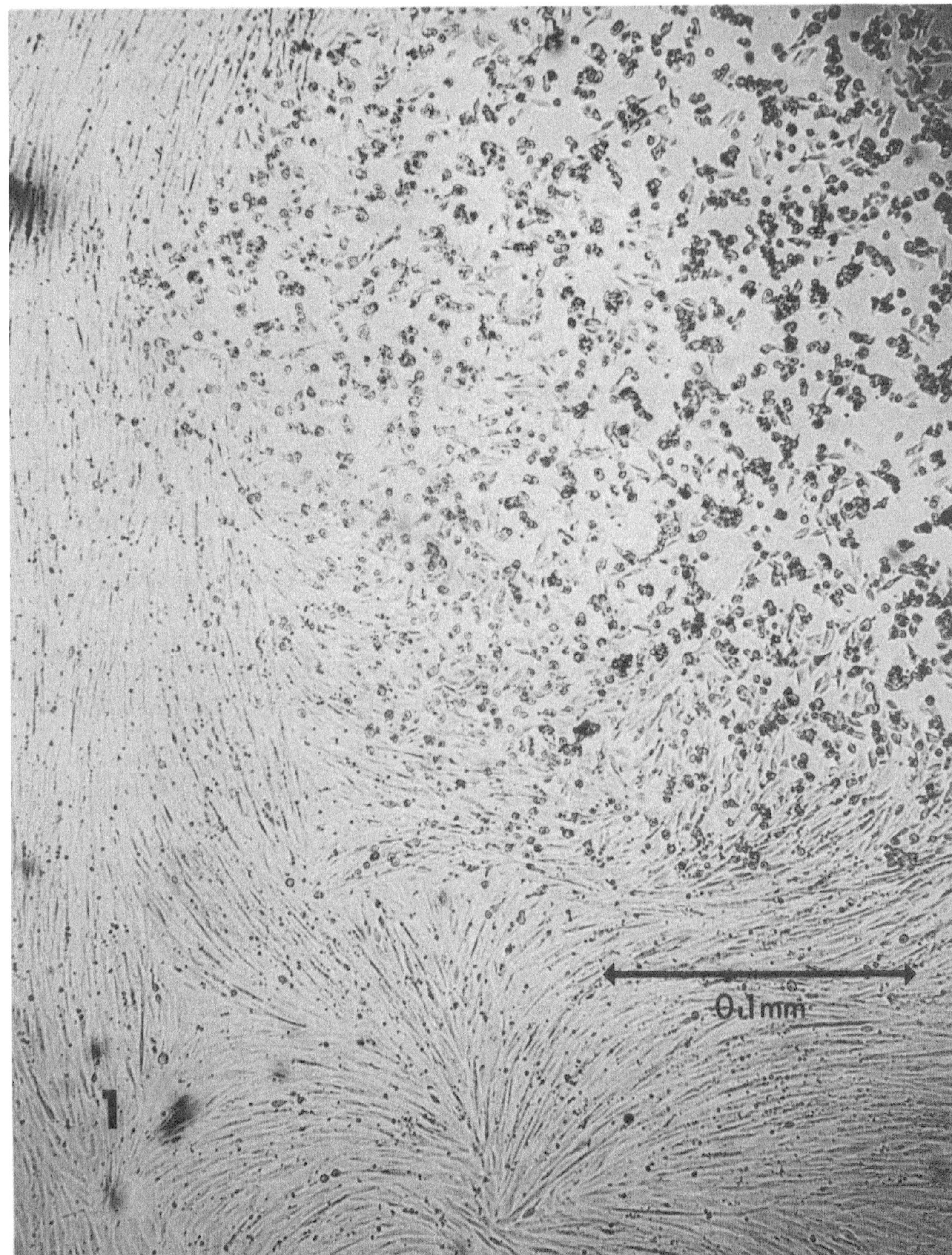
0.1mm
1

Lasfargues and Moore (1971) found that in such instances the rapidly growing fibroblasts may polymerize collagen on the epithelial-like cells and smother them. They prevented this in normal tissues by the use of collagenase in the growth medium. In our laboratory, this finding has been expanded in the growth of cancer cells in mixed cultures and will be discussed in Section 3.

2.5. *Discussion*

Most of the methods used for the isolation of malignant cells from solid tumors, with the exception of the spillout techniques, are the same as for "normal" tissues (Parker, 1961).

In our laboratory, we have attempted to expand on the spillout technique of Lasfargues and Ozzello (1958) for breast tumors and apply variations of this method to all solid tumors. In an effort to keep the stromal cells released to a minimum, the following schedule is used:

1. Spillout technique (Lasfargues and Ozzello, 1958): All tissue slicing is done in the presence of complete growth medium (see Table 1). The larger the specimen, the more apt one is to obtain adequate numbers of viable cancer cells for culture. The trypan blue exclusion test (Hanks and Wallace, 1958) indicates such yields to contain highly variable numbers of viable cells, from less than 1% to about 50%. On the average, only about 10–20% of the cells exclude the trypan blue. Many of these cells may be incapable of proliferating, as badly injured cells may still exclude the trypan blue (DeLuca, 1965). Ideally, 5×10^5 cells are desired for the 30-ml Falcon flask or 2×10^6 cells for the 250-ml flask, although successful outgrowths have been obtained with many fewer cells.
2. The spinner spillout technique (Leibovitz *et al.*, 1973*a*): The minces are retrieved from the spillout technique and placed in a 50-ml spinner flask (Bellco) containing 30 ml of growth medium. The minces are spun at about 200 rpm for 20 min. This method has been found to increase the yield from five- to tenfold. Contamination with stromal cells is more evident in this method, but usually they are present in small numbers.
3. The trypsin–versene spillout technique (Leibovitz *et al.*, 1973*a, b*): If adequate numbers of cells are not obtained by the above two

FIG. 2. Scattered clusters of "cancer cells" appearing in a 1-month-old culture on collagenase medium of an adenocarcinoma of the ovary that had metastasized to the peritoneum (accession No. SW-419). The scattered clusters of "cancer cells" are more commonly seen than the clones noted in Fig. 1.

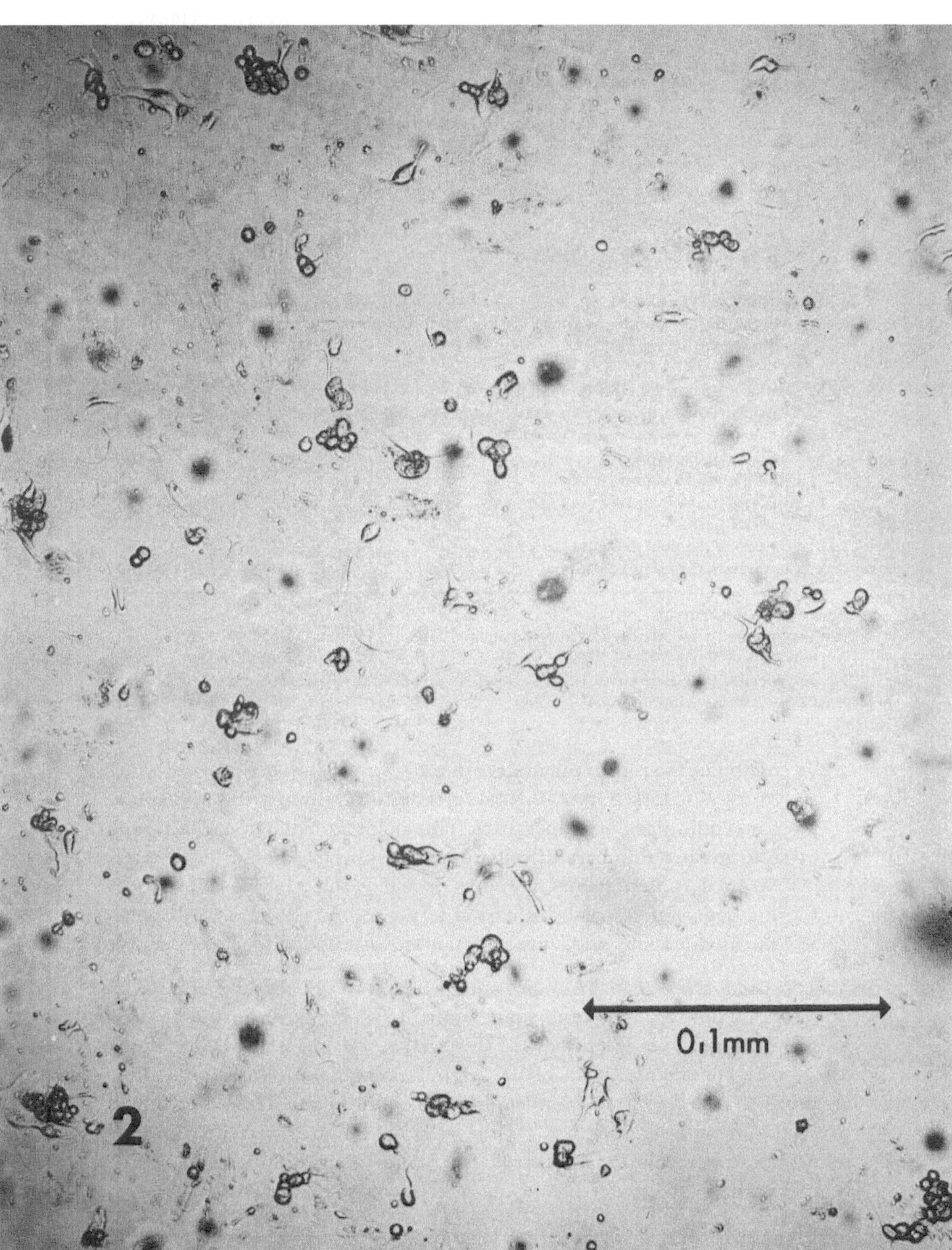
0,1mm
2

TABLE 1

"PAP" Medium for the Cultivation of Newly Isolated Human Cancer Cells

To 800 ml H_2O add the following:	
1. 1 pkg medium L-15 (Grand Island powder, 1-liter pkg)	
2. L-Aspartic acid[a]	50.00 mg
3. L-Proline[a]	50.00 mg
Sterilize by Millipore filter method	
Add the following sterile solutions:	
1. Hydracortisone sodium succinate (Solu-cortef, Upjohn), diluted in sterile H_2O to 10 mg/ml	1.00 ml
2. Insulin, 40 u/ml (Lilly)	0.25 ml
3. Methocel, 15 cps, 2% (Dow Chemical)	100.00 ml
4. Yeastolate (Difco)–agarose (Pharmacia) supplement[bc]	12.50 ml[c]
5. Na polypectate[a]–sucrose supplement[bd]	2.50 ml[d]
6. Catalase, 50,000 u/ml[a]	1.00 ml
7. Glutathione,[a] 15 mg/ml	1.00 ml
8. PVP,[a] GMW 360,000, 10%	10.00 ml
9. Fetal calf serum	100.00 ml
10. Fungazone (Squibb), 5 mg/ml	0.25 ml
11. Gentamycin (Schering), 50 mg/ml	1.00 ml

[a]Nutritional Biochemical.
[b]Both supplements are sterilized by autoclaving at 121°C for 15 min.
[c]Yeastolate, 1.00%; Agarose, 0.25%.
[d]Na polypectate, 1.00%; surcrose, 10.00%. Note: Na polypectate will go into solution only in at least a 3 × sucrose solution.

methods, the remaining minces in the spinner flask are covered with 30 ml of 0.25% trypsin–0.10% versene (Gray Industries) and spun for 30 min at room temperature. This yields from ten- to a thousand-fold greater numbers of cells than the spinner spillout technique. Stromal contamination is more probable than in the above two methods, but, as will be discussed in the following section, collagenase medium may make the stromal cells useful as a feeder layer.

Collagenase Dispersion: The above methods may fail to yield adequate numbers of desired cells from some tumor tissues rich in fibrous tissue, e.g., some lung and breast tumors. If this occurs, the minces are collected in a test tube containing 10 ml of 0.5 mg/ml collagenase (Nutritional Biochemical, Worthington) in complete growth medium and allowed to stand overnight at room temperature. If the cells have not dispersed from the tissue, the tissue minces are stirred for ½ h at about 200 rpm at room temperature.

FIG. 3. Tight clusters of "cancer cells" noted in a 1-month-old culture of collagenase medium of an adenocarcinoma of the transverse colon (SW-48).

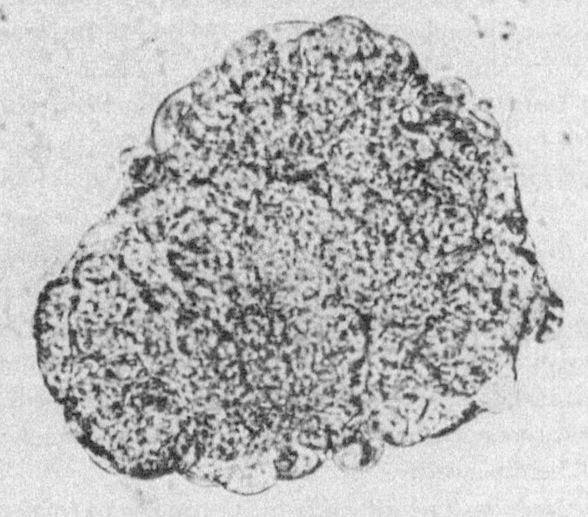
0,1 mm
3

At the present time, we are evaluating the above methods for both efficiency and yield. Indications are that the trypsin–versene spillout method is the best single method in obtaining ample supplies of cells. As the spillout method is used in slicing the tissues for the trypsinization technique, comparative studies of these two methods can be done with little extra effort.

3. *Development of Media for the Cultivation of Cancer Cells*

The trend in media for tissue cell cultures has been from the complete body fluid (Harrison, 1907) to the complete synthetic media (White, 1946, 1949). Over 100 different media have been advocated in the last 60 years (Waymouth, 1972) for both general and special needs. Most media in use today for tissue cell cultivation are a blend of body fluids, usually serum, and synthetic ingredients. Only a small number of laboratory-adapted tissue cell lines have been completely weaned from the need for exogenous macromolecules for proliferation (Evans *et al.*, 1956; Waymouth, 1956, 1959; Tribble and Higuchi, 1963; Ham, 1965; Ling *et al.*, 1968). However, these media soon contain macromolecules released by the growing cells and/or dead cells (Temin *et al.*, 1972). Thus tissue culture media design is still essentially empirical. Excellent reviews of the advances made in tissue culture media have been published (Waymouth, 1954, 1960, 1965, 1968, 1972; Morgan, 1958). A survey of formulations of commercially available media was recently compiled (Morton, 1970). As this chapter is solely concerned with the cultivation of newly isolated cancer cells, only selected articles will be reviewed.

Design of Medium: The difficulty in attempting to write this chapter is that no medium devised, to date, has consistently established long-term cultures of newly isolated cancer cells, whereas permanent cell lines have been established using a wide variety of media and procedures. Therefore, the establishment of such cell lines is considered fortuitous and not due to any given technique or medium (Whitescarver *et al.*, 1968; Bassin *et al.*, 1972). Eagle (1955*a*, 1959) devised the simplest synthetic media that, when supplemented by serum, would support the growth of both normal and "altered" cells. Other investigators noted the need for additional nutrients for specific cell lines under study (Neuman and Tytell, 1960; Neuman and McCoy, 1956; Haff and Swim, 1956). Leibovitz (1963) went to the other extreme of Eagle's findings and used the maximum amount of each amino

---

FIG. 4. Development of the tight clusters of "cancer cells" shown in Fig. 3 into grapelike clusters. These grapelike clusters persisted for from 2 to 7 months of *in vitro* life (SW-48).

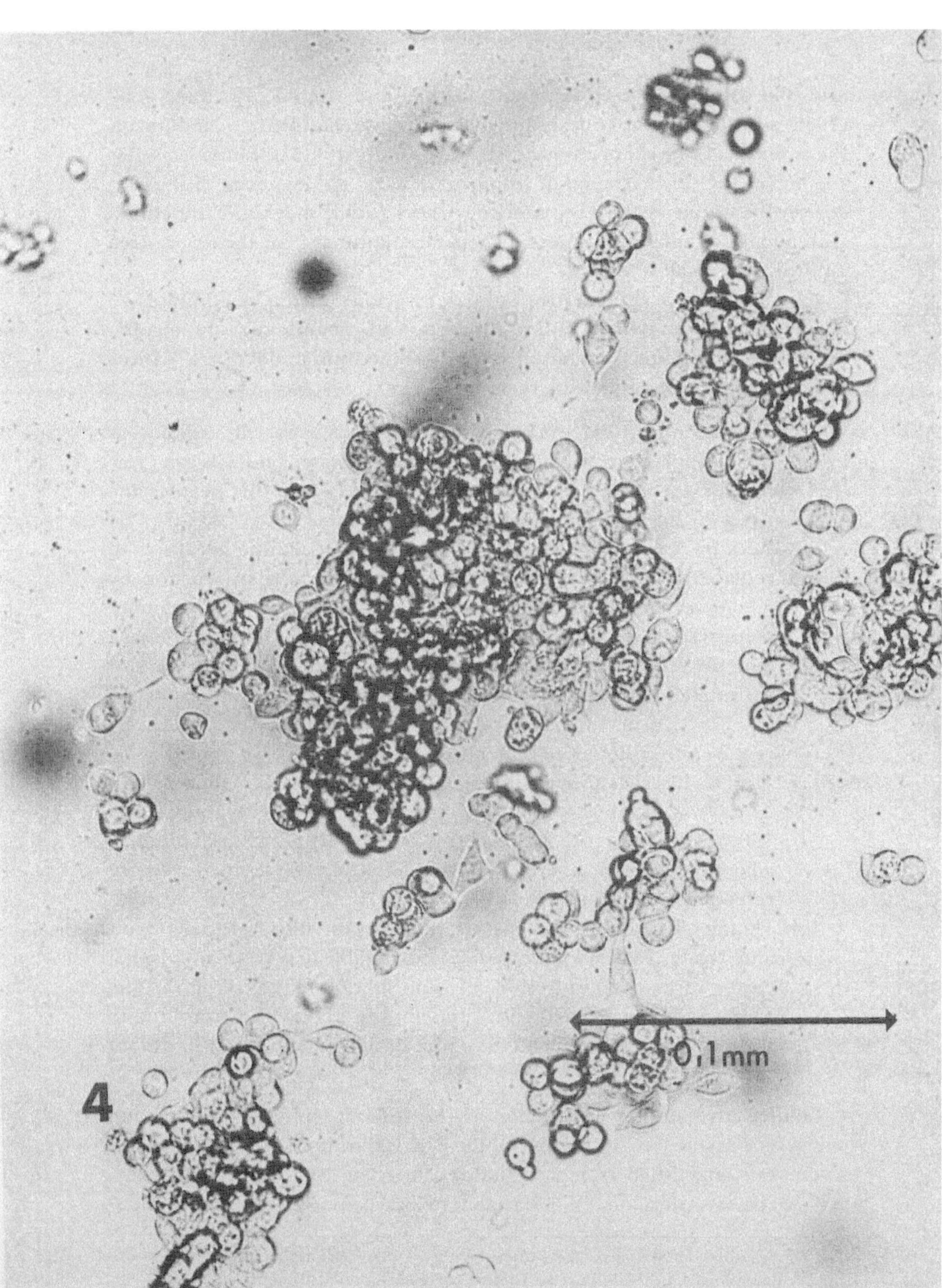
0,1mm
4

acid that would not be toxic to both normal and altered cells. Ling *et al.* (1968) adjusted the amino acid content even higher, basing their medium on the amino acid content of animal tissues instead of serum. Of interest is that the higher the concentration of amino acids used, the less need of the cells for serum supplements. Ling and coworkers found that using a medium with 54 mM of amino acids per liter was near optimum for the serum-free cultures they established.

Initially, after a comparative study of various media, medium L-15 (Leibovitz, 1963), fortified with 9–10% fetal calf serum, 0.01 u/ml insulin, and 10 μg/ml cortisol, was chosen as the base medium to develop a "cancer cell" medium for the following reasons:

1. The medium utilizes the free base amino acids, especially arginine, as the buffer system instead of sodium bicarbonate. The cells can grow in free gas exchange with the atmosphere, and this negates the necessity for special incubators.
2. Because galactose, sodium pyruvate, and *dl*-alanine are used to replace glucose as the energy source, lactic acid production by metabolizing cells is about one-tenth that in glucose-containing media (Eagle *et al.*, 1958; Leibovitz, 1963; Baugh and Tytell, 1967). The pH remains in the optimal range for tissue cell growth without the rapid fluctuations experienced with glucose media (Mackenzie *et al.*, 1961). Even in closed containers, highly glycolytic cells rarely require refeeding more than once per week.
3. Most tissue cells can be maintained over a long period of time, at least 21 days, without refeeding (Richardson and Leibovitz, 1965; Rose, 1969). This is not true, however, for the rapidly growing laboratory-adapted strains of altered cells as HeLa or HEp-2; these require refeeding at least once per week.
4. Plating efficiency is excellent. We disperse 10,000 SW-13 cells (Scott and White No. 13, epithelial-like cells established from an adrenal cortex carcinoma) in 5 ml of medium in a 30-ml Falcon flask. The well-isolated single cells show doubling in about 24 h, continue to form colonies, and then fill the entire flask in about 1 month without refeeding.

Comparative studies were made of the spillout, spinner spillout, and minces technique (see Section 2). Of the first 100 tumor tissues studied, cell lines were established from five (nasopharyngeal, SW-5; adrenal cortex, SW-13; transverse colon, SW-48; rhabdomyosarcoma, SW-80; and a metas-

FIG. 5. Transition of the grapelike clusters of Fig. 4 (SW-48) into small islands of two-dimensional epithelial-like cells. These occurred after about 7 months *in vitro*.

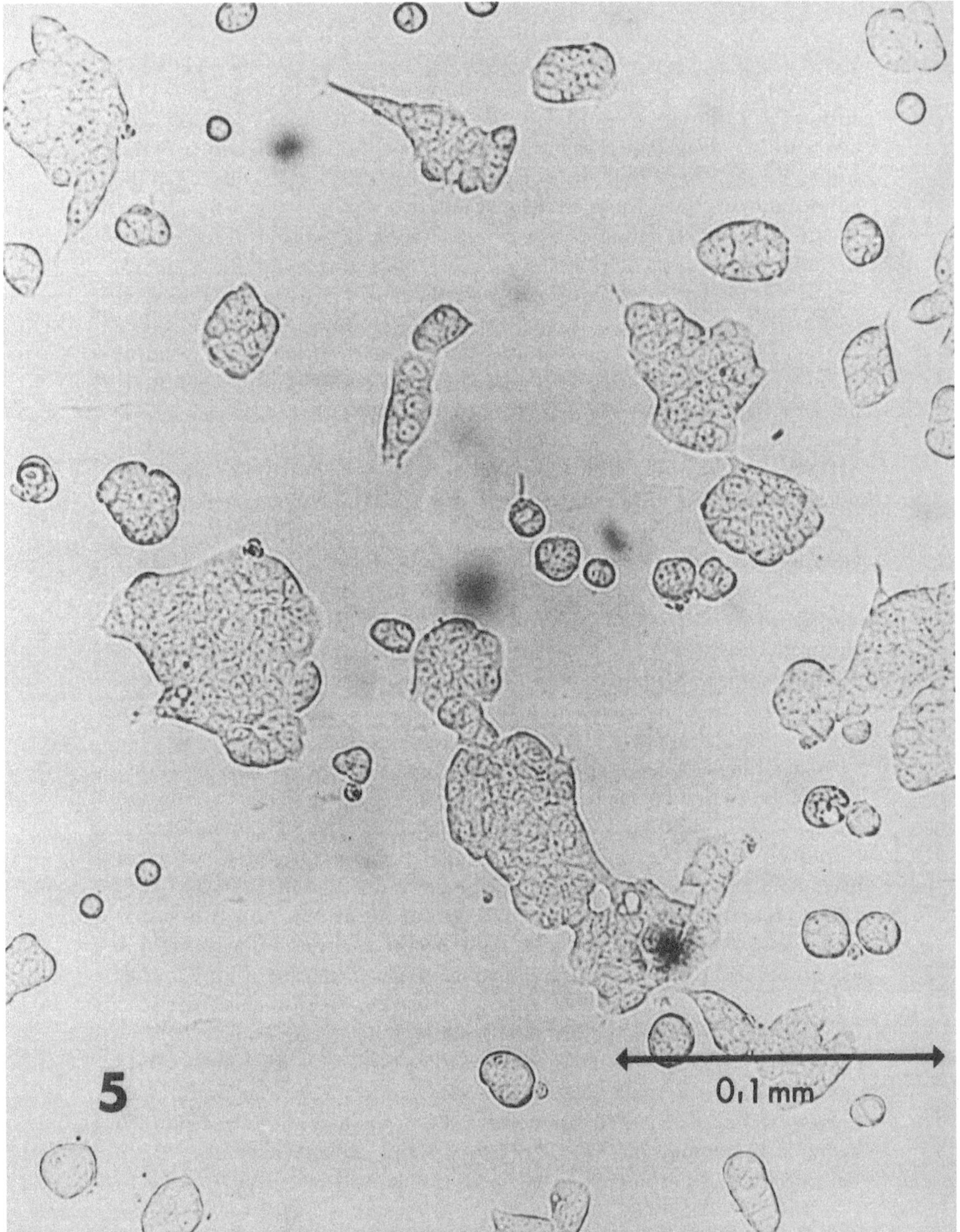
5
0,1 mm

tasis to the liver from an adrenal tumor, SW-47). These were all isolated by the various spillout techniques. This medium permitted luxuriant growth of stromal cells (fibroblasts), and several of the lines established were salvaged by the use of collagenase (Lasfargues and Moore, 1971). In the course of this study, it was noted that the collagenase had little or no effect on the epithelial-like cells and many elongated cells that were not typical fibroblasts. We then put mixed cultures on long-term use of collagenase instead of the periodic use advocated by Lasfargues and Moore. Ideally, this medium would permit both the fibroblasts and the cancer cells to proliferate as cocultures with the possibility that the cancer cells would obtain essential nutrients from the fibroblasts until they could be self-sustaining. Growth of fibroblast-like cells would be self-limited by contact inhibition and their finite life span. Our experience is that fibroblasts usually start to die after several months of *in vitro* life. The collagenase medium is prepared by adding 0.5 mg per milliter of growth medium and is used only when fibroblast-like cells start to dominate the culture and is continued until they start to die. The emergence of epithelial-like cells in this system is shown in Figs. 1 and 2. Occasionally, the desired cells remain as tight clusters (Fig. 3) which may detach from the plastic surface after variable periods of incubation. These can be retrieved from the supernatant and established as fibroblast-free cultures. The transition of such clusters to a monolayer is shown in Figs. 3–6 for cancer cells isolated from an adenocarcinoma of the transverse colon (accession No. SW-48); this *in vitro* adaptation slowly evolved over a 7-month period.

During the past year, we have been investigating various compounds that may be useful as detoxifiers and/or as growth stimulants. The reagents that we have found useful to date are listed in Table 1; the code name for this formula is "PAP." We wanted to use collagen because this glycoprotein had been found useful in the growing of fastidious cells (Ehrmann and Gey, 1956; McLimans *et al.*, 1966), but it would be useless once we added collagenase. We therefore are testing the pectin compounds, because these glycoproteins appear to have a similar function in the plant kingdom as collagen in the animal kingdom. Agarose is used in very low concentrations for a possible structural lattice; microbiologists have long known that low concentrations of agar facilitate the growth of fastidious organisms in fluid media. Catalase is used to neutralize peroxidases after the findings of Lieberman and Ove (1959). Methocel and polyvinylpyrrolidine are known detoxifiers, although their mode of action is unknown (Waymouth, 1972). Yeastolate is used essentially as a growth stimulant (Robertson *et al.*, 1955;

FIG. 6. Final transition of SW-48 into a complete monolayer of epithelial-like cells. This culture had been passed 15 times in 18 months.

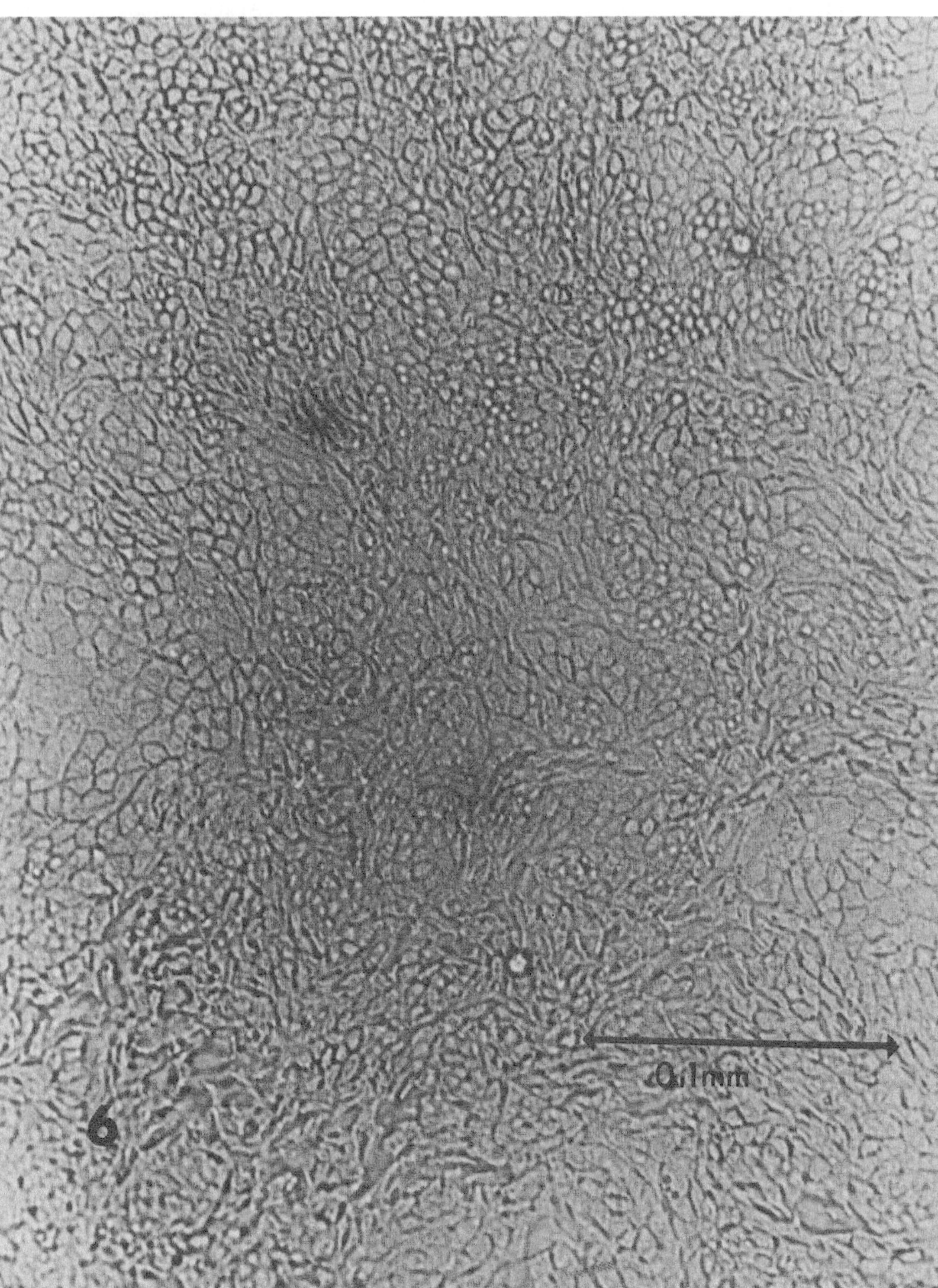
0.1mm
6

Føgh and Lund, 1957). PAP medium appears to enchance the growth and longevity of cancer-like cells; an unexpected dividend is that fibroblasts grow slower in this medium than in previous formulas. However, collagenase medium is still necessary when they start to dominate the culture.

Our attempts to develop a medium for the growth of newly isolated cancer cells are empirical at this stage. Too often, we still note clusters of cancer cells that fail to proliferate or have limited *in vitro* survival. A moderate number of specimens, although appearing to have large numbers of tissue cells on original processing, have only lymphocyte-like cells remaining after 24–72 h culture. Studies are in progress to prevent lymphocyte cytolysis. Although PAP medium is only a step toward the goal of developing a medium for the cultivation of newly isolated cancer cells, we have a number of cultures that appear to be developing into permanent cell lines; these still require the test of time and characterization. Isolates that have had at least a year of *in vitro* life, in addition to those listed on p. 40, include SW-156 (kidney carcinoma), SW-161 (alveolar cell carcinoma), SW-193 (endometrial carcinoma of the uterus), SW-213 (squamous carcinoma mass from the neck), and SW-267 (chemodectoma of the organ of Zuckerkandl).

4. *References*

Aaronson, S. A., Todaro, G. J., and Freeman, A. E., 1970, Human sarcoma cells in culture: Identification by colony-forming ability on monolayers of normal cells, *Exp. Cell Res.* **61**:1.

Allison, A. C., and Law, L. W., 1968, Effects of antilymphocyte serum on virus oncogenesis, *Proc. Soc. Exp. Biol. Med.* **127**:207.

Anderson, N. G., 1953, The mass isolation of whole cells from rat liver, *Science* **117**:627.

Anigstein, L., Anigstein, D. M., and Rennels, E. G., 1965, Effect of neonatal inoculation of thymus antiserum on growth of Sarcoma 180 in mice, *Texas Rep. Biol. Med.* **23**:705.

Anigstein, L., Anigstein, D. M., Rennels, E. G., and O'Steen, W. K., 1966, Induced alteration of resistance to transplantable mammary adenocarcinoma in mice neonatally inoculated with rat thymus antiserum, *Cancer Res.* **26**:1867.

Auersperg, N., 1964, Long term culture of hypodiploid human tumor cells, *J. Natl. Cancer Inst.* **32**:135.

Baron, S., and Rabson, A. S., 1957, A culture strain (LAC) of human epithelial-like cells from an adenocarcinoma of the lung, *Proc. Soc. Exp. Biol. Med.* **96**:515.

Bassin, R. H., Plata, E. J., Gerwin, B. I., Mattern, C. F., Haapala, D. K., and Chu, E. W., 1972, Isolation of a continuous epithelioid cell line, HBT-3, from a human breast carcinoma, *Proc. Soc. Exp. Biol. Med.* **141**:673.

Baugh, C. L., and Tytell, A. A., 1967, Propagation of the human diploid cell WI-38 in galactose medium, *Life Sci.* **6**:371.

Berman, L., and Stulberg, C. S., 1956, Eight culture strains (Detroit) of human epithelial-like cells, *Proc. Soc. Exp. Biol. Med.* **92**:730.

Beynish-Melnick, M., Fernbach, D. J., and Lewis, R. T., 1963, Studies on human leukemia. I. Spontaneous lymphoblastoid transformation of fibroblastic bone marrow cultures derived from leukemic and non-leukemic children, *J. Natl. Cancer Inst.* **31**:1311.

Bichel, J., 1938, Dauerzuchtüng von leukämischen Zellen *in vitro*, *Z. Krebsforsch.* **48**:92.

Burlington, H., 1959, Enzyme patterns in cultured kidney cells, *Am. J. Physiol.* **197**:68.

Burrows, M. T., 1910, The cultivation of tissues of the chick-embryo outside the body, *JAMA* **55**:2057.

Cailleau, R., 1960, The establishment of a cell strain (MAC-21) from a mucoid adenocarcinoma of the human lung, *Cancer Res.* **20**:837.

Cameron, G., and Chambers, R., 1937, Neoplasm studies. III. Organization of cells of human tumors in tissue culture, *Am. J. Cancer* **30**:115.

Carrel, A., 1923, A method for the physiological study of tissues *in vitro*, *J. Exp. Med.* **38**:407.

Chang, R. S., 1954, Continuous subcultivation of epithelial-like cells from normal human tissues, *Proc. Soc. Exp. Biol. Med.* **87**:440.

Cobb, J. P., Walker, D. G., and Wright, J. C., 1961, Comparative chemotherapy studies on primary short term cultures of human normal, benign, and malignant tumor tissues—A five year study, *Cancer Res.* **21**:583.

Coman, D. R., 1942, Human neoplasms in tissue culture, *Cancer Res.* **2**:618.

Costachel, O., Fadei, L., and Badea, E., 1969, Tumor cell suspension culture on non-adhesive substratum, *Z. Krebsforsch.* **72**:24.

Debruyn, W. M., Korteweg, R., and Van Waveren, E. K., 1949, Transplantable mouse lymphosarcoma T86157 (M.B.) studied *in vitro* and at autopsy, *Cancer Res.* **9**:282.

DeLuca, L., 1965, The use of trypsin for the determination of cellular viability, *Exp. Cell Res.* **40**:186.

Eagle, H., 1955*a*, The specific amino acid requirements of a human carcinoma cell (strain HeLa) in tissue culture, *J. Exp. Med.* **102**:37.

Eagle, H., 1955*b*, Propagation in fluid medium of a human epidermoid carcinoma, strain K. B., *Proc. Soc. Exp. Biol. Med.* **89**:362.

Eagle, H., 1958–1959, Metabolic studies with normal and malignant human cells in culture, in: *The Harvey Lectures*, pp. 156–175, Academic Press, New York, 1960.

Eagle, H., 1959, Amino acid metabolism in mammalian cell cultures, *Science* **130**:432.

Eagle, H., and Foley, G. E., 1958, Cytotoxicity in human cell cultures as a primary screen for the detection of anti-tumor agents, *Cancer Res.* **18**:1017.

Eagle, H., and Piez, K., 1962, The population-dependent requirement by cultured mammalian cells for metabolites which they can synthesize, *J. Exp. Med.* **116**:29.

Eagle, H., Barban, S., Levy, M., and Schulze, H. O., 1958, The utilization of carbohydrates by human cell cultures, *J. Biol. Chem.* **233**:551.

Ebeling, A. H., 1921, Fibrin and serum as a culture medium, *J. Exp. Med.* **33**:641.

Ehrmann, R. L., and Gey, G. O., 1956, The growth of cells on a transparent gel of reconstituted rat-tail collagen, *J. Natl. Cancer Inst.* **16**:1375.

Evans, V. J., and Earle, W. R., 1947, The use of perforated cellophane for the growth of cells in tissue culture, *J. Natl. Cancer Inst.* **8**:103.

Evans, V. J., Bryant, J. C., Fioramonti, M. D., McQuilkin, W. T., Sanford, K. K., and Earle, W. R., 1956, Studies of a nutrient media for tissue cells *in vitro*, I. A protein-free chemically defined medium for cultivation of strain L cells, *Cancer Res.* **16**:77.

Evans, V. J., Bryant, J. C., Kerr, H. A., and Shilling, E. L., 1964, Chemically defined media for cultivation of long-term cell strains from four mammalian species, *Exp. Cell Res.* **36**:439.

Fawcett, D. W., and Vallee, B. L., 1952, Studies on the separation of cell types in serosanguinous fluids, blood, and vaginal fluids by flotation on bovine plasma albumin, *J. Lab. Clin. Med.* **39**:354.

Fawcett, D. W., Vallee, B. L., and Soule, M. H., 1950, A method for concentration and segregation of malignant cells from bloody, pleural and peritoneal fluids, *Science* **111**:34.

Feller, W. F., Stewart, S. E., and Kantor, J., 1972, Primary tissue culture explants of human breast cancer, *J. Natl. Cancer Inst.* **48**:1117.

Ferrebee, J. W., and Geiman, Q. M., 1946, Studies on malarial parasites. III. A procedure for preparing concentrates of *Plasmodium vivax*, *J. Infect. Dis.* **78**:173.

Fjelde, A., 1955, Human tumor cells in tissue culture, *Cancer* **8**:845.

Føgh, J., and Lund, R., 1957, Continuous cultivation of epithelial-cell strain (FL) from human amniotic membrane, *Proc. Soc. Exp. Biol. Med.* **94:**532.

Foley, J. F., 1973, Acid mucopolysaccharide production of human fibroblasts *in vitro*, presented at Central States Branch Tissue Culture Association Meeting, Ardmore, Okla., May.

Foley, J. F., and Aftonomos, 1965, Growth of human breast neoplasms in cell culture, *J. Natl. Cancer Inst.* **34:**217.

Foulds, L., 1954, The experimental study of tumor progression: A review, *Cancer Res.* **14:**327.

Frisch, A. W., Jentoft, V., Burger, R., and Losli, E. J., 1955, A human epithelial-like cell (MABEN) derived from an adenocarcinoma of lung: Isolation, continuous propagation and effects of selected viruses, *Am. J. Clin. Pathol.* **25:**1107.

Gaugas, J. M., Chesterman, F. C., Hirsch, M. S., Rees, R. J. W., Harvey, J. J., and Gilchrist, C., 1969, Unexpected high incidence of tumors in thymectomized mice treated with antilymphocytic globulin and *Mycobacterium leprae, Nature (Lond.)* **222:**1033.

Gey, G. O., 1933, An improved technique for massive tissue culture, *Am. J. Cancer* **17:**752.

Gey, G. O., 1954–1955, Some aspects of the constitution and behaviour of normal and malignant cells contained in continuous culture, in: *The Harvey Lectures,* Series L, pp. 154–229, Academic Press, New York, 1956.

Gey, G. O., and Gey, M. K., 1936, The maintenance of human normal cells and tumor cells in continuous culture. I. Preliminary report: Cultivation of mesoblastic tumors and normal tissue and notes on methods of cultivation, *Am. J. Cancer* **27:**45.

Gey, G. O., Coffman, W. D., and Kubicek, W. T., 1952, Tissue culture studies of the proliferate capacity of cervical carcinoma and normal epithelium, *Cancer Res.* **12:**264.

Ginsberg, H. S., 1957, Discussion, Properties acquired by cells maintained in continuous culture, in: Cellular Biology, Nucleic Acids, and Viruses, *Ann. N.Y. Acad. Sci. Spec. Publ. V,* pp. 362–363.

Gwatkin, R. B. L., and Thomsen, J. L., 1964, A new method for dispersing the cells of mammalian tissues, *Nature (Lond.)* **201:**1242.

Haff, R. F., and Swim, H. E., 1956, Amino acid requirements of rabbit fibroblasts, strain RM3, *Fed. Proc.* **15:**591.

Ham, R. G., 1963, Albumin replacement by fatty acids in clonal growth of mammalian cells, *Science* **140:**802.

Ham, R. G., 1965, Clonal growth of mammalian cells in a chemically defined, synthetic medium, *Proc. Natl. Acad. Sci.* **53:**288.

Hanks, J. H., and Wallace, J. H., 1958, Determination of cell viability, *Proc. Soc. Exp. Biol. Med.* **98:**188.

Harrison, R. G., 1907, Observations on the living developing nerve fiber, *Proc. Soc. Exp. Biol. Med.* **4:**140.

Henle, G., and Deinhardt, F., 1957, The establishment of strains of human cells in tissue culture, *J. Immunol.* **79:**54.

Hertz, R., 1959, Choriocarcinoma of women maintained in serial passage in hamsters and rats, *Proc. Soc. Exp. Biol. Med.* **102:**77.

Hibbs, J. B., Lambert, L. H., and Remington, J. S., 1972, Control of carcinogenesis: A possible role for the activated macrophage, *Science* **177:**998.

Hinz, R. W., and Syverton, J. T., 1959, Mammalian cell cultures for the study of influenza virus. I. Preparation of monolayer cultures with collagenase, *Proc. Soc. Exp. Biol. Med.* **101:**19.

Houba, V., 1967, The use of pronase for dispersing cells, *Experientia* **23:**372.

Hsu, T. C., and Kellog, D. S., 1960, Primary cultivation and continuous propagation *in vitro* of tissues from small biopsy specimens, *J. Natl. Cancer Inst.* **25:**221.

Ioachim, H. L., 1970, Tissue culture of human tumors: Its use and prospects, *Pathol. Ann.* **5:**217.

Jensen, F. C., and Castellano, G. A., 1960, The long term maintenance of tumor explants, *Cancer Chemother. Rep.* **8:**135.

Jensen, F. C., Gwatkin, R. B. L., and Biggers, D., 1964, A simple organ culture method which allows simultaneous isolation of specific types of cells, *Exp. Cell Res.* **34:**440.

Jordan, W., 1956, Human nasal cells in continuous cultures; establishment of two lines of epithelial-like cells, *Proc. Soc. Exp. Biol. Med.* **92:**867.

Kalant, H., and Young, F., 1957, Metabolic behaviour of isolated liver and kidney cells, *Nature (Lond.)* **179:**816.

Kaltenbach, J. P., 1954, The preparation and utilization of whole cell suspensions obtained from solid mammalian tissues, *Exp. Cell Res.* **7:**568.

Kohler, P. O., Bridson, W. E., Hammond, J. M., Weintraub, F., Kirschner, M. A., and Van Thiel, D. H., 1971, Clonal lines of human choriocarcinoma cells in culture, in: *In vitro Methods in Reproductive Cell Biology*, p. 137, Karolinska Symposia on Research Methods in Reproductive Endocrinology, 3rd Symposium.

Kraemer, P. M., 1972, Complex carbohydrates of mammalian cells in culture, in: *Growth, Nutrition, and Metabolism of Cells in Culture*, Vol. 1 (G. H. Rothblat, and V. J. Cristofalo, eds.), pp. 371–426, Academic Press, New York.

Lasfargues, E. Y., 1957, Cultivation and behavior *in vitro* of the normal mammary epithelium of the adult mouse, *Exp. Cell Res.* **13:**553.

Lasfargues, E. Y., and Moore, D. H., 1971, A method for the continuous cultivation of mammary epithelium, *In vitro* **7:**21.

Lasfargues, E. Y., and Ozzello, L., 1958, Cultivation of human breast carcinomas, *J. Natl. Cancer Inst.* **21:**1131.

Lasfargues, E. Y., Coutinho, W. G., and Moore, D. H.,1972, Pitfalls in the isolation of a human breast carcinoma virus in tissue culture, *J. Natl. Cancer Inst.* **48:**1101.

Lata, G., and Reinerston, J., 1957, Cholesterol synthesis by isolated rat liver cells, *Nature (Lond.)* **178:**47.

Laws, J., and Strickland, L., 1956, Metabolism of isolated liver cells, *Nature (Lond.)* **178:**309.

Lazarus, H., Tegeler, W., Mazzono, H. M., Leroy, J. G., Boone, B. A., and Foley, G. E., 1966, Determination of sensitivity of individual biopsy specimens to potential inhibitory agents: Evaluation of some explant culture methods as assay systems, *Cancer Chemother. Rep.* **50:**543.

Leibovitz, A., 1963, The growth and maintenance of tissue-cell cultures in free gas exchange with the atmosphere, *Am. J. Hyg.* **78:**173.

Leibovitz, A., McCombs, W. B., III, Johnston, D., McCoy, C. E., and Stinson, J. C., 1973*a*, Two new human cancer cell lines, presented at Tissue Culture Association Meeting, Boston.

Leibovitz, A., McCombs, W. B., III, Johnston, D., McCoy, C. E., and Stinson, J. C., 1973*b*, New human cancer cell culture lines. I. SW-13, small cell carcinoma of the adrenal cortex, *J. Natl. Cancer Inst.* **51:**691.

Leighton, J., 1954, Studies on human cancer using sponge matrix tissue culture. I. The growth patterns of a malignant melanoma, adenocarcinoma of the parotid gland, papillary adenocarcinoma of the thyroid gland, adenocarcinoma of the pancreas, and epidermoid carcinoma of the uterine cervix (Gey's HeLa strain), *Texas Rep. Biol. Med.* **12:**847.

Leighton, J., 1957*a*, Appraisal of the malignant properties of human cells in continuous culture: A discussion, in: Cellular Biology, Nucleic Acids, and Viruses, *Ann. N.Y. Acad. Sci. Spec. Publ. V*, pp. 356–361.

Leighton, J., 1957*b*, Contributions of tissue culture studies to the understanding of the biology of cancer: A review, *Cancer Res.* **17:**929.

Leighton, J., Kline, I., Belkin, M., Legallais, F., and Orr, H. C., 1957, The similarity in histological appearance of some human "cancer" and "normal" cell strains in sponge-matrix tissue culture, *Cancer Res.* **17:**359.

Levintow, L., and Eagle, H., 1961, Biochemistry of cultured mammalian cells, in: *Annual Review of Biochemistry*, Vol. 30 (J. M. Luck, F. W. Allen, and G. Mackinney, eds.) pp. 605–640, Annual Reviews, Palo Alto, Calif.

Lieberman, I., and Ove, P., 1959, Growth factors for mammalian cells in culture, *J. Biol. Chem.* **234:**2754.

Ling, C. T., Gey, G. O., and Richters, V., 1968, Chemically characterized concentrated corodies for continuous cell culture (the 7C's media), *Exp. Cell Res.* **52:**469.

Lockhart, R. Z., Jr., and Eagle, H., 1959, Requirements for growth of single human cells, *Science* **129:**252.

Mackenzie, C. G., Mackenzie, J. B., and Beck, P., 1961, The effect of pH on growth, protein synthesis, and lipid-rich particles of cultured mammalian cells, *J. Biophys. Biochem. Cytol.* **9:**141.

Macpherson, I., and Montagnier, L., 1964, Agar suspension culture for the selective assay of cells transformed by polyoma virus, *Virology* **23:**291.

McAllister, R. M., and Reed, G., 1968, Colonial growth in agar of cells derived from neoplastic and non-neoplastic tissues of children, *Pediat. Res.* **2:**356.

McLimans, W. F., Mount, D. T., Bogitch, S., Crouse, E. J., Harris, G., and Moore, G. E., 1966, A controlled environment system for study of mammalian cell physiology, *Ann. N.Y. Acad. Sci.* **139:**190.

Moore, A. E., Sabachewsky, L., and Toolan, H. M., 1955, Culture characteristics of four permanent cell lines of human cancer cells, *Cancer Res.* **15:**598.

Morgan, J. F., 1958, Tissue culture nutrition, *Bacteriol. Rev.* **22:**20.

Morton, H. J., 1970, A survey of commercially available tissue culture media, *In Vitro* **6:**89.

Moscona, A., 1952, Cell suspensions from organ rudiments of chick embryos, *Exp. Cell Res.* **3:**535.

Neuman, R. E., and McCoy, T. A., 1956, Dual requirement of Walker carcinosarcoma 256 *in vitro* for asparagine and glutamine, *Science* **124:**124.

Neuman, R. E., and Tytell, A. A., 1960, Amino acid requirements for growth of avian lung cultures, *Proc. Soc. Exp. Biol. Med.* **103:**71.

Ozzello, L., and Speer, F. D., 1958, The mucopolysaccharides in the normal and the diseased breast, *Am. J. Pathol.* **34:**993.

Ozzello, L., Lasfargues, E. Y., and Murray, M. R., 1960, Growth promoting activity of acid muco-polysaccharides on a strain of human mammary carcinoma cells, *Cancer Res.* **20:**600.

Parker, R. C., 1961, *Methods of Tissue Culture*, 3rd ed., Hoeber, New York.

Pattillo, R. A., and Gey, G. O., 1968, The establishment of a cell line of human hormone-synthesizing trophoblastic cells *in vitro, Cancer Res.* **28:**1231.

Patuleia, M. D., and Friend, C., 1967, Tissue culture studies on murine virus-induced leukemia cells: Isolation of single cells in agar–liquid medium, *Cancer Res.* **27:**726.

Pierce, G. B., and Johnson, L. D., 1971, Differentiation and cancer, *In Vitro* **7:**140.

Pious, D. A., Hamburger, R. N., and Mills, S. E., 1963, Clonal analysis of primary human cultures, *Fed. Proc.* **22:**382.

Pomerat, C. M., Nowinski, W. W., and Rose, G. G., 1950, Tissue culture of cells from body fluids, *Texas Rep. Biol. Med.* **8:**521.

Puck, T., and Marcus, P. I., 1955, A rapid method for viable cell titration in tissue culture: The use of X-irradiated cells to supply conditioning factors, *Proc. Natl. Acad. Sci.* **41:**432.

Puck, T., Marcus, P. I., and Cieciura, S. J., 1956, Clonal growth of mammalian cells *in vitro*: Growth characteristics of colonies from single HeLa cells with and without a feeder layer, *J. Exp. Med.* **103:**653.

Reed, M. V., and Gey, G. O., 1962, Cultivation of normal and malignant lung tissue: The establishment of three adenocarcinoma cell strains, *Lab. Invest.* **11:**638.

Richardson, H. B., and Leibovitz, A., 1965, Hand, foot, and mouth disease in children, *J. Pediat.* **67:**6.

Rightsel, W. A., Schultz, P., Muething, D., and McLean, I. W., 1956, Use of vinyl plastic containers in tissue culture for viral assays, *J. Immunol.* **76:**464.

Rinaldini, L. M., 1958, The isolation of living cells from animal tissues, *Int. Rev. Cytol.* **7:**587.

Rinaldini, L. M., 1959, An improved method for the isolation and quantitative cultivation of embryonic cells, *Exp. Cell Res.* **16:**477.

Robertson, H. E., Brunner, K. T., and Syverton, J. T., 1955, Propagation *in vitro* of poliomyelitis viruses. III. pH change of HeLa cell cultures for assay, *Proc. Soc. Exp. Biol. Med.* **88:**119.

Rose, H. M., 1969, Adenoviruses, in: *Diagnostic Procedures for Viral and Rickettsial Infections*, (E. H. Lennette, and N. J. Schmidt, eds.), pp. 205–226, American Public Health Association, New York.

Rothblat, G. H., and Cristofalo, V. J. (eds.), 1972, *Growth, Nutrition and Metabolism of Cells in Culture*, Vols. 1 and 2, Academic Press, New York.

Rous, P., and Jones, F. A., 1916, A method of obtaining suspensions of living cells from the fixed tissues and for the plating out of individual cells, *J. Exp. Med.* **23:**555.

Royle, J. G., 1946, Some cultural and cytological characteristics of human tumors *in vitro*, *Cancer Res.* **6:**225.

Rubin, H., 1965–1966, The behavior of cells before and after virus-induced malignant transformation, *The Harvey Lecture Series 61*, Academic Press, New York, 1967.

Sanders, F. K., and Burford, B. O., 1964, Ascites tumors from BHK 21 cells transformed *in vitro* by polyoma virus, *Nature (Lond.)* **201:**786.

Santesson, L., 1935, Characteristics of epithelial mouse tumor cells *in vitro* and tumor structures *in vivo*: A comparative study. *Acta Pathol. Microbiol. Scand. Suppl.* **24:**1.

Sinkovics, J. G., Dreyer, D. A,, Shirato, E., Cabiness, J. R., and Shellenberger, C. C., 1971, Cytotoxic lymphocytes. I. Destruction of neoplastic cells in cultures of human origin, *Texas Rep. Biol. Med.* **29:**227.

Sinkovics, J. G., Cabiness, J. R., and Shullenberger, C. C., 1972, Monitoring *in vitro* of immune reactions to solid tumors, *Frontiers Radiat. Ther. Oncol.* **7:**99.

Southam, C. M., 1954, Growth of human adenocarcinoma cells in tissue culture, *Cancer* **7:**394.

Southam, C. M., and Goettler, P. J., 1953, Growth of human epidermoid carcinoma cells in tissue culture, *Cancer* **6:**809.

Sumegi, I., and Rajka, G., 1972, Amyloid-like substance surrounding mammary cancer and basal cell carcinoma, *Acta. Pathol. Microbiol. Scand. Sect. A* **80:**185.

Sumegi, I., Goreczky, L., and Roth, I., 1954, Recent studies on the amyloid in malignant tumors, *Acta. Morphol. Acad. Sci. Hungary* **4:**463.

Syverton, J. T., and McLaren, L. C., 1957, Human cells in continuous culture. I. Derivation of cell strains from esophagus, palate, liver and lung, *Cancer Res.* **17:**923.

Temin, H. M., Pierson, R. W., Jr., and Dulak, N. C., 1972, The role of serum in the control of multiplication of avian and mammalian cells in culture, in: *Growth, Nutrition, and Metabolism of Cells in Culture*, Vol. 1 (G. H. Rothblat, and V. J. Cristofalo, eds.), pp. 49–81, Academic Press, New York.

Therkelsen, A. J., 1964, "Sandwich" technique for the establishment of cultures of human skin for chromosome investigation, *Acta Pathol. Microbiol. Scand.* **61:**317.

Toolan, H. W., 1953, Growth of human tumors in cortisone-treated laboratory animals: The possibility of obtaining permanently transplantable human tumors, *Cancer Res.* **13:**389.

Toolan, W. H., 1954, Transplantable human neoplasms maintained in cortisone-treated laboratory animals: H. S. No. 1, H. Ep. No. 1, H. Ep. No. 2, H. Ep. No. 3, and H. Emb. Rh No. 1, *Cancer Res.* **14:**660.

Toolan, W. H., 1957, Permanently transplantable human tumors maintained in conditioned heterologous hosts: H. Chon. No. 1, H. Ep. No. 4, and H. Ad. No. 1, *Cancer Res.* **17:**418.

Traub, R. N., 1972, Mechanism of immunosuppression by antilymphocyte antibody, *Pathobiol. Ann.* **2:**129.

Tribble, H. R., and Higuchi, K., 1963, Studies on nutrition and metabolism of animal cells in serum-free medium. II. Cultivation of cells in suspension, *J. Infect. Dis.* **112:**221.

Trowell, O. A., 1953, The action of cortisone on lymphocytes *in vitro*, *J. Physiol. (Lond.)* **119:**274.

Trowell, O. A., 1959, The culture of mature organs in a synthetic medium, *Exp. Cell Res.* **16:**118.

Vaage, J., 1968, A mechanical technique for obtaining high yields of viable dispersed tumor cells, *Transplantation* **6:**137.

Walker, D. G., Lyons, M. M., and Wright, J. C., 1965, Observation on primary short-term cultures of human tumors: A second 5-year study, *Eur. J. Cancer* **1:**265.

Waymouth, C., 1954, The nutrition of animal cells, *Int. Rev. Cytol.* **3:**1.

Waymouth, C., 1956, A serum-free nutrient solution sustaining rapid and continuous proliferation of strain L (Earle) mouse cells, *J. Natl. Cancer Inst.* **17:**315.

Waymouth, C., 1959, Rapid proliferation of sublines of NCTC clone 929 (strain L) mouse cells in a simple chemically defined medium (MB 752/1), *J. Natl. Cancer Inst.* **22:**1003.

Waymouth, C., 1960, Growth in tissue culture, in: *Fundamental Aspects of Normal and Malignant Growth* (W. W. Nowinski, ed.), pp. 546–587, Elsevier, Amsterdam.

Waymouth, C., 1965, Construction and use of synthetic media, in: *Cells and Tissues in Culture,* Vol. 1 (E. N. Wilmer, ed.), pp. 99–142, Academic Press, New York.

Waymouth, C., 1967, Somatic cells *in vitro*: Their relationship to progenitive cells and to artificial milieux, *Natl. Cancer Inst. Monogr.* **26:**1.

Waymouth, C., 1968, Tissue culture media: Animal cells, in: *Metabolism* (P. L. Altman, and D. S. Dittmer, eds.), pp. 180–187, FASEB, Washington, D.C.

Waymouth, C., 1972, Construction of tissue culture media, in: *Growth, Nutrition and Metabolism of Cells in Culture,* Vol. 1 (G. H. Rothblat, and V. J. Cristofalo, eds.), pp. 11–47, Academic Press, New York.

Weinhouse, S., 1972, Glycolysis, respiration, and anomalous gene expression in experimental hepatomas: G.H.A., Clowes memorial lecture, *Cancer Res.* **32:**2007.

Wespic, H. T., 1970, Separation of viable tumor cells from nonviable tumor cells by flotation on bovine serum albumin: A short communication, *J. Natl. Cancer Inst.* **45:**1031.

White, P. R., 1946, Cultivation of animal tissues *in vitro* in nutrients of precisely known constitution, *Growth* **10:**231.

White, P. R., 1949, Prolonged survival of excised animal tissues *in vitro* in nutrients of known composition, *J. Cell Comp. Physiol.* **34:**221.

Whitescarver, J., Recher, L., Sykes, J. A., and Briggs, L., 1968, Problems involved in culturing human breast tissue, *Texas Rep. Biol. Med.* **26:**613.

Williams, E. D., Brown, C. L., and Doniach, I., 1966, Pathological and clinical findings in a series of 67 cases of medullary cancer of the thyroid, *J. Clin. Pathol.* **19:**103.

Wilson, B. W., and Lau, T. L., 1963, Dissociation and cultivation of chick embryo cells with an actinomycete protease, *Proc. Soc. Exp. Biol. Med.* **114:**651.

Wolff, E., 1956*a*, La culture de cellules tumorales sur de explants d'organes *in vitro, Experientia* **12:**321.

Wolff, E., 1956*b*, La culture des tumeurs sur des organes embryonaires explantes *in vitro, Rev. Med. (Bruxells)* **36:**2235.

Yohn, D. S., McD. Hammon, W., Atchison, R. W., and Castro, B. C., 1962, Serial heterotransplantation of human adenocarcinoma No. 1 in the cheek pouch of unconditioned adult Syrian hamsters, *Cancer Res.* **22:**443.

Zaroff, L., Sato, G., and Mills, S. E., 1961, Single cell platings from freshly isolated mammalian tissue, *Exp. Cell Res.* **23:**565.

Zimmerman, M., Devlin, T., and Pruss, M., 1960, Anaerobic glycolysis of dispersed cell suspensions from normal and malignant tissues, *Nature (Lond.)* **185:**315.

New Approaches to the Cultivation of Human Breast Carcinomas

3

ETIENNE Y. LASFARGUES*

1. Introduction

Despite many attempts, the cultivation of human breast tumors still remains a challenging problem. Attention to these neoplasms has increased since the discovery of a virus-like particle morphologically comparable to the mouse mammary tumor virus (MTV) in the milk of patients with a history of breast cancer (Moore *et al.*, 1969, 1971). The mouse mammary tumor virus discovered by Bittner (1936) reproduces exclusively in epithelial cells and induces tumors in the mammary gland only (Lasfargues and Moore, 1966). If a comparable mechanism is valid for human breast tumors, a similar virus might be produced by the epithelial cells derived from these carcinomas, hence the sudden interest in their cultivation and the mounting awareness of the difficulties involved.

Mouse mammary tumors grow well in tissue culture, but human breast tumors do not; under the most favorable conditions, fragments of breast carcinomas yield short-lived epithelial cells and fibroblasts which grow vigorously. Considering that the epithelial cell is the prime target, the

*Supported by Public Health Service grant CA-08515, contract NIH-NCI-72-3868, General Research support grant FR-5582 from the NIH, and grant-in-aid M-43 from the state of New Jersey.

ETIENNE Y. LASFARGUES Institute for Medical Research, Camden, New Jersey presence of fibroblasts in the cultures is undesirable. In a pioneering work, Cameron and Chambers (1937) stressed the importance of the epithelium and recommended special procedures for its isolation. They observed that the epithelial cells do not form a monolayer as readily as the fibroblasts but cohere in small islets which later develop into larger acinar formations. Similar observations were made by Coman (1942, 1944), who attributed the mobility of the cancer cells and their ability to form loose aggregates to their decreased cohesiveness. On the basis of these observations, Lasfargues and Ozzello (1958) explanted the cells spilling freely from sliced mammary carcinomas and obtained small, independent colonies of pure epithelial cells. Eventually, a cell line (BT-20) derived from a multicentric primary carcinoma was established and has been serially subcultured to date.

As a rule, human breast cancer cells *in vitro* are overgrown by the fibroblasts of the tumor stroma. In early attempts, Gey and Gey (1936), Royle (1946), Orr and McSwain (1955), Foley and Aftonomos (1965), and Whitescarver *et al.* (1968) obtained by conventional techniques a higher percentage of fibroblasts than epithelium. For this reason, the establishment of a cell line has been a rare event. To avoid the fibroblasts, Reed and Gey (1962) explanted a breast tumor metastatic to the lungs and obtained a cell line (AlAb) which grows as pure epithelium. Two other cell lines, one derived from the pleural fluid (Lev III) and the other from the ascites fluid (Sal III) of patients with breast cancer, have a lymphoblastic morphology and grow only in suspension (Giraldo, 1970).

The desirability of growing human breast cancer cells is great. It is evident that if cells from a number of tumors could be isolated from patients and be propagated to larger populations in tissue culture, several tests would become available to the treating physician. Furthermore, if the viral etiology of mammary cancers is eventually demonstrated in man, such cell lines could become a source of replicating virus for the preparation of vaccines. The following pages describe some personal observations and recently developed techniques which might help to solve some of the problems concerning the cultivation of these tumors.

2. *Methods of Explantation*

2.1. *Importance of the Tumor Morphology*

Human mammary tumors vary widely in morphology, ranging from a solid mass of tumor cells to a very fibrous, almost acellular lump. Each type demands a different technique in handling, processing, and culturing. The choice of an adequate method is therefore directed by the appearance of the biopsy specimen, which can roughly be classified as belonging to one of three types: (1) cystic hyperplasia, (2) fibroadenoma, or (3) carcinoma. Of these, the first two are considered benign tumors while the third, subdivided into several groups, includes scirrhous, medullary, and intraductal carcinomas.

2.1.1. Benign Tumors

a. Cystic Hyperplasia. Cystic hyperplasia is the most common structural lesion which occurs in the breast of middle-aged women. The cysts usually derive from hyperplastic ducts which have not undergone complete involution; they are lined by ductal epithelium and may be tensely filled with fluid. In some circumstances, the living epithelium may proliferate in papillary formations that fill the entire cyst. In either case, the overall lesion is tough, of a rubbery consistency, even more so when connective tissue hyperplasia happens to increase the thickness of the cystic envelopes.

Obviously the chances of success in explanting such a lesion greatly depend on the extent of the papillary outgrowth and on the relative thickness of the surrounding envelopes, whose pressure may induce necrosis of the epithelial cells.

b. Fibroadenoma. Fibroadenoma occurs most often in young women. This tumor is characterized by a hyperplasia of the loose connective tissue surrounding the lactiferous ducts and acini as well as by a hyperplasia of the ductal epithelium. It is well encapsulated and of soft consistency even though of mesenchymal origin; the cut surface may show cross-sectioning of many ducts. This type of material is not neoplastic but has in recent years become more and more available from operating rooms.

Fibroadenomas do not present any tissue culture problems; they grow well following trypsinization and can eventually give rise to an extensive growth of the epithelium.

2.1.2. Carcinomas

a. Scirrhous Carcinomas. Scirrhous carcinomas are the most frequent and the most dangerously malignant of breast cancers. The tumor is usually well circumscribed and hard. The epithelial cells deeply embedded in a dense and abundant fibrous stroma may be arranged in single file lying within lymph spaces; they are polygonal, compressed by the fibrous tissue which they appear to infiltrate and in which they survive under relatively anaerobic conditions. Thus the scirrhous quality of a tumor can be regarded as a defense mechanism by which the organism apposes barriers of interlacing collagen fibers to cell penetration. The presence of mitotic figures is rare among the neoplastic cells, which otherwise are quite resilient to physical hardships.

The cultivation of a scirrhous carcinoma depends on how successfully one can extricate the neoplastic cells from their fibrous casing. Explantation of tumor fragments is more likely to result in overgrowth of fibroblasts than of epithelium, which emerges only from small areas in the cut surface. In this particular situation, enzymatic digestion of the collagen and interfibrillary cement offers a gentle way of liberating the strands of cancer cells. Collagenase has been found particularly efficient in dissociating such tumors.

b. Medullary Carcinomas. Medullary carcinomas differ from the preceding group in texture and general appearance. This type of tumor is usually well circumscribed, round, 4–6 cm in diameter, and soft. The tumor is formed by voluminous masses of epithelial cells with an abundant cytoplasm and large vesicular nuclei; many mitoses occur among these cells, which are loosely connected with each other. Since the tumor stroma is almost nonexistent, the medullary carcinoma is ideal for tissue culture. Enzymatic dissociation is not necessary because slicing provides an abundance of cell aggregates spilling freely into the surrounding medium. These aggregates, about 90% epithelial, are immediately explantable.

c. Intraductal Carcinomas. Intraductal Carcinomas or "comedo carcinomas" are another type of lesion particularly favorable for cultivation. The tumor may originate from a duct papilloma, and, even though confined within the walls of the ducts, the progression of the tumor cells is more diffuse than in a circumscribed medullary carcinoma. When the tumor is sliced, wormlike casts can be expressed from the cut surface; these are formed by neoplastic epithelial cells that can be readily explanted.

Scirrhous carcinomas are 30 times more common than medullary and comedo carcinomas. This explains why success in the cultivation of breast carcinoma, usually dependent on the availability of highly cellular tumors, is so rare.

2.2. *Techniques of Cultivation*

Since the morphology of the biopsy specimen is a determining factor, the efficiency of tissue culture techniques involving tumor fragment explantation is variable. However, organ cultures which rely on fragment morphology remain the method of choice for study of the influence of hormones and chemical compounds on cell interactions and function.

Cell cultures, on the other hand, have improved with the availability of new methods that permit the gathering of cells otherwise inaccessible in tumor fragments. The cell populations obtained by enzymatic dispersion are more homogeneous and whether grown in monolayer or in suspension offer enough flexibility to be used in the development of a wide variety of tests.

2.2.1. Organ Cultures

Unlike monolayer cell cultures, organ cultures retain the anatomical relationships between cell types and reproduce to some extent the physiological reactions expressed in the organism. Because organ cultures are maintained for only 1 or 2 weeks, chemically defined media can be used: medium 199 (Morgan *et al.*, 1950), CMRL-1066 (Parker *et al.*, 1957), NCTC-109 (Evans *et al.*, 1964), and Waymouth's MB 752/1 (Waymouth, 1959) are the most frequently employed.

Method: The organ culture method is essentially the watchglass technique described by H. B. Fell (1951). In order to limit the outgrowth of undifferentiated cells and to promote organization, the explants are not immersed in the medium but rather placed on a nutritive gel (Gaillard, 1953; Wolff, 1952) or on a raft floating on liquid medium (Chen, 1954). Two to four fragments, about 3 mm^2 in size, are exposed to the ambient atmosphere of the culture dish and draw their nutrients by capillarity at the medium interface.

Organ cultures have been simplified by the availability of commercial sterile, plastic culture dishes (Falcon Plastics, Oxnard, Calif.). These are small petri dishes 6 cm in diameter with a built-in center well in which 1 ml of culture medium is placed. Around the well is a groove with a ringshaped absorbing pad onto which 5 ml of sterile distilled water is poured to condition the humidity of the chamber. The tissue fragments themselves are placed on a fine mesh stainless steel grid laid down on top of the well so that it comes in direct contact with the culture medium. The whole system is incubated at 37°C under a controlled 5% CO_2 atmosphere in air (Fig. 1).

The culture medium can be pipetted off and replaced every 2 or 3 days; at the end of the experiment the tissue fragments are fixed, embedded in paraffin or epon, and processed by routine histological procedures.

Merits of the Method: From a theoretical point of view, organ cultures appear to be ideally adapted to the study of breast tumors. The periodic removal of the culture medium permits a survey of the metabolites released and assessment of the sensitivity of the tumor fragments to various hormonal groups. With this system, a thorough analysis of the hormonal requirements of normal mammary glands of mice and rats has been made (Elias, 1957; Prop, 1959; Lasfargues and Murray, 1959; Rivera, 1964; Dilley and Nandi, 1968) and the physiological mechanisms regulating the secretory function of the mammary cell have been probed (Banerjee and Banerjee, 1971; Oka and Topper, 1972; Turkington, 1972).

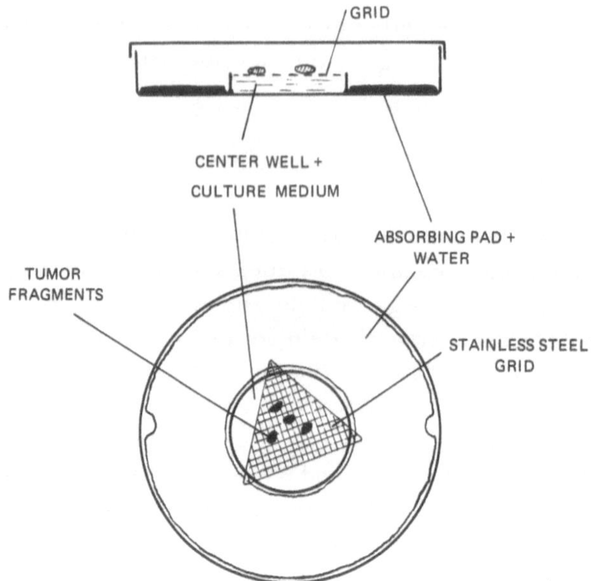

FIG. 1. Falcon plastic organ culture dish.

With human tumors, however, no two cultures placed in an identical situation produce the same results. As pointed out by Stoll (1970), the major problem of the organ culture method is the heterogeneity of the tumor fragments; when the specimen is very fibrous the nutritive exchanges between the viable tumor cells inside the explant and the surrounding medium do not take place properly. If, by comparison, a soft tumor is explanted, the fragments disaggregate spontaneously and thus fail to generate a protective membrane. Wolff and Wolff (1966) circumvented this difficulty by wrapping tumor fragments in a chicken vitelline membrane and succeeded in passing the tumor cells through several generations of cultures. In general, significant conclusions are difficult to reach from organ cultures unless statistical evaluations are made on a large number of fragments.

2.2.2. Cell Cultures

An alternative to organ cultures are cell cultures, which can be initiated from the enzymatic digest of tumors or from spilled cells.

a. Enzymatic Dissociation. To liberate the neoplastic cells enmeshed in the fibrous stroma of scirrhous carcinoma, an enzymatic dissociation is the best approach. Trypsin and versene, however, should not be selected for the primary dissociation of breast tumors. Even though they are a choice combination for the dispersion of many types of cells, they do not attack collagen, which is a major component of these neoplasms. The long exposure of the few liberated cells to trypsin, which results from the tough resistance of the collagen structure, induces breakdown of the proteins coating the cell membrane and irreversible damage. Versene* sequesters the calcium ions participating in the linkage of cell membranes. Like trypsin, it requires a calcium-magnesium-free saline solution for maximum efficiency. Over long periods of dissociation, such an environment does not provide the optimal physiological conditions for survival and very few of the harvested cells recover.

Collagenase,† by comparison, has a maximum efficiency in isotonic solutions containing both calcium and magnesium ions; it also hydrolyzes collagen (Table 1). Low concentrations of 5–10% serum do not reduce its

TABLE 1

Some Comparative Properties of Trypsin and Collagenase

Trypsin	*Collagenase*
Optimum activity at pH 7.8–8.7	Optimum activity at pH 6.5–7.8
Active in calcium-magnesium-free saline solutions	Active in aqueous solutions containing calcium and magnesium
Dependent on time and concentration	*Not* dependent on time or concentration
Does not attack collagen but does attack intercellular mucoproteins	Hydrolyzes collagen, reticulin, cartilage, gelatin
Damages cell membrane	Does *not* damage cell membrane

activity, which is highest in a pH range from 6.5 to 7.8. This allows the use of collagenase in complete culture media, in which it dissolves well. Collagenase solutions are sterilized through a 0.45-μm millipore filter and should be prepared fresh for every specimen. Because collagenase is not cytotoxic, one is not restricted with respect to time and concentrations as with trypsin. Tumors with a heavy collagen matrix can be incubated for several hours in complete culture medium containing the desired concentration of enzyme with minimal damage to the cells.

*Versene: ethylenediaminetetraacetate, or EDTA.

†Collagenase is obtained from *Clostridium histolyticum.* The CLS tissue culture grade manufactured by the Worthington Biochemical Corporation, Freehold, N.J., is quite satisfactory for dissociation of mammary tissues. It has an average titer of 150 u/mg. A unit is the amount of enzyme required to liberate 1 mM leucine equivalents from purified collagen in 18 h at 37°C.

Procedure: An appropriate fragment of breast tumor cut aseptically in the operating room by the surgeon is immediately placed in a sterile jar with a small volume of culture medium. Eagle's minimum essential medium with 5% fetal calf serum and a battery of antibiotics (penicillin, 1000 u/ml; neomycin, 500 μg/ml; tetracycline, 5 μg/ml) is most frequently used. The specimen can then be kept at room temperature for as long as 24 h.

In the tissue culture laboratory, the tumor is trimmed under the dissecting scope, washed rapidly in Hank's–Eagle's medium, then sliced in a petri dish containing 5–10 ml of complete, serum-supplemented culture medium (Fig. 2). In turn, the slices are cut into small fragments 2 or 4 mm^2 in size. One of two courses of action is then available, depending on whether the consistency of the tumor is soft or hard.

A semisoft tumor can be dissociated in 1 h or less. The cut fragments, drained from the medium, are placed in a 50-ml Erlenmeyer flask containing 10-ml of Hank's–Eagle's MEM with 1 mg collagenase per milliliter. The whole is incubated at 37°C with mild magnetic stirring (100 rpm). When dissociation is completed, the suspension is transferred to a conical centrifuge tube and allowed to sediment.

A very hard tumor is dissociated over a much longer period of time. The drained fragments are transferred to 10 ml of Eagle's MEM supplemented with 5% fetal bovine serum and 0.5–1 mg collagenase per milliliter. The whole is incubated at 37°C overnight or for 24 h without agitation; in time, the fragments appear swollen and break apart on gentle pipetting. Because of the length of the enzymatic action, some serum is necessary not only to supply minimum nutritional requirements but also to protect the cell morphology and physiology. As above, the cell suspension is collected in a conical tube and allowed to sediment.

From this point on, the handling of the cells is the same: the supernatant is carefully withdrawn with a Pasteur pipette, and the cells washed in fresh Hank's–Eagle's solution are resuspended in complete culture medium, then distributed in aliquot portions into the chosen culture vessels.

b. Spilled-Cells Technique. When a tumor specimen is sliced in culture medium, there are always some cells escaping from the stroma. Observed by direct light microscopy, these appear globular and are often aggregated in small groups of five to ten cells. The cell suspension may be extremely abundant if the tumor is a medullary or comedo carcinoma. In that case, enzymatic dissociation is not necessary. On slicing, the tumor stroma empties itself into the surrounding medium, which takes on a milky appearance from the many floating tumor cells. This suspension, aspirated with a Pasteur pipette, is passed through three layers of sterile gauze and collected in a conical centrifuge tube, and the cells are allowed to sediment (Fig. 2).

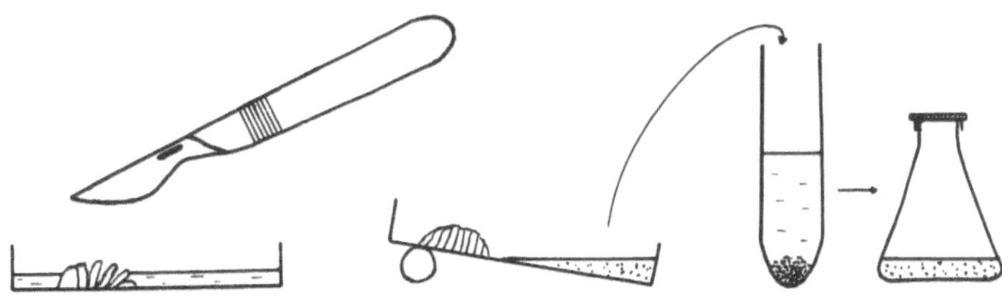

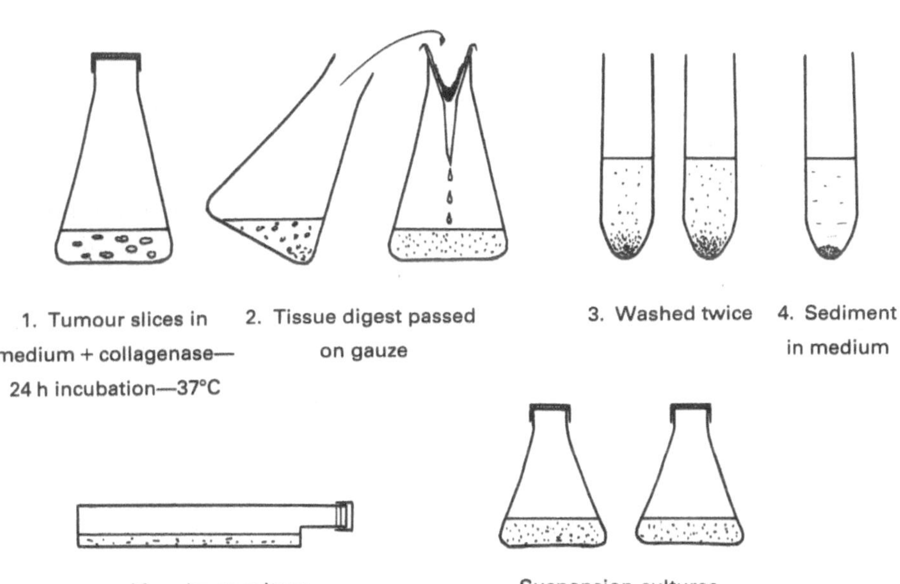

FIG. 2. Procedures for collecting and explanting human breast tumor cells. Following collections of cells by enzymatic dissociation or the "spilling" technique, they are grown in a 75-cm^2 Falcon flask as a monolayer or in a 50-ml Erlenmeyer flask in suspension.

The viable cells, very refringent when observed by direct light microscopy (Fig. 3), sediment rapidly. By comparison, the debris, fibers and dead cells do not scatter light, and they sediment more slowly. These can therefore be partly separated from the viable cells by withdrawal of the supernatant. The pellet of viable cells resuspended in complete culture medium is then distributed into the appropriate culture flasks.

c. Monolayer Culture. The cell suspensions obtained either by enzymatic dissociation or by the "spilling" technique can be mechanically induced to form monolayers on a plasma film (Lasfargues and Ozzello, 1958) or on a coat of reconstituted collagen (Ehrmann and Gey, 1956; Whitescarver *et al.*, 1968). More simply, the cells can be placed in contact with the plastic or the glass of the culture vessel by spreading them on the entire area in a minimum volume of culture medium. The amount of medium must be sufficient to maintain moisture between the aggregates while not enough to allow them to float. Surface tension keeps the cells in close contact with the floor of the flask on which their cytoplasm attaches.

Attachment is usually slow and depends on the concentration of serum. If the cultures remain undisturbed for at least 48 h 20–40% serum is favorable to the attachment of cells. The attached cells are then rapidly washed and refed with complete nutritive medium.

The epithelial cells are the major cell type in the aggregates; they spread out of the original clump to form thin sheets with a smooth border membrane. The "spilled cells" originate epithelial colonies almost exclusively; they do not become confluent or show mitotic activity even though they remain healthy for several days or weeks. Eventually the outside rim of the colony curls up and is slowly pulled back towards the original clump; this is shortly followed by cell breakdown and autolysis.

Following collagenase dissociation, fibroblasts are often interspersed between the epithelial colonies (Fig. 4). When they are present, their active replication enables them to rapidly fill the spaces between the epithelial colonies. Eventually the cell population has to be split; this is done by trypsinization.

d. Suspension Culture. When cells obtained from a tumor either by collagenase dissociation or by the spilling method are explanted, many of them float in the medium, while others rapidly attach to the floor of the culture flask. If the free-floating cells are plated on a thin plasma film, they form epithelial colonies, but the cells which primarily attach to the floor of the culture flask are fibroblasts and lymphoid cells. Evidently the epithelial cells attach poorly, and this offers an opportunity to separate them from the

---

FIG. 3. Three-day-old culture of spilled cell aggregates collected from a highly cellular breast tumor. Many single cells shed from the original clumps. The bar on the lower left corner represents 100 μm.

FIG. 4. A week-old monolayer culture made from the enzymatic digest of a scirrhous carcinoma. Epithelial cells are seen in the upper left corner and around the more compact aggregates. Many fibroblasts expand in between. Scale bar: 100 μm.

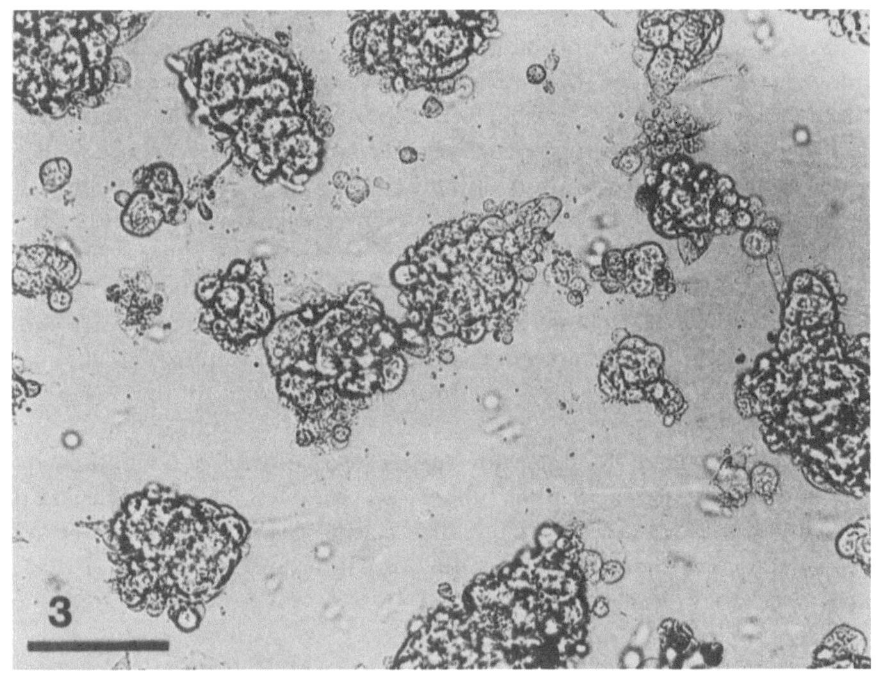
3

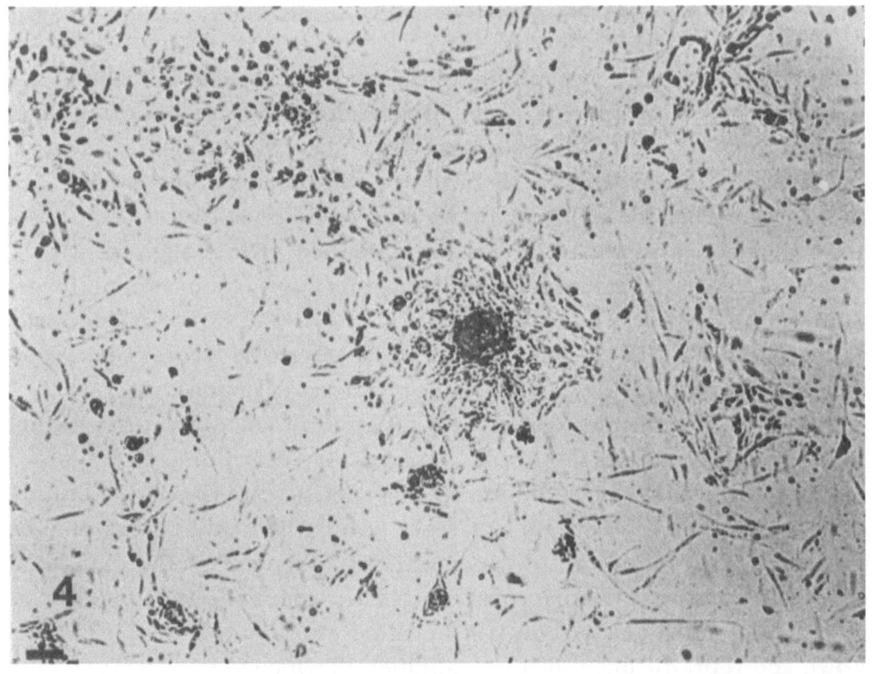
4

other cell types. It also suggests that a state of permanent suspension might be more appropriate for keeping the epithelium in culture. This can be achieved by reducing the concentration of serum in the medium. Every 24 h a brisk twirl of the culture resuspends the clumps which may have started to stick to the glass. Placing the cultures permanently on a rotary shaker regulated at a low number of revolutions per minute is not recommended; breast tumor cells often break down if they are too frequently disturbed.

Spilled cells remain easily in suspension, but cultures obtained by collagenase dispersion often show the formation of a heavy fibroblastic layer at the bottom of the flask. These cells, which originate from the tumor stroma, settle down regardless of the serum concentration. Some epithelial cells may eventually get trapped with the fibroblasts but most of them remain free-floating.

A most convenient container for suspension cultures is a small 50-ml Erlenmeyer flask with a snap-on rubber cap (Kimble). The cells harvested from tumors either after collagenase dissociation or by the spilling method are resuspended in 10–20 ml of culture medium and incubated in these flasks at 37°C.

2.3. Maintenance and Subcultivation

The maintenance and replication of breast cancer cells in culture are dominated by the complexity of mammary physiology. It has often been assumed that following conversion to malignancy cells can acquire a degree of independence which allows them to grow in much simpler media than normal cells. This does not seem to be true with breast cancer cells. Also, specific hormones do not appear to stimulate their growth significantly.

Many media have been used to set up primary cultures of human breast tumors. Among these are medium 199, NCTC-109, McCoy's 5A (McCoy *et al.*, 1959), Eagle's MEM (Eagle, 1959), and RPMI-1640 (Moore *et al.*, 1966). These media enriched with 20–40% concentrations of serum and a variety of hormones give conflicting results with respect to their growth-promoting activity on primary breast tumor cells. It seems that, depending on the tumor of origin, the cultures react differently to a specific experimental medium. Some are inhibited, others do not react at all, while still others may be stimulated. Apparently the physiological dependencies of the explanted cells are responsible for such inconsistencies. In order to design a medium of fundamental nutritional activity it is therefore essential to have a cell line of known and reproducible growth capabilities on which to test various media depleted of ingredients such as hormones or serum.

2.3.1. Evaluation of Culture Media

The BT-20 cell line, derived from a human breast carcinoma and maintained for several years in tissue culture, is particularly well suited to serve as a reference cell for this type of study. BT-20 cells have been freed from mycoplasma by the method of Fogh and Fogh (1969);* they are hormone independent and have a population doubling time of 36 h in Eagle's MEM with 10% fetal calf serum.

By keeping the concentration of serum constant, several of the chemically defined commercial media were tested; one of them, RPMI-1640, reduced the doubling population time of BT-20 cells to 30 h and therefore was selected as the basic salt and amino acid mixture with which the nutritive value of other ingredients was to be measured.

2.3.2. Serum Substitute

An important variable of the culture medium is the serum. Usually, large concentrations of human cord or fetal calf serum are added as a nutritive complement to primary breast cultures. However, the serum contains large amounts of hormones which influence cell growth. In a quantitative study, Esber *et al.* (1973) reported the presence of relatively high levels of insulin, estrogens, progesterone, and testosterone in commercial samples of bovine sera (Fig. 5). The finding of testosterone in pools of commercial sera might explain their inhibiting effect on some breast tumor cells, but estrogens and progesterone can induce similar inhibition (Rivera *et al.*, 1963).

The serum is also a potential source of contamination: bovine syncytial virus (BSV) is common in calf serum, while infectious hepatitis virus and mycoplasma are found in many high-speed pellets of human serum. For these reasons, the development of a hormone-free serum substitute offering good nutritive qualities and stable enough to be autoclaved was undertaken (Lasfargues *et al.*, 1973).

Peptones, already successfully used to supplement synthetic media (Waymouth, 1956; Pumper, 1958; Merchant and Hellman, 1962), lactalbumin hydrolysate, and yeastolate were selected as the basic nutrients for a serum substitute. All three are heat stable and known to promote cell growth. Polyvinylpyrrolidone (PVP),† an inert nontoxic polymer currently used intravenously for the treatment of hypovolemic shock, was also added

*Until 1972, several sublines of BT-20 were found to be chronically infected by a slow-growing anaerobic form of mycoplasma of human origin: *Mycoplasma orali* type I. Following treatment of the cells in the laboratory of Dr. J. Fogh, Sloan-Kettering Institute, New York, a mycoplasma-free subline was obtained which is now available.

†Polyvinylpyrrolidones (PVP) are manufactured by GAF Corporation, New York, N.Y. Information concerning the properties of these compounds can be found in GAF technical bulletins 7543-018 and AP-123.

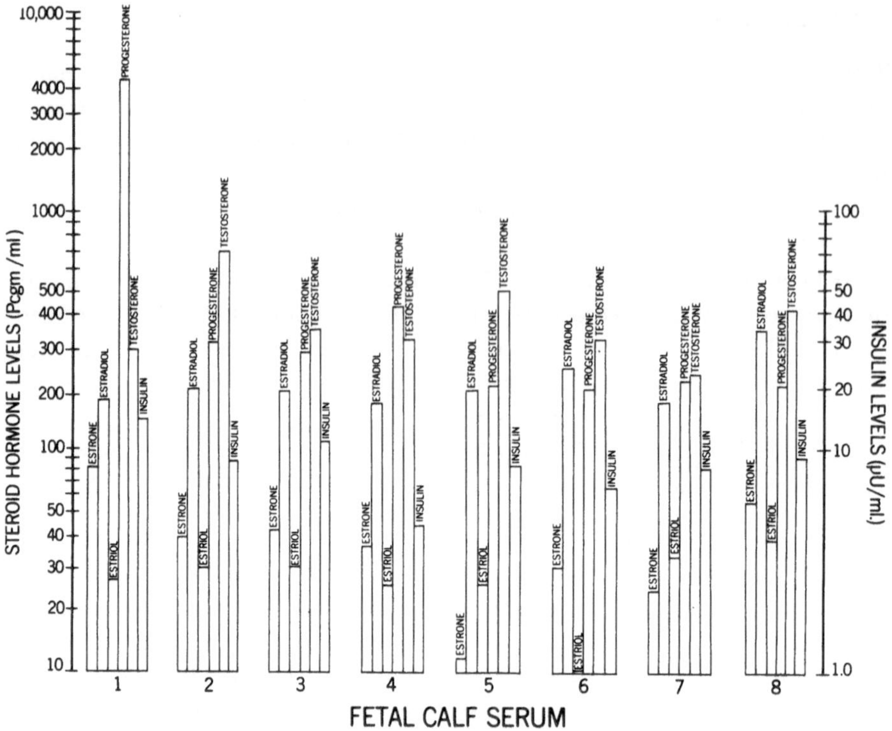

FIG. 5. Amount of hormones found in eight samples of commercial fetal calf serum. Reproduced from Esber *et al.* (1973) through the courtesy of Dr. H. J. Esber.

because it has physical properties comparable to those of plasma proteins. PVP K-90 has a molecular weight of 360,000 and at a concentration of 3.5% the same viscosity as serum. The composition of the serum substitute per 100 ml of triple-distilled pyrogen-free water is therefore as follows:*

> Bactopeptone (Difco), 5 g; PVP K-90, 3.5 g; dextrose, 0.5 g; lactalbumin hydrolysate, 2.5 g; yeastolate, 0.5 g.

This is a clear solution of amber color very similar to serum in its physical and nutritional qualities. It can be sterilized by autoclave at 10 lb pressure for 20 min. At a concentration of 10% (v/v) in RPMI-1640 or Eagle's MEM, this mixture maintains the growth of various cell lines indefinitely (Lasfargues *et al.*, 1973).

If, as described above, BT-20 is taken as the reference cell line for measurement of the nutritional value of the serum substitute in RPMI-1640, it is found that the doubling time of the cell population is about 50 h (Fig. 6).

*This description of the composition and preparation of the serum substitute is reproduced from *In Vitro* by permission of the Tissue Culture Association, Inc.

Because the serum substitute is autoclaved, it is free of the adventitious viruses and mycoplasma; because it is hormone free, it can be used efficiently to evaluate the role of specific hormones on the physiology of human breast cells in culture.

2.3.3. Hormonal Influences

The stimulation of the growth of breast tumor cells by specific hormones in tissue culture remains a matter of controversy.

From the experimental results obtained with tissues from laboratory animals, it has been established that normal mammary glands in culture respond directly and specifically to hormones by an increase in growth, differentiation, and secretory activity. Tumor tissues, however, react differently. Wellings and Jentoft (1972) found that, in general, cultures of breast biopsies do better without hormonal or serum complementation and that high concentrations of estradiol can be toxic. With improved techniques permitting a better selection of viable tissues, Flaxman and Lasfargues

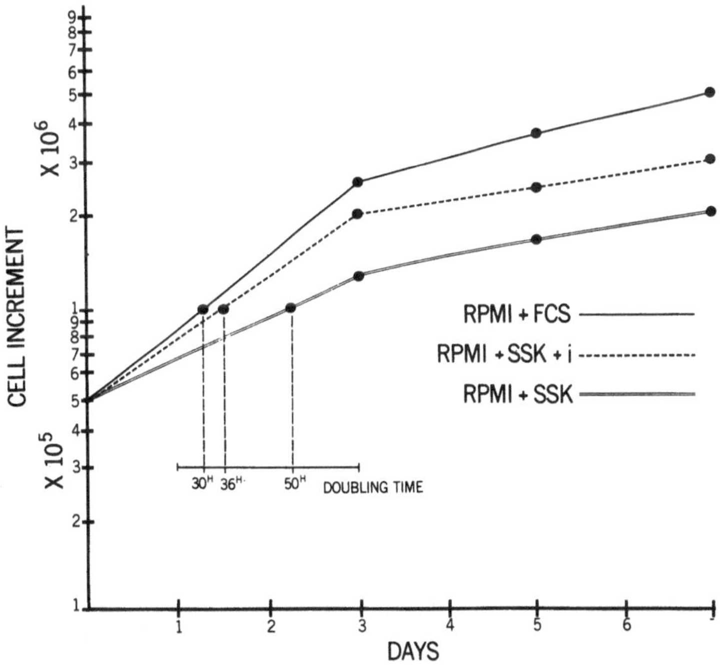

FIG. 6. Growth curves of BT-20 cells over a 7-day period. RPMI, Roswell Park Memorial Institute medium 1640; SSK, serum substitute with PVP K-90; *i*, insulin.

(1973) have observed that the human mammary epithelium in culture is somewhat independent of hormonal or serum factors but that insulin increases the rate of DNA synthesis.

Barker *et al.* (1964) had previously reported that serum is not absolutely essential to the survival of the cultures but that insulin is a good growth stimulant. Insulin was long thought to have a direct effect on the replication of mammary epithelial cells. This stimulation, however, is not specific since cells from organs other than the mammary gland can show increased mitotic activity in its presence (Gey and Thalimer, 1924; von Haam and Cappel, 1940; Bullough, 1954). This activity appears to occur through a binding of the hormone to the lipoproteins of the cell membrane, whose enhanced permeability and pinocytosis favor a rapid intake of the nutritional elements of the medium.

Elias (1972) reported that human ductal epithelium in dysplasias and fibroadenomas can form "pearls" of squamous metaplastic growth under the effect of insulin at concentrations of 5–20 μg/ml. He estimated that the minimal requirements of human mammary tissues for insulin were ten times higher than for the mouse.

From the above observations, insulin emerges as an essential growth factor for normal as well as for neoplastic mammary cells. The lack of stimulation reported by Feller *et al.* (1972) probably resulted from the inhibiting effect of other hormones present in the serum or experimentally added.

Observations that insulin maintains ribosome function and can to some extent replace the serum (Schwartz and Amos, 1968) prompted its incorporation as a permanent ingredient in a serum-free medium. Effectively, addition of insulin at a concentration of 0.02 u/ml in RPMI-1640 supplemented with 10% serum substitute resulted in a 36-h population doubling time for BT-20 cells (Fig. 6); this is about the same as with Eagle's medium and fetal calf serum.

2.3.4. Tissue Interactions

Following collagenase dissociation of scirrhous carcinoma, the fibroblasts grow more rapidly than the epithelium. The epithelium, however, can be kept in serial subcultures, along with the fibroblasts, if collagenase is added to the culture medium in a concentration of 0.5 mg/ml, at least once a month, for the duration of one feeding. The epithelial cells, cleaned by this treatment from the native collagen that polymerizes on their outer membrane, can then be maintained in culture for several months.

It seems, therefore, that the limiting action exerted by the fibroblasts is mainly due to the production of collagen. Under the stimulation of the proteolytic enzymes released by the tumor cells, fibroblasts derived from the tumor stroma are particularly apt to produce large amounts of native collagen which coats the epithelium. In the culture medium, however, fibroblasts release metabolites which permit maintenance of the epithelial cells for a longer period.

Fibroblasts of embryonic origin are fast growing, but, unlike tumor fibroblasts, they produce minimum amounts of collagen. When they are associated with epithelial aggregates collected from a primary breast tumor, a symbiotic type of culture results in which the neoplastic cells can proliferate (Fig. 7). If the embryonic fibroblasts are derived from a male embryo, it is possible to distinguish them from the tumor cells in later passages by the sex chromosome.

The system of cocultivation used in our laboratory consists of mixing, in a small Erlenmeyer flask, 1×10^6 embryonic cells with the epithelial aggregates newly harvested from a breast carcinoma. The embryonic fibroblasts settle down in a few hours, but most of the tumor cells continue to float. If some of them are trapped with the fibroblasts, they can expand freely because they are not inhibited by excessive amounts of newly formed collagen.

According to the type of tumor explanted, one of the three following situations can be observed: (1) tumor and embryonic cells coexist in perfect symbiosis—these cultures can be subcultivated when confluence is achieved; (2) the tumor cells feed on the embryonic ones—the fibroblasts gradually vanish from the culture and have to be replaced by new cells; (3) the tumor cells give out toxic substances—these kill the embryonic elements and the tumor cells themselves may become necrotic (Figs. 8–10).

There is some indication that such variations in cell-to-cell relationships are somewhat related to the malignancy of the tumor cells: most fibroadenomas conform to the first category while many scirrhous carcinomas show toxic effects.

2.3.5. Role of Physical Factors

The growth and maintenance of breast carcinoma cells in culture are to some extent influenced by the type of substrate on which they are more likely to spread; for monolayer cultures, plastic surfaces are more efficient than glass. Acrylamide gels currently used for electrophoresis have been found favorable for the epithelium (Haskill, 1973) but not for fibroblasts. This property is used to separate the neoplastic epithelium from the tumor stroma.

When epithelial cells are induced to spread out in a monolayer, their life span is always short, but if they are kept as aggregates, in suspension, they can live for 6–7 months. It seems, therefore, that mammary cells, which have a natural tendency to assume a semialveolar structure, need this type of organization to survive. Withdrawal of the serum and a slight hypotonicity of the culture medium can do much to keep the cells in suspension. In hypotonic media, the cells become spherical and acquire a tensile peripheral membrane that is not likely to attach to solid surfaces; the preparation of the serum substitute in water provides such a hypotonic condition plus a degree of viscosity comparable to that of serum. Viscosity, which favors clumping of cells, is obtained by addition of polyvinylpyrrolidone (PVP).

2.3.6. *Maintenance and Splitting of Cultures*

The method which presently gives the best results for the long-term maintenance of primary breast tumor cells is a suspension culture in RPMI-1640 medium, 10% serum substitute, and 0.02 u/ml insulin. Every 3 days the Erlenmeyer flasks in which the cells are kept in suspension are placed on a rack at a 45° angle. After 5 min the cells sediment in the angle formed by the floor and wall of the flask. With a Pasteur pipette three-fourths of the supernatant is then aspirated without disturbing the sediment and replaced by an equal volume of fresh medium. If the pH of the medium remains higher than 7, only half of the supernatant is replaced once a week.

Three established human breast carcinoma cell lines, BT-20, AlAb, and 734B, grow continuously in this medium when explanted at a multiplicity of 1×10^6 cells in 10 ml of culture fluid.

These cell lines, BT-20 in particular, may form large aggregates which require enzymatic dispersion and splitting after 8–10 days. For this purpose, the cell clumps are gathered by sedimentation at low-speed centrifugation and the supernatant is completely removed. The sediment is first rapidly washed in 2–4 ml of a calcium-magnesium-free saline* solution containing 0.0002% EDTA; it is centrifuged at low speed, then exposed for 5 min to the same solution but with 0.0416% trypsin. The clumps are totally dispersed by gentle pipetting. The single cells, sedimented again at low-speed centrifugation, are resuspended in complete culture medium and distributed in 1×10^6 aliquots into new culture flasks.

*The calcium-magnesium-free saline used is the one recommended by Pucks: NaCl, 8g; KCl, 0.4 g; $NaHCO_3$, 0.35 g; glucose, 1 g; distilled, pyrogen-free water, 1000 ml.

FIG. 7. Symbiotic cocultivation of spilled breast carcinoma cells with human embryonic fibroblasts. The epithelial cells infiltrate the parallel arrays of fibroblasts quite freely. Scale bar: 100 μm.

FIG. 8. Circumscribed colonies of tumor cells lysing the fibroblastic layer around them. Scale bar: 100 μm.

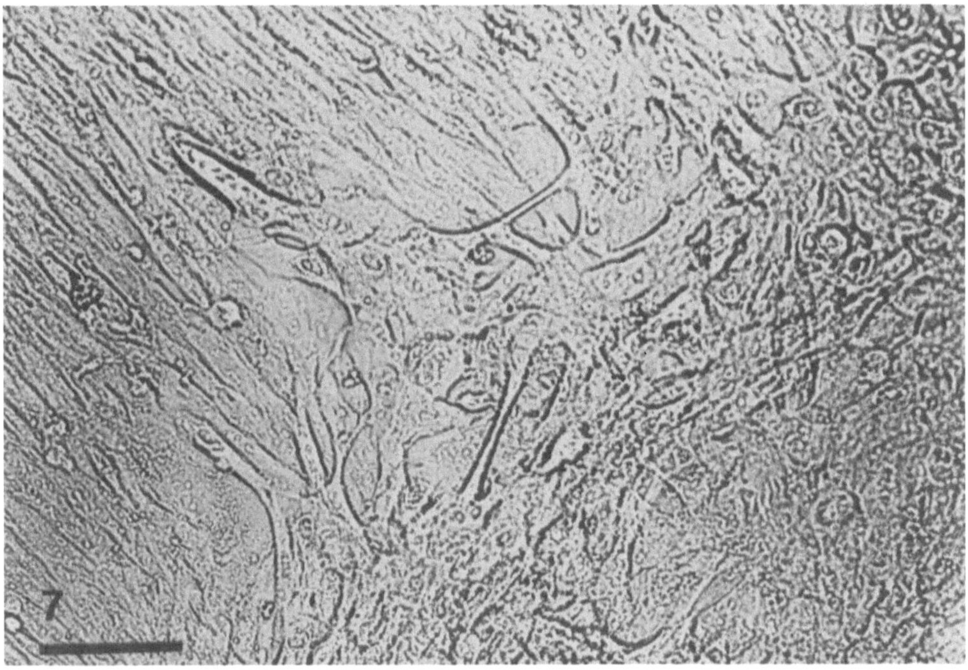

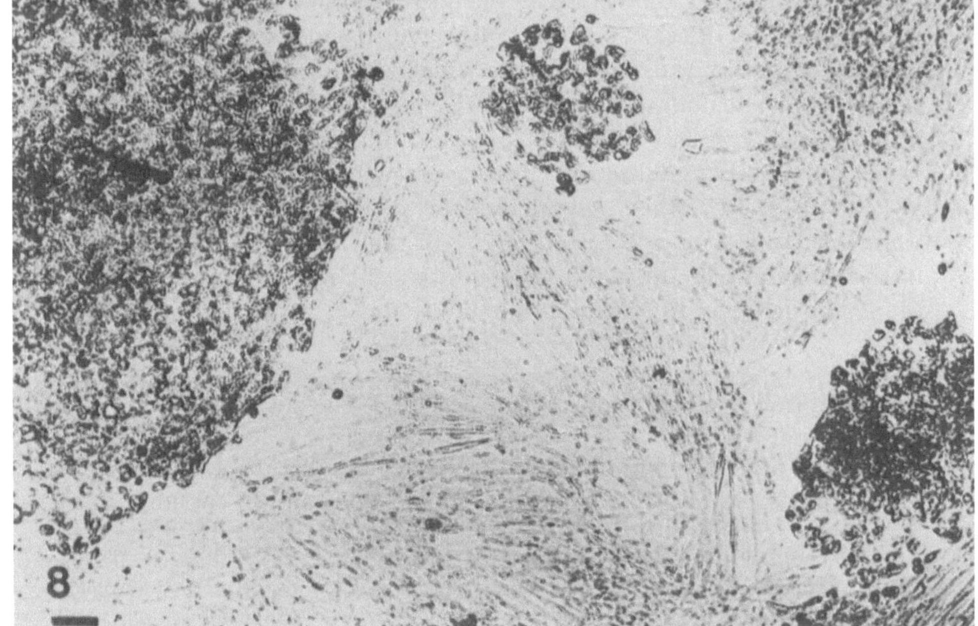
8

Cocultures: Since normal fibroblasts settle down rapidly and proliferate as a feeder layer on the bottom of the flask, passages are done in two steps: (1) the free-floating aggregates are first sedimented in a conical tube and the supernatant is replaced by fresh medium; (2) the layer of normal cells is trypsinized in a versene–trypsin solution as described above, 5×10^5 cells are added to the epithelial aggregates, and the mixture is passed to a new flask. When the primary aggregates are large and compact with a dense core suggesting necrosis, they should be dissociated in the same way as the BT–20 aggregates.

2.4. *Causes for Failure*

The procedures which have been described have reduced failure in the cultivation of human breast tumors to such causes as the size of the specimen, the morphology of the tumor, and previous therapeutic treatment of the cancer patient. All these causes are unrelated to technical deficiencies: a small tumor nodule, for instance, might not yield enough cells replicating at a rate rapid enough to upset the normal amount of cell autolysis; a very sclerotic carcinoma might be deficient for the same reason; previous hormonal, radiotherapeutic, or chemotherapeutic treatment of the patient might also be conducive to large masses of necrotic cells unfit for cultivation.

Unexpectedly, the time lapse between surgery and cultivation does not appear to be as critical as was once suspected. If the tumor is immediately placed in an adequate tissue culture medium containing antibiotics, it can be stored for several hours before being processed. Slices of breast carcinomas in Eagle's MEM with 10% fetal calf serum, 1000 u/ml penicillin, 500 μg/ml neomycin, and 10 μg/ml tetracycline have originated viable cultures after 48 h storage at 4°C. Others, kept in the same medium at room temperature, were still viable 3 days after surgery. This has made possible long-term dissociation of hard tumors in collagenase as well as long-distance shipment of biopsy specimens in insulated containers.

3. *Applications of Cell Cultures to Breast Cancer Research*

Because of the difficulties in growing primary tumors and because of the present rarity of available cell lines, applications of the tissue culture

FIG. 9. Details of a colony of tumor cells lysing the surrounding fibroblasts. Scale bar: 100 μm.

FIG. 10. Epithelial aggregate producing proteolytic enzymes that destroy normal fibroblasts. Necrotic cells and cell debris are seen in the center and right side of the photograph. Large, refringent tumor cells infiltrate the healthy fibroblasts. Scale bar: 100 μm.

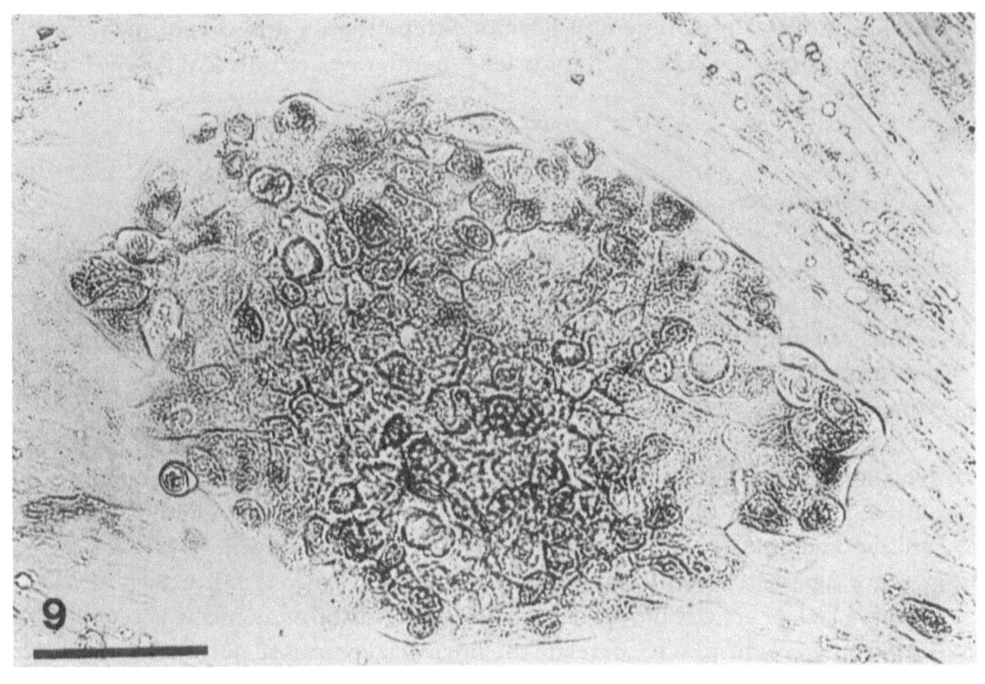
9

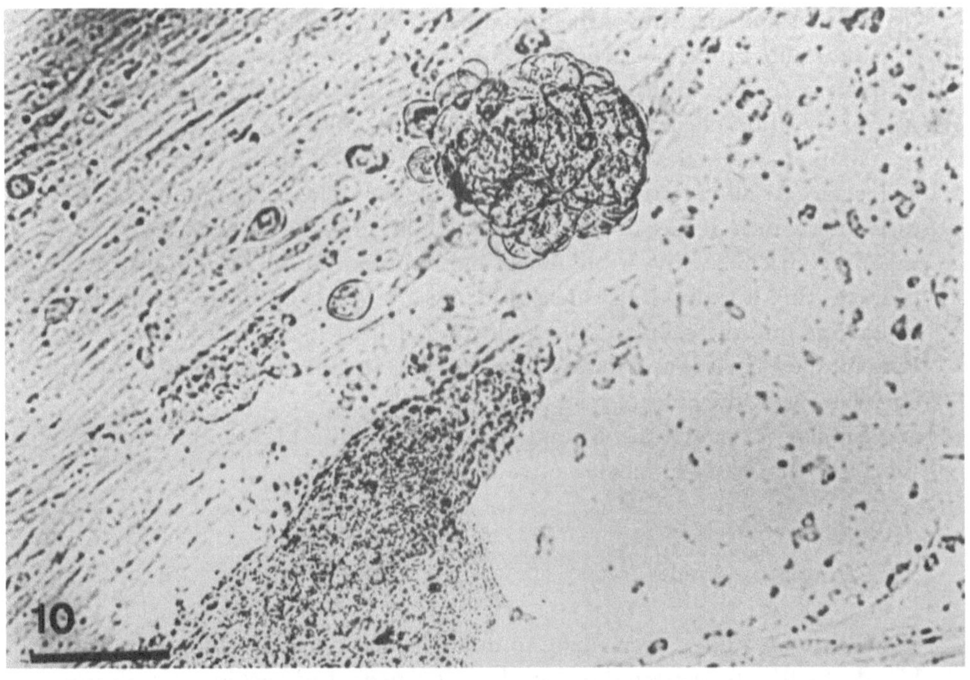
10

methods to the development of hormone-dependency and diagnostic tests have been very few. The attempts briefly mentioned are only guidelines for further research.

3.1. Detection of Hormone Dependency

Several attempts have been made to detect the sensitivity of fresh tumor biopsies to hormones by the organ culture method. However, the large number of explants required and the length of the histological procedures are serious drawbacks to this technique. More direct approaches have been considered; among these were measurement of oxygen consumption by cells maintained in Warburg flasks (Rienets, 1959), determination of estrogen-sensitive isocitric dehydrogenase (Hollander *et al.*, 1959), incorporation of ^{14}C-leucine (Henson and Legros, 1963), and measurement of glucose utilization and lactic acid production (Barker and Richmond, 1971).

Once again, the results have been conflicting; steroid hormones have shown a lack of activity if not an inhibiting effect. Mioduszewska *et al.* (1968), however, were the first to correlate the hormonal response of tumor cells in culture with the condition of the patients over a 2-yr period. They found that lack of response to prolactin but stimulation of the cultures by hydrocortisone indicated an unfavorable prognosis; the patients in this group had a 90% mortality rate. The reverse, i.e., stimulation by prolactin and inhibition by hydrocortisone, indicated a good prognosis; all patients lived beyond the 2-yr observation period.

A simpler system developed by Burstein (1971) makes use of the epithelial aggregates spilling out of the tumor stroma. The suspended cells are distributed in a series of culture tubes containing a chemically defined medium enriched with various hormonal combinations. The response of the cells to the hormones is measured by the incorporation of tritiated thymidine into the cellular DNA following a short-term cultivation period. Patients have been found to respond to hormone therapy in a manner which correlates with the culture results.

A similar method can be used to detect specific high-affinity estrogen receptors that bind ^{3}H-labeled estradiol on the cell surface.

3.2. Diagnostic Procedures

A few attempts have been made to detect specific tumor antibodies in the blood of patients suspected to have breast cancer. Indirect immunofluorescence is a choice technique when a standard cell line, well characterized as a human breast carcinoma, can be used as the antigen on which the patient's serum is tested. However, the method is delicate because of the natural presence in all sera of a variety of heterophil, nonspecific antibodies that require exhaustive absorptions. Using primary cell cultures of human breast tumors, Edynak *et al.* (1972) have shown the presence of specific antibodies in 91% of the sera from patients following surgery but in only 20% of normal donors. Priori *et al.* (1972) have used mouse mammary tumor cell lines producing type B and C virus particles to react with the serum of human patients on the assumption that a common virus antigen would be detectable; the results have been inconclusive. There is, however, possibility that the isolation of new, highly antigenic cell lines from human breast carcinoma might help in the development of a practical immunofluorescence test.

Cell lines could also be useful for the detection of lymphocytic interactions. Pathologists agree that a heavy lymphocytic infiltration in mammary tumors is a favorable prognosis. As revealed by time-lapse photomicrography, emperipolesis followed by death of the cancer cells is a common effect of lymphocyte activity (Sherwin and Richters, 1972). The mechanisms of this lymphocytic tropism might be immunochemical in nature. Among the circulating lymphocytes of patients with breast cancer there seem to be a number of cells that become sensitized to tumor antigens, then react to contact with the carcinoma cells by promptly destroying them. There also exist, in the serum of patients with growing tumors, circulating antigen–antibody complexes which can block lymphocytic cytotoxicity by coating the tumor antigens at the cell membrane (Helström *et al.*, 1969). A demonstration of these blocking factors was obtained by exposing BT-20 cells to the heat-inactivated serum of breast cancer patients. Sensitized lymphocytes which usually destroyed BT-20 cells lost their cytotoxic effect on contact with the serum-treated cells (Sinkovics *et al.*, 1972). These results even though preliminary are encouraging and should spur further efforts to develop better diagnostic tests.

4. *Conclusions*

The technical progress made in the cultivation of human breast tumors over the past years is dominated by the possibility of isolating large numbers of neoplastic epithelial cells from the tumor stroma by collagenase dispersion or by the "spilling" method. The availability of nontoxic collagenase whose activity remains highest in complete culture media has been a turning point in the development of the present methods of explantation.

The suspension form appears to be the most favorable type of culture for the epithelial aggregates, which have a natural tendency to develop as three-dimensional structures. The suspension system also permits separation of fibroblasts from epithelial cells because of their differential rates of sedimentation and attachment.

Chemically defined media complemented with a serum substitute containing nutritive heat-resistant polypeptides have maintained primary breast tumor cells 3–5 months longer than the same media complemented with serum and various hormone combinations.

Insulin emerges as an essential factor for the maintenance and growth of human breast tissues. It does not act as a specific hormone influencing one particular phase of the mammary gland cycle but as a general modifier of the cell membrane favoring better nutritional exchanges with the environment. RPMI-1640 complemented with 10% serum substitute and 0.02 u/ml insulin has maintained the viability of human carcinoma cells for about 12 months. The lack of cell division suggests a basic nutritional deficiency.

Besides the BT-20 cell line, only two others are known to have been directly isolated from mammary tumors: HBT-3, reported by Bassin *et al.* (1972), was derived from an adenocarcinoma; the most recent one, HBT-39, obtained by Plata *et al.* (1973) from a duct cell carcinoma, was cloned into three sublines, two of which are epithelial. A number of other cell lines lately derived from pleural effusions are included in the list of human tumor cell lines presented in Chapter 5.

However, it is necessary that all the cell lines derived from pleural effusions be characterized as breast tumor cells. Many of them grow actively in suspension but cannot be converted to monolayer cultures. Since epithelial lung cells and lymphocytes can be obtained from pleural fluids, the breast origin of these cultures remains questionable. For this reason, it seems that greater efforts should be made to isolate neoplastic cells from the tumor itself.

The deficiency of culture media to support cell replication of primary breast carcinoma cells is another problem which might be overcome either by cocultivation techniques or by use of conditioned media. Human embryonic cells are being used with some success as feeder layers; also, the filtered cell-free medium collected from stock human embryo cell cultures appears to supply the tumor cells with some missing metabolites. Under these conditions, several primary breast tumor cells which have sustained a limited number of passages may eventually emerge as established lines.

5. *References*

Banerjee, M. R., and Banerjee, D. N., 1971, Hormonal regulation of RNA synthesis and membrane ultrastructures in mouse mammary gland, *Exp. Cell Res.* **64**:307.

Barker, B. E., Fanger, H., and Farnes, P., 1964, Human mammary slices in organ culture. I. Method of culture and preliminary observations on the effect of insulin, *Exp. Cell Res.* **35**:437.

Barker, J. R., and Richmond, C., 1971, Human breast carcinoma culture: The effects of hormones, *Brit. J. Surg.* **58**:732.

Bassin, H. B., Plata, E. J., Gerwin, B. I., Mattern, C. F., Haapola, D. K., and Chu, E. W., 1972, Isolation of a continuous epithelioid cell line, HBT-3, from a human breast carcinoma, *Proc. Soc. Exp. Biol. Med.* **141**:673.

Bittner, J. J., 1936, Some possible effects of nursing on the mammary gland tumor incidence in mice, *Science* **84**:162.

Bullough, W. S., 1954, A study of the hormonal relations of epidermal mitotic activity *in vitro*. II. Insulin and pituitary growth hormone, *Exp. Cell Res.* **17**:186.

Burstein, N. A., 1971, Human carcinoma of the breast *in vitro:* The effect of hormones, *Cancer* **27**:1112.

Cameron, G., and Chambers, R., 1937, Neoplasm studies, organization of cells of human tumors in tissue culture, *Am. J. Cancer* **30**:115.

Chen, J. M., 1954, The cultivation in fluid medium of organized liver, pancreas, and other tissues of foetal rats, *Exp. Cell Res.* **7**:518.

Coman, D. R., 1942, Human neoplasms in tissue culture, *Cancer Res.* **2**:618.

Coman, D. R., 1944, Decreased mutual adhesiveness, a property of cells from squamous cell carcinoma, *Cancer res.* **4**:625.

Dilley, W. G., and Nandi, S., 1968, Rat mammary gland differentiation *in vitro* in the absence of steroids, *Science* **161**:59.

Eagle, H., 1959, Amino acid metabolism in mammalian cell cultures, *Science* **130**:432.

Edynak, E. M., Hirshaut, Y., Bernhard, M., and Trempe, G., 1972, Fluorescent antibody studies of human breast cancer, *J. Natl. Cancer Inst.* **48**:1137.

Ehrmann, R. L., and Gey, G. O., 1956, The growth of cells on a transparent gel of reconstituted collagen, *J. Natl. Cancer Inst.* **16**:1375.

Elias, J. J., 1957, Cultivation of adult mouse mammary gland in hormone enriched synthetic medium, *Science* **126**:842.

Elias, J. J., 1972, Response of human mammary dysplasias and fibroadenomas in organ culture, presented at Workshop on Culture of Human Mammary Tissues, Asilomar, August 1–3.

Esber, H. J., Payne, J. I., and Bogden, A. E., 1973, Variability of hormone concentrations and ratios in commercial sera used for tissue culture, *J. Natl. Cancer Inst.* **50**:559.

Evans, V. J., Bryant, J. C., Kerr, H. A., and Schilling, E. L., 1964, Chemically defined media for cultivation of long-term cell strains from four mammalian species, *Exp. Cell Res.* **36**:439.

Fell, H. B., 1951, Methods for study of organized growth *in vitro:* Techniques of bone cultivation, in: *Methods in Medical Research* (M. B. Visscher, ed.), pp. 234–237, Year Book Publishers, Chicago.

Feller, W. F., Stewart, S. E., and Kantor, J., 1972, Primary tissue culture explants of human breast cancer, *J. Natl. Cancer Inst.* **48**:1117.

Flaxman, B. A., and Lasfargues, E. Y., 1973, Hormone-independent DNA synthesis by epithelial cells of human mammary gland in organ culture, *Proc. Soc. Exp. Biol. Med.* **143**:371.

Fogh, J., and Fogh, H., 1969, Procedures for control of mycoplasma contamination of tissue cultures, *Ann. N.Y. Acad. Sci.* **172**:15.

Foley, J. F., and Aftonomos, B. T., 1965, Growth of human breast neoplasms in cell culture, *J. Natl. Cancer Inst.* **34**:217.

Gaillard, P. J., 1953, Growth and differentiation of explanted tissues, *Int. Rev. Cytol.* **2**:331.

Gey, G. O., and Gey, M. K., 1936, The maintenance of human normal cells and tumor cells in continuous culture, *Am. J. Cancer* **27**:45.

Gey, G. O., and Thalimer, W., 1924, Observations on insulin introduced into the medium of tissue culture, *JAMA* **82**:1609.

Giraldo, G., Beth, E., Hirshaut, Y., Aoki, T., Old, L. J., Boyse, E. A., and Chopra, H. C., 1971, Human sarcomas in culture: Foci of altered cells and a common antigen in human fibroblast cultures by filtrates, *J. Exp. Med.* **133:**454.

Haskill, J. S., 1973, A micro acrylamide culture method for colony inhibition and cloning solid tumors, *J. Nat. Cancer Inst.*, submitted.

Hellström, I., Hellström, K. E., Evans, C. H., Heppner, G. H., Pierce, G. E., and Yang, J. P. S., 1969, Serum mediated protection of neoplastic cells from inhibition by lymphocytes immune to their tumor specific antigens, *Proc. Natl. Acad. Sci.* **62:**362.

Henson, J. C., and Legros, N., 1963, *In vitro* effect of testosterone and 17β-estradiol on L-leucine ^{14}C incorporation into human breast cancer tissue, *Cancer* **16:**404.

Hollander, V. P., Smith, D. E., and Adamson, T. E., 1959, Studies on estrogen sensitive transhydrogenase: The effect of estradiol 17β and α-ketoglutarate production on non-cancerous and cancerous breast tissue, *Cancer* **12:**135.

Lasfargues, E. Y., and Moore, D. H., 1966, Cell transformation by the mammary tumor virus *in vitro*, in: *Symposium on Malignant Transformation by viruses* (W. H. Kirsten, ed.), pp. 44–59, Springer-Verlag, New York.

Lasfargues, E. Y., and Murray, M. R., 1959, Hormonal influences on the differentiation and growth of embryonic mouse mammary glands in organ culture, *Develop. Biol.* **1:**413.

Lasfargues, E. Y., and Ozzello, L., 1958, Cultivation of human breast carcinomas, *J. Natl. Cancer Inst.* **21:**1131.

Lasfargues, E. Y., Coutinho, W. G., Lasfargues, J. C., and Moore, D. H., 1973, A serum substitute that can support the continuous growth of mammary tumor cells, *in vitro.* **8:**494.

McCoy, T. A., Maxwell, M., and Kruse, P. F., 1959, Amino acid requirements of the Novikoff lepatoma *in vitro, Proc. Soc. Exp. Biol. Med.* **100:**115.

Merchant, D. J., and Hellman, K. B., 1962, Growth of L-M strain mouse cells in a chemically defined medium, *Proc. Soc. Exp. Biol. Med.* **110:**194.

Mioduszewska, O., Koszarowski, T., and Gorski, C., 1968, Influence of hormones on mammary carcinoma *in vitro* and on the clinical course of the disease, *Pol. Tyg. Lek.* **23:**965.

Moore, D. H., Sarkar, N. H., Kelly, C. E., Pillsbury, N., and Charney, J., 1969, Type B particles in human milk, *Texas Rep. Biol. Med.* **27:**1029.

Moore, D. H., Charney, J., Kramarsky, B., Lasfargues, E. Y., Sarkar, N. H., Brennan, M. J., Burrows, J. H., Sirsat, S. M., Paymaster, J. C., and Vaidya, A. B., 1971, Search for a human breast cancer, *Nature (Lond.)* **229:**611.

Moore, G. E., Sandberg, A. A., and Ulrich, K., 1966, Suspension cell culture and *in vivo* and *in vitro* chromosome constitution of mouse leukemia L1210, *J. Natl. Cancer Inst.* **36:**405.

Morgan, J. F., Morton, H. J., and Parker, R. C., 1950, Nutrition of animal cells in tissue culture. I. Initial studies on a synthetic medium, *Proc. Soc. Exp. Biol. Med.* **73:**1.

Oka, T., and Topper, J. Y., 1972, Hormone-dependent accumulation of rough endoplasmic reticulum in mouse mammary epithelial cells *in vitro, J. Natl. Cancer Inst.* **48:**1225.

Orr, M. F., and McSwain, B., 1955, Tissue culture of human breast carcinoma, *Am. J. Pathol.* **31:**125.

Parker, R. C., Castor, L. N., and McCulloch, E. A., 1957, Altered cell strains in continuous culture: A general survey, in: Cellular Biology, Nucleic Acids and Viruses (O. V. St. Whitelock, ed), *N.Y. Acad. Sci. Spec. Publ. V,* pp. 303–313.

Plata, E. J., Aoki, T., Robertson, D. D., Chu, E. W., and Gerwin, B. I., 1973, An established cultured cell line (HBT-39) from human breast carcinoma, *J. Natl. Cancer Inst.* **50:**849.

Priori, E. S., Anderson, D. E., Williams, W. C., and Dmochowski, L., 1972, Immunological studies on human breast carcinoma and mouse mammary tumors, *J. Natl. Cancer Inst.* **48:**1131.

Prop, F. J., 1959, Organ cultures of total mammary glands of the mouse, *Nature (Lond.)* **184:**379.

Pumper, R. W., 1958, Adaptation of tissue culture cells to a serum-free medium, *Science* **128:**363.

Reed, M. V., and Gey, G. O., 1962, Cultivation of normal and malignant human lung tissue. I. The establishment of three adenocarcinoma cell strains, *Lab. Invest.* **11**:638.

Rienets, K. G., 1959, The effects of estrone and testosterone on respiration of human mammary cancer *in vitro, Cancer* **12**:958.

Rivera, E. M., 1964, Differential responsiveness to hormones of C3H and A mouse mammary tissues in organ culture, *Endocrinology* **74**:853.

Rivera, E. M., Elias, J. J., Bern, H. A., Napalkov, N. P., and Pitelka, D. R., 1963, Toxic effects of steroid hormones on organ cultures of mouse mammary tumors, with a comment on the occurrence of viral inclusion bodies, *J. Natl. Cancer Inst.* **31**:671.

Royle, J. G., 1946, Some cultural and cytological characteristics of human tumors *in vitro, Cancer res.* **6**:225.

Schwartz, A., and Amos, H., 1968, Partial restoration of ribosome function by insulin, *in vitro* **3**:190.

Sherwin, R. P., and Richters, A., 1972, Pathobiologic nature of lymphocyte interaction with human breast cancer, *J. Natl. Cancer Inst.* **48**:1111.

Sinkovics, J. G., Reeves, W. J., and Cabiness, J. R., 1972, Cell and antibody mediated immune reactions of patients to cultured cells of breast carcinoma, *J. Natl. Cancer Inst.* **48**:1145.

Stoll, B. A., 1970, Investigation of organ culture as an aid to the hormonal management of breast cancer, *Cancer* **25**:1228.

Turkington, W. R., 1972, Regulation of gene expression in normal and neoplastic mammary cells: a review, *J. Natl. Cancer Inst.* **48**:1231.

von Haam, E., and Cappel, L., 1940, Effects of hormones on cells grown *in vitro*. I. The effects of sex hormones on fibroblasts, *Am. J. Cancer* **39**:354.

Waymouth, C., 1956, A serum-free nutrient solution sustaining rapid and continuous proliferation of strain-L (Earle) mouse cells, *J. Natl. Cancer Inst.* **17**:315.

Waymouth, C., 1959, Rapid proliferation of sublines of NCTC clone 929 (strain L) mouse cells in a simple chemically defined medium (MB 752/1), *J. Natl. Cancer Inst.* **22**:1003.

Wellings, S. R., and Jentoft, V. L., 1972, Organ cultures of normal, dysplastic, hyperplastic and neoplastic human mammary tissues, *J. Natl. Cancer Inst.* **49**:329.

Whitescarver, J., Recher, L., Sykes, J. A., and Briggs, L., 1968, Problems involved in culturing human breast tissues, *Texas Rep. Biol. Med.* **26**:613.

Wolff, E., 1952, La culture d'organes embryonnaires *in vitro, Rev. Sci.* **90**:189.

Wolff, E., and Wolff, E., 1966, Cultures organotypiques de longue durée de deux tumeurs humaines du tube digestif, *Eur. J. Cancer* **2**:93.

Old and New Problems in Human Tumor Cell Cultivation 4

RELDA M. CAILLEAU

1. Introduction

There are really no new problems in the cultivation of human tumor cells, merely a greater awareness of some of the old ones, an increased understanding of what they are. In general, the difficulties lie in obtaining tumor cells from the patient and growing or maintaining them *in vitro* without adding any "foreign" living substance. It is equally difficult to separate the tumor cells from extraneous normal cells or tissues and to demonstrate that the cells growing in tissue culture are identical to the neoplastic cells found in the host.

These difficulties usually have been overcome without too much trouble in experiments carried out on other mammals: mouse, rat, guinea pig, hamster, and rabbit. Such studies have yielded abundant cultures and cell lines of neoplastic origin. But these laboratory animals are often highly inbred strains, carefully selected as to age, sex, food, environment, genetic background, and response to chemical challenge under controlled conditions. Experiments can be duplicated or modified by injection or treatment of litter mates or inbred hosts. Conditions approaching those needed to fulfill Koch's postulates can be produced.

RELDA M. CAILLEAU Department of Medicine, M. D. Anderson Hospital and Tumor Institute, University of Texas at Houston, Houston, Texas

Human subjects, on the other hand, are far from uniform in all these respects. Each individual, if not each tumor, exists as a separate biological and genetic entity, and it is utterly impossible to duplicate an experiment by injection of tumor cells into an allogeneic host. To control our experiments by identifying the tumor, removing it, culturing it *in vitro* or transferring it to another human host, and reproducing the same series of events is neither feasible, practical, nor routinely sanctioned.

Viral agents, present in many types of rodent tumors (leukemia and mammary tumors), have been studied under carefully controlled conditions and have been definitely linked with the respective neoplastic diseases. While viruses have been hunted relentlessly as the causative agent of all human tumors, they have only infrequently been found. In a great number of human tumors, either viruses are not present or their presence is in serious doubt, controversial, or undetectable. This subject is discussed fully in Chapter 15 and incidentally in Chapter 14.

Rather than generalize on all types of tumor cell cultivation, I have decided to emphasize the difficulties encountered in trying to grow human mammary carcinoma cells or tissue. This tumor material serves as an example of just about all the difficulties and frustrations one can encounter. To date, only a handful of long-term cell lines of epithelial origin and appearance have been established from human breast tumor tissue (Plata *et al.*, 1973; Bassin *et al.*, 1972; Dobrynin, 1963; Lasfargues and Ozzello, 1958). Another line established for over 10 months (at the time of publication) by Martorelli *et al.* (1969) seems to be less epithelial-like in appearance and is of doubtful origin. A few established lines have been isolated from metastatic lesions or pleural effusions (Young *et al.*, 1974; Giraldo *et al.*, 1971; Reed and Gey, 1962). Trempe and Fogh (1973) also mention the establishment of a line from a breast carcinoma.

Other lines have been reported from breast tumor tissue or pleural effusions: some are possibly lymphoblastoid (Feller *et al.*, 1970, 1972), and some have been short-lived (Foley and Aftonomos, 1965) or both short-lived and overrun by fibroblasts (Gewant and Goldenberg, 1970).

In discussing the difficulties in obtaining, growing, and identifying human cancer cells *in vitro*, it is necessary to mention many topics elaborated on in other chapters. Rather than repeat the references which the other writers have fully covered, I shall mention only the main reviews or general articles dealing with each topic, certain particularly pertinent studies which illustrate our discussion, and relatively recent references which may have appeared in foreign-languages or in obscure journals. The plethora of books, articles, reviews, and proceedings of symposia and conferences published in the last 5–10 years on each subject has become so overwhelming that it is impossible to keep abreast of all such information whether it is easily available or not. I therefore apologize beforehand for any omissions.

Following are some of the general references published prior to 1968 that should provide excellent background material: *A Bibliography of the Research in Tissue Culture, 1884–1950* (1953), *Cells and Tissues in Culture* 3 vols. (Willmer, 1965, 1966), *National Cancer Institute Monograph*, Vol. 26 (1967), and *Cancer Cells in Culture* (Katsuta, 1968). Another book on this general subject is *Growth, Nutrition, and Metabolism of Cells in Culture* (Rothblat and Cristofalo, eds., 1972). Two recent and important publications on chromosome banding techniques by Hsu are *Mammalian Chromosome Newsletter* (1972) and "Longitudinal Differentiation of Chromosomes" (1973).

2. Types of Cells Found in Human Breast Carcinomas and Pleural Effusions

In almost every tumor surgically removed from a patient and placed in culture, a variety of cells are present in different amounts and degrees of viability. If the tumor cells predominate and are vigorous and mitotically active, they may persist, outlive the usual accompanying fibroblasts or other normal cell types, and slowly or rapidly adapt to the culture medium. These tumors then may become established as a cell line or strain.

In human mammary carcinomas, the invasive mass usually includes a hard fibrous matrix (except in rare cases of comedo carcinoma and some medullary or mucinous carcinomas). This matrix can also contain fatty tissue, blood, lymphocytes, and other cells not always easily identified. Frequently the majority of the tumor cells are necrotic, degenerating, or dead by the time the tissue reaches the laboratory. When maximum cooperation between surgeon, pathologist, and technician exists, the tissue may be in culture within 1–2 h after the excision of the tumor. But after studying more than 200 breast tumors and pleural effusions we have reached the conclusion that in most tumors with a high percentage of necrotic or dead tumor cells, the majority of these cells were probably degenerating or dead *in vivo*. This viewpoint is shared by Cooper (1973).

The use of pleural fluid from patients with primary or metastatic breast cancer eliminates two of the main difficulties associated with cultures obtained directly from the solid breast tumor tissue: fibroblasts and necrosis. The prevailing fast-growing, enveloping fibroblasts are practically nonexistent in pleural effusions, while the tumor cells present are generally 75–99% viable. This contrasts with a tumor cell viability of 5–10% in the majority of the breast tumors we have handled. Another advantage to using pleural effusions is that a large number of cells can be concentrated out of 500–2000 ml of fluid, and the tumor cells exist in suspension as single cells or small clumps or clusters of cells. A third advantage lies in the possibility of obtaining, from the same patient, multiple effusions over a period of several months. This is equivalent to running an experiment in triplicate or better. Multiple sampling may show the influence of any treatment the patient receives on the amount, type, and viability of cells obtained from pleural effusions.

However, while solid breast tumors are "contaminated" with fibroblasts which tend to outgrow and overrun the tumor cells, the pleural exudates may contain considerable numbers of other cell types such as lymphocytes and mesothelial-like cells. Thus the first problem is the identification of the cell types present and their multiplication or establishment in culture. Too many people have "cultured" breast tumor cells only to find that the cell which finally predominates is a mesothelial-like or fibroblast-like cell rather than the original epithelial tumor cell.

2.1. *Fibroblasts*

Fibroblasts are the most ubiquitous cell contaminant observed in breast tumor tissue. They grow more rapidly than tumor cells, surround them, and literally seem to smother them. If not eliminated or checked by one or more of the various methods recommended for their control, they will usually eliminate the tumor cells before their own demise after 3–6 months of *in vitro* growth. The other most frequently observed cell type in breast carcinoma explants is the lymphocyte. Occasionally histiocytes and fat cells appear in cultures but normally do not survive or multiply for any appreciable length of time.

In pleural effusions, fibroblasts are rarely seen during the first few days or weeks *in vitro* but fibroblast-like cells may appear and even dominate after one or more months of culture. Often these fibroblast-like cells are atypical, and chromosome and electron microscopic studies may be required to determine whether they are of malignant epithelial or normal fibroblast origin (Lichtiger *et al.*, 1970; Lasfargues and Ozzello, 1958; Leighton *et al.*, 1956) (Figs. 1–4).

2.2. *Mesothelial-like Cells*

While the fibroblast is the *bête noire* of solid tumor explants, another cell type pervades the cultures of pleural effusions. These cells are large, generally

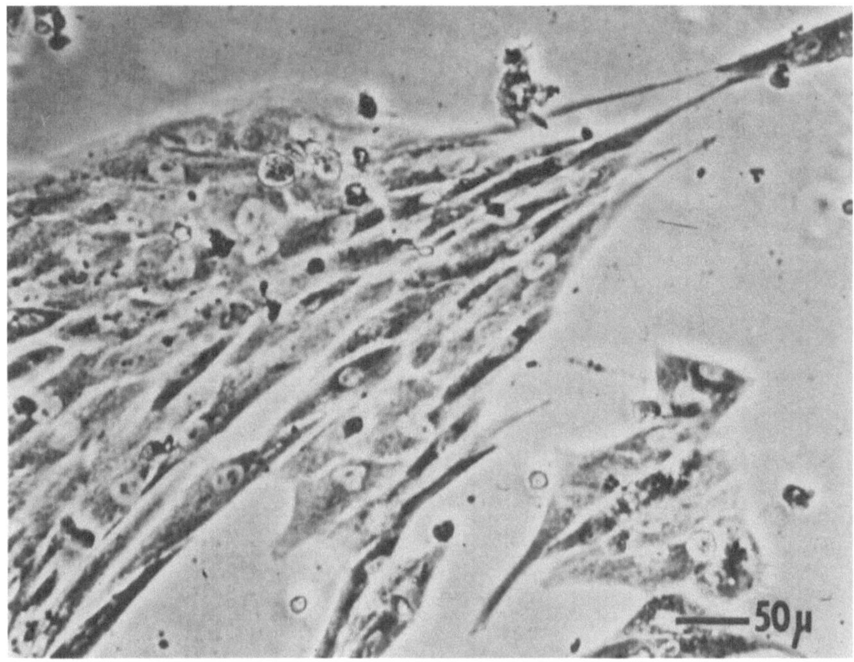

FIG. 1. Phase contrast micrograph of cells from a pleural effusion showing fibroblast-like appearance, 21 days in culture.

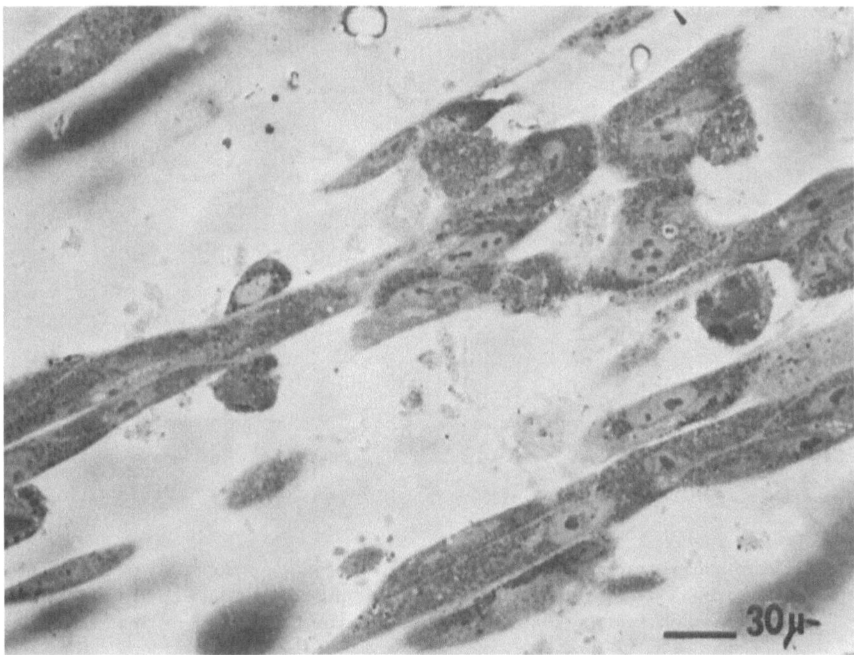

FIG. 2. Similar cells to those in Fig. 1, Epon-embedded 1-μm section. Note elongated shape with distinctly granular cytoplasm. Methylene blue–azur II stain.

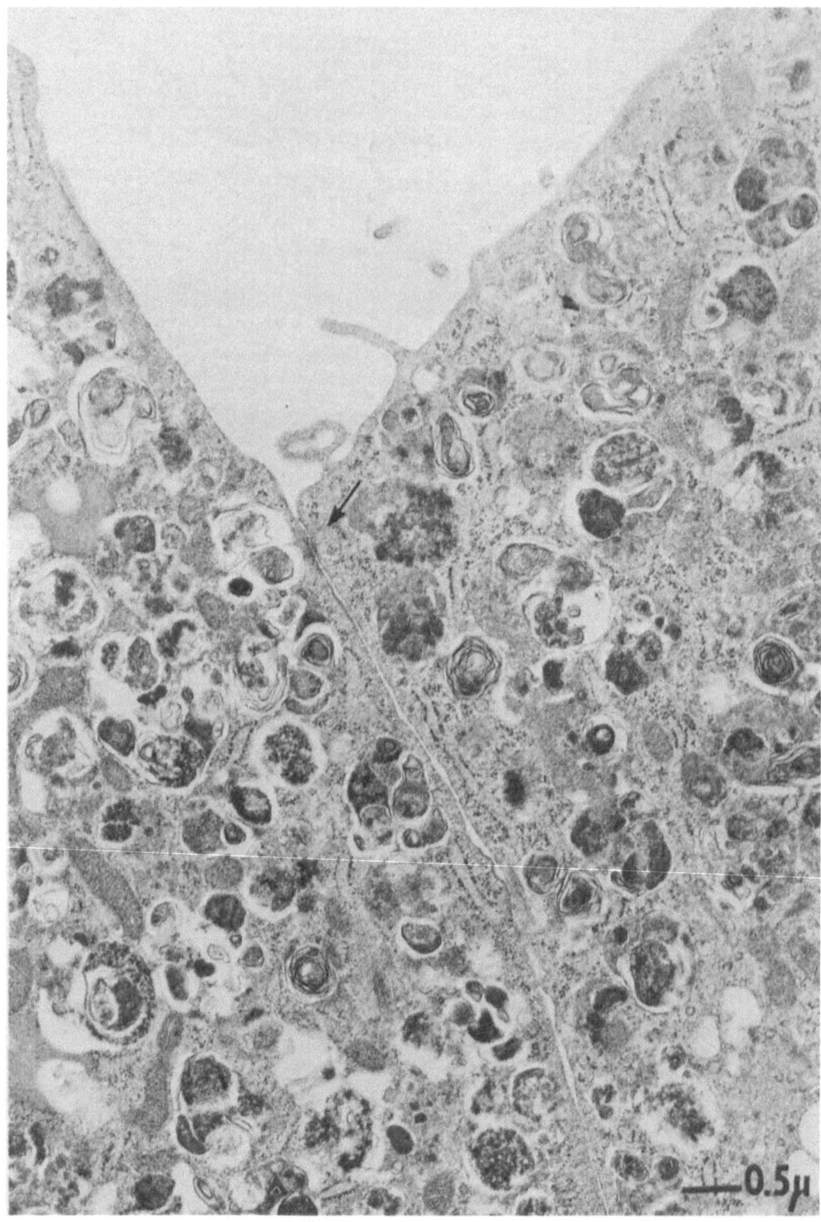

FIG. 3. Electron micrograph of material fixed in Fig. 2 showing portions of two cells. Arrow indicates a site of thickening of the membranes resembling a poorly developed desmosome. Granular cytoplasm is due to numerous lysosomes and electron-dense material.

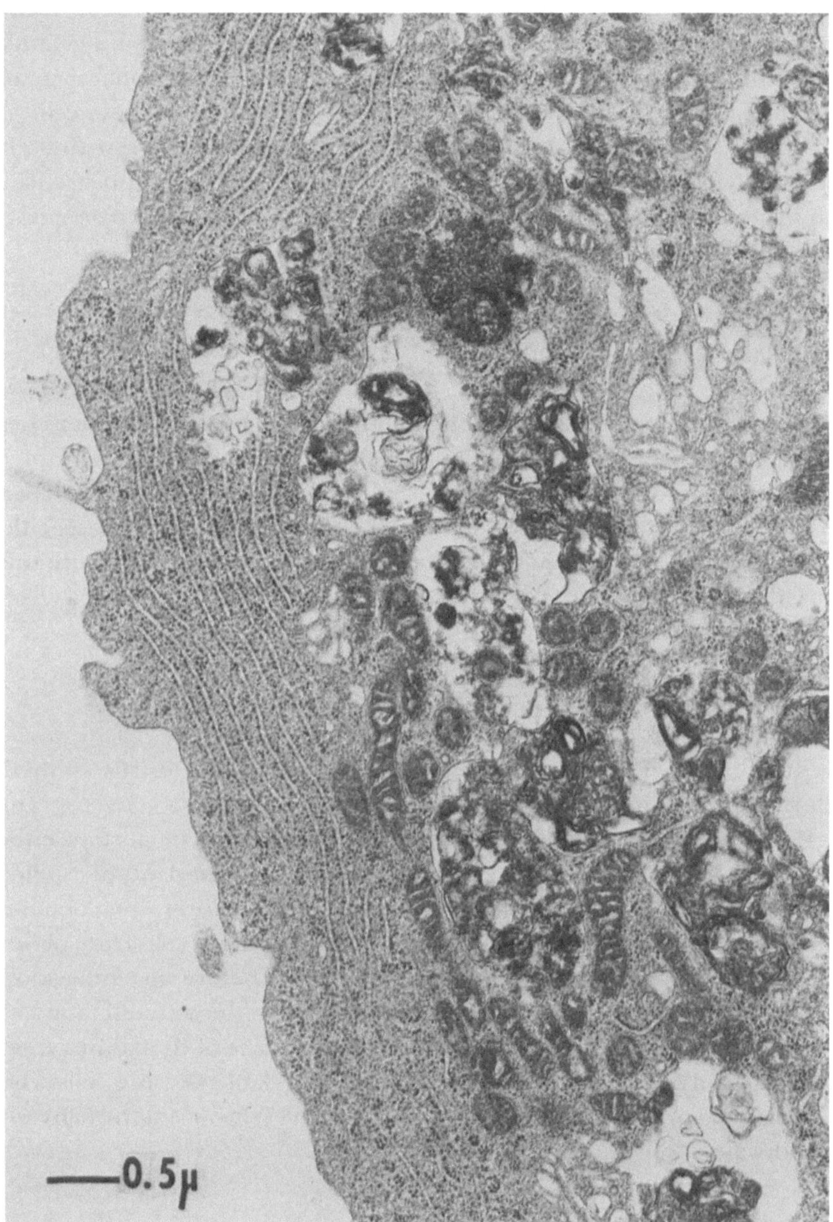

FIG. 4. Border of another cell from the same preparation as in Fig. 3 showing part of the free margin of the cell. Subjacent to the cell membrane are several layers of slender cisternae of ribosome-bearing endoplasmic reticulum arranged in parallel.

appearing as scattered individual cells which settle rapidly on the surface of the flask. The shape is usually ovoid; the cytoplasm is dense and granular around the nucleus and on one side of the cell, while the peripheral area of the cytoplasm is thin and clear. We do not know whether these cells are monocytes, macrophages, or mesothelial cells but have chosen the term "mesothelial-like" to designate them. Figures 5–7 show their appearance as seen by phase contrast photography of the living cells and electron microscopic studies of the fixed material.

2.3. Other Cells

Besides the nontumor cells mentioned above, many other cell types appear in our cultures. The majority of them merely survive, migrate, or multiply to a limited extent for a few weeks. The identification of these cells has not been completed, so in Fig. 8 are shown some of the types most frequently seen that we have labeled with the nonscientific names which help us to recognize them (dendritic, ladybug, round floating cell, etc.).

2.4. Tumor Cells

The tumor cells are generally recognizable by the characteristic epithelial pattern of the living culture (Figs. 9 and 10) and that in electron micrographs (Figs. 11 and 12). They tend to clump or grow in patches or clusters, either on the surface of the flask when obtained from tumor explants of "spilled" cells or in balls or grapelike clusters floating in the medium when obtained from pleural effusions (Fig. 13). This ability of some tumor cells from pleural effusions to remain in suspension for several days before attaching to the substrate can be useful in separating such cells from the contaminating cell types which attach readily to the plastic or glass surface of the culture vessel. It is always advisable to check every culture for viable floating cells when discarding old or used medium so that one doesn't "throw out the baby with the bathwater."

3. Means of Separating the Various Cell Types Present

To try to separate tumor cells, which are presumably distinguishable from the other cell types present, a great variety of ingenious methods have been recommended. They range from the simplest, such as transferring the

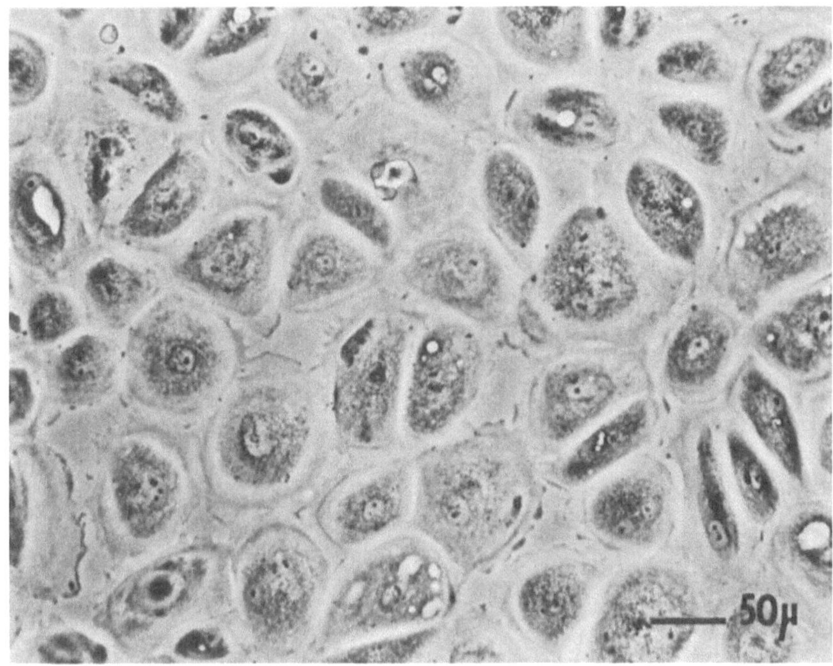

FIG. 5. Phase contrast photomicrograph of mesothelial-like cells grown from pleural effusion, 77 days in culture.

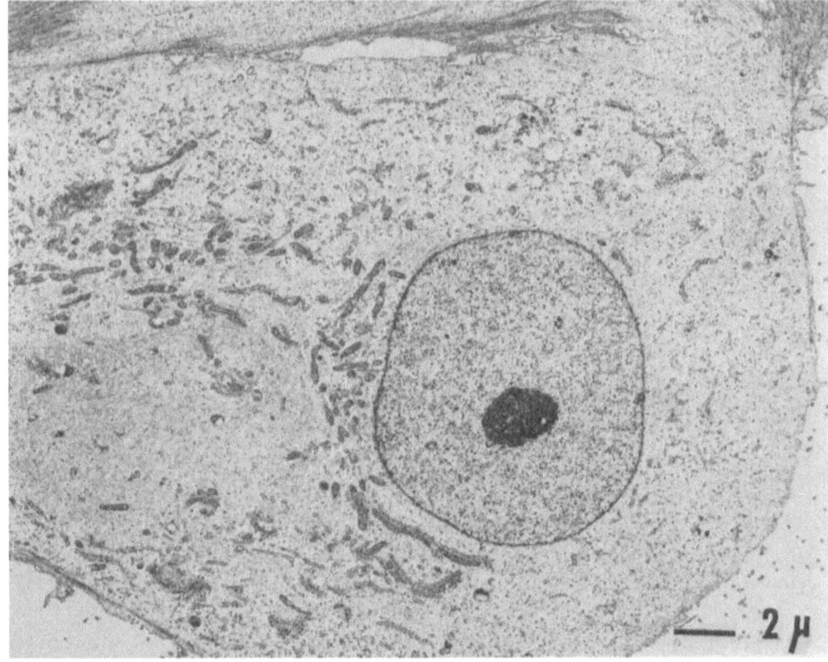

FIG. 6. Electron micrograph of one of the cells shown in Fig. 5.

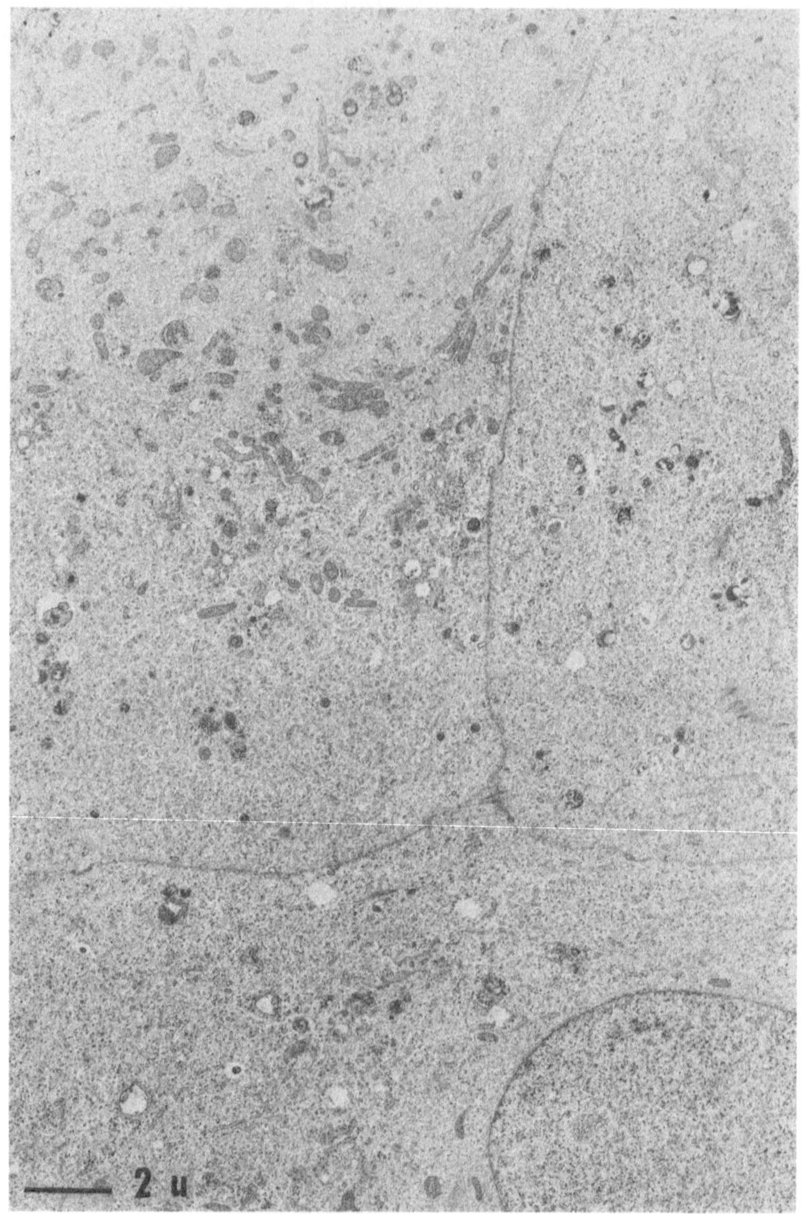

FIG. 7. Electron micrograph of adjacent cells shown in Fig. 5. The overall density of the cytoplasm is uniform and the nucleus has a bland appearance with diffuse distribution of the chromatin material.

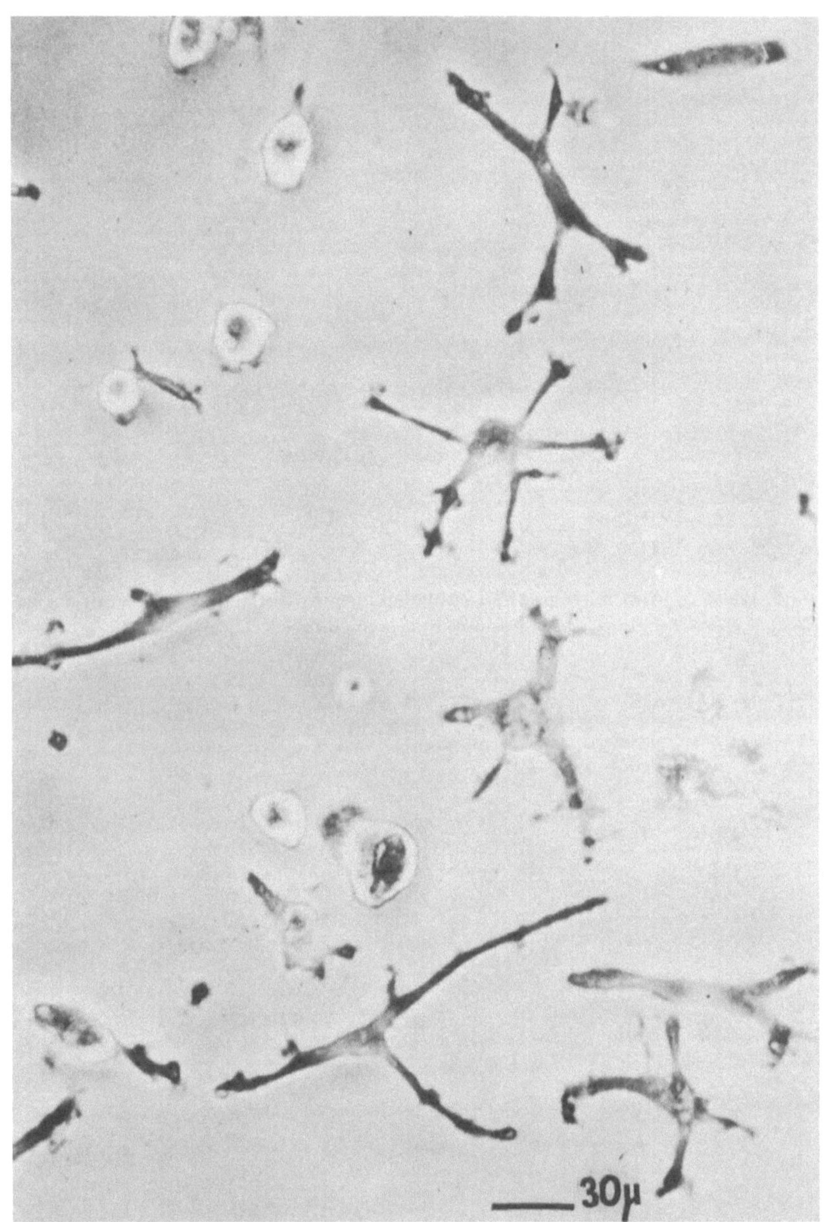

FIG. 8. Phase contrast micrograph of "dendritic" and "ladybug" cells from a malignant pleural effusion, 52 days in culture.

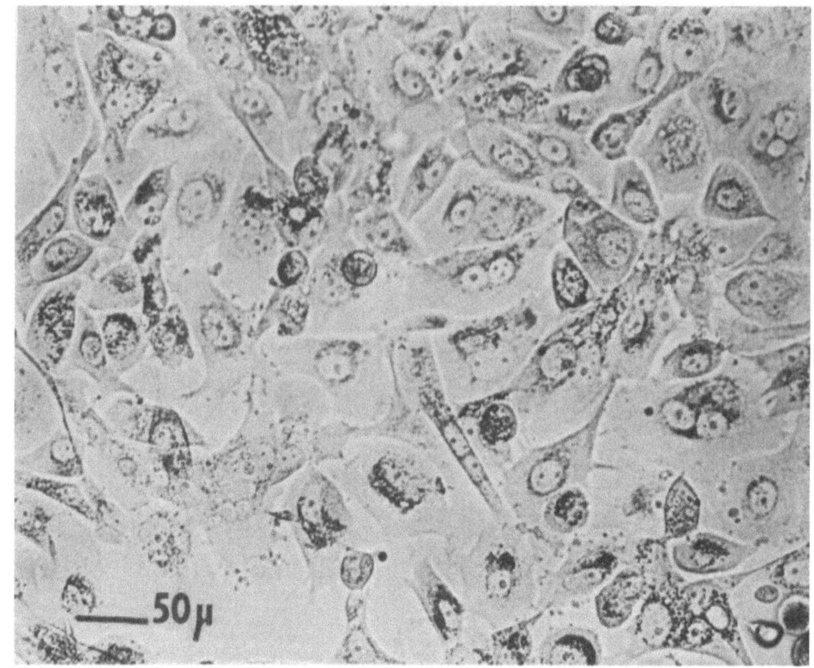

FIG. 9. Phase contrast micrograph of epithelial outgrowth from an explant of a solid breast tumor, 8 days in culture.

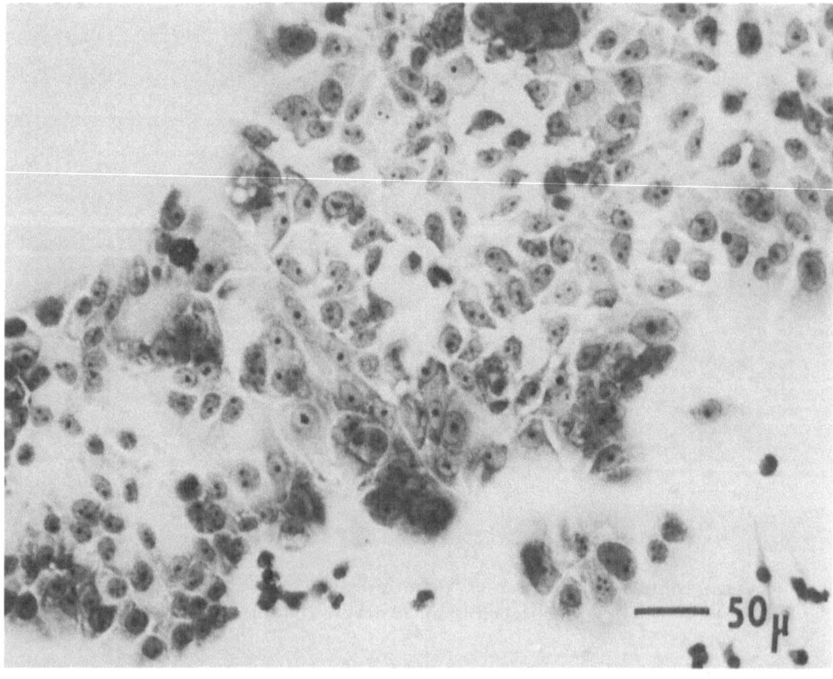

FIG. 10. Coverslip preparation of tumor cells from a pleural effusion, 4 days in culture. Giemsa stain.

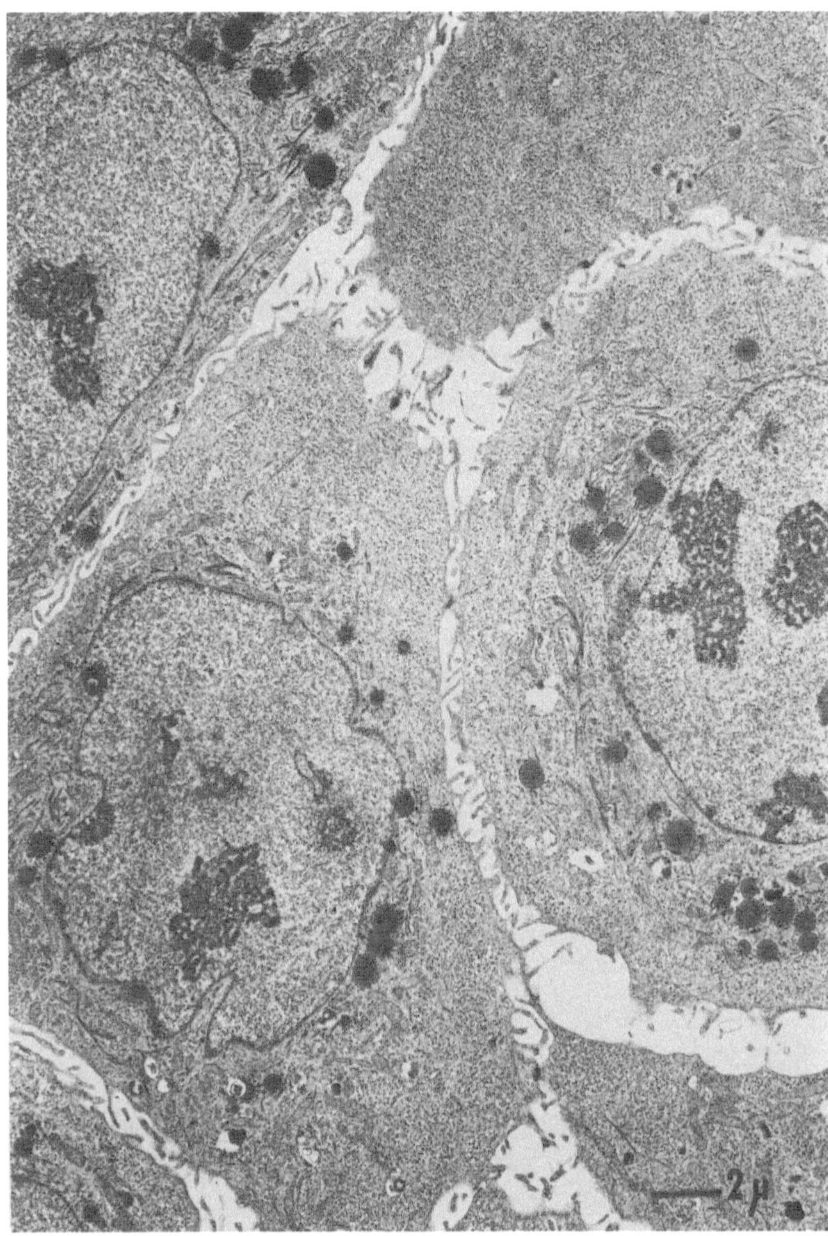

FIG. 11. Electron micrograph of solid tumor seen in Fig. 9. The moderately high nuclear cytoplasmic ratio is evident. The nuclei have irregular profiles, nucleoli are multiple and prominent.

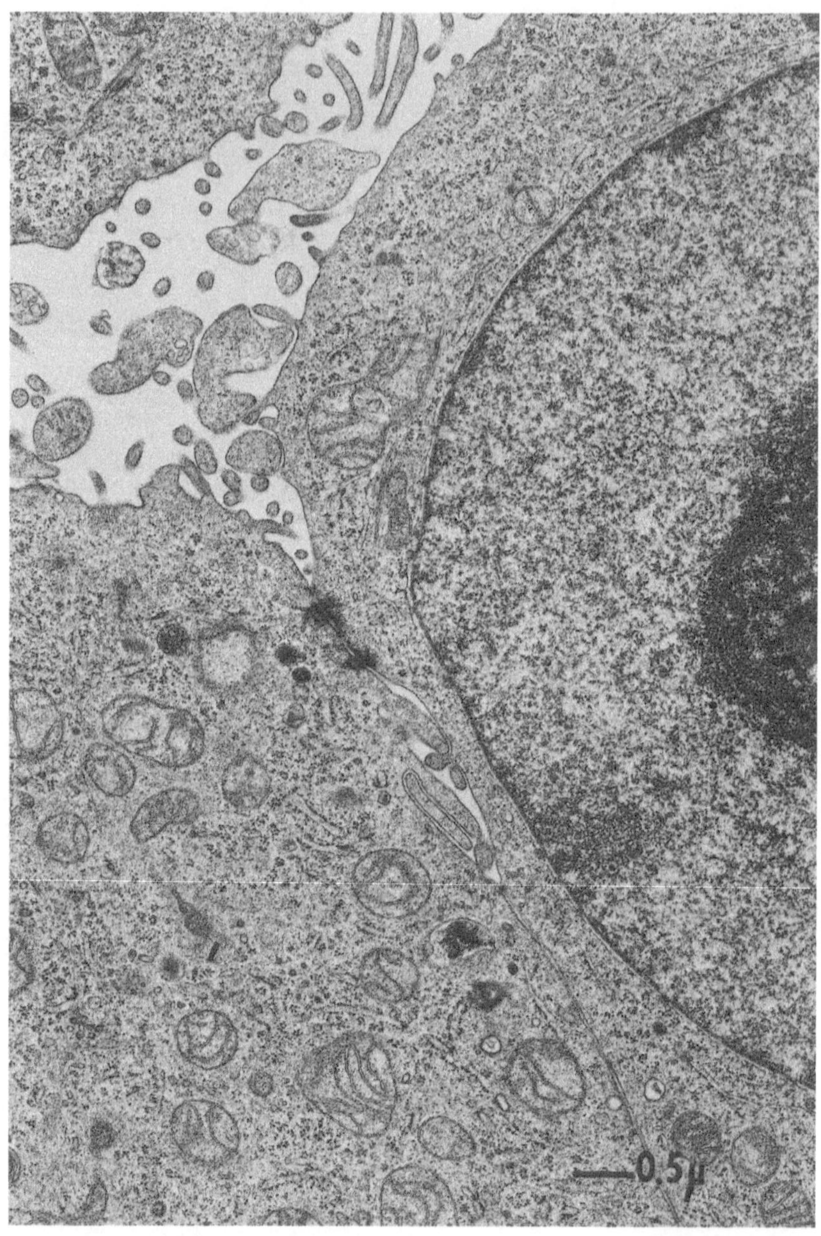

FIG. 12. Electron micrograph of MDA-MB-157 tumor cells from a tissue culture. Note scattered mitochondria and numerous ribosomes free within the cytoplasm and attached to short, narrow cisternae of endoplasmic reticulum. Two desmosomes and numerous microvilli at the periphery of the cells are present.

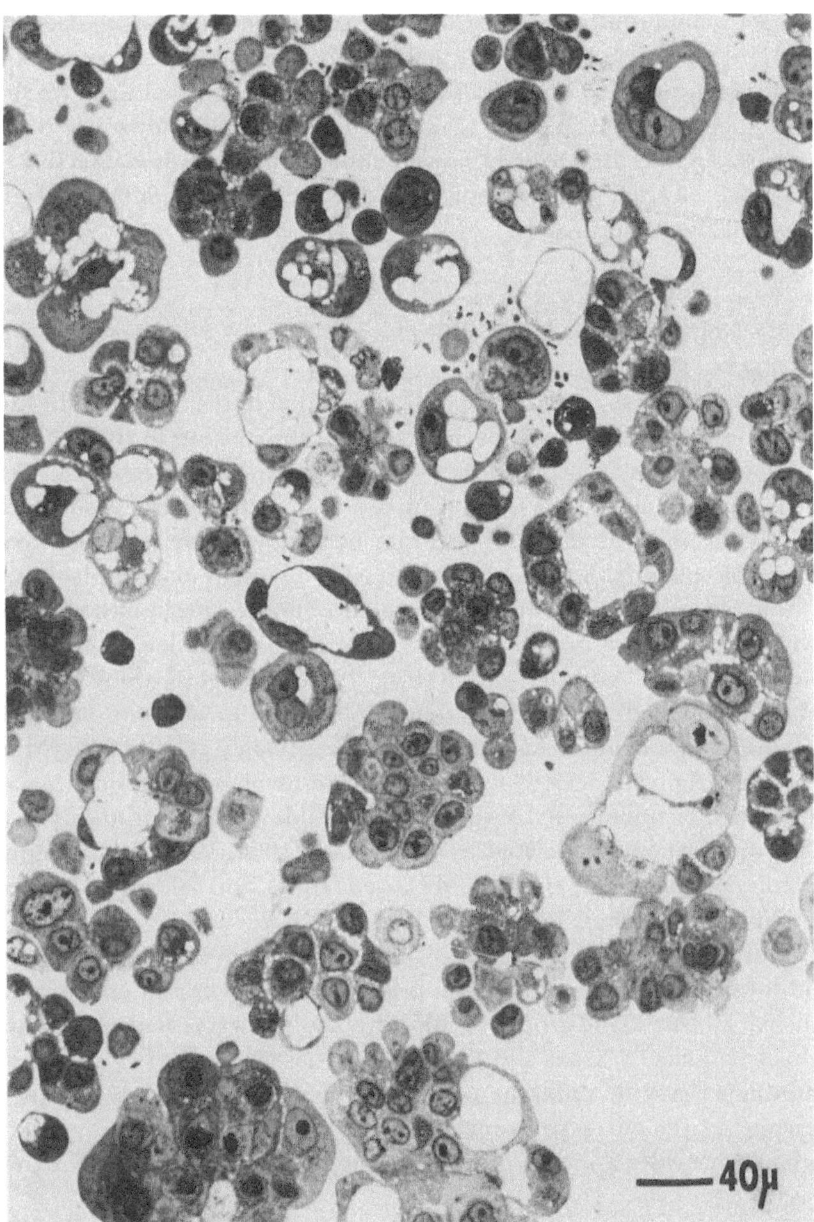

FIG. 13. One-micrometer section of an Epon-embedded pellet of hemolyzed pleural fluid showing numerous epithelial cells in "balls" or clusters of varying size. Methylene blue–azur II stain.

supernatant fluid containing balls of tumor cells to another flask and leaving the majority of the nontumor cells behind, to systems of great complexity. Because no one method is applicable to all types of cells or cultures, we shall list here some examples of many of the methods that have shown a degree of success. Again, it cannot be emphasized enough that a method effective for one type of cell from one organ or from one species may not be successful when applied to other tissues.

3.1. *Mechanical, Physical, and Physiological*

As mentioned above, transferring cells suspended in the supernatant fluid by pouring or pipetting and leaving behind cells sticking to the substrate serves as a crude way of separation. Even inadvertantly placing a flask in the incubator upside down for a few days may accomplish the same result, but is not really recommended! Fibroblasts may be scraped away with a gel-foam pledget or a rubber policeman, or, conversely, the tumor mass or plaque can be dislodged or scraped and transferred to another flask. Other simple mechanical means of separation use glass beads (Wöhler *et al.*, 1972; Rabinowitz, 1965; Aronson and Kessel, 1960) and glass wool filtration combined with dextran centrifugation (Morrison, 1967). A more complex method employs countercurrent distribution (Walter *et al.*, 1969). Many techniques originally devised to separate various blood components have been applied to tumor cells as well. These include the discontinuous Ficoll density gradient system devised by Sykes *et al.* (1964, 1970), beef albumin gradients (Wespic, 1970; Zucker and Cassen, 1969), and velocity sedimentation (Miller and Phillips, 1969).

Several methods have used simple variations in the depth of the overlying liquid layer as a means of depressing fibroblast growth and encouraging epithelial growth (Sandstrom, 1966). The use of perforated cellophane, originally applied by Evans and Earle (1947), has also served as a means of separating cells with different oxygen requirements or as a means of restricting movement, separating two types of cells or conditioning media. Chapter 9 provides a more complete discussion and bibliography of this subject.

Osgood and Krippaehne (1955) devised a simple, ingenious method of varying the depth of medium covering the cells to produce a gradient in the gas (O_2, CO_2) phase affecting the cells. Some of the most interesting work on this subject has been done by McLimans and his collaborators (McLimans *et al.*, 1968*a,b*; Tunnah *et al.*, 1968; Harris *et al.*, 1966) and comprehensively reviewed by McLimans (1969, 1972). Other studies on oxygen requirement have been applied to submerged cultures (Radlett *et al.*, 1972), cloning of cells (Richter *et al.*, 1972), and organ or tumor culture in hyperbaric oxygen (Stier and Halasz, 1966) as a means of overcoming anoxic central necrosis. The toxic effects of ozone (Pace *et al.*, 1969) were tested on human and mouse cell lines. The use of perfusion chambers for high-density suspension cultures (Kruse *et al.*, 1970) or circumfusion systems (Rose *et al.*, 1970) for cultivation of cells under special conditions also requires rigorous control of the gas phase. Katsuta *et al.* (1968) and Katsuta and Takaota (1961*a,b*, 1964) have employed parabiotic cultures to study the influence of one cell type on another through medium exchange. Studies on tissue explants or organ cultures have employed a sponge matrix or a collagen-coated cellulose sponge as a substrate (Kalus *et al.*, 1968; Leighton, 1951). Some complex methods applied to organ culture or small pieces of tumor have been designed to regulate the gas phase or oxygen tension to try to separate fibroblasts from epithelial cells (McLimans, 1972; Trowell, 1954, 1959, 1966; Jensen *et al.*, 1964). Other variations in suspension culture systems have been designed to study large numbers of cells and their metabolic products under continuously controlled or monitored conditions (Himmelfarb *et al.*, 1969; Moore *et al.*, 1963). Another system of organ-type culture combined with embryonic mesonephrose has given excellent results in the hands of Wolff and his coworkers and is discussed at length in Chapter 8 and also in Chapter 6. Mention should be made of some early studies by Parshley and Simms (1950), who noted that chick epithelial cells proliferated better than fibroblasts when the pH was slightly acid (6.9), the calcium concentration reduced, and the phosphate concentration raised in the culture medium. However, this approach seems to have been neglected except in relation to enzyme treatment of cells.

Some cell types grow better on glass, others on plastic, and it is advisable when trying to culture new tumors to use at least one flask of each type per experiment. It has also been found helpful in initiating tumor cultures to use "conditioned" medium, or the pleural fluid from the same patient as part of the medium. We have found that most plastic ware tends to be quite alkaline and can raise the pH of some media to levels above 8.0. When this occurs, it is often critical and gassing the cultures with a 5–10% CO_2-in-air mixture is required to bring the pH down to the normal range.

Another subject touched on by Waymouth (1970) is the importance of knowing or controlling the osmolality of the media in cell cultures.

3.2. Enzymatic

In most studies on breast tumor explants, it has been found advisable to treat the pieces of tissue with one or more of a number of enzymes for various times and at various temperatures. These enzymes have been used primarily as a means of loosening or destroying the fibrin-like matrix which surrounds or encapsulates the tumor cells, particularly in scirrhous carcinoma.

Trypsin was one of the first enzymes used and has been extensively employed for all types of cells with a fair degree of success. It is still used by most workers to obtain single cell suspensions from established cultures which stick to the surface of the flask. However, Levan and Biesele (1958), among others, showed that trypsin treatment increases chromosome alterations as well as produces deleterious effects on the cells. This latter effect was used by DeLuca (1965) to increase the sensitivity of cultured cells to cytotoxic agents.

Early in his studies on mammary tissue culture, Lasfargues (1957) found collagenase useful in dissociating mouse mammary tissue and he has continued to use it in his present studies. In this book, both Lasfargues (Chapter 3) and Leibovitz (Chapter 2) discuss in detail their use of collagenase as a means of initially separating tumor cells from the surrounding stroma. Both authors have studied collagenase as an additive to the culture medium as a means of controlling or discouraging fibroblastic growth (Lasfargues, 1972).

In experiments using mouse and chick embryonic organs and tissue, adverse effects of collagenase treatment were observed by Wessells and Cohen (1968). They found that morphological structure was affected and morphogenesis arrested. Similar effects were observed by Grobstein and Cohen (1965). These authors also found crystalline collagenase to be 10–50 times more potent than the crude collagenase preparations.

Pronase has been found by several workers (Houba, 1967; Sullivan and Schafer, 1966; Gwatkin and Thomson, 1964) to be superior to trypsin in dispersing cells, and it does not appear to harm the cells or affect their viability or their ability to attach to glass.

Elastase has been recommended as an enzyme to replace trypsin, since it was noted by Phillips (1972) to be a small but active fraction of many trypsin preparations, which would explain why crude trypsin seems to be more effective than purified trypsin or chymotrypsin.

All these enzymes succeed totally or partially in producing single cell suspensions from tumors composed of a mixture of cell types, but they do not achieve complete success in separating the epithelial or tumor cells from the nonmalignant cells or fibroblasts which are present. A combination of many methods seems to be necessary to achieve this goal.

3.3. Modifications in Media

The chemical, enzymatic or hormonal composition of the medium in which cells can be grown has been recognized as an important factor in the survival of the tissue or the establishment of a cell line since the earliest tissue culture studies. The variations studied and the number of articles which have appeared are legion, and will be discussed here only in a few pertinent instances. For an in-depth treatment of the subject, see Chapter 2. Most tissue culture workers are familiar enough with the names of the formulas, such as 199, MEM, NCTC-109, RPMI-1640, F-10, MB-752/1, and L-15, to associate them with the laboratories or workers who devised them; prominent investigators are Healy *et al.* (1971), Morgan *et al.* (1950, 1955), Ham (1962, 1965), Evans *et al.* (1964), Leibovitz (1963), Sanford *et al.* (1963), Waymouth (1959), Eagle (1955). This list mentions only a few of those who have provided us with the major media used for many cell lines or useful in attempts to isolate and establish new ones. Waymouth (1965, 1967) has written several reviews covering most aspects of this subject.

The use of chick embryo extract or feeder layers allowed propagation of many cells that could not have been studied by other means. But the unknown factors supplied by these substrates often compounded the difficulties in recognizing the growth properties or metabolism of the cells being studied. Irradiated HeLa cells, or normal cells with the inability to continue to divide, have been used as a feeder layer to propagate other cell types (Puck and Marcus, 1955). The use of these techniques has gradually decreased as the composition of the media used has become more sophisticated, although they may be useful in initiating the culture of certain types of cells. The dangers of viral or other contamination, as well as increased confusion as to the role of the living cells introduced in the substrate, have resulted in the abandonment of most of these substances. A comprehensive review of these methods is presented by various authors in Willmer's (1965, 1966) three-volume treatise, *Cells and Tissues in Culture.*

Even these complex media, supplemented with serum from various sources, have proven unsuccessful with many tumors, and it has been necessary to add other substances. The use of "conditioned" media in which embryonic or similar cells have grown has been found useful. Breast cancer cultures in particular, whether from mouse tissue or human, have shown the need for various hormones. Insulin is considered essential, at least for the initiation of these cultures (Ceriani *et al.*, 1972; Koyama *et al.*, 1972; Turkington, 1969; Barnawell, 1965; Barker *et al.*, 1964; Rivera, 1964*a,b*; Lasfargues, 1962; Elias, 1959; Elias and Rivera, 1959; Lasfargues and Murray, 1959).

The necessity of other hormones is somewhat controversial, as most of the studies have been done with mouse mammary tissue in organ-type culture. The favorable influence of cortisol, aldosterone, somatotropin, estrogen, prolactin, progesterone, or 17β-estradiol has been recognized by most of the abovementioned workers. Others have found cortisone useful in maintaining organ cultures of mouse skin (Gillette *et al.*, 1961) and in influencing adhesiveness to glass (Aujard and Chany, 1966), or cortisol helpful in growth hormone synthesis (Kohler *et al.*, 1969).

The presence or absence of certain chemical compounds in the medium may be necessary for the proliferation of one or more cell types, or may function in the transformation of a "normal" cell into a malignant form (Benyesh-Melnick *et al.*, 1963). Ross *et al.* (1962) have written an excellent review of this subject.

Ling *et al.* (1968) have modified the proportions of practically all the essential components in the usual recommended media and devised a serum-free one which seems adequate for some mouse and rat cell lines. The presence of certain steroids proved necessary for mouse mammary tumor in culture (Smith and King, 1972), while tests by MacDougall *et al.* (1965) showed that cholesterol and related derivatives were toxic to organ cultures of rabbit aorta. The variable effects of vitamins A and C on cultured cells and tissue have been reviewed by Fell and Rinaldini (1965). The effect of vitamin E on cultured cells was found to be dependent on the substrate used (Corwin and Humphrey, 1972). Biotin and B_{12} were found to be essential for certain cells grown in chemically defined media (Sanford *et al.*, 1963). The growth-promoting or toxic effect of a vitamin, hormone, or serum varies with other conditions and with the type of cell or serum utilized (Evans *et al.*, 1972; Sanford *et al.*, 1972*a,b*; Sanford, 1967; Cailleau and Kirk, 1954, 1957).

Not only does the effect of the hormone, vitamin, serum, etc., vary with the cell type in question, but within narrow limits the enzymatic constitution of the culture may be altered. The cell may be transformed from malignant to nonmalignant, from nonmalignant to malignant, from epithelioid to fibroblast-like, or from fibroblastoid to epithelial-like. The chromosome stemline can be changed and a new sensitive or resistant line established (Ioachim, 1970; Auersperg, 1969; German *et al.*, 1964).

The danger of viral, mycoplasmal, and other contamination and the toxic effects or variable results found with serum or biological fluids from different sources have forced many workers to turn to serum substitutes. These substitutes can be obtained in powdered form and are uniform in quality or can be autoclaved to insure sterility. Some products used in the early days of bacteriology such as peptones, casein, whey or lactalbumin hydrolysates, and yeast autolysates are again appearing on the menu (Habeshaw, 1972; Taylor *et al.*, 1972; Yamane *et al.*, 1968; Holmes, 1967; Lépine *et al.*, 1956; Ginsberg *et al.*, 1955). These are just a few of the variety of substances being used as substitutes for biological nonautoclavable culture components.

Certain advantages exist in media which allow cells to grow in suspension and, combined with the necessary growth factors, inhibitors, or enzymes, permit epithelial cells and fibroblasts to develop at different rates or in different areas in the container. Various concentrations of agar, collagen, or methylcellulose, in particular, have been used to this purpose (Masurovsky and Peterson, 1973; Bryant, 1969; Costăchel *et al.*, 1969; Patuleia and Friend, 1967; Schindler, 1964; Tribble and Higuchi, 1963).

Conversely, Rappaport and Bishop (1960) indicate that chemical treatment of pyrex glass is necessary to increase cell attachment when synthetic medium is used. Fisher *et al.* (1958) found that fetuin has a similar function in cell attachment.

All these methods are devised with the purpose of fostering the growth of one cell type at the expense of another, of providing adequate or ideal growth conditions for the cell being studied, and of eliminating, if possible, all outside sources of contamination, particularly mycoplasmas and viruses.

4. *Presence or Absence of Mycoplasmas, Viruses, and Other Contaminants: Implications*

The subject of contamination is discussed at length in other chapters in this volume, but there is a need to mention the less obvious mycoplasmal and viral types of contamination of cell cultures. Methods are now available (immunofluorescence, cytotoxic effects, electron microscopic examination) to identify these particles if they are present. The presence of virus particles may either alter or destroy the cultures or allow them to propagate better than in the absence of the virus. Similarly, if the cultures are infected with mycoplasma, particularly when antibiotics are present in the medium, little or no toxic effect may occur. Under other conditions and with other cell strains, mycoplasmal contamination can be fatal.

Much has been written on the viral etiology of cancer in humans, and I leave the discussion of this subject to the other, more qualified authors. However, in relation to human breast carcinoma cultures, although many workers are able to find virus particles in cultures of human mammary carcinomas (Feller *et al.*, 1970; Seman *et al.*, 1969), others have been unable to detect any virus by electron microscopic or other techniques in primary cultures of established cell lines (Plata *et al.*, 1973; Calafat and Hageman, 1972; Sykes *et al.*, 1968).

Studies on fetal calf serum used in culturing most cell lines or tumor material have shown that viruses, as well as mycoplasmas, may be present in the commercial serum used (Boone *et al.*, 1971; Molander *et al.*, 1971) and thus lead to erroneous conclusions as to their possible origin in the tumor being cultured (Federoff *et al.*, 1971) or in the patient.

The significance of the identification of mycoplasmas or viruses in cultured cells cannot be overemphasized. The presence of one or the other may be the additional factor which allows the cells to multiply *in vitro*. It is of primary importance to know whether this material is truly the causative agent of the tumor and present in the host. If not, it must be determined whether it is incidental to the host, or contamination introduced by laboratory procedures or by use of certain biological products in the media. Viruses and mycoplasmas, when added to uncontaminated cultures, frequently produce morphological, chemical, and chromosomal changes in the cells, another reason for identifying the source of these entities and determining whether they were present initially *in vivo* and, if not, how they got into cultures.

5. *Identification of Cultured Cells*

5.1. *Pathology*

The ultimate identification of the tumor (using breast carcinoma as our example) is made by microscopic examination of a piece of the tissue which has been fixed and stained and examined by a qualified pathologist who has excised the malignant area. This has been the basic procedure for many years and is considered reliable for the identification of a tumor obtained from *in vivo* or surgical sources. But once the tumor cells have been suspended in culture medium and maintained for even a few hours in a tube or flask, their appearance may be quite altered and totally foreign to most anatomists or pathologists who have never seen or studied living cells in culture. Cells, as they spread out and grow on a glass or plastic substrate, may change size and shape, develop or lose granules or vacuoles, and alter their genetic configuration and enzyme composition.

5.2. *Staining and Photography*

It therefore becomes necessary to be able to identify each type of cell, as it was in the host and as it survives, adapts, or multiplies *in vitro*. To do this, it is necessary to study the gross microscopic appearance of the usual hematoxylin and eosin stained sections of the tumor, and also to follow the outgrowths from explants of the tissue or cells from pleural effusions using one or more of a variety of other stains (Papanicolaou, Giemsa, fluorescent antibody, etc.). Frequent photographs of the growing material using ordinary bright-field or phase contrast microscopy or time-lapse cinematography, etc., are extremely useful in identifying cell types present and noting changes which occur with time and other variables. Whenever possible, electron microscope sections should be made and pictures taken of aliquots of the same original material and of cultured cells which have been photographed in a living condition immediately before fixation.

5.3. *Enzymatic Differences*

Enzymatic studies (Farnes, 1967; Fortelius, 1963), while less frequently used in the identification of tumors of primary origin, may be invaluable in determining whether a so-called cell line is truly what it is claimed to be, or possibly "contaminated" by some other cell line of human or even nonhuman origin. Many cell lines thought to be of different origins have turned out to be HeLa or mouse L-cells after careful enzymatic (Gartler, 1967; Simpson and Stulberg, 1963; Brand and Syverton, 1960) or chromosome analysis (Herrick *et al.*, 1970; Hsu, 1961).

5.4. *Chromosomes*

The chromosome count, karyotype, or radioautography picture can be an excellent way to identify human cells, and with the new banding techniques chromosome staining may soon be as accurate as fingerprinting (Comings *et al.*, 1973; Shiraishi and Yosida, 1972; Drets and Shaw, 1971; Schnedl, 1971*a,b*; Sumner *et al.*, 1971). These methods are applicable with established cultures and somewhat less feasible with fresh tumor material. However, study of the chromosome pattern has proven most useful in indicating that great care must be exercised to avoid a mixture of cell lines in the culture tube.

5.5. *Transplantation*

The presumptive criterion of malignancy is the production of a similar or identical tumor in an acceptable host, such as the hamster cheek pouch or rabbit cornea. But the lack of a tumor formation comparable to the initial tumor does not necessarily prove that the cultured cells were not of malignant origin. Many experiments with human and mouse cultures derived from tumor cells have shown that loss of malignancy or transplantability may occur fairly early during *in vitro* growth. This was demonstrated by attempts to transplant a recently isolated mucoid adenocarcinoma line from a human lung into the hamster cheek pouch (Cailleau, 1960). Similar experiments with a breast carcinoma line (Dobrynin, 1963) gave identical results: first inoculations produced tumors but subsequent attempts failed. Many other studies have been carried out with mouse cell lines and show a similar loss of "virulence" or transplantability even when the cells still contain the virus found in the *in vivo* line (Sandford *et al.*, 1972*b*; Price *et al.*, 1971; Cailleau and Dirksen, 1968; Evans and Andresen, 1968; Foley and Drolet, 1964). In studies with Ehrlich ascites carcinoma in tissue culture, this property has been utilized to provide immunoprotection against the corresponding virulent mouse line (Morgan *et al.*, 1970; Cailleau and Costa, 1961). Obviously the application of these procedures in humans is somewhat more difficult to study or control.

6. *Proof that Cells Cultured Are the Tumor Cells of Origin*

The crux of the situation, the ultimate goal of our studies, is to identify the tumor material in the cancerous organ or fluid. This is usually done by the clinician, pathologist, and surgeon. Then the tissue or fluid must be placed in the growth medium, which, it is hoped, does not contain any of the various contaminating, deleterious, or toxic agents listed previously. This medium does contain, it is hoped, all the necessary factors (chemical, biological, physical, physiological, etc.) needed for the growth of the tumor cells. But, unfortunately, with rare exceptions, the tissue or fluid that is cultured contains more than one type of cell. By judicious dispersion of the tissue or cells using any one or more of the various methods mentioned earlier, certain cell types appear rather consistently in breast tumors or fluids and seem to be identifiable, at least in the early stages of *in vitro* culture.

This discussion will be limited to the cells present in pleural exudates from persons with mammary carcinomas. The subject of solid breast tumors is presented in detail in Chapter 3.

Of the 30 or more fluids that we have studied to date (June 1973), only one has yielded a cell line (Young *et al.*, 1974). Several other pleural effusions have contained "tumor" cells or clusters, or plaques of cells which have persisted and multiplied for 3–6 months. But their growth rate has been very slow and the tumor cells have either died out or been overgrown by cells whose morphological appearance is quite different from that of the cells originally diagnosed as "tumor." What must be determined is whether the larger "mesothelial-like" cell which seems to grow concurrently with the "tumor" cell is another cell type or merely an adaptation or type of pleomorphism which can occur during prolonged cultivation in certain media. Similarly, the cells with an uncharacteristic fibroblast-like appearance which appear in older cultures of pleural effusions may or may not be fibroblasts. Several of our cultures had cells which were thought to be fibroblasts when examined by light microscopy but were considered to be epithelial on electron microscopic examination (Figs. 2–4).

Other cell types which appear frequently in our pleural effusions have, as yet, not been identified. In lieu of the correct scientific name, we have called them "dendritic" and "ladybug" because of their characteristic shapes (Fig. 8).

One more cell type has appeared in pleural fluids from two different patients on several occasions. This cell is relatively small and round, and it tends to form small balls or grapelike clusters floating in the medium. Very few settle down on the surface of the flask, so they can easily be poured off with the supernatant fluid as a means of separating them from the other types of cells mentioned above, all of which attach firmly to the glass. These floating clusters seem to multiply for a few weeks before reaching a stationary phase, after which they slowly degenerate.

Identification of the larger "mesothelial-like" cell type found in most of our pleural fluid cultures remains difficult. While certain characteristics resemble those of mesothelial cells as recognized by other tissue culture workers, the published literature on mesothelial cells is scanty and often contradictory. Stoebner *et al.* (1970) have compared the electron microscopic structures of hyperplastic and malignant mesothelium. Their pictures show types ranging from epithelial or cuboidal to fibroblastoid, with many variations in the ultrastructure of the cell. Castor and Naylor (1969) have compared the morphological and biochemical properties of normal and malignant mesothelial cells and found no major differences.

Apparently, mesothelial cells, monocytes, and macrophages and even tumor cells of epithelial origin can change shape, size, and even biochemical structure as well as chromosome pattern under the influence of prolonged *in vitro* cultivation and variations in growth conditions. An excellent study of the different forms assumed by cultured monocytes is presented by Sutton (1967). In spite of constant surveillance throughout the culture cycle, it may still be impossible to certify the origin of the cell type which emerges. Morphological, electron microscopic, enzymatic, hormonal, immunological, and chromosomal criteria will probably all be needed to authenticate the origins or the types of cells eventually established in culture from many breast tumor tissues or pleural fluids. Certain other tumor types are easier to identify, and to grow. This is especially true of melanomas, where the presence of pigment may be sufficient in itself to establish the origin of the cells in culture (Oettgen *et al.*, 1968). One of the relatively recent methods used in identifying or classifying some human mammary tumors is based on a specific estrogen-binding capacity (Korsten and Persijn, 1972). The application of these methods to cultures of tumor tissue or pleural effusions is not yet feasible, and the accuracy of present methods must be improved.

Immunofluorescent staining may provide another technique by which cells of different types or species can be identified. The fluorescent antibody technique is helpful in determining many types of contamination, especially viral. Its use in detecting differences between normal and malignant cells may become increasingly important. A review by Beutner (1961) discusses most of the early studies, while Lasfargues in his chapter emphasizes some of the recent applications in relation to breast tumors.

7. *Isolation of a Metastatic Breast Tumor Cell Line from Pleural Effusion*

The tumor cell line MDA-MB-157 was obtained and established in culture under conditions as diametrically opposite as possible from our usual procedure (Young *et al.*, 1974). Normally pleural effusions were used only from patients who had not undergone radiotherapy and had *not* received chemotherapy. The fluids were drawn in a vacuum bottle, heparinized, and handled as rapidly as possible after thoracentesis. This time the fluid was received at 4.30 P.M., December 29, 1972, and (for obvious reasons) was allowed to stand at room temperature until January 2, 1973. Then one of us decided to process it anyway. Cell counts (using trypan blue) showed less than 5% viable cells, in contrast to 75–95% in most of our pleural effusion samples. Four T-30 flasks were made and rather neglected for about 2 wk. As they showed little pH change, they were handled only once or twice during the first month of culture just to add fresh medium and to pour off the dead cells, debris, etc., that floated in the fluid. After about 1 month in culture, a few very small foci or plaques of epithelioid cells were found in one flask of the original four. After 6 wk, these plaques had grown more abundant and increased in size. The culture became sufficiently heavy by March 9, 1973, so that two additional flasks could be started from floating cells shaken off from the cell sheet that now covered the original flask. All three flasks were ready for additional subculture after 2 wk. Since that time, the cultures have been divided 1:2 to 1:10 every 3–7 days, grown in several kinds of media less complicated than our initial hormone (insulin, cortisol, decadron) enriched medium, and studied by us and several collaborators. While a few other cells of various types were present at the beginning, by the time the first subcultures were made only one type remained (Fig. 14). Chromosome counts show characteristic aneuploidy and range from 56 to 66 with a mean value of 64 (Fig. 15). The cell line was considered established

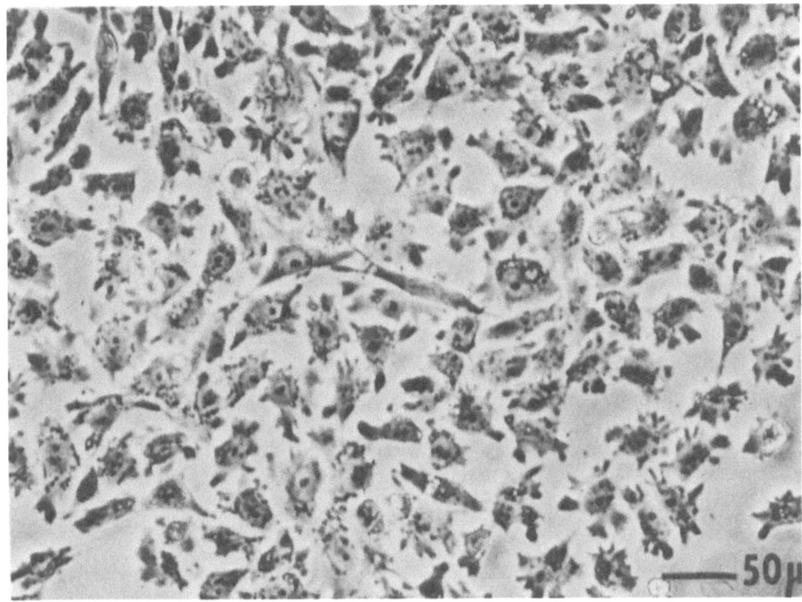

FIG. 14. Phase contrast micrograph of MDA-MB-157 cells after 50 days in culture. The scalloped or frilled periphery of the cells is characteristic of this line.

within 3 months because of the selective way in which it grew and the characteristic electron microscopic picture (Fig. 16). It started from very few cells, which took nearly 2 months to proliferate. A few other cell types present did not persist and died out quickly. Once started, the growth rate has accelerated instead of slowing down. It now grows on simple media such as F-10 plus 20% fetal calf serum, or RPMI-1640 plus 10% fetal calf serum, as well as on one of our initial complicated media of L-15 plus 10% fetal calf serum plus glutathione, insulin, cortisol, decadron, and added sterile-filtered pleural effusion from the same subject or another patient with mammary carcinoma.

This unorthodox system happened to work in this one case. Unfortunately, repeated attempts with other pleural effusions left standing for several days have not been successful. In general, our best results, with cultures containing abundant viable tumor cells with variable amounts and kinds of other cell types present, have been obtained following our standard technique of handling the fluid as rapidly as possible, hemolyzing the red blood cells (if present), and inoculating the flasks fairly heavily (about 1×10^6/ml), then removing the supernatant fluid with floating cells to another flask after a few hours or at 24-h intervals.

Fractionation on an albumin density gradient (1.065) also seems to be helpful in partially separating cell types present in pleural effusions so that fewer "mesothelial" cells remain in the portion containing the tumor cells.

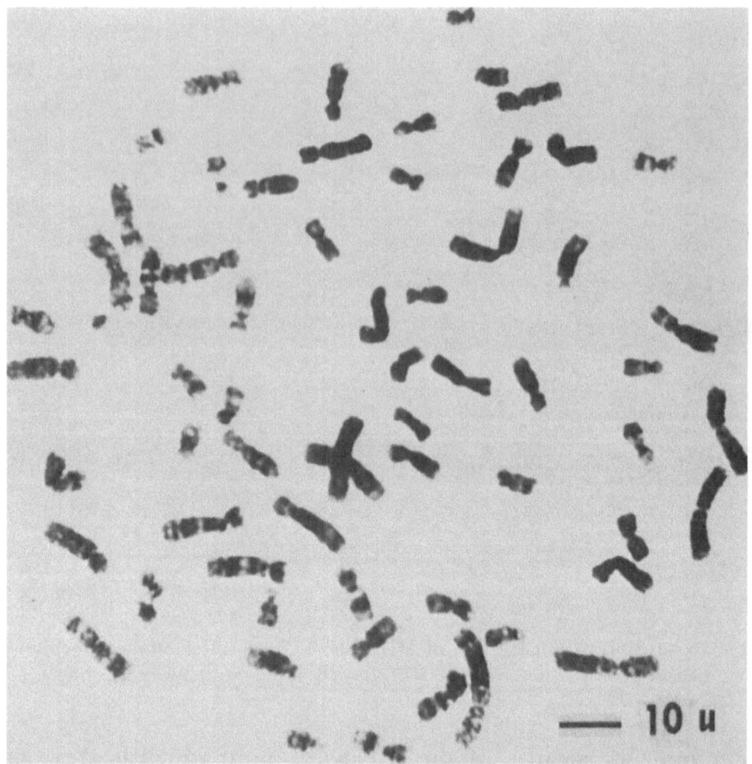

FIG. 15. Banded chromosomes from cell line MDA-MB-157, 65 chromosomes. Giemsa stain.

8. Conclusion

Obviously, the routine establishment of tumor cell lines in tissue culture from most tumors and pleural effusions is not yet a reality.

Difficulties still not recognized or completely understood are (a) presence (or absence) of other needed or deleterious cell types in the cultures; (b) insufficiencies in the growth media; (c) the mutation, adaptation, or transformation of the tumor cell in culture necessary to permit its multiplication or survival *in vitro*; (d) recognition of each cell type present in tissue culture with respect to its origin and the possibility of pleomorphism. It is extremely important to recognize these possibilities, for only by doing so can one devise the methods necessary to prove the origin of established cell lines derived from a mixed cell population.

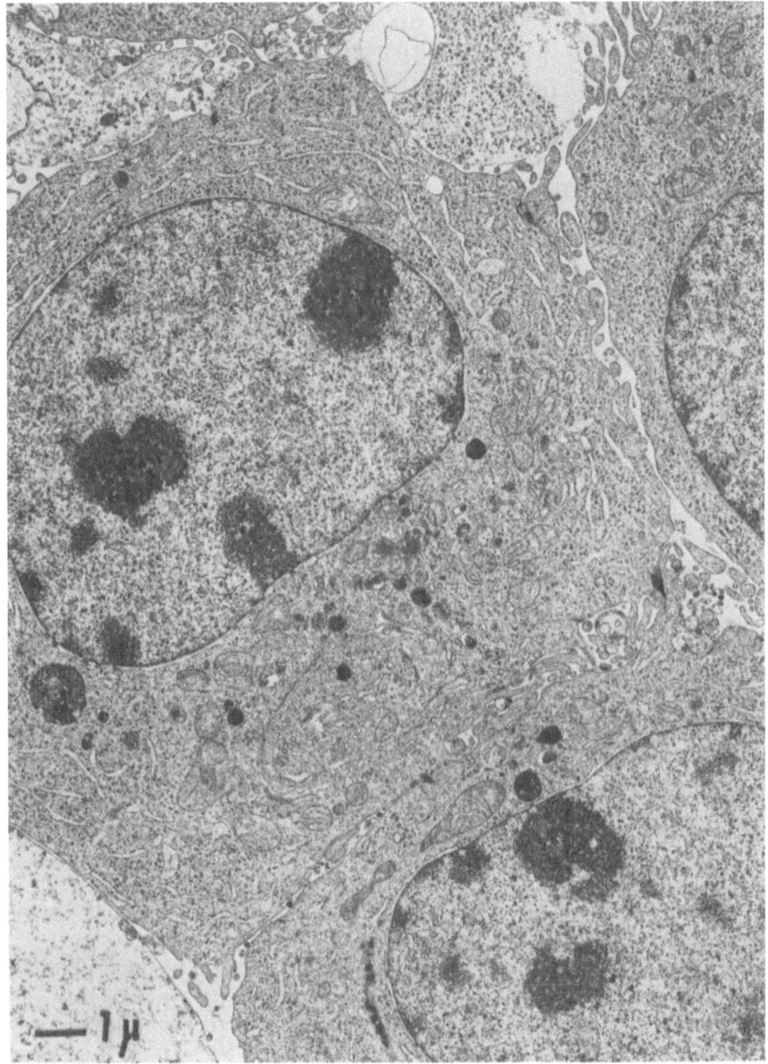

FIG. 16. Electron micrograph of cells from cell line MDA-MB-157 showing characteristic epithelial features.

9. Addendum

Since submitting this chapter for publication, we have obtained three more breast tumor cell lines from pleural effusions (Cailleau *et al.*, 1974). They are as follows: MDA-MB-134, containing 41–45 chromosomes with a mean of 43 or 44; MDA-MB-175, with a mean of 49 chromosomes; and MDA-MB-231, with a chromosome number approximately triploid, ranging between 60 and 72 with a mean of 68. All three lines are visibly different from each other and from our first line, MDA-MB-157. No viruses have been observed and no contamination with mycoplasma has been detected. Line 231 grows very rapidly, and it could be transferred at a 1 : 10 dilution every 5–10 days within 3 months of isolation. Line 175 grows very slowly in tight epithelial clusters or clumps and is transferred only at 1 : 2 to 1 : 5 dilutions every 3–4 wk. Line 134 is composed of small cells, almost lymphocytic in appearance, which settle loosely on the glass surface, remain round or form small spindles, and are easily shaken off the surface of the flask.

10. References

A Bibliography of the Research in Tissue Culture, 1884–1950, 1953, Vols. 1 and 2, (prepared by M. R. Murray and G. Kopach), Academic Press, New York.

Aronson, M., and Kessel, R. W. I., 1960, New method for manipulation, maintenance, and cloning of single mammalian cells *in vitro, Science* **131:**1376–1377.

Auersperg, N., 1969, Histogenetic behavior of tumors. II. Roles of cellular and environmental factors in the *in vitro* growth of carcinoma cells, *J. Natl. Cancer Inst.* **43:**175–190.

Aujard, C., and Chany, E., 1966, Effet de l'hydrocortisone sur la morphologie et l'adhésivité mutuelle ou au verre de cellules en culture (souche KB), *Exp. Cell Res.* **44:**53–65.

Barker, B. E., Fanger, H., and Farnes, P., 1964, Human mammary slices in organ culture, *Exp. Cell Res.* **35:**437–448.

Barnawell, E. B., 1965, A comparative study of the responses of mammary tissues from several mammalian species to hormones *in vitro, J. Exp. Zool.* **160:**189–206.

Bassin, R. H., Plata, E. J., Gerwin, B. I., Mattern, C. F., Haapala, D. K., and Chu, E. W., 1972, Isolation of a continuous epithelioid cell line, HBT-3, from a human breast carcinoma, *Proc. Soc. Exp. Biol. Med.* **141:**673–680.

Benyesh-Melnick, M., Fernback, D. J., and Lewis, R. T., 1963, Studies on human leukemia. I. Spontaneous lymphoblastoid transformation of fibroblastic bone marrow cultures derived from leukemic and nonleukemic children, *J. Natl. Cancer Inst.* **31:**1311–1331.

Beutner, E. H., 1961, Immunofluorescent staining: The fluorescent antibody method, *Bacteriol. Rev.* **25:**49–76.

Boone, C. W., Mantel, N., Caruso, T. D., Jr., Kazam, E., and Stevenson, R. E., 1971, Quality control studies on fetal bovine serum used in tissue culture, *In Vitro* **7:**174–189.

Brand, K. G., and Syverton, J. T., 1960, Immunology of cultivated mammalian cells. I. Species specificity determined by hemagglutination, *J. Natl. Cancer Inst.* **24:**1007–1019.

Bryant, J. C., 1969, Methylcellulose effect on cell proliferation and glucose utilization in chemically defined medium in large stationary cultures, *Biotechnol. Bioeng.* **11:**155–179.

Cailleau, R., 1960, The establishment of a cell strain (MAC-21) from a mucoid adenocarcinoma of the human lung, *Cancer Res.* **20:**837–840.

Cailleau, R., and Costa, F., 1961, Long-term *in vitro* cultivation of some mouse ascites tumors: Ehrlich ascites carcinoma, *J. Natl. Cancer Inst.* **26:**271–281.

Cailleau, R., and Dirksen, E. R., 1968, Chromosomes, virulence and virus in AKR leukemia, in: *Cancer Cells in Culture* (H. Katsuta, ed.), pp. 195–204, University Park Press, University Park, Pa.

Cailleau, R., and Kirk, P. L., 1954, The influence of various culture media on the growth of Earle's strain L cells and chick-heart fibroblasts *in vitro, J. Natl. Cancer Inst.* **15:**295–303.

Cailleau, R., and Kirk, P. L., 1957, Some factors affecting the growth-promoting properties of serum in tissue culture, *Tex. Rep. Biol. Med.* **15:**237–249.

Cailleau, R., Young, R., Olivé, M., and Reeves, W. J. Jr., 1974, Breast tumor cell lines from pleural effusions, *J. Natl. Cancer Inst.* **53:**661–714.

Calafat, J., and Hageman, P. C., 1972, Attempts to detect a mammary tumour virus in human material, in: *Fundamental Research on Mammary Tumors* (J. Mouriquand, ed.), INSERM, Paris.

Castor, C. W., and Naylor, B., 1969, Characteristics of normal and malignant human mesothelial cells studied *in vitro*, *Lab. Invest.* **20:**437–443.

Ceriani, R. L., Contesso, G. P., and Nataf, B. M., 1972, Hormone requirement for growth and differentiation of the human mammary gland in organ culture, *Cancer Res.* **32:**2190–2196.

Comings, D. E., Avelino, E., Okada, T. A., and Wyandt, H. E., 1973, The mechanism of C- and G-banding of chromosomes, *Exp. Cell Res.* **77:**469–493.

Cooper, E. H., 1973, The biology of cell death in tumours, *Cell Tissue Kinet.* **6:**87–95.

Corwin, L. M., and Humphrey, L. P., 1972, Vitamin E: Substrate-dependent growth effect on cells in culture, *Proc. Soc. Exp. Biol. Med.* **141:**609–612.

Costăchel, O., Fadei, L., and Badea, E., 1969, Tumor cell suspension culture on non adhesive substratum, *Z. Krebsforsch.* **72:**24–31.

Decennial Review Conference on Cell, Tissue and Organ Culture, 1966, *Natl. Cancer Inst. Monogr.*, Vol. 26 (1967).

DeLuca, C., 1965, The use of trypsin for the determination of cellular viability, *Exp. Cell Res.* **40:**186–188.

Dobrynin, Y. V., 1963, Establishment and characteristics of cell strains from some epithelial tumors of human origin, *J. Natl. Cancer Inst.* **31:**1173–1196.

Drets, M. E., and Shaw, M. W., 1971, Specific banding patterns of human chromosomes, *Proc. Natl. Acad. Sci.* **68:**2073–2077.

Eagle, H., 1955, The specific amino acid requirements of a mammalian cell (strain L) in tissue culture, *J. Biol. Chem.* **214:**839–852.

Elias, J. J., 1959, Effect of insulin and cortisol on organ cultures of adult mouse mammary gland, *Proc. Soc. Exp. Biol. Med.* **101:**500–502.

Elias, J. J., and Rivera, E., 1959, Comparison of the response of normal, precancerous and neoplastic mouse mammary tissues to hormones *in vitro*, *Cancer Res.* **19:**505–511.

Evans, V. J., and Andresen, W. F., 1968, Spontaneous neoplastic transformations in C3H mouse cells *in vitro*, in: *Cancer Cells in Culture* (H. Katsuta, ed.), pp. 263–280, University Park Press, University Park, Pa.

Evans, V. J., and Earle, W. R., 1947, The use of perforated cellophane for the growth of cells in tissue culture, *J. Natl. Cancer Inst.* **8:**103–119.

Evans, V. J., Bryant, J. C., Kerr, H. A., and Schilling, E. L., 1964, Chemically defined media for cultivation of long-term cell strains from four mammalian species, *Exp. Cell Res.* **36:**439–474.

Evans, V. J., Price, F. M., Sanford, K. K., Kerr, H. A., and Handleman, S. L., 1972, Comparative effects of mare, stallion, gelding horse, and fetal bovine sera on neoplastic transformation *in vitro*, *J. Natl. Cancer Inst.* **49:**505–511.

Farnes, P., 1967, Histochemical approaches to cell characterization *in vitro*, in: Second Decennial Review Conference on Cell, Tissue and Organ Culture, 1966, *Natl. Cancer Inst. Monogr.* **26:**199–228.

Federoff, S., Evans, V. J., Hopps, H. E., Sanford, K. K., and Boone, C. W., 1971, Summary of proceedings of a workshop on serum for tissue culture purposes, *In Vitro* **7:**161–167.

Fell, H. B., and Rinaldini, L. M., 1965, The effects of vitamins A and C on cells and tissues in culture, in: *Cells and Tissues in Culture: Methods, Biology and Physiology*, Vol. 1 (E. N. Willmer, ed.), pp. 659–699, Academic Press, New York.

Feller, W. F., Old, L., and Beth, E., 1970, Type-C particles in an established cell line of human origin, *Proc. Am. Assoc. Cancer Res.* **11:**25 (abst.).

Feller, W. F., Stewart, S. E., and Kantor, J., 1972, Primary tissue culture explants of human breast cancer, *J. Natl. Cancer Inst.* **48:**1117–1120.

Fisher, H. W., Puck, T. T., and Sato, G., 1958, Molecular growth requirements of single mammalian cells: The action of fetuin in promoting cell attachment to glass, *Proc. Natl. Acad. Sci.* **44:**4–10.

Foley, G. E., and Drolet, B. P., 1964, Loss of neoplastic properties *in vitro*. I. Observations with S-180 cell lines, *Cancer Res.* **24:**1461–1467.

Foley, J. F., and Aftonomos, B. T., 1965, Growth of human breast neoplasms in cell culture, *J. Natl. Cancer Inst.* **34:**217–229.

Fortelius, P., 1963, Enzyme activity in cultured cells under various influences, a cytochemical approach, *Acta Pathol. Microbiol. Scand.* **164:**1–94.

Gartler, S. M., 1967, Genetic markers as tracers in cell culture, in: Decennial Review Conference on Cell, Tissue and Organ Culture, 1966, *Natl. Cancer Inst. Monogr.* **26:**167–195.

German, J. L., III, Evans, V. J., Cortner, J. A., and Westfall, B. B., 1964, Characterization of three human cell lines by chromosomal complement and by certain biochemical parameters: Reversible alteration of isozyme patterns by different media, *J. Natl. Cancer Inst.* **32:**681–707.

Gewant, W. C., and Goldenberg, I. S., 1970, Techniques of human breast neoplasm cell culture, *Eur. Surg. Res.* **2:**392–400.

Gillette, R. W., Findley, A., and Conway, H., 1961, Effect of cortisone on skin maintained in organ culture, *J. Natl. Cancer Inst.* **27:**1285–1309.

Ginsberg, H. S., Gold, E., and Jordan, W. S., Jr., 1955, Tryptose phosphate broth as supplementary factor for maintenance of HeLa cell tissue cultures, *Proc. Soc. Exp. Biol. Med.* **89:**66–71.

Giraldo, G., Beth, E., Hirshaut, Y., Aoki, T., Old, L. J., Boyse, E. A., and Chopra, H. C., 1971, Human sarcomas in culture: Foci of altered cells and a common antigen; induction of foci and antigen in human fibroblast cultures by filtrates, *J. Exp. Med.* **133:**454–478.

Grobstein, C., and Cohen, J., 1965, Collagenase: Effect on the morphogenesis of embryonic salivary epithelium, *Science* **150:**626.

Gwatkin, R. B. L., and Thomson, J. L., 1964, A new method for dispersing the cells of mammalian tissues, *Nature (Lond.)* **201:**1242–1243.

Habeshaw, J. A., 1972, A serum-protein-free medium for the culture of macrophages and related cells, *J. Pathol.* **108:**95–96.

Ham, R. G., 1962, Clonal growth of diploid Chinese hamster cells in a synthetic medium supplemented with purified protein fractions, *Exp. Cell Res.* **28:**489–500.

Ham, R. G., 1965, Clonal growth of mammalian cells in a chemically defined, synthetic medium, *Proc. Natl. Acad. Sci.* **53:**288–293.

Harris, G., Mount, D. T., McLimans, W. F., Tunnah, K., Scheele, S., and Moore, G. E., 1966, Gas monitor and control unit for cell culture systems, *Biotechnol. Bioeng.* **8:**489–509.

Healy, G. M., and Parker, R. C., 1966, Cultivation of mammalian cells in defined media with protein and nonprotein supplements, *J. Cell Biol.* **30:**539–553.

Healy, G. M., Teleki, S., von Seefried, A., Walton, M. J., and Macmorine, H. G., 1971, Improved chemically defined basal medium (CMRL-1969) for primary monkey kidney and human diploid cells, *Appl. Microbiol.* **21:**1–5.

Herrick, P. R., Baumann, G. W., Merchant, D. J., Shearer, M. C., Shipman, C., Jr., and Brackett, R. G., 1970, Serologic and karyologic evidence of incorrect identity of an animal cell line (guinea pig spleen), *In Vitro* **6:**143–147.

Himmelfarb, P., Thayer, P. S., and Martin, H. E., 1969, Spin filter culture: The propagation of mammalian cells in suspension, *Science* **164:**555–557.

Holmes, R., 1967, Preparation from human serum of an alpha-one protein which induces the immediate growth of unadapted cells *in vitro*, *J. Cell Biol.* **32:**297–308.

Houba, V., 1967, The use of pronase for dispersing cells, *Experientia* **23:**572.

Hsu, T. C., 1961, Chromosomal evolution in cell populations, *Int. Rev. Cytol.* **12:**69–161.

Hsu, T. C., 1972, *Mammalian Chromosome Newsletter*, Vol. 13, No. 1, January 1972, arranged by the Section of Cell Biology, The University of Texas M. D. Anderson Hospital and Tumor Institute at Houston.

Hsu, T. C., 1974, Longitudinal differentiation of chromosomes, *Ann. Rev. Genet.*, **7:**153–176.

Ioachim, H. L., 1970, Tissue culture of human tumors, in: *Pathology Annual 1970* (S. C. Sommers, series ed.), pp. 217–256, Appleton-Century-Crofts, New York.

Jensen, E. V., Block, G. E., Smith, S., Kyser, K., and DeSombre, E. R., 1970, Estrogen receptors and breast cancer response to adrenalectomy, in: Prediction of Response in Cancer Therapy, *Natl. Cancer Inst. Monogr.*, Vol. 34.

Jensen, F. C., Gwatkin, R. B. L., and Biggers, J. D., 1964, A simple organ culture method which allows simultaneous isolation of specific types of cells, *Exp. Cell Res.* **34:**440–447.

Kalus, M., Ghidoni, J. J., and O'Neal, R. M., 1968, The growth of tumors in matrix cultures, *Cancer* **22:**507–516.

Katsuta, H., 1968, *Cancer Cells in Culture* (H. Katsuta, ed.), University Park Press, University Park, Pa.

Katsuta, H., and Takaota, T., 1961*a*, Parabiotic cell culture. II. Interaction between cell lines, *Jap. J. Exp. Med.* **31:**225–235.

Katsuta, H., and Takaota, T., 1961*b*, Parabiotic cell culture. III. Further investigation on the interaction between cell lines, *Jap. J. Exp. Med.* **31:**307–319.

Katsuta, H., and Takaota, T., 1964, Parabiotic cell culture. IV. Interaction between normal and ascites tumor cells of rats, *Jap. J. Exp. Med.* **32:**963–980.

Katsuta, H., Takaota, T., and Nagai, Y., 1968, Interaction in culture between normal and tumor cells of rats, in: *Cancer Cells in Culture* (H. Katsuta, ed.), pp. 157–168, University Park Press, University Park, Pa.

Kohler, P. O., Frohman, L. A., Bridson, W. E., Vanha-Perttula, T., and Hammond, J. M., 1969, Cortisol induction of growth hormone synthesis in a clonal line of rat pituitary tumor cells in culture, *Science* **166:**633–634.

Korsten, C. B., and Persijn, J.-P., 1972, A simple assay for specific estrogen binding capacity in human mammary tumours, *Z. Klin. Chem. Klin. Biochem.* **10:**502–508.

Koyama, H., Sinha, D., and Dao, T. L., 1972, Effects of hormones and 7,12-dimethylbenz(*a*)anthracene on rat mammary tissue grown in organ culture, *J. Natl. Cancer Inst.* **48:**1671–1680.

Kruse, P. F., Jr., Keen, L. N., and Whittle, W. L., 1970, Some distinctive characteristics of high density perfusion cultures of diverse cell types, *In Vitro* **6:**75–88.

Lasfargues, E. Y., 1957, Cultivation and behavior *in vitro* of the normal mammary epithelium of the adult mouse. II. Observations on the secretory activity, *Exp. Cell Res.* **13:**553–562.

Lasfargues, E. Y., 1962, Concerning the role of insulin in the differentiation and functional activity of mouse mammary tissues, *Exp. Cell Res.* **28:**531–542.

Lasfargues, E. Y., 1972, Collagenase as a cell dispersion agent in tissue cultures, in: *Collagenase* (I. Mandl, ed.), pp. 83–89, Gordon and Breach, New York.

Lasfargues, E. Y., and Murray, M. R., 1959, Hormonal influences on the differentiation and growth of embryonic mouse mammary glands in organ culture, *Develop. Biol.* **1:**413–435.

Lasfargues, E. Y., and Ozzello, L., 1958, Cultivation of human breast carcinomas, *J. Natl. Cancer Inst.* **21:**1131–1147.

Leibovitz, A., 1963, The growth and maintenance of tissue-cell cultures in free gas exchange with the atmosphere, *Am. J. Hyg.* **78:**173–180.

Leighton, J., 1951, A sponge matrix method for tissue culture: Formation of organized aggregates of cells *in vitro*, *J. Natl. Cancer Inst.* **12:**545–561.

Leighton, J., Kline, I., and Orr, H. C., 1956, Transformation of normal human fibroblasts into histologically malignant tissue *in vitro*, *Science* **123:**502–503.

Lépine, P., Slizewicz, P., Daniel, P., and Paccaud, M., 1956, Cultures cellulaires dans un milieu utilisant l'hydrolysat de caséine comme source d'acides aminés, *Ann. Inst. Pasteur* **90:**654.

Levan, A., and Biesele, J. J., 1958, Role of chromosomes in cancerogenesis, as studied in serial tissue culture of mammalian cells, *Ann. N.Y. Acad. Sci.* **71:**1022–1053.

Lichtiger, B., Mackay, B., and Tessmer, C. F., 1970, Spindle-cell variant of squamous carcinoma, *Cancer* **26:**1311–1320.

Ling, C. T., Gey, G. O., and Richters, V., 1968, Chemically characterized concentrated corodies for continuous cell culture (the 7C's culture media), *Exp. Cell Res.* **52:**469–489.

MacDougall, J. D. B., Biswas, S., and Cook, R. P., 1965, The effects of certain C_{27} steroids on organ cultures of rabbit aorta, *Brit. J. Exp. Pathol.* **46:**549–553.

Martorelli, B., Jr., Parshley, M. S., and Moore, J. G., 1969, Effects of chemotherapeutic agents on two lines of human breast carcinomas in tissue culture, *Surg. Gynecol. Obstet.*, pp. 1001–1006.

Masurovsky, E. B., and Peterson, E. R., 1973, Photo-reconstituted collagen gel for tissue culture substrates, *Exp. Cell Res.* **76:**447–448.

McLimans, W. F., 1969, Physiology of the cultured mammalian cell, in: *Anemic Mammalian Cell Reactions* (G. L. Tritsch, ed.), pp. 307–367, Marcel Dekker, New York.

McLimans, W. F., 1972, The gaseous environment of the mammalian cell in culture, in: *Growth, Nutrition, and Metabolism of Cells in Culture* (G. H. Rothblat and V. J. Cristofalo, ed.), pp. 137–170, Academic Press, New York.

McLimans, W. F., Blumenson, L. E., and Tunnah, K. V., 1968*a*, Kinetics of gas diffusion in mammalian cell culture systems. II. Theory, *Biotechnol. Bioeng.* **10:**741–763.

McLimans, W. F., Crouse, E. J., Tunnah, K. V., and Moore, G. E., 1968*b*, Kinetics of gas diffusion in mammalian cell culture systems. I. Experimental, *Biotechnol. Bioeng.* **10:**725–740.

Miller, R. G., and Phillips, R. A., 1969, Separation of cells by velocity sedimentation, *J. Cell Physiol.* **73:**191–202.

Molander, C. W., Kniazeff, A. J., Boone, C. W., Paley, A., and Imagawa, D. T., 1971, Isolation and characterization of viruses from fetal calf serum, *In Vitro* **7:**168–173.

Moore, G. E., Mount, D., Tara, G., and Schwartz, N., 1963, Growth of human tumor cells in suspension cultures, *Cancer Res.* **23:**1735–1741.

Morgan, J. F., Campbell, M. E., and Morton, H. J., 1955, The nutrition of animal tissues cultivated in vitro. I. A survey of natural materials as supplements to synthetic medium 199, *J. Natl. Cancer Inst.* **16:**557–567.

Morgan, J. F., Eng, C. P., Heuchert, M. D., and Kirk, H. D., 1970, Loss of transplantability and induction of immunoprotection by mouse ascites tumor cells in tissue culture, *Proc. Soc. Exp. Biol. Med.* **134:**305–308.

Morgan, J. F., Morton, H. J., and Parker, R. C., 1950, Nutrition of animal cells in tissue culture. I. Initial studies on a synthetic medium, *Proc. Soc. Exper. Biol. Med.* **73:**1–8.

Morrison, J. H., 1967, Separation of lymphocytes of rat bone marrow by combined glass-wool filtration and dextran-gradient centrifugation, *Brit. J. Haematol.* **13:**229–235.

Oettgen, H. F., Aoki, T., Old, L. J., Boyse, E. A., DeHarven, E., and Mills, G. M., 1968, Suspension culture of a pigment-producing cell line derived from a human malignant melanoma, *J. Natl. Cancer Inst.* **41:**827–843.

Osgood, E. E., and Krippaehne, M. L., 1955, The gradient tissue method, *Exp. Cell Res.* **9:**116–127.

Pace, D. M., Landolt, P. A., and Aftonomos, B. T., 1969, Effects of ozone on cells *in vitro, Arch. Environ. Health* **18:**165–170.

Parshley, M. S., and Simms, H. S., 1950, Cultivation of adult skin epithelial cells (chicken and human) *in vitro, Am. J. Anat.* **86:**163–189.

Patuleia, M. C., and Friend, C., 1967, Tissue culture studies on murine virus–induced leukemia cells: Isolation of single cells in agar–liquid medium, *Cancer Res.* **27:**726–730.

Phillips, H. J., 1972, Dissociation of single cells from lung or kidney tissue with elastase, *In Vitro* **8:**101–105.

Plata, E. J., Aoki, T., Robertson, D. D., Chu, E. W., and Gerwin, B. I., 1973, An established cultured cell line HBT-39 from human breast carcinoma, *J. Natl. Cancer Inst.* **50:**849–862.

Price, F. M., Gantt, R. R., and Evans, V. J., 1971, Effect of fractions of horse and fetal bovine serum on neoplastic conversion of C3H mouse cells in tissue culture, *In Vitro* **6:**437–440.

Puck, T. T., and Marcus, P. I., 1955, A rapid method for viable cell titration and clone production with HeLa cells in tissue culture: The use of X-irradiated cells to supply the conditioning factors, *Proc. Natl. Acad. Sci.* **41:**432.

Rabinowitz, Y., 1965, Adherence and separation of leukemic cells on glass bead columns, *Blood* **26:**100–103.

Radlett, P. J., Telling, R. C., Whitside, J. P., and Maskell, M. A., 1972, The supply of oxygen to submerged cultures of BHK 21 cells, *Biotechnol. Bioeng.* **14:**437–445.

Rappaport, C., and Bishop, C. B., 1960, Improved method for treating glass to produce surfaces suitable for the growth of certain mammalian cells in synthetic medium, *Exp. Cell. Res.* **20:**580–584.

Reed, M. V., and Gey, G. O., 1962, Cultivation of normal and malignant human lung tissue. I. The establishment of three adenocarcinoma cell strains, *Lab. Invest.* **11:**638–653.

Richter, A., Sanford, K. K., and Evans, V. J., 1972, Influence of oxygen and culture media on plating efficiency of some mammalian tissue cells, *J. Natl. Cancer Inst.* **49:**1705–1712.

Rivera, E. M., 1964*a*, Differential responsiveness to hormones of C3H and A mouse mammary tissues in organ culture, *Endocrinology* **74:**853–864.

Rivera, E. M., 1964*b*, Maintenance and development of whole mammary glands of mice in organ culture, *J. Endocrinol.* **30:**33–39.

Rose, G. G., Kumegawa, M., Nikai, H., Bracho, M., and Cattoni, M., 1970, The dual-rotary circumfusion system for mark II culture chambers, *Microvasc. Res.* **2:**24–60.

Ross, J. D., Treadwell, P. E., and Syverton, J. T., 1962, Cultural characterization of animal cells, *Ann. Rev. Microbiol.* **16:**141–188.

Rothblat, G. H., and Cristofalo, V. J., (eds.), 1972, *Growth, Nutrition, and Metabolism of Cells in Culture,* Academic Press, New York.

Ryan, G. B., Grobéty, J., and Majno, G., 1973, Mesothelial injury and recovery, *Am. J. Pathol.* **71:**93–112.

Sandstrom, B., 1966, Studies on cultivated liver cells: Some approaches to the study of the liver cell with the aid of tissue culture, in: *Abstracts of Uppsala Dissertations in Medicine,* Vol. 29, Almqvist and Wiksell, Stockholm.

Sanford, K. K., 1967, "Spontaneous" neoplastic transformation of cells *In vitro*: Some facts and theories, in: Decennial Review Conference on Cell, Tissue and Organ Culture, 1966, *Natl. Cancer Inst. Monogr.* **26:**387–418.

Sandford, K. K., Dupree, L. T., and Covalesky, A. B., 1963, Biotin, B_{12} and other vitamin requirements of a strain of mammalian cells grown in chemically defined medium, *Exp. Cell Res.* **31:**345–375.

Sanford, K. K., Burris, J. F., and Handleman, S. R., 1972*a*, Chemical analyses of sera influencing neoplastic transformation *in vitro, J. Natl. Cancer Inst.* **49:**1553–1561.

Sanford, K. K., Jackson, J. L., Parshad, R., and Gantt, R. R., 1972*b*, Evidence for an inhibiting influence of fetal bovine serum on "spontaneous" neoplastic transformation *in vitro, J. Natl. Cancer Inst.* **49:**513–518.

Schindler, R., 1964, Quantitative colonial growth of mammalian cells in fibrin gels, *Exp. Cell Res.* **34:**595–598.

Schnedl, W., 1971*a*, Analysis of the human karyotype using a reassociation technique, *Chromosoma* **34:**448–454.

Schnedl, W., 1971*b*, Banding pattern of human chromosomes, *Nature New Biol.* **233:**93–94.

Seman, G., Myers, B., Williams, W. C., Gallager, H. S., and Dmochowski, L., 1969, Studies on the relationship of viruses to the origin of human breast cancer. II. Viruslike particles in human breast tumors, *Tex. Rep. Biol. Med.* **27:**839–866.

Shiraishi, Y., and Yosida, T. H., 1972, Banding pattern analysis of human chromosomes by use of a urea treatment technique, *Chromosoma* **37:**75–83.

Simpson, W. F., and Stulberg, C. S., 1963, Species identification of animal cell strains by immunofluorescence, *Nature (Lond.)* **199:**616–617.

Smith, J. A., and King, R. J. B., 1972, Effects of steroids on growth of an androgen-dependant mouse mammary carcinoma in cell culture, *Exp. Cell Res.* **73:**351–359.

Stier, H. A., and Halasz, N. A., 1966, Organ culture and tumor culture in hyperbaric oxygen, *Am. J. Med. Sci.* **252:**391–393.

Stoebner, P., Miech, G., Sengel, A., and Witz, J. P., 1970, Notions d'ultrastructure pleurale. I. L'hyperplasie mésothéliale. II. Les mésothéliomes, *Presse Med.* **78:**1179–1184, 1403–1408.

Sullivan, J. C., and Schafer, I. A., 1966, Survival of pronase-treated cells in tissue culture, *Exp. Cell Res.* **43:**676.

Sumner, A. T., Evans, H. J., and Buckland, R. A., 1971, New technique for distinguishing between human chromosomes, *Nature New Biol.* **232:**31–32.

Sutton, J. S., 1967, Ultrastructural aspects of *in vitro* development of monocytes into macrophages, epithelioid cells, and multinucleated giant cells, in: Decennial Review Conference on Cell, Tissue and Organ Culture, 1966, *Natl. Cancer Inst. Monogr.* **26:**71–141.

Sykes, J. A., Grey, C. E., Scanlon, M., Young, L., and Dmochowski, L., 1964, Density gradient centrifugation studies of the Bittner virus, *Tex. Rep. Biol. Med.* **22:**609–627.

Sykes, J. A., Recher, L., Jernstrom, P. H., and Whitescarver, J., 1968, Morphological investigation of human breast cancer, *J. Natl. Cancer Inst.* **40:**195–223.

Sykes, J. A., Whitescarver, J., Briggs, L., and Anson, J. H., 1970, Separation of tumor cells from fibroblasts with use of discontinuous density gradients, *J. Natl. Cancer Inst.* **44:**855–864.

Taylor, W. G., Dworkin, R. A., Pumper, R. W., and Evans, V. J., 1972, Biological efficacy of several commercially available peptones for mammalian cells in culture, *Exp. Cell Res.* **74:**275–279.

Trempe, G., and Fogh, J., 1973, Variation in characteristics of human tumor cell lines derived from similar tumors, *In Vitro* **8:**433 (abst.).

Tribble, H. R., Jr., and Higuchi, K., 1963, Studies on the nutrition and metabolism of animal cells in serum-free media. II. Cultivation of cells in suspension, *J. Infect. Dis.* **112:**221–225.

Trowell, O. A., 1954, A modified technique for organ culture *in vitro, Exp. Cell Res.* **6:**246–248.

Trowell, O. A., 1959, The culture of mature organs in a synthetic medium, *Exp. Cell Res.* **16:**118–147.

Trowell, O. A., 1966, Tissue culture in radiobiology, in: *Cells and Tissues in Culture: Methods, Biology and Physiology,* Vol. 3, (E. N. Willmer, ed.), pp. 64–149, Academic Press, New York.

Tunnah, K. V., McLimans, W. F., and Moore, G. E., 1968, Rocker cell culture incubator, *Biotechnol. Bioeng.* **10:**698–706.

Turkington, R. W., 1969, Hormonal regulation of cell proliferation in breast cancer cells *in vitro, N.Y. State J. Med.* **69:**2649–2655.

Walter, H., Krob, E. J., and Ascher, G. S., 1969, Separation of lymphocytes and polymorphonuclear leukocytes by countercurrent distribution in aqueous two-polymer phase systems, *Exp. Cell Res.* **55:**279–283.

Waymouth, C., 1959, Rapid proliferation of sublines of NCTC clone 929 (strain L) mouse cells in a simple chemically defined medium (MB 752/1), *J. Natl. Cancer Inst.* **22:**1003–1017.

Waymouth, C., 1965, Construction and use of synthetic media, in: *Cells and Tissues in Culture: Methods, Biology and Physiology,* Vol. 1 (E. N. Willmer, ed.), pp. 99–142, Academic Press, New York.

Waymouth, C., 1967, Somatic cells in vitro: Their relationship to progenitive cells and to artificial milieux, in: Decennial Review Conference on Cell, Tissue and Organ Culture, 1966, *Natl. Cancer Inst. Monogr.* **26:**1–21.

Waymouth, C., 1970, Osmolality of mammalian blood and of media for culture of mammalian cells, *In Vitro* **6:**109–127.

Wepsic, H. T., 1970, Separation of viable tumor cells from nonviable tumor cells by flotation on bovine serum albumin: A short communication, *J. Natl. Cancer Inst.* **45:**1031–1034.

Wessells, N. K., and Cohen, J. H., 1968, Effects of collagenase on developing epithelia *in vitro*: Lung, ureteric bud, and pancreas, *Develop. Biol.* **18:**294–309.

Willmer, E. N. (ed.), 1965, 1966, *Cells and Tissues in Culture: Methods, Biology and Physiology,* Vols. 1, 2, 3, Academic Press, New York.

Wöhler, W., Rüdiger, H. W., and Passarge, E., 1972, Large scale culturing of normal diploid cells on glass beads using a novel type of culture vessel, *Exp. Cell Res.* **74:**571–573.

Yamane, I., Matsuya, Y., and Jimbo, K., 1968, An autoclavable powdered culture medium for mammalian cells, *Proc. Soc. Exp. Biol. Med.* **127:**335–336.

Young, R., Cailleau, R., Mackay, B., and Reeves, W. J., Jr., 1974, Establishment of cell line MDA-MB-157 from a pleural effusion from a human breast carcinoma, *In Vitro* **9:**239–245.

Zucker, R. M., and Cassen, B., 1969, The separation of normal human leukocytes by density and classification by size, *Blood* **34:**591–600.

New Human Tumor Cell Lines 5

JØRGEN FOGH AND GERMAIN TREMPE

1. *Introduction*

There has been a feeling of frustration among many investigators trying to establish cell lines of human tumor cells. Numerous unsuccessful attempts, many of which have remained unpublished, have led to the conclusion that cell line establishment is controlled by the rare occurrence of a tumor with a built-in potential for long-term *in vitro* growth and by the application of intriguing culture techniques. The results given in the present chapter may, at least in part, contradict these conclusions. With techniques which in no particular way stand out as unusual, and by using medium and serum combinations, and in some cases added hormones, which are generally known to everyone involved in tissue culture, we have, during a rather short period of time, established a high number of new cell lines. These have originated from primary or metastatic human tumors, solid or effusions. In all fairness, many of our attempts to establish continuous lines have failed. However, the total number of attempts over successes is not truly representative of the frequency with which lines might be established. Many variations must be considered in this respect, including the choice of material, collection procedures, lapse of time between the clinical procedure and preparation for tissue culture, technical competence of assistants, and incidental factors known to everyone working in tissue culture. One thing, however, stands out as a conclusion: the *careful* attention to all the minute

JØRGEN FOGH AND GERMAIN TREMPE Memorial Sloan-Kettering Cancer Center, New York, N.Y.

details provided by the dedicated tissue culturist seems to be the most important of all factors and cannot well be substituted for by special recipes or fancy equipment.

This chapter presents 31 new cell lines derived from tumors of 30 patients. We shall summarize and comment briefly on the methods of collection of tumor tissue, preparation for culture, nutrition, and initial and continuous cultivation procedures which led to the establishment of these lines. In addition, some of the growth characteristics, the cell morphology, chromosome abnormalities, tumor-producing capacity, and ultrastructural aspects of the lines will be reported and compared with characteristics of previously reported cell lines. Additional characterization is desirable, in particular with methods which may serve to identify cell lines with the types of tumor of origin.

There is plenty of evidence that the same type of tumor, based on the pathologist's diagnosis, may yield established cell lines with different characteristics. This is an essential aspect of the problem of cancer. In research with such cells it poses the problem that one cell line may not give sufficient representation of a particular type of tumor. For full evaluation, many cell lines derived from tumors of similar histopathological appearance may be necessary in the various cancer research disciplines in which cultured human tumor cells are essential. We are well on the way to establishing a sizable collection of well-characterized, contamination-free human tumor cell lines representing numerous tumor types. The latter part of this chapter deals with this subject.

2. *Methods of Collection of Tumor Specimens*

2.1. *Solid Tumors or Metastases*

Substantial comparative studies on the various aspects of collection and procurement are lacking. Obviously, sterility is important, and the surgical personnel with which we work have been instructed to exercise care in this respect, as well as to avoid any contact between tumor specimen and disinfectants used in surgical procedures. Some specimens, particularly those from skin, oro- and nasopharynx, esophagus, gastrointestinal tract, and lung, as well as gynecological and genitourinary specimens, usually harbor microbial flora. If culture can be initiated within 1 h after surgery, the specimen is collected without medium in a petri dish. Prior to cultivation, medium with antibiotics is added for $\frac{1}{2}$ h. If longer periods are required, the specimen is collected in a jar of tissue culture medium with penicillin and streptomycin, and sometimes fungizone. If processing for culture is delayed beyond a few hours, the specimen is kept at 4°C; otherwise, it is kept at room temperature. We have evidence that the shortest possible time between collection and processing is advantageous for obtaining growth of tumor cells in culture.

Since first priority has to be given to the pathology diagnosis, proper amounts of the tumor must be provided for this purpose, and since many tumors removed at surgery are very small, our cultivation attempts have often been hampered by the limited size of the specimen we receive. A larger piece obviously increases the possibility of successful culture growth. Selection of the part of the surgical specimen most suitable for culture may be difficult. Chances for successful growth increase with the number of tumor cells available. We have found it extremely important to have a trained pathologist select the proper part and/or to have part of the specimen received in our laboratory processed for independent examination by the pathologist. According to the second method, after removal of bloody areas and necrotic tissue we select the portion which appears macroscopically to be tumor. When there is doubt, two or several portions are dealt with independently, in terms of both pathology and cultivation. Diagnosis is obtained from the pathologist within 48 h, and it is then decided whether to continue or discard the individual cultures. Special training of the personnel responsible for the choice of the part used for cultivation is also pertinent. Much time may be used needlessly when cultivation is initiated from a nonmalignant portion, and, even worse, long-term cultures under such conditions may incorrectly be assumed to consist of, and be used in research as, tumor cells. Absolute certainty in this respect is obtained only when microscopic observations by the pathologist confirm that the actual specimen used for culture consists mainly of tumor cells.

Further studies are necessary to evaluate, under strictly controlled conditions, variables in the individual steps of collection of tumor material, including containers, instruments, solutions, selection and separation of specimens, temperature, and time between supply and culture. It is also very likely that other combinations of antibiotics are preferable to those we have used in the past. The studies should include a sufficient number of samples of individual types of tumors to provide significant information on this important aspect of human tumor cell culture work.

2.2. *Effusions*

For collection of malignant effusions, special containers with attached tubing are available. The presterilized, closed needle-valve–syringe–tubing–bottle system brings the fluid directly from the pleura or abdominal cavity to the receiving bottle. From the tissue culture laboratory, the cytology department is immediately provided with a sample of that effusion for confirmation of diagnosis.

2.3. *Normal Tissue*

Whenever possible, specimens of skin are collected from the surgical incision at the time of surgery. Methods of collection are similar to those for tumor tissue.

3. *Methods of Preparation and Initial Culture*

The following methods were those that resulted in cultures from which established lines, in many cases, were derived.

3.1. *Solid Tumors*

Under sterile conditions, the tumor specimen, after removal of fat and necrotic parts, was washed in medium and minced into pieces of approximately 1 mm^3 size. After several additional washings with medium, the specimen was treated as follows: (1) Part of it was treated with trypsin, 0.25% at 37°C, until a sufficient number of cells was suspended. These were seeded in culture containers, usually at a concentration of $3–5 \times 10^5$ cells/ml in the medium–serum combination of choice (Tryps, Table 1). (2) Other tumor pieces were placed on the glass surface of culture containers in various numbers for initiation of fragment cultures (Fragm, Table 1). (3) Cells spilled in the medium while the fragments were being cut were collected, centrifuged, and seeded separately (Spill, Table 1). Certain fragment cultures were grown (4) in plasma clot (Clot, Table 1) or (5) on collagen (Coll, Table 1). Occasionally, cultures were initiated by planting fragments or by inoculating trypsinized cell suspension (6) onto established monolayers of primary human amnion cells (Amn, Table 1).

3.2. *Effusions*

Pleural or ascitic fluids were centrifuged at 125 *g* for 10 min in order to recover the tumor cells. When the fluids were more than lightly hemorrhagic, erythrocytes were separated and removed, either by slow-speed centrifugation or by the following technique: The pellet resulting from centrifugation was resuspended in 9 vol. of sterile distilled water for 60 s with constant stirring. One volume of 10× concentrated phosphate-buffered saline was added. This suspension was immediately centrifuged at 125 *g* for 10 min. After the fluid had been decanted, the cells in the pellet were seeded in one of the medium–serum combinations of choice, usually at concentrations of 5×10^5 to 1×10^6 cells/ml.

3.3. *Normal Tissue*

Cultures of skin cells were initiated as fragment cultures, usually in McCoy's medium 5A (McCoy *et al.*, 1959) with 15% fetal bovine serum.

3.4. *Nutrition*

As shown in Tables 1 and 2, different media were used during initial culture, as well as later for the various established cell lines. These included 512 (Fogh *et al.*, 1969); McCoy's; Waymouth's (Waymouth, 1959); Eagle's MEM (Eagle, 1959); L-15 (Leibovitz, 1963); RPMI-1640 (Moore *et al.*, 1967); PAP (Leibovitz, Chapter 2); and LY (Fogh and Lund, 1957). Fetal calf serum (Microbiological Associates or Difco) was filtered through Millipore filters in our laboratory by the method previously described (Fogh and Fogh, 1969). Human serum was freshly collected, processed, and filtered in our laboratory. All sera were stored for 2 wk at 4°C prior to use. A mixture of insulin, hydrocortisone, and prolactin, each at a concentration of 5μg/ml, was added to some of the initial cultures. All cultures were grown in T-flasks. Penicillin, 100 units/ml, and streptomycin, 100 μg/ml, were added to all media.

4. *Thirty-One New Cell Lines*

4.1. *General Characteristics*

The cell line designation, tumor or metastasis of origin, preparation and initial culture technique, period of time between initial cultivation and indication of establishment, cell morphology, medium and serum used for

TABLE 1

General Characteristics of Established Human Cell Lines Derived from Solid Tumors[a]

Cell line	Tumor	I/M	Sex	Age	Race	Blood type	Culture Technique	Initial medium[b]	Time of establishment (wk)	Cell morphology[c]	Continuous cult medium[b]	Highest present passage
HT-3	Carcinoma, uterine cervix	M to lymph node	F	58	C	A+	Fragm	(a)	8	E	(b)	145
HT-29	Adenocarcinoma, colon	I	F	44	C	A+	Fragm	(a)	8	E	(b)	130
Caki-1	Adenocarcinoma, kidney	M to skin	M	49	C	O–	Spill	(b)	1	E	(b)	18
Caki-2	Adenocarcinoma, kidney	I	M	69	C	A–	Spill	(b)	8	E	(b)	28
Calu-1	Carcinoma, lung	M to pleura	M	47	C	A+	Tryps	(b)	8	E	(b)	38
Casa-1	Carcinoma, mucoepidermoid of submaxillary gland	M to lung	M	61	C	O+	Spill/Amn	(c)	8	E	(b)	9
Caov-1	Papillary serous cystadenocarcinoma, ovary	M to omentum	F	47	C	O+	Fragm/Tryps	(b,i)	4	E	(b)	4
SK-LMS-1	Leiomyosarcoma, vulva	I	F	43	C	O+	Tryps	(f)	2	F	(e)	32
Saos-1	Sarcoma, chondro/osteogenic	M to chest wall	F	17	C	A+	Fragm/Tryps	(b)	5	F	(b)	12
SK-OS-10	Sarcoma, osteogenic	M to lung	M	13	C	A+	Tryps	(f)	6	F	(e)	15
Saos-2	Sarcoma, osteogenic	I	F	11	C	B+	Fragm/Spill/Tryps	(b,e,i,l)	4	E	(b)	22
Safi-1	Fibrosarcoma, recurrent	I	M	68	C	O+	Fragm/Tryps	(e,i,k)	4	F	(b)	9

Ast-1	Astrocytoma	I	F	62	N	O+	Fragm/ Spill/ Tryps	(b)	2	S	(b)	12
Ins-1	Adenoma, islet cell, pancreas	I	M	50	C	O+	Fragm/ Clot	(g)	8	E	(h)	39
HT-144	Melanoma	M to subcutaneous tissue	M	29	C	O+	Fragm	(a)	6	E	(b)	77
SK-MEL-2	Melanoma	M to skin	M	60	C	A+	Spill	(d)	20	E	(e)	28
SK-MEL-3	Melanoma	M to lymph node	F	42	C	O+	Tryps	(b)	32	F	(d)	20
Malme-3M	Melanoma	M to lung	M	43	C	AB+	Fragm/ Spill/ Tryps	(b,i)	1	E	(i)	24
Malme-3S	Melanoma	M to lung	M	43	C	AB+	Fragm/ Spill/ Tryps	(b,i)	1	S	(j)	7
SK-UT-1	Mesodermal mixed tumor, uterus	I	F	75	C	B+	Tryps	(f)	2	E	(e)	24
Tera-1	Teratoma, malignant	M to lung	M	47	C	B−	Fragm/ Tryps Coll	(b)	27	E	(b)	38
Tera-2	Teratoma, malignant	M to lung	M	22	C	A+	Fragm/ Tryps Coll	(b)	8	E	(b)	38

[a] Abbreviations: I, primary tumor; M, metastasis; Fragm, fragment culture; Spill, spilled cells technique; Tryps, trypsinization; Amn, seeded on culture of primary amnion cells; Clot, plasma clot; Coll, collagen substrate.

[b] Media: (a) 512, 15% fetal calf serum; (b) McCoy's 5a, 15% fetal calf serum; (c) Waymouth's, 15% fetal calf serum; (d) Eagle's MEM, 10% fetal calf serum; (e) Eagle's MEM, 15% fetal calf serum; (f) Eagle's MEM, 20% fetal calf serum; (g) LY, 40% human serum; (h) LY, 20% human serum; (i) L-15, 15% fetal calf serum; (j) RPMI-1640, 15% fetal calf serum; (k) McCoy's, 20% fetal calf serum; (l) PAP, 15% fetal calf serum.

[c] Cell morphology: E, epithelial-like; F, fibroblast-like; S, stellate.

TABLE 2

General Characteristics of Established Human Cell Lines Derived from Malignant Effusions

Cell line	Tumor	Effusion	Sex	Age	Race	Blood type	Initial medium[a]	Time of establishment (wk)	Cell morphology[b]	Continuous culture medium[a]	Highest present passage
SK-BR-3	Adenocarcinoma of breast	Pleural	F	43	C	A+	(d)	8	E	(e)	36
SK-CO-1	Adenocarcinoma of colon	Ascitic	M	65	C	O+	(m)	6	E	(e)	28
SK-NEP-1	Nephroblastoma	Pleural	F	25	C	A+	(m)	6	Sph	(b)	24
SK-HEP-1	Adenocarcinoma of liver	Ascitic	M	52	C	—	(m)	1	E	(e)	20
SK-MES-1	Carcinoma, squamous, lung	Pleural	M	65	C	O+	(m)	4	E	(d)	24
SK-OV-1	Adenocarcinoma, primary site unknown, clinically either breast or ovary	Pleural	F	65	C	O+	(m)	22	E	(m)	30
SK-OV-3	Adenocarcinoma of ovary	Ascitic	F	64	C	B+	(m)	23	E	(d)	19
SK-SC-1	Melanoma (presumably)	Pleural	M	74	C	—	(m)	6	E	(e)	26
SK-HD-1	Hodgkin's disease	Pleural	F	22	C	O+	(m)	7	St	(b)	13

[a] Media: (b) McCoy's 5a, 15% fetal calf serum; (d) Eagle's MEM, 10% fetal calf serum; (e) Eagle's MEM, 15% fetal calf serum; (m) Eagle's MEM, 10% fetal calf serum, 10% human serum, hormones.

[b] Cell morphology: E, epithelial-like; Sph, spherical (suspension culture); St, stellate.

continuous culture, and highest passage level obtained to date are shown for 22 new cell lines from solid tumors or metastases in Table 1. Similar data are shown for nine cell lines derived from cells in malignant effusions in Table 2. The patient's sex, age, race, and blood type are indicated for each case.

With the exception of the Ins-1 line, derived from an insulinoma, the origins in all cases were malignant tumors. Malme-3M and Malme-3S are established lines, of the monolayer and suspension type, respectively, derived from the same tumor. Among the solid tumors shown in Table 1, eight were primary tumors and 13 were metastases. Taking Malme-3M and Malme-3S as one case, 27% of tumors from which lines were established in this material were primary; 73% were metastases or effusions.

In most cases, several initial culture techniques were attempted. Table 1 lists the technique or techniques which resulted in cultures from which the cell lines from solid tumors or metastases were established. In the attempts with these specimens, three such cultures were initiated with fragments, three with spilled cells, and five with trypsinized cells. For the remaining tumors, the cultures which eventually resulted in lines were initiated either by a combination of methods or by pooling cultures resulting from several methods during the subsequent transfers. Tables 1 and 2 show that medium and serum combinations, with or without added hormones, used in cultures which subsequently led to established lines varied considerably. No particular pattern is indicated; the material is not extensive enough to depict significant trends.

With one exception, Saos-2, the morphology of the cultured cells (Tables 1 and 2) was that to be expected from the tumor of origin. Thus all established lines derived from carcinomas contained cells of epithelial-like morphology; the sarcoma lines contained cells of fibroblast-like morphology. Cells of the Ins-1 line are of epithelial-like morphology. The only two suspension-type lines, Malme-3M and SK-NEP-1, consist of spherical cells. Ast-1, derived from an astrocytoma, and SK-HD-1, derived from Hodgkin's disease, contain cells of stellate morphology. Photomicrographs of hematoxylin-eosin stained cells of 30 of the lines and a Nomarski micrograph of one cell line are shown in Fig. 1–31.

The "times of establishment," shown as the number of weeks after initiation of culture in Tables 1 and 2, indicate the times at which several experienced tissue culturists agreed that the cultures exhibited all the apparent "potentials" of continuous growth. No exact measurements were made at these times. The number of culture passages (last column of Tables 1 and 2) has confirmed that all (but a few) new lines were capable of cell division over long periods of time. The few lines with low passage numbers are presently being carried in the laboratory in the hope that the cells, as expected, will continue to divide in many successive passages.

4.2. *Increase in Cell Population*

In many approaches in cancer research, it is advantageous to work with a cell line capable of producing a sizable population within a limited period of time. This is not always possible. Rates of cell division among the new cell lines presented here differ greatly. This has also been the case for the many other cell lines established from human tumors by others with which we have worked. As shown in Table 3 (data established from our experience with the cells), even cell lines derived from tumors of the same tissues vary considerably in their rates of growth. The transfer factors shown are not truly comparable since the types of medium and serum in which the cell lines were cultured vary. However, for each line the supposedly best medium–serum combination in terms of rapidity of growth was chosen. Among the breast and colon carcinoma lines, the weekly transfer factor varied from 1.5 to 10; for the cervix carcinoma lines, between 4 and 20. Kidney carcinoma lines differed in weekly transfer factor between 2 and 5, lung carcinoma lines between 2 and 30, and lines derived from carcinoma of the ovary varied from 1.5 to 5. Among the many lines derived from melanomas, as well as those from osteogenic sarcomas, the weekly transfer factor varied only between 2 and 5.

For the other new lines presented here, this factor was as follows: Tera-1 (1.5); Tera-2 (2); SK-UT-1 (5.5); Casa-1 (1.1); SK-LMS-1 (3.5); Saos-2 (4); Safi-1 (2); Ast-1 (3.5); Ins-1 (20); SK-HEP-1 (4); SK-MES-1 (3); and SK-HD-1 (4). The data were obtained from cultures grown in the media listed in Tables 1 and 2 as continuous culture media.

4.3. *Chromosome Analysis*

A summary of chromosome data for the 31 new lines is shown in Table 4. The analysis, carried out by Helle Fogh, included exact determination of chromosome numbers and estimation of the frequencies of abnormalities such as dicentrics, translocational exchanges, breaks and gaps, acentric fragments, ring chromosomes, pulverization, etc., and the occurrence of marker chromosomes. There is considerable variation among all the cell lines; also among the metaphases within each line. Some of the lines have pronounced modal numbers, others not. The SK-OV-1 line, for example,

---

FIGS. 1–31. Cell lines established from human tumors. Figures 1–18 and 20–31 are fixed preparations, stained with hematoxylin and eosin. Figure 19 shows a living culture observed by interference contrast (Nomarski) microscopy. All magnifications, except Fig. 19, are ×320. Figure 19 is magnified ×800.

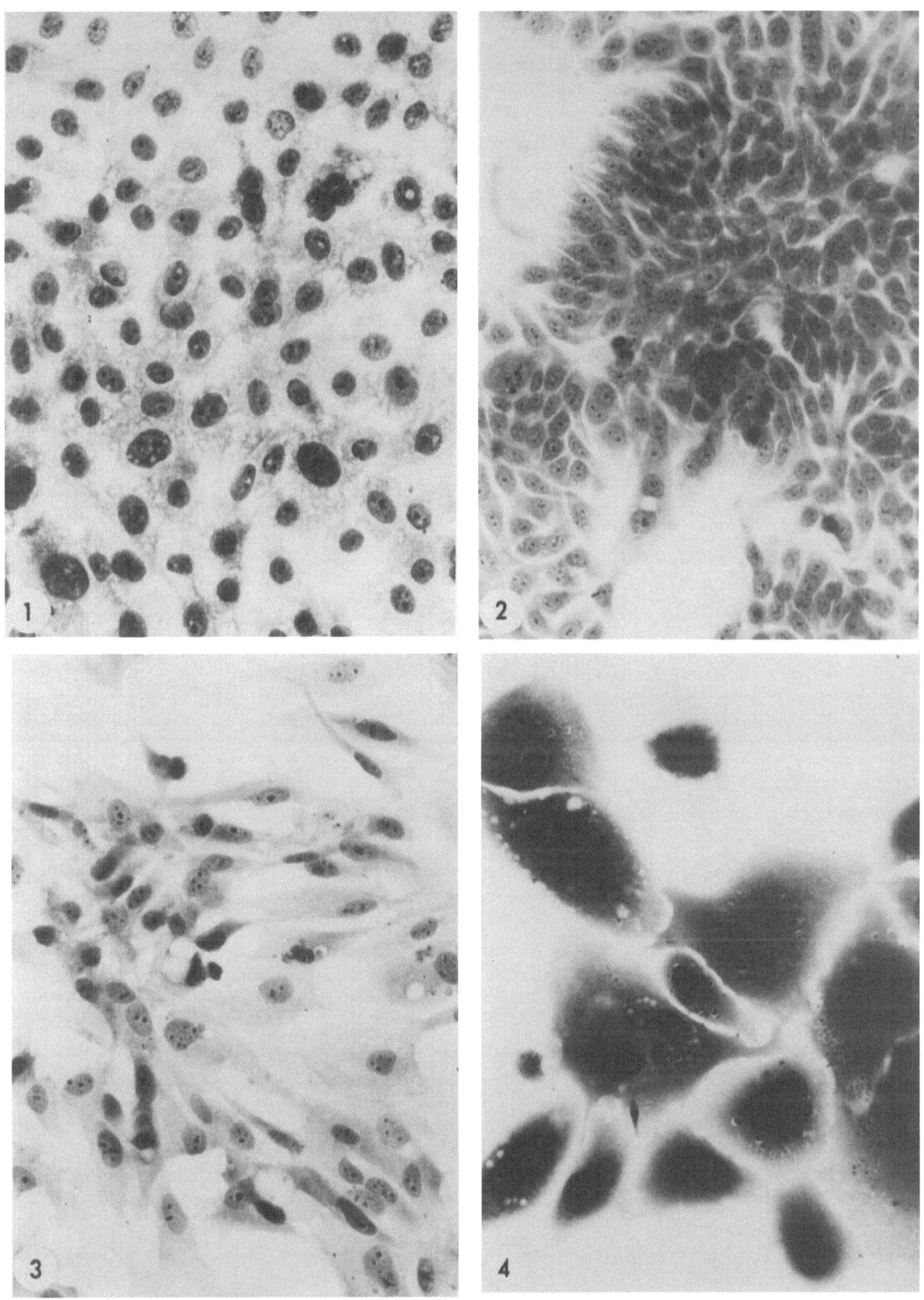

FIGS. 1–4. (1) HT-3; carcinoma, uterine cervix. (2) HT-29; adenocarcinoma, colon. (3) Caki-1; adenocarcinoma, kidney. (4) Caki-2; adenocarcinoma, kidney.

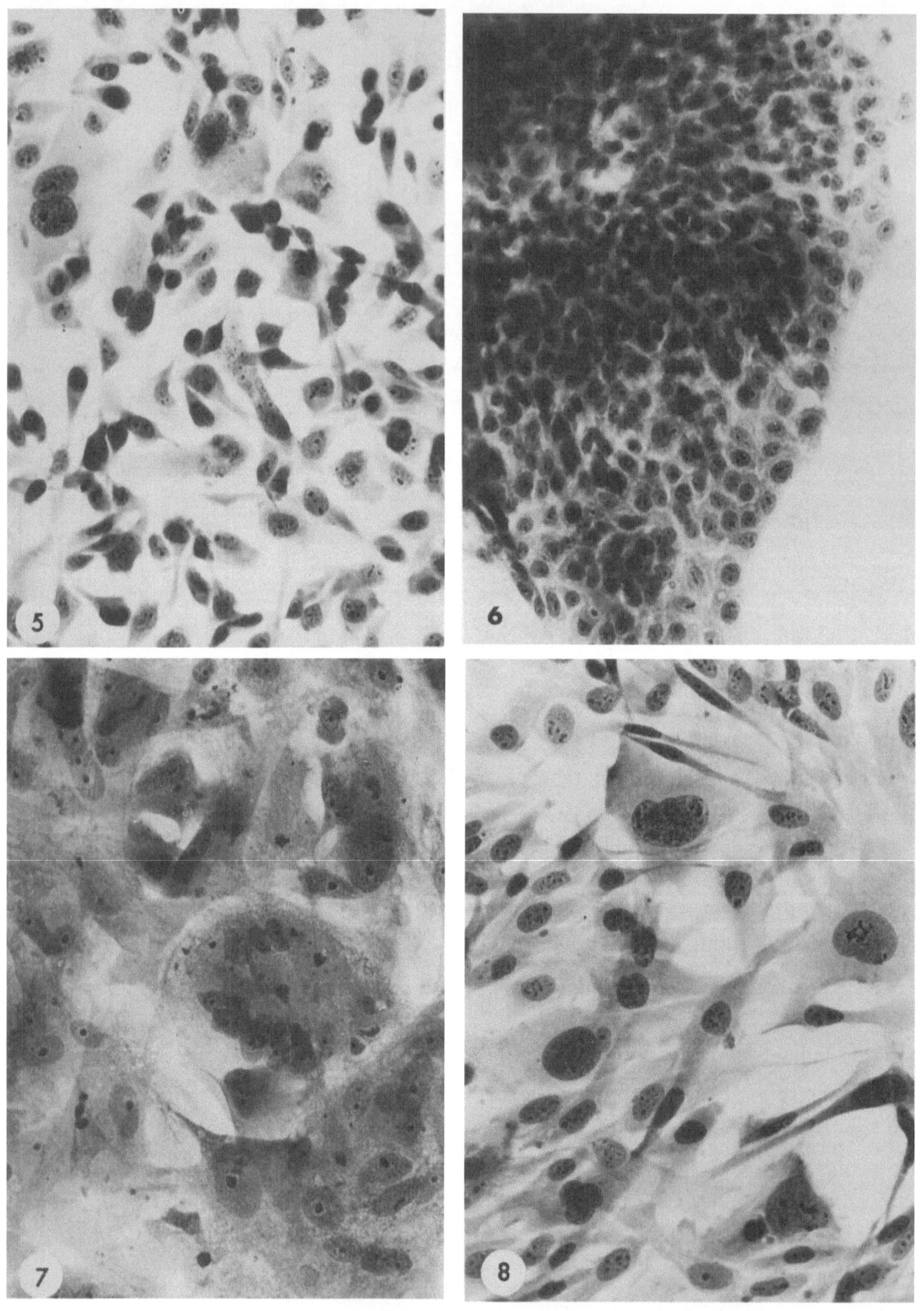

FIGS. 5–8. (5) Calu-1; carcinoma, lung. (6) Casa-1; mucoepidermoid carcinoma of submaxillary gland. (7) Caov-1; papillary serous cystadenocarcinoma, ovary. (8) SK-LMS-1; leiomyosarcoma, vulva.

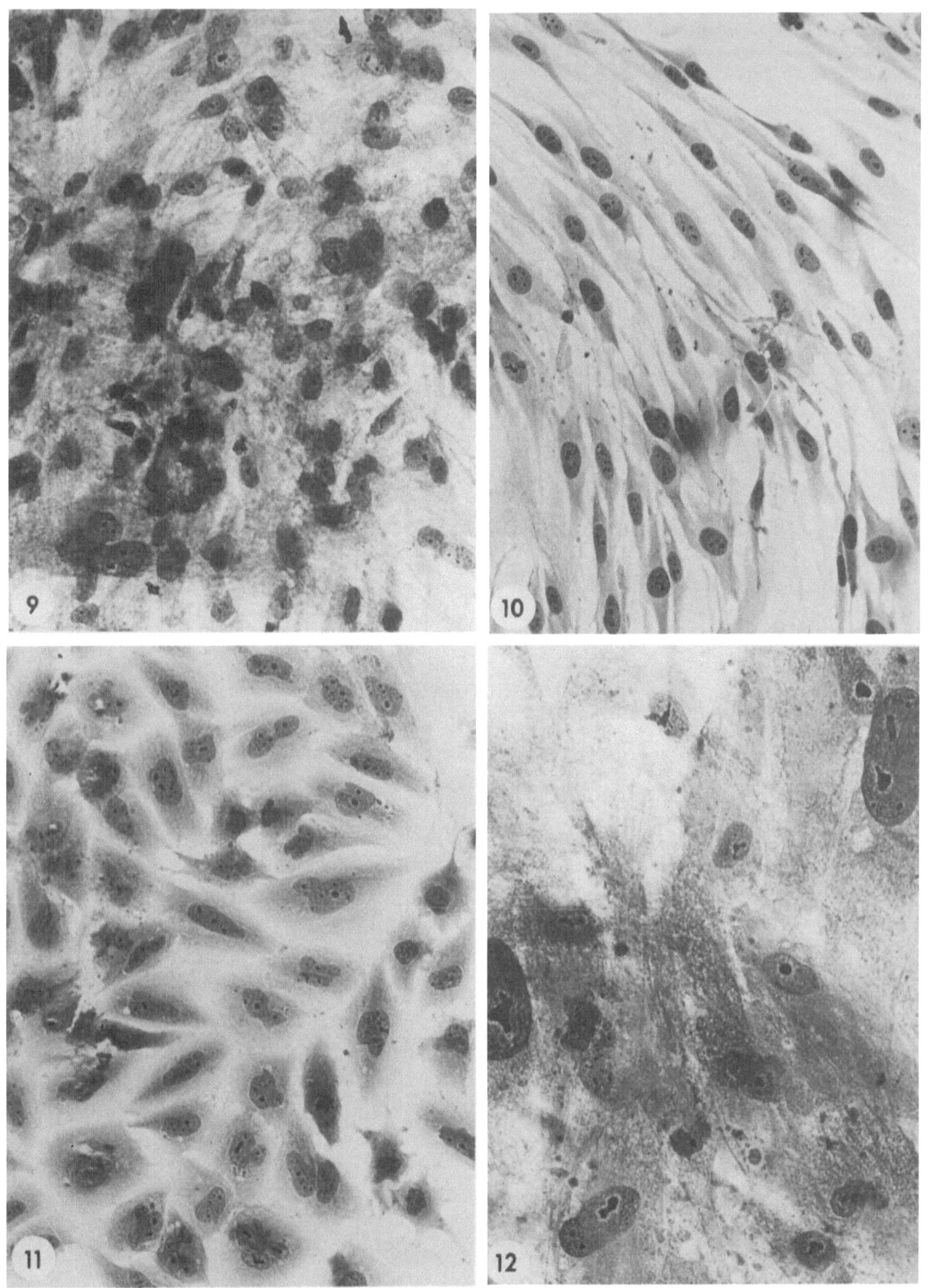

FIGS. 9–12. (9) Saos-1; sarcoma, chondro/osteogenic. (10) SK-OS-10; sarcoma, osteogenic. (11) Saos-2; sarcoma, osteogenic. (12) Safi-1; fibrosarcoma, recurrent.

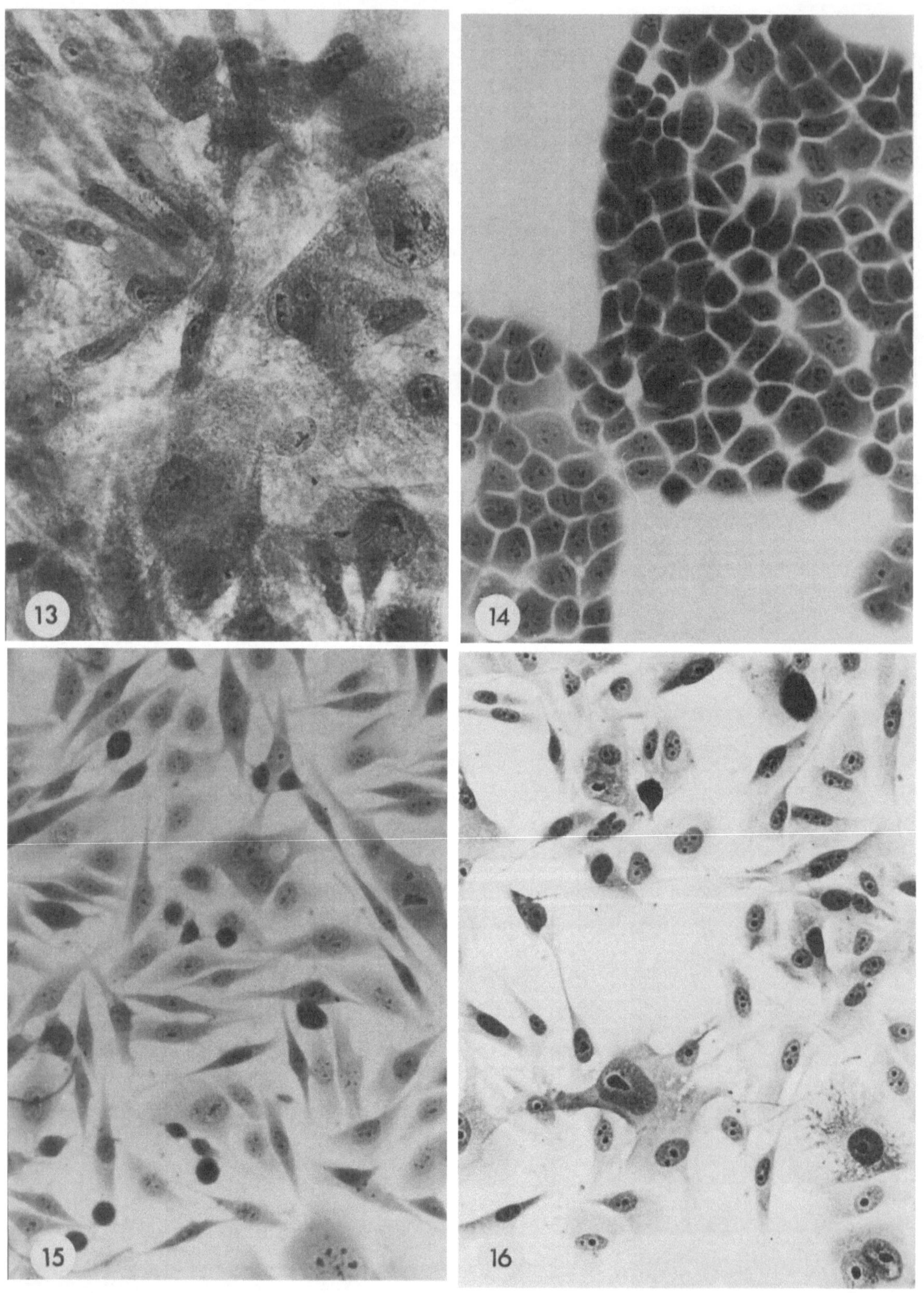

FIGS. 13–16. (13) Ast-1; astrocytoma. (14) Ins-1; adenoma, islet cell, pancreas. (15) HT-144; melanoma. (16) SK-MEL-2; melanoma.

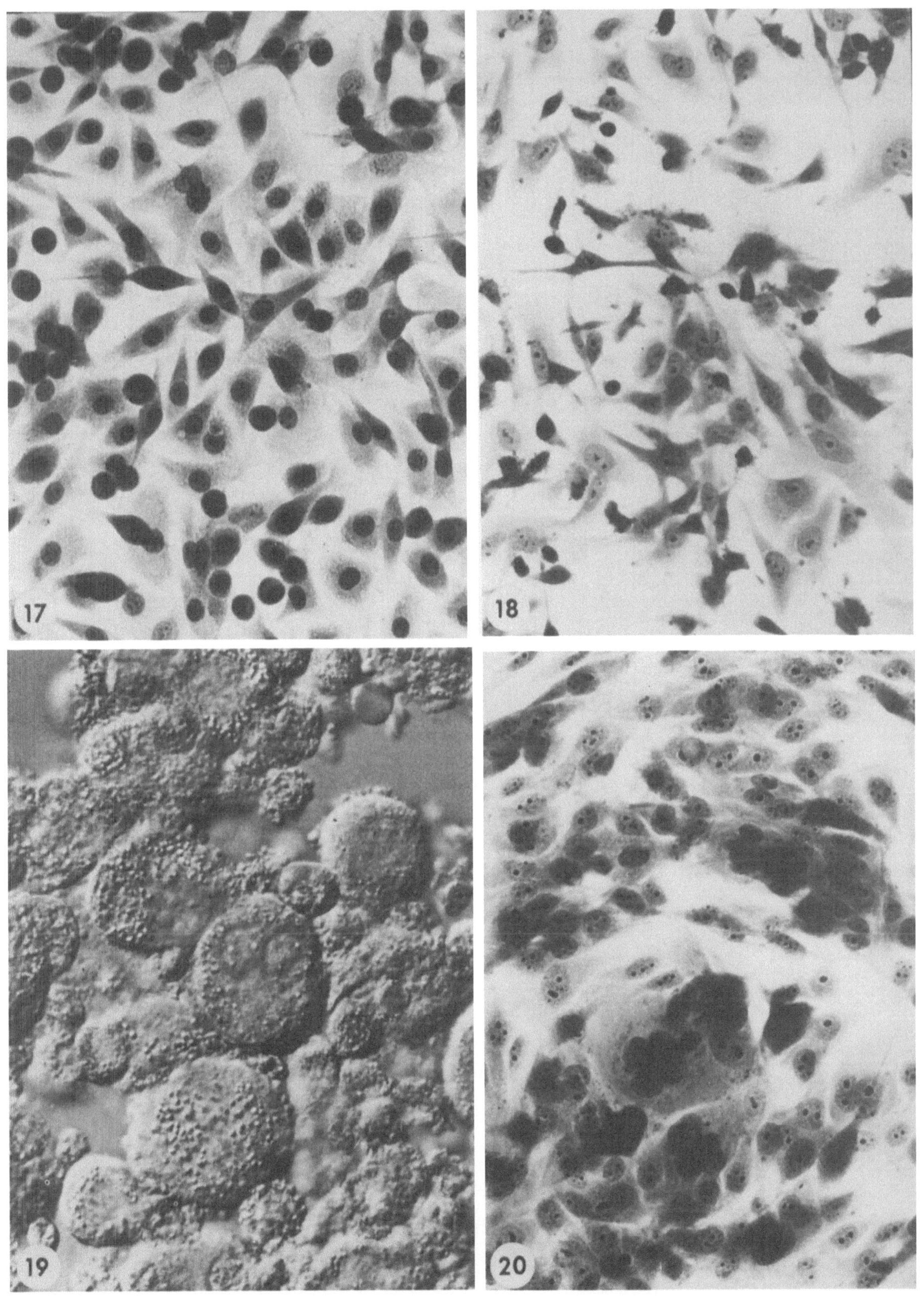

FIGS. 17–20. (17) SK-MEL-3; melanoma. (18) Malme-3M; melanoma. (19) Malme-3S; melanoma. (20) SK-UT-1; mesodermal mixed tumor, uterus.

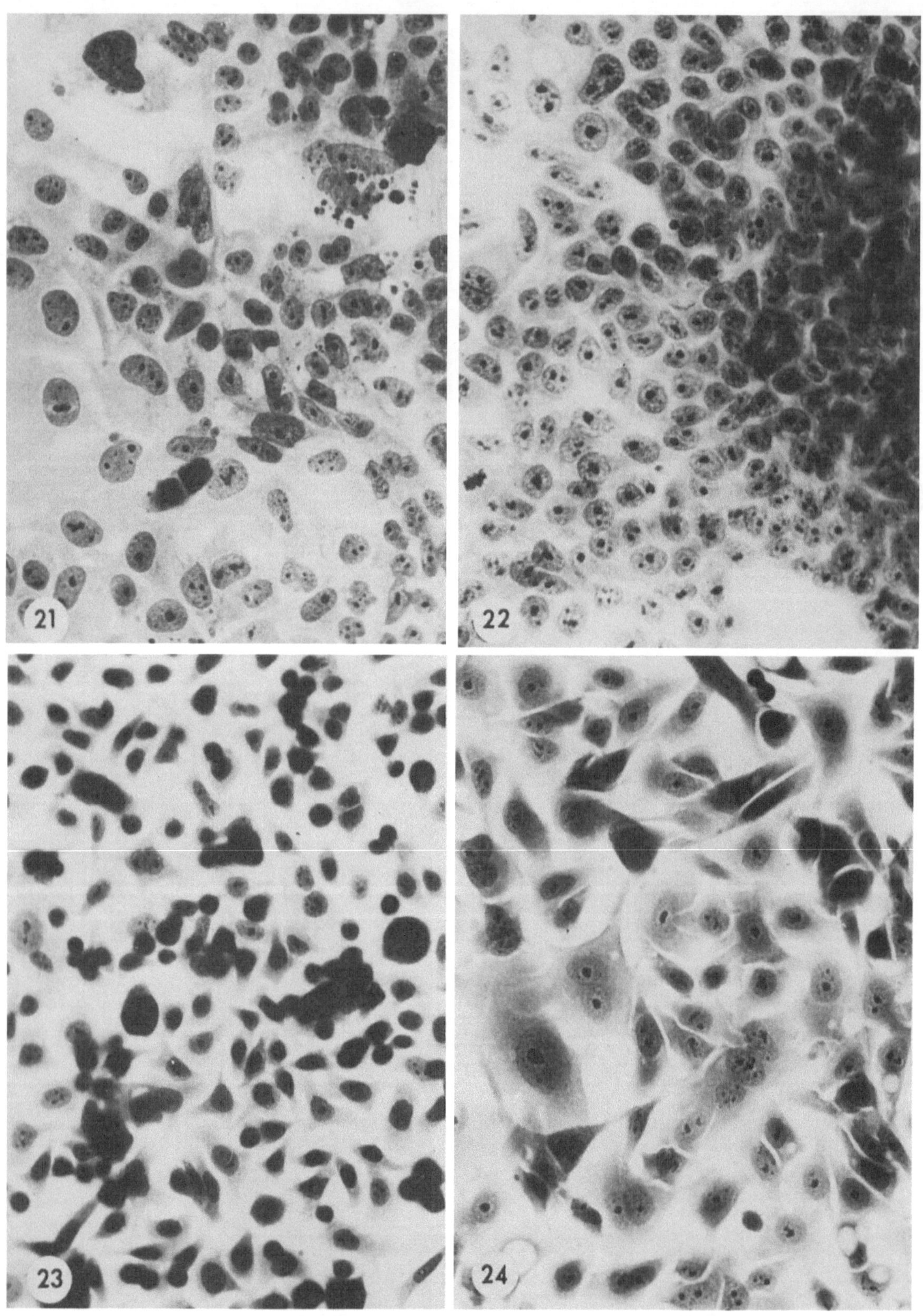

FIGS. 21–24. (21) Tera-1; teratoma, malignant. (22) Tera-2; teratoma, malignant. (23) SK-BR-3; adenocarcinoma, breast. (24) SK-CO-1; adenocarcinoma, colon.

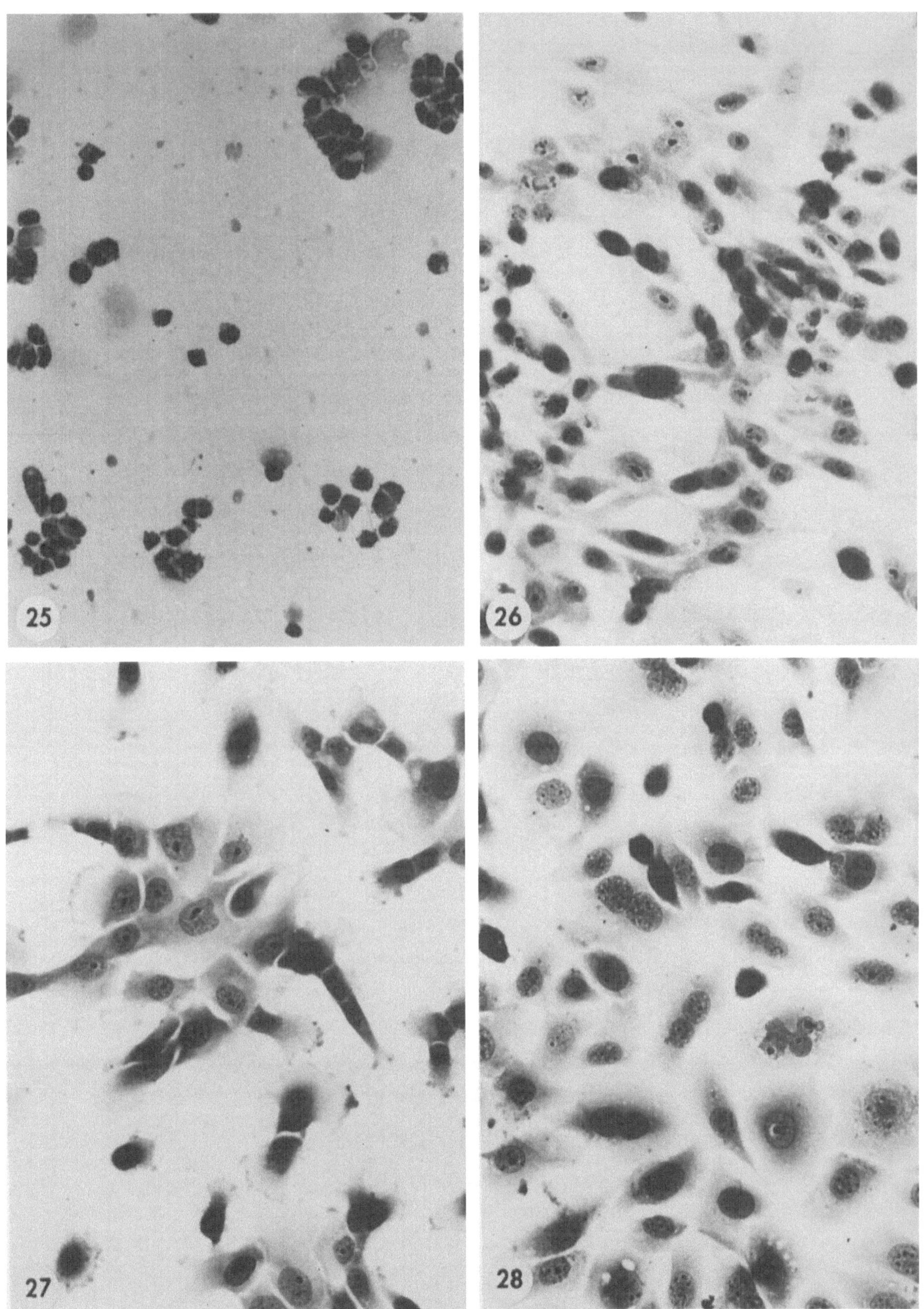

FIGS. 25–28. (25) SK-NEP-1; nephroblastoma. (26) SK-HEP-1; adenocarcinoma, liver. (27) SK-MES-1; carcinoma, squamous, lung. (28) SK-OV-1; adenocarcinoma, primary site unknown, clinically either breast or ovary.

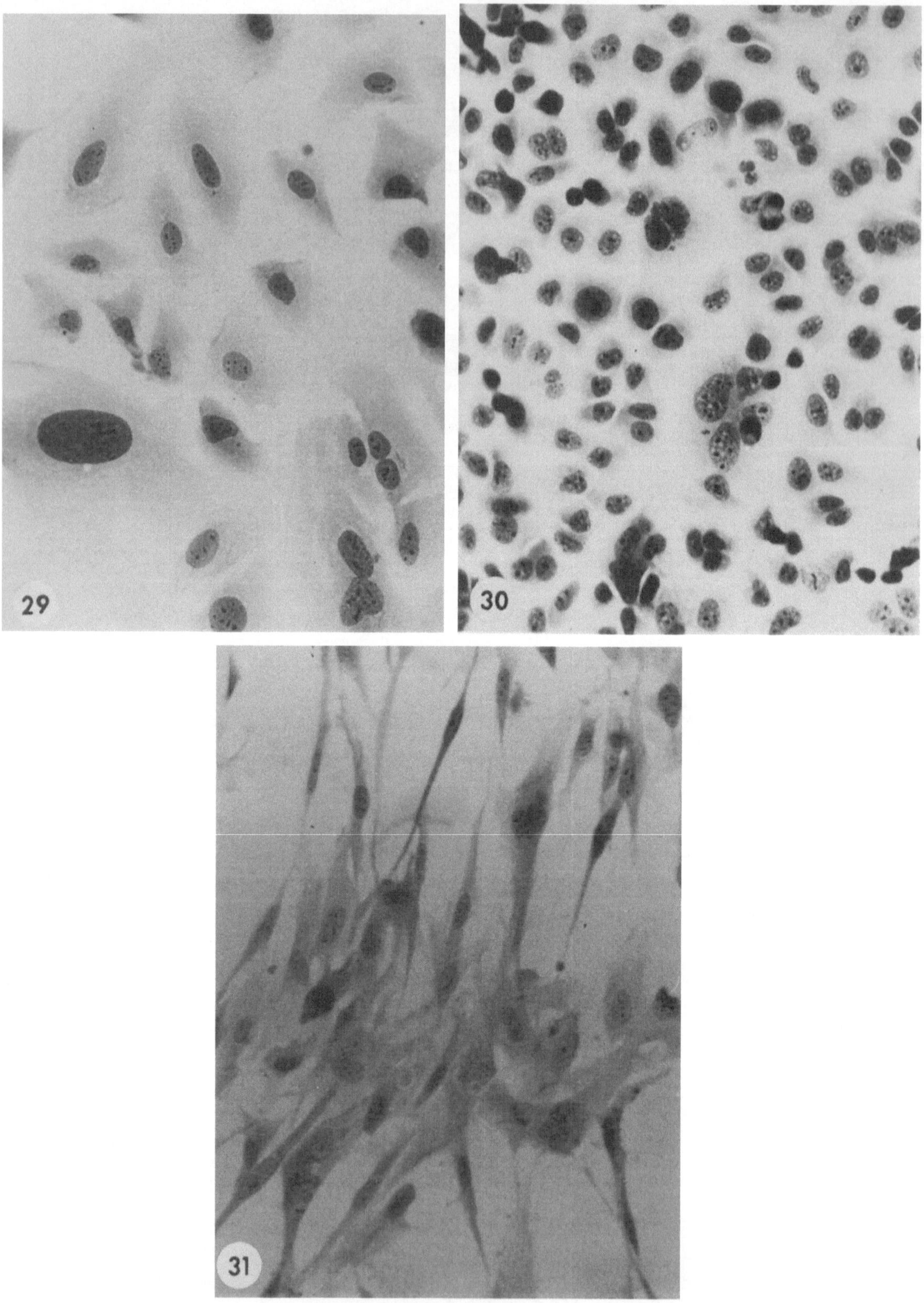

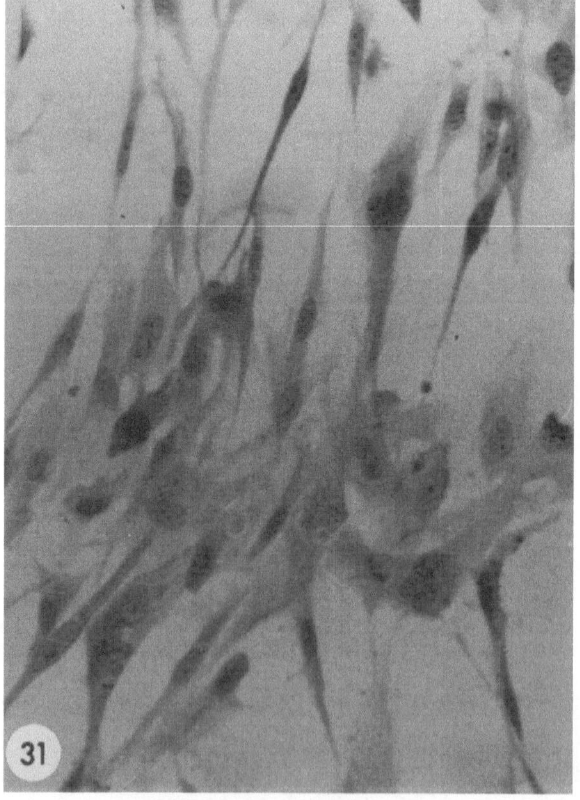

FIGS. 29–31. (29) SK-OV-3; adenocarcinoma, ovary. (30) SK-SC-1; melanoma (presumably). (31) SK-HD-1; Hodgkin's disease.

contains cells with chromosome numbers distributed over a very wide range. With one exception, abnormalities were observed in cells of all the lines; however, frequencies and degrees of abnormalities varied considerably. Marker chromosomes were characteristic of most lines. The following types of markers were seen: large metacentric or polycentric, large submetacentric, and large subtelocentric. In addition, a double ring marker chromosome was observed in the SK-OV-1 line. Two different marker chromosomes were present, at varied frequencies, in many lines. All 31 lines showed departure from diploidy either in regard to chromosome number or chromosome morphology or in terms of the number of chromosomes per classification group according to karyotypic analysis.

4.4. *Tumor Production in Nude Mice*

A number of the cell lines presented here have been tested for tumor-producing capacity in athymic (*Nu/Nu*) mice. At this time, the following lines have produced tumors: HT-3, HT-29, Caki-1, Caki-2, Calu-1, SK-LMS-1, Ins-1, SK-MEL-3, SK-UT-1, SK-CO-1, SK-HEP-1, and SK-HD-1. The tumors are presently under study to ascertain their degree of similarity to the patient's tumor of origin.

4.5. *Electron Microscopy*

Many of the present cell lines have also been examined by electron microscopy by Dr. N. H. Sarkar of this Institute. They include HT-3, HT-29, Caki-1, Caki-2, Calu-1, Casa-1, SK-LMS-1, Ins-1, HT-144, SK-UT-1, Tera-1, Tera-2, SK-BR-3, SK-CO-1, SK-NEP-1, SK-HEP-1, SK-MES-1, SK-OV-1, SK-SC-1, and SK-HD-1. In spite of extensive searching, no particles which definitely can be characterized as type B or C particles have been observed in any of these lines.

5. *Discussion*

During our work with the cell lines, those reported here as well as those established by other investigators, we have searched for similarities and differences in characteristics. Certain general similarities were to be expected since all the cultured cells were derived from tumor cells, and there

TABLE 3

Weekly Cell Population Increase for Cell Lines Derived from Human Tumors[a,b]

Weekly transfer factor	Carcinoma						Melanoma	Osteogenic sarcoma
	Breast	Cervix	Colon	Kidney	Lung	Ovary		
1.5	SK-OV-1[p] MDA-MB-134[q] MDA-MB-175[q]		SW-403[s][3]			SK-OV-3[b] Caov-1[b]		
2	Sal III[b]		SW-48[r]	Caki-2[b] SW-156[r]	SW-161[s]		SK-MEL-1[d] RPMI-7931[e] RPMI-7986[e][4] SK-MEL-2[e] SH-4[e][2] T-40[k][7]	Kooning's[e][5]
3	Lev III[j]		SK-CO-1[e]	Caki-1[b]	SK-MES-1[d] Chelo-1[b] Calu-1[b]		SK-MEL-3[b] LeCa 26-5[b] SW-489[s][3]	SK-OS-3B[e]
4	BT-20[n] AlAb[b] SK-BR-3[b] MDA-MB-157[o]	HT-3[b] ME-180[b] ŚzC[e]	HT-29[b]		SK-LU-1[b]		RPMI-4445[e][4] RPMI-7262[e][4] SK-SC-1[e] HT-144[b] RPMI-8252[e][4]	SK-OS-5[e] 393 OS (393 T)[e]

5			RPMI-4788[(e)]	SK-NEP-1[(b)] A-498[(e)]		A-549[(e)]	RPMI-7031[(e)(4)] RPMI-7041[(e)(4)] RPMI-7951[(e)(4)] RPMI-5966[(e)] RPMI-8072[(e)(4)] A 101 D[(e)(6)] A 375[(e)(6)] Malme-3M[(i)] Malme(3S[(j)]	RPMI-41[(b)] RPMI-5959[(e)(4)] Saos-1[(b)] 2 OS (2T)[(b)] MT[(b)] SK-OS-10[(e)]
10	G-11[(e)(1)] SH-3[(e)(2)]	SiHa[(f)]	CMP[(d)] SW-480[(s)(3)]		MAC-21[(e)]			
20		HeLa[(h)]						
30					9812[(e)]			

[a]Originator: (1) established by E. J. Plata, obtained from G. Cannon; (2) established by and obtained from G. Seman; (3) established by and obtained from A. Leibovitz; (4) established by and obtained from G. E. Moore; (5) established by and obtained from Y. Hirshaut; (6) established by D. Giard and obtained from W. Nelson-Rees; (7) established by and obtained from A. J. Dalton.

[b]Media: (b) McCoy's 5a, 15% fetal calf serum; (d) Eagle's MEM, 10% fetal calf serum; (e) Eagle's MEM, 15% fetal calf serum; (f) Eagle's MEM, 20% fetal calf serum; (h) LY, 20% human serum; (i) L-15, 15% fetal calf serum; (j) 1640, 15% fetal calf serum; (k) McCoy's, 20% fetal calf serum; (n) MEM, 10% fetal calf serum, insulin; (o) L-15, 20% fetal calf serum; (p) Eagle's MEM, 10% human serum, 10% fetal calf serum; (q) L-15, 10% fetal calf serum, 10% beef amniotic fluid, cortisone, insulin; (r) L-15, 10% fetal calf serum, cortisone and insulin; (s) PAP, 10% fetal calf serum.

TABLE 4

Chromosome Data for Cell Lines Derived from Human Tumors or Malignant Effusions

Cell line	Modal range	Abnormalities[a]	Markers
HT-3	Hypo- to hypertriploid	+++	Large subtelocentric;, large submetacentric
HT-29	Hypo- to hypertriploid	++	Large submetacentric, large meta- or polycentric
Caki-1	Hypertriploid	++	Large meta- or polycentric
Caki-2	Hypopenta- to hypohexaploid	++	Large subtelocentric
Calu-1	Hypotriploid	++	Large subtelocentric, large submetacentric
Casa-1	Hypo- to hyperdiploid	+	None
Caov-1	Hypo- to hyperdiploid	+	None
SK-LMS-1	Hypo- to hypertriploid	++	Large submetacentric
Saos-1	Hypo- to hypertriploid	0	None
SK-OS-10	Hypodiploid to diploid	++	None
Saos-2	Hyperdiploid to hypopentaploid	++	Minute
Safi-1	Hypo- to hyperdiploid	0	None
Ast-1	Hypo- to hyperdiploid	+	None
Ins-1	Hypo- to hypertriploid	++	Large submetacentric

HT-144	Hypo- to hypertriploid	++	Large submetacentric, large subtelocentric, minute
SK-MEL-2	Hyperdiploid to hypertetraploid	++	Large telocentric
SK-MEL-3	Hypo- to hypertetraploid	++	None
Malme-3M	Hypertriploid to hypotetraploid	+	Large submetacentric
Malme-3S	Hypertriploid to hypotetraploid	+	Large submetacentric
SK-UT-1	Hypo- to hyperdiploid	++	None
Tera-1	Hypotriploid	++	Large metacentric
Tera-2	Hypotriploid	+	None
SK-BR-3	Hypertriploid to hypotetraploid	+++	Large submetacentric
SK-CO-1	Hypertriploid to hypotetraploid	+++	Large submetacentric
SK-NEP-1	Hypo- to hypertriploid	+	Large subtelocentric
SK-HEP-1	Hyperdiploid to hypotriploid	++	Large subtelocentric, large submetacentric
SK-MES-1	Hyperdiploid to hypotriploid	++	Large submetacentric
SK-OV-1	Hypodiploid to hypertetraploid	+++	Large submetacentric, double ring
SK-OV-3	Hypodiploid to hypotetraploid	++	None
SK-SC-1	Hyperdiploid	++	Large subtelocentric
SK-HD-1	Hypo- to hyperdiploid	++	Large submetacentric

[a] 0, +, ++, +++ indicate the relative frequencies and the degree of structural changes.

were similarities. However, many different types of tumors (based on pathology) were involved in the comparison, and one could assume that the characteristics would vary among the groups of cell lines derived from different tumors. This was indeed the case. Perhaps less expected were the pronounced differences in many of the properties and characteristics observed among cell lines originating from the same type of tumor. No two established cell lines appeared to be identical on the basis of presently available characterization; with further characterization, the differences among the lines will undoubtedly increase in magnitude. Data shown in Tables 3 and 4 demonstrate this point.

The chromosome analysis was pertinent in regard to the following three questions: (1) Were there chromosomal characteristics which associated the cells of the different lines with the type of cancer cell from which they were supposedly derived? (2) Did the chromosome patterns resemble those previously reported for other lines derived from similar tumors? (3) Did the cells differ from normal cells to the extent that their malignancy was established?

In addition, chromosomal characterizations served as identification in terms of species and cell line distinction.

Since the actual tumors used for our cultivation were not submitted to chromosome analysis, the comparison necessary to answer the first question must be based on data obtained by others on similar tumors. For example, carcinomas of the cervix, breast, lung, liver, and ovary have been studied by several investigators, along with other cancers. The results have shown that there is no characteristic chromosome picture for any of the tumors. Chromosome numbers varied greatly. Of 70 primary tumors, distribution of modal number was pseudodiploid in 62.9% of the cases, pseudotriploid in 30.3%, and pseudotetraploid in 6.8%. For 121 metastatic tumors, the same distributions were 45.1, 41.5, and 13.4% (Sandberg and Yamada, 1965). Among 22 cervix tumors, chromosome numbers ranged from 44.7 to 94.4, with 57.8 the mean of all cases (Wakonig-Vaartaja and Hughes, 1967). Our HT-3 cervix line was in the higher part of this range, as was our SK-BR-3 line, when compared to the breast carcinoma data of Makino *et al.* (1964) and in particular to the apparently diploid case reported by Miles (1967). However, the numbers for a hepatoma (65–83, with a remarkable modal of 75) (Makino *et al.*, 1964), were higher than those of our SK-HEP-1 line. A pronounced variation also in chromosome abnormalities and in the presence of marker chromosomes, even among tumors from the same organ, has been characteristic of all analyses reported (Sandberg and Yamada, 1965; Wakonig-Vaartaja and Hughes, 1967; Makino *et al.*, 1959, 1964; Miles, 1967; Yamada *et al.*, 1966). It seems highly unlikely, therefore, that identification of a cell line with these tumor types is possible by the classical chromosome techniques. It is hoped that the new banding techniques may pinpoint intrachromosomal changes and that some of those will be specific for the cells of a particular type of tumor.

Regarding the second point, when averages were established from analysis of many cells certain features appeared to be characteristic of the individual cell lines, in terms of numbers, aberrations, new chromosomes, and karyotypes. Yet there were pronounced variations in these respects among the lines derived from the same types of tumors.

The present analysis has proven without doubt that our cell lines cannot be characterized as normal. They have the typical chromosome picture of cancer cells. Even for the Casa-1 line, although chromosome numbers were close to diploid, abnormalities were limited, and no markers were seen, changes were observed in the karyotypes. It might be premature, based on chromosome analysis alone, to characterize Casa-1 cells as malignant. Further evaluation is pending upon studies of the type of tumor (salivary gland carcinoma) from which the cell line was derived, as well as other cell lines derived from this type of tumor. From literature reviews, from data obtained directly from the cell line originators, and from our own experience, we have attempted to find distinguishing clinical data, characteristics of the tumor material, special culture media or nutritional factors, as well as methods of cultivation which might be the basis for the successful establishment of continuous tumor cell lines. In essence, the search has been negative. No one factor or combination of factors appears to be common.

6. *Establishment of a Human Tumor Cell Line Collection*

As previously mentioned, many investigators have encountered great difficulties in establishing cell lines from human tumors, in spite of numerous attempts. It is now apparent that some tumors can be cultured quite frequently. Other types, however, have not yet yielded cell lines. Cultures assumed and/or claimed to consist of cells derived from tumor cells often appear to represent other components of the tumor (e.g., stromal tissue or reticuloendothelial cells) or normal epithelium. Handling through many culture passages, often by several laboratories, increases the risk of contamination, not only with bacteria, fungi, mycoplasmas, viruses, and perhaps parasites, but also with extraneous cells, human or nonhuman. There is therefore an obvious risk, and indeed existing evidence, that cell lines used in research may bear only slight resemblance, if any, to the original tumor cells. Work with such cells leads to erroneous results.

The answer to these problems appears to be (1) to establish new, additional cell lines, under strictly controlled conditions, with ample characterization in regard to origin and malignancy along the various stages of cultivation, and with storage of cultures in liquid nitrogen as early as possible after the establishment; (2) to carry out a thorough characterization study of already available cell lines, aiming at identification in regard to species, tumor type, malignancy, etc. The particular need for well-characterized cell lines capable of yielding large amounts of cells has been pointed out in several chapters of this book as it relates to many techniques in cancer research. Therefore, our laboratory at Sloan-Kettering Institute has for some time been involved in collecting cell lines derived from many different tumors. To make this collection as complete and representative as possible, within a limited period of time, our efforts have been directed simultaneously toward the development of new cell lines in our own laboratory and toward the collection and characterization of lines established by others. Part of this effort has emphasized the types of tumors from which cell lines have not previously been established. Some of the methods which have led to the successful establishment of lines have been summarized above. New methods, based on experience gained and present experimentation, appear promising.

As part of this effort we have prepared an inventory of published cell lines, established either from human tumor material or from patients with hematopoietic malignancies (see Section 9). Other contributors to this book were requested to comment on and add to this list in order to make it as complete as possible. Despite all these efforts, we cannot guarantee that omissions have not occurred. If so, we apologize to those whose contributions we did not recognize. It is possible that some of the cell lines listed do not exist anymore. However, we are trying to acquire as many of these as possible. If they are free of contamination and if they qualify as human tumor cell lines after proper characterization in our laboratory (and not before then), we intend to make them available to other investigators. Because of the increasing emphasis on experimental human cancer cell research, and because the ultimate conquest of human cancer obviously must be accomplished from work with human systems, this type of material should be of incomparable value in further efforts in cancer research.

Acknowledgments

Part of this work was supported by Sloan-Kettering Institute Grant NCI-CA-08748; part by NIH contract NOI-CB-43854. Dr. Lloyd J. Old's interest in this program has been most encouraging. We appreciate the help given by Drs. Stephen S. Sternberg and Steven I. Hajdu in establishing tumor diagnoses. A number of the tumor specimens were obtained from the

Procurement Service (Dr. Yashar Hirshaut). Excellent technical assistance, most recently by Ellen Møllgaard, is acknowledged. Shirley DeVore and Gwendolyn Holmes have contributed much in order to make the list of published cell lines as complete as possible.

7. *References*

Eagle, H., 1959, Amino acid metabolism in mammalian cell cultures, *Science* **130**:432.

Fogh, J., and Fogh, H., 1969, Procedures for control of mycoplasma contamination of tissue cultures, *Ann. N.Y. Acad. Sci.* **172**:15 (Art. 2).

Fogh, J., and Lund, R. O., 1957, Continuous cultivation of epithelial cell strain (FL) from human amniotic membrane, *Proc. Soc. Exp. Biol. Med.* **94**:532.

Fogh, J., Ramos, L., and Fogh, H., 1969, Transformation of primary human amnion cells with simian virus 40, *in: Axenic Mammalian Cell Reactions* (G. L. Tritsch, ed.), p.59, Marcel Dekker, New York.

Leibovitz, A., 1963, The growth and maintenance of tissue-cell cultures in free gas exchange with the atmosphere, *Am. J. Hyg.* **78**:173.

Makino, S., Ishihara, T., and Tonomura, A., 1959, Cytological studies of tumors. XXVII. The chromosomes of thirty human tumors, *Z. Krebsforsch.* **63**:184.

Makino, S., Sasaki, M., and Tonomura, A., 1964, Chromosome studies in fifty-two human tumors, *J. Natl. Cancer Inst.* **32**:741.

McCoy, T., Maxwell, M., and Kruse, P., 1959, Amino acid requirements of the Novikoff hepatoma *in vitro*, *Proc. Soc. Exp. Biol. Med.* **100**:115.

Miles, C. P., 1967, Chromosome analysis of solid tumors. II. Twenty-six epithelial tumors, *Cancer* **20**:1274.

Moore, G., Gerner, R., and Franklin, H., 1967, Culture of normal human leukocytes, *JAMA* **199**:519.

Sandberg, A. A., and Yamada, K., 1965, Chromosomes and cancer, *CA* **15**:58.

Wakonig-Vaartaja, R., and Hughes, D. T., 1967, Chromosome studies in 36 gynaecological tumors: of the cervix, corpus uteri, ovary, vagina and vulva, *Eur. J. Cancer* **3**:263.

Waymouth, C., 1959, Rapid proliferation of sublines of NCTC clone 929 (strain L) mouse cells in a simple chemically defined medium (MB 752/1), *J. Natl. Cancer Inst.* **22**:1003.

Yamada, K., Takagi, N., and Sandberg, A. A., 1966, Chromosomes and causation of human cancer and leukemia. II. Karyotypes of human solid tumors, *Cancer* **19**:1879.

8. *Appendix: Published Cell Lines Established from Human Tumors*

8.1. *Carcinomas*

Tissue of origin	Cell line designation	Originator(s)	Year	Reference
Adrenal	SW-13	Leibovitz, A.	1971	Leibovitz, A., *et al.*, *In Vitro 8*:433, 1973
	SW-47	Leibovitz, A.	1971	Leibovitz, A., Chapter 2, this volume
Bladder		Yajima, T.	1967	Yajima, T., *Jap. J. Urol. 61*:805, 1970
	RT4 128	Rigby, C.	1968	Rigby, C., and Franks, L. M., *Brit. J. Cancer 24*:746, 1970
	T24	Bubenik, J.	1970	Bubenik, J., *et al.*, *Int. J. Cancer 11*:765, 1973
Breast	BT-20	Lasfargues, E., Ozzello, L.	1958	Lasfargues, E., and Ozzello, L., *J. Natl. Cancer Inst. 21*:1131, 1958
	AlAb	Reed, M., Gey, G.	1958	Reed, M., and Gey, G., *Lab. Invest. 2*:638, 1962
	CaMa	Dobrynin, Y.	1959	Dobrynin, Y., *J. Natl. Cancer Inst. 31*:1173, 1963
	Lev III	Beth, E., Old, L. J.	1967	Giraldo, G., *et al.*, *J. Exp. Med. 133*:454, 1971
	Sal III	Beth, E., Old, L. J.	1967	Giraldo, G., *et al.*, *J. Exp. Med. 133*:454, 1971
	M-1	Martorelli, B.	1968	Martorelli, B., *et al.*, *Surg. Gynecol. Obstet. 128*:1001, 1969
	SK-BR-3	Trempe, G., Old, L. J.	1970	Fogh, J., and Trempe, G., this chapter
	734B	Brennan, M.	1970	Lasfargues, E., *et al.*, *Proc. Am. Assoc. Cancer Res. 13*:42, 1972
	HBT-3	Plata, E.	1971	Bassin, R., *et al.*, *Proc. Soc. Exp. Biol. Med. 141*:673, 1972
	HBT-39	Plata, E.	1972	Plata, E., *et al.*, *J. Natl. Cancer Inst. 50*:849, 1973

Breast (cont'd)	MDA-MB-157	Young, R., Cailleau, R., Mackay, B., Reeves, W. J.	1973	Young, R., *et al.*, *In Vitro 9*:239, 1974
	MDA-MB-134	Cailleau, R.	1973	Cailleau, R., Chapter 4, this volume
	MDA-MB-175	Cailleau, R.	1974	
	MDA-MB-231	Cailleau, R.	1974	
Cervix	HeLa	Gey, G., Gey, M.	1951	Gey, G., *et al.*, *Cancer Res. 12*:264, 1952
	HEp-1	Fjelde, A.	1953	Fjelde, A., *Cancer 8*:845, 1955
	C3-II	Norrby, K.	1959	Norrby, K., *et al.*, *Cancer Res. 22*:147, 1962
	C-4 I and II	Auersperg, N.	1960	Auersperg, N., *J. Natl. Cancer Inst. 32*:135, 1964
	C-27		1962	
	C-33 I and II		1962	
	HT-3	Fogh, J.	1963	Fogh, J., and Trempe, G., this chapter
	ME-180	Sykes, J.	1967	Sykes, J., *et al.*, *J. Natl. Cancer Inst. 45*:107, 1970
	OG	Ogawa, I.	1967	Ogawa, I., *Nippon Sanka-Fujinka Gakkai Zasshi 19*:1086, 1967
	SiHa	Ito, Y.	1968	Friedl, F., *et al.*, *Proc. Soc. Exp. Biol. Med. 135*:543, 1970
	SzC	Bloom, E.	1971	Bloom, E., *et al.*, *Int. J. Cancer 12*:21, 1973
Colon	RPMI-4788	Moore, G.	1961	Tanigaki, N., *et al.*, *J. Immunol. 97*:634, 1966
	Z 516[a]	Wolff, Et., Wolff, Em.	1963	Wolff, Et., and Wolff, Em., *Eur. J. Cancer 2*:93, 1966
	HT-29	Fogh, J.	1964	Fogh, J., and Trempe, G., this chapter
	Az 110[a]	Wolff, Et., Wolff, Em.	1969	Wolff, Em., *et al.*, *C. R. Acad. Sci. Paris 274*:341, 1972

[a]Organotypic culture.

8.1. *Carcinomas (cont'd)*

Tissue of origin	Cell line designation	Originator(s)	Year	Reference
Colon (Cont'd)	CMP	Rounds, D.	1969	Rounds, D., *Cancer Res. 30*:2847, 1970
	SK-CO-1	Trempe, G., Old, L. J.	1972	Fogh, J., and Trempe, G., this chapter
	SW-48	Leibovitz, A.	1972	Leibovitz, A., Chapter 2, this volume
	Led-WIDR	Wallace, R.	1972	Petricciani, J., *et al.*, *Cancer Res. 34*:105, 1974
Gall bladder	RPMI-0191	Moore, G.	1958	Ishihara, T., *et al.*, *Cancer Res. 22*:375, 1962
Kidney	CCRF-6	Foley, G.	1956	Foley, G., *et al.*, *Cancer Res. 20*:930, 1960
	RPMI-1938	Moore, G.	1960	Ishihara, T., *et al.*, *Cancer Res. 22*:375, 1962
	TuWi	Dobrynin, Y.	1962	Dobrynin, Y., *J. Natl. Cancer Inst. 31*:1173, 1963
	Caki-1, Caki-2	Fogh, J.	1971	Fogh, J., and Trempe, G., this chapter
	SK-NEP-1	Trempe, G., Old, L. J.	1971	Fogh, J., and Trempe, G., this chapter
	A-498, A-704	Giard, D. J.	1972, 1973	Giard, D. J., *et al.*, *J. Natl. Cancer Inst. 51*:417, 1973
	SW-156	Leibovitz, A.	1973	Leibovitz, A., Chapter 2, this volume
Larynx	HEp-2	Fjelde, A.	1952	Moore, A., *et al.*, *Cancer Res. 15*:598, 1955
	CCRF-108	Foley, G.	1956	Foley, G., *et al.*, *Cancer Res. 20*:930, 1960
Liver	L-16	Chen, J.	1960	Chen, J., *et al.*, *VIII Int. Cancer Congr. Moscow*, p.136, 1962

Liver (cont'd)	SK-HEP-1	Trempe, G., Old, L. J.	1971	Fogh, J., and Trempe, G., this chapter
Lung	Maben	Frisch, A.	1953	Frisch, A., *et al.*, *Am. J. Clin. Pathol.* *25*:1107, 1955
	LAC	Baron, S.	1955	Baron, S., and Rabson, A., *Proc. Soc. Exp. Biol. Med.* *96*:515, 1957
	ThoCu, SaBa	Reed, M., Gey, G.	1958	Reed, M., and Gey, G., *Lab. Invest.* *2*:638, 1962
	MAC-21	Cailleau, R.	1959	Cailleau, R., *Cancer Res.* *20*:837, 1960
	MEP	Ho, S.	1959	Ho, S., *et al.*, *VIII Int. Cancer Congr. Moscow*, p.135, 1962
	9812	Price, P.	1969	Aaronson, S., *et al.*, *Exp. Cell Res.* *61*:1, 1970
	Chelo-1	Coalson, R., Nordquist, R.	1969	Coalson R., *et al.*, *Lab. Invest.* *28*:38, 1973
	SK-MES-1	Trempe, G., Old, L. J.	1970	Fogh, J., and Trempe, G., this chapter
	OAT	Oboshi, S.	1970	Oboshi, S., *et al.*, *Gann* *62*:505, 1971
	Calu-1	Fogh, J.	1971	Fogh, J., and Trempe, G., this chapter
	ChaGo	Rabson, A.	1971	Rabson, A., *et al.*, *J. Natl. Cancer Inst.* *50*:669, 1973
	A-549, A-427	Giard, D.	1972	Giard, D., *et al.*, *J. Natl. Cancer Inst.* *51*:417, 1973
	SW-161	Leibovitz, A.	1973	Leibovitz, A., Chapter 2, this volume
Mouth	HEp-3	Moore, A.	1952	Toolan, H., *Cancer Res.* *14*:660, 1954
	KB	Eagle, H.	1954	Eagle, H., *Proc. Soc. Exp. Biol. Med.* *89*:362, 1955
Nasal septum	RPMI-2650	Moore, G.	1962	Tanigaki, N., *et al.*, *J. Immunol.* *97*:634, 1966
Neck	A-253, A-388	Giard, D.	1972	Giard, D., *et al.*, *J. Natl. Cancer Inst.* *51*:417, 1973
	SW-213	Leibovitz, A.	1973	Leibovitz, A., Chapter 2, this volume

8.1. Carcinomas (cont'd)

Tissue of origin	Cell line designation	Originator(s)	Year	Reference
Ovary	RPMI-131	Moore, G.	1959	Ishihara, T., *et al.*, *Cancer Res. 22*:375, 1962
	SK-OV-1	Trempe, G., Old, L. J.	1970	Fogh, J., and Trempe, G., this chapter
	Caov-1	Fogh, J.		
	SK-OV-3	Trempe, G., Old, L. J.	1973	
Pancreas	CaPa	Dobrynin, Y.	1959	Dobrynin, Y., *J. Natl. Cancer Inst. 31*:1173, 1963
Pharynx	Detroit 562	Peterson, W.	1968	Peterson, W., *et al.*, *Proc. Soc. Exp. Biol. Med. 136*:1187, 1971
	FaDu	Rangan, S.	1968	Rangan, S., *Cancer 29*:117, 1972
Placenta	BeWo	Pattillo, R., Gey, G.	1966	Pattillo, R., *et al.*, *Science 159*:1467, 1968
	JEG-1,-2,-3, -4,-7,-8	Kohler, P., Bridson, W.	1968	Kohler, P., and Bridson, W., *J. Clin. Endocrinol. Metab. 32*:683, 1971
Rectum	AZ 432[a]	Wolff, Et., Wolff, Em.	1972	Wolff, Et., and Wolff, Em., *C.R. Acad. Sci. Paris*
Salivary Gland	558	Timofeyevsky, A.	1961	Dobrynin, Y., *J. Natl. Cancer Inst. 31*:1173, 1963
	Nagoya-78	Muragishi, H.	1966	Muragishi, H., *Nagoya Iagaku (J. Nagoya Med. Assoc.) 92*:373, 1969
	Casa-1	Fogh, J.	1972	Fogh, J., and Trempe, G., this chapter
Stomach	CaVe	Dobrynin, Y.	1959	Dobrynin, Y., *J. Natl. Cancer Inst. 31*:1173, 1963

Stomach (cont'd)	Za 200[a]	Wolff, Et., Wolff, Em.	1962	Wolff, Et., and Wolff, Em., *Eur. J. Cancer* *2*:93, 1966
Thyroid	PS,TR,TS	Hirose, M.	1966	Hirose, M., *Acta Med. Okayama 22*:185, 1968
	—	Jones, G. W.	1967	Jones, G. W., *et al., Proc. Soc. Exp. Biol. Med. 126*:426, 1967
Uterus	AN_3CA	Dawe, C. J.	1962	Dawe, C. J., *et al., J. Natl. Cancer Inst.* *33*:441, 1964
	HEC-1	Notake, Y., Kuramoto, H.	1969	Kuramoto, H., *Acta Obstet. Gynaecol. Jap.* *19*:47, 1972
	SW-193	Leibovitz, A.	1973	Leibovitz, A., Chapter 2, this volume
Vulva	A-431	Giard, D.	1973	Giard, D., *et al., J. Natl. Cancer Inst.* *51*:417, 1973

[a]Organotypic culture.

8.2. *Sarcomas*

Tissue of origin	Cell line designation	Originator(s)	Year	Reference
Ewing sarcoma	SK-ES-1	Bloom, E.	1971	Bloom, E., *Cancer Res. 32*:960, 1972
Fibrosarcoma	HFS_9	Ranadive, K.	1957	Ranadive, K., *et al., Pathol. Biol. 9*:549, 1961
	8387	Price, P.	1966	Aaronson, S., *et al., Exp. Cell Res. 61*:1, 1970
	Safi-1	Fogh, J.	1973	Fogh, J., and Trempe, G., this chapter
	HT-1080	Rasheed, S.	1973	Rasheed, S., *et al., Cancer 33*:1027, 1974
Kaposi sarcoma	Kap 9, Kap 13, Kap 16, Kap 19, Kap 22	Giraldo, G.	1970	Giraldo, G., *et al., J. Natl. Cancer Inst. 49*:1495, 1972
Leiomyosarcoma	SK-LMS-1	Trempe, G., Old, L. J.	1971	Fogh, J., and Trempe, G., this chapter
Liposarcoma	HLS_2	Gangal, S.	1957	Gangal, S., *et al., Indian J. Med. Res. 49*:756, 1961
	RPMI-1922	Moore, G.	1960	Ishihara, T., *et al., Cancer Res. 22*:375, 1962
	SA-4	Morton, D.	1968	Aaronson, S., *et al., Exp. Cell Res. 61*:1, 1970
	SK-LS-4	Beth, E., Old, L. J.	1969	Giraldo, G., *et al., J. Exp. Med. 133*:454, 1971
Neurosarcoma	T_2	Trujillo, J.	1966	Trujillo, J., *et al., Cancer Res. 32*:1066, 1972
Osteogenic-sarcoma	RPMI-41	Moore, G.	1959	Ishihara, T., *et al., Cancer Res. 22*:375, 1962

Osteogenic-sarcoma (cont'd)	2 OS (2 T)	Pontén, J., Saksela, E.	1964	Pontén, J., and Saksela, E., *Int. J. Cancer* *2*:434, 1967
	MT	McAllister, R.	1968	McAllister, R., *et al.*, *Cancer 27*:397, 1971
	SK-OS-3B	Beth, E., Old, L. J.	1968	Giraldo, G., *et al.*, *J. Exp. Med. 133*:454, 1971
	MC-1	McAllister, R.	1968	Aaronson, S., *et al.*, *Exp. Cell Res.* *61*:1, 1970
	C-584	Morton, D.	1968	Aaronson, S., *et al.*, *Exp. Cell Res.* *61*:1, 1970
	SK-OS-5	Beth, E., Old, L. J.	1969	Giraldo, G., *et al.*, *J. Exp. Med. 133*:454, 1971
	393 OS (393 T)	Pontén, J.	1969	Pontén, J., Chapter 7, this volume
	T 187	Maunoury, R.	1970	Maunoury, R., *et al.*, *Pathol. Biol. 20*:369, 1972
	SK-OS-10	Trempe, G., Old, L. J.	1972	Fogh, J., and Trempe, G., this chapter
	Saos-2	Fogh, J.	1973	Fogh, J., and Trempe, G., this chapter
Osteo/chondro-sarcoma	Saos-1	Fogh, J.	1973	Fogh, J., and Trempe, G., this chapter
Rhabdomyo-sarcoma	RD-2	McAllister, R.	1968	McAllister, R., *et al.*, *Cancer 24*:520, 1969
	SW-80	Leibovitz, A.	1971	Leibovitz, A., Chapter 2, this volume
	T-35	Dalton, A., Szakacs, J.	1971	Dalton, A., *et al.*, *J. Natl. Cancer Inst. 50*:879, 1973
	A-204	Giard, D.	1972	Giard, D., *et al.*, *J. Natl. Cancer Inst.* *51*:417, 1973
	A-673	Giard, D.	1972	Giard, D., *et al.*, *J. Natl. Cancer Inst.* *51*:417, 1973
Sarcoma		Stewart, S.	1970	Stewart, S., *et al.*, *J. Natl. Cancer Inst.* *48*:273, 1972

8.3. *Nerve Tumors*

Type	Cell line designation	Originator(s)	Year	Reference
Astrocytoma	CHB	Lightbody, J.	1968	Lightbody, J., *et al.*, *J. Neurobiol. 1*:411, 1970
	GL VI GL XVII GL XVIII	Chapekar, T., Talwar, G.	1971	Chapekar, T., *et al.*, *Indian J. Med. Res 60*:1186, 1972
	A-382	Giard, D.	1972	Giard, D., *et al.*, *J. Natl. Cancer Inst. 51*:417, 1973
	Ast-1	Fogh, J.	1973	Fogh, J., and Trempe, G., this chapter
Glioblastoma	22 lines designated TC No. 178, 224, 307, 342, 359, 377, 386, 406, 469, 470, 477, 504, 507, 513, 516, 517, 526, 532, 533, 549, 584, 593	Manuelidis, E. E.	1957–1965	Manuelidis, E. E., *J. Neurosurg. 22*:368, 1965
	87MG 105 MG 118 MG 138 MG	Pontén, J.	1966	Pontén, J., *et al.*, *Acta Pathol. Microbiol. Scand. 74*: 465, 1968
	178 MG 251 MG	Pontén, J.	1967 1968	Beckman, G., *et al.*, *Hum. Hered.21*: 238, 1971
	C356	Pinkerton, H.	1968	Pinkerton, H., *et al.*, *Cancer Res. 31*:1483 1971

Glioblastoma (cont'd)	343 MG, 348 MG, 372 MG, 373 MG, 399 MG	Westermark, B.	1969, 1969, 1969, 1969, 1970	Beckman, G., *et al.*, *Hum. Hered.* *21*:238, 1971
	410 MG	Westermark, B.	1970	Westermark, B., and Hugosson, R., *Acta pathol. Microbiol. Scand.*, in press
	489 MG, 495 MG	Westermark, B.	1970	Beckman, G., *et al.*, *Hum. Hered.* *21*:238, 1971
	539 MG, 563 MG	Westermark, B.	1971	Pontén, J., Chapter 7, this volume
	692 MG, 716 MG	Westermark, B.	1972	Pontén, J., Chapter 7, this volume
	A 172	Giard, D.	1972	Giard, D., *et al.*, *J. Natl. Cancer Inst.* *51*:417, 1973
Neuroblastoma	NJB	Goldstein, M.	1966	Goldstein, M., *J. Pediat. Surg.* *3*:166, 1968
	IMR-32	Tumilowicz, J.	1967	Tumilowicz, J., *et al.*, *Cancer Res.* *30*:2110, 1970
	SK-N-SH, SK-N-MC	Biedler, J.	1970, 1971	Spengler, B., *et al.*, *In Vitro* *8*:410, 1973
	Fj-1NB, Fj-2NB	Fjelde, A.	1971	Fjelde, A., *et al.*, *Proc. Am. Assoc. Cancer Res.* *14*:108, 1973
	Fj-3NB, Fj-4NB, Fj-5NB	Fjelde, A.	1972	Fjelde, A., *et al.*, *Proc. Am. Assoc. Cancer Res.* *14*:108, 1973
	SK-N-BE	Biedler, J.	1972	Biedler, J., *et al.*, *In Vitro* *8*:410, 1973
	Fj-6NB	Fjelde, A.	1973	Fjelde, A., *et al.*, *Proc. Am. Assoc. Cancer Res.* *14*:108, 1973
Paraganglioma	T-13	Dalton, A., Szakacs, J.	1971	Heine, U., *et al.*, *Cancer Res.* *31*:542, 1971

8.4. *Melanomas*

Cell line designation	Originator(s)	Year	Reference
CCRF-105 CCRF-104 CCRF-107	Foley, G.	1956 1957 1957	Foley, G., *et al.*, *Cancer Res. 20*:930, 1960
RPMI-3236	Moore, G.	1962	Toshima, S., *et al.*, *Cancer 21*:202, 1968
LeCa 26-5	Romsdahl, M.	1965	Romsdahl, M., and Hsu, T., *Surg. Forum 18*:78, 1967
HT-144	Fogh, J.	1966	Fogh, J., and Trempe, G., this chapter
SK-MEL-1	Oettgen, H.	1966	Oettgen, H., *et al.*, *J. Natl. Cancer Inst. 41*:827, 1968
RPMI-5966	Moore, G.	1966	Toshima, S., *et al.*, *Cancer 21*:202, 1968
MeGo	Maul, G., Romsdahl, M.	1969	Maul, G., and Romsdahl, M., *Cancer Res. 30*:2782, 1970
SK-SC-1	Trempe, G., Old, L. J.	1971	Fogh, J., and Trempe, G., this chapter
T-40	Dalton, A., Szakacs, J.	1971	Dalton, A., *et al.*, *J. Natl. Cancer Inst. 50*:879, 1973
A-375	Giard, D.	1972	Giard, D., *et al.*, *J. Natl. Cancer Inst. 51*:417, 1973
SK-MEL-2 SK-MEL-3	Trempe, G., Old, L. J.	1972	Fogh, J., and Trempe, G., this chapter
A-875	Giard, D.	1973	Giard, D., *et al.*, *J. Natl. Cancer Inst. 51*:417, 1973
Malme-3M and -3S	Fogh, J.	1973	Fogh, J., and Trempe, G., this chapter

8.5. *Miscellaneous Tumors*

Type	Cell line designation	Originator(s)	Year	Reference
Chemodectoma	SW-267	Leibovitz, A.	1973	Leibovitz, A., Chapter 2, this volume
Insulinoma	Ins-1	Fogh, J.	1959	Fogh, J., and Trempe, G., this chapter
Mesodermal Mixed tumor cultures	SK-UT-1 and -1B	Trempe, G., Old, L. J.	1972	Fogh, J., and Trempe, G., this chapter
Mesothelioma	RPMI-212	Moore, G.	1959	Ishihara, T., *et al., Cancer Res.* 22:375, 1962
	SK-MES-1	Trempe, G., Old, L. J.	1970	Fogh, J., and Trempe, G., this chapter
Teratoma	Tera-1, Tera-2	Fogh, J.	1970, 1971	Fogh, J., and Trempe, G., this chapter

8.6. *Patients with Hematopoietic Malignancies*

Diagnosis	Source	Cell line designation	Originator(s)	Year	Reference
Leukemias					
Acute					
lymphoblastic	Blood	CCRF-CEM	Foley, G.	1964	Foley, G., *et al.*, *Cancer 18*:522, 1965
		SK-L2	Clarkson, B.	1965	Clarkson, B., *et al.*, *Cancer 20*:926, 1967
		LK 1D LK 60	Armstrong, D.	1966	Armstrong, D., *Proc. Soc. Exp. Biol. Med. 122*:475, 1966
		LK 63	Armstrong, D.	1966	Miles, C., *et al.*, *Cancer Res. 28*:481, 1968
		SK-L6	Clarkson, B.	1966	Clarkson, B., *et al.*, *Cancer 20*:926, 1967
		RPMI-8382 RPMI-8392 RPMI-8402 RPMI-8412 RPMI-8422 RPMI-8432 RPMI-8442 RPMI-8452	Moore, G.[a]	1972	Moore, G., *et al.*, *In Vitro 8*:434, 1973
		MOLT	Minowada, J.	1971	Minowada, J., *et al.*, *J. Natl. Cancer Inst. 49*:891, 1972
Acute lymphocytic	Lymph node	F-89	Jensen, E.	1966	Jensen, E., *et al.*, *J. Natl. Cancer Inst. 39*:745, 1967
Chronic lymphocytic	Lymph node	F-137			

Acute myelogenous	Blood	RPMI-8866	Moore, G.	1965	Shevach, E., *et al.*, *J. Clin. Invest.* *51*:1933, 1972
		RPMI-5328, RPMI-1537	Moore, G.	1966, 1967	Huang, C., *et al.*, *J. Natl. Cancer Inst.* *43*:1129, 1969
		OUMS-12	Miyoshi, I.	1970	Miyoshi, I., *et al.*, *Gann* *62*:413, 1971
Acute myeloblastic	Blood	RPMI-6410, RPMI-9154	Moore, G.	1964	Moore, G., *et al.*, *Cancer* *19*:713, 1966
		(RPMI-8195, -8205, -8235)	Moore, G.	1965	
		SK-L4, SK-L5	Clarkson, B.	1966	Clarkson, B., *et al.*, *Cancer* *20*:926, 1967
		LK 57	Armstrong, D.	1966	Armstrong, D., *Proc. Soc. Exp. Biol. Med.* *122*:475, 1966
Acute myelomonocytic	Blood	SK-L1, SK-L3	Clarkson, B.	1965	Clarkson, B., *Cancer* *20*:926, 1967
		SK-L7, SK-L8	Clarkson, B.	1966	
		SK-L10	Clarkson, B.	1967	Southam, C., *Cancer* *23*:281, 1969
	Bone marrow	F-49	Jensen, E.	1965	Jensen, E., *et al.*, *J. Natl. Cancer Inst.* *39*:745, 1967
Chronic myelogenous	Blood	M2	Lucas, L.	1964	Lucas, L., *et al.*, *J. Natl. Cancer Inst.* *37*:753, 1966
		RPMI-1115, RPMI-1210, RPMI-1245, RPMI-1285	Moore, G.	1965	Tanigaki, N., *et al.*, *J. Immunol.* *97*:634, 1966
		(RPMI-4265, -7865, 1694, -1695)	Moore, G.	1965	Moore, G., *et al.*, *Cancer* *19*:713, 1966)

[a]Other lines established by Dr. G. E. Moore are listed on p. 301.

8.6. *Patients with Hematopoietic Malignancies (cont'd)*

Diagnosis	Source	Cell line designation	Originator(s)	Year	Reference
Chronic myelogenous (cont'd)	Blood	G-6	Chandra, S.	1968	Chandra, S., *et al.*, *Cancer Res.* *31*:441, 1971
		Cy-LMC-1	deGrouchy, J.	1969	deGrouchy, J., *et al.*, *Ann. Genet.* *13*:157, 1970
		LAHL1	Possnerova, V.	1969	Possnerova, V., *et al.*, *Neoplasma* *17*:513, 1970
	Spleen	SK-L9	Clarkson, B.	1967	Clarkson, B., *Cancer* *20*:926, 1967
Chronic myeloblastic	Blood	LK 87A LK 91	Armstrong, D.	1966	Miles, C., *et al.*, *Cancer Res.* *28*:481, 1968
Myelomas					
Multiple myeloma	Blood	RPMI-8226	Moore, G.	1966	Matsuoka, Y., *et al.*, *Proc. Soc. Expl. Biol. Med.* *125:* 1246, 1967
	Blood Bone marrow	266 Bl 255 Bm 268 Bm	Nilsson, K.	1968	Nilsson, K., *et al.*, *Clin. Exp. Immunol.* *7*:477, 1970
		IM-9	Buell, D.	1967	Buell, D., *et al.*, in: *Develop. Aspects Cell Cycle* (Cameron *et al.*, eds.), 1971
	Blood	IM-10	Buell, D.	1969	Shevach, E., *et al.*, *J. Clin. Invest.* *51*:1933, 1972
		RPMI-5286	Moore, G.	1966	Huang, C., *et al.*, *J. Natl. Cancer Inst.* *43*:1129, 1969

Lymphomas					
Reticulum cell sarcoma	Lymph node	F-132, F-148	Jensen, E.	1966	Jensen, E., *et al.*, *J. Natl. Cancer Inst. 39*:745, 1967
	Ilium	27M	Pontén, J.	1966	Pontén, J., *Int. J. Cancer 2*:311, 1967
	Blood	SK-RCS-1	Clarkson, B.	1967	Clarkson, B., *et al., Cancer Res. 29*:823, 1969
Lymphosarcoma	Lymph node	CCRF-100	Foley, G.	1957	Foley, G., *et al., Cancer Res. 20*:930, 1960
	Biopsy	CCRF-106			
	Lymph node	25M, 40M	Pontén, J.	1966	Pontén, J., *Int. J. Cancer 2*:311, 1967
		109M	Nilsson, K.	1967	Nilsson, K., *et al., Int. J. Cancer 3*:183, 1968
(Lymphocytic lymphoma)	Lymph node		Trujillo, J.	1964	Trujillo, J., *et al., Nature 209*:310, 1966
Follicular lymphoma (?)	Lymph node	139M	Nilsson, K.	1967	Nilsson, K., *et al., Int. J. Cancer 3*:183, 1968
Hodgkin's disease	Biopsy	SS_5	Stewart, S.	1967	Stewart, S., *et al., J. Natl. Cancer Inst. 43*:1, 1969
	Blood	SK-HD-1	Trempe, G., Old, L. J.	1971	Fogh, J., and Trempe, G., this chapter
	Lymph node	31M, 61M, 82M	Pontén, J.	1966	Pontén, J., *Int. J. Cancer 2*:311, 1967
(Pre-Hodgkin)					
Hodgkin's disease		129M, 130M, 134M	Nilsson, K.	1967	Nilsson, K., *et al., Int. J. Cancer 3*:183, 1968
		SK-HNF-5	Eisinger, M.	1970	Eisinger, M., *et al., Nature 233*:104, 1971

8.6. *Patients with Hematopoietic Malignancies (cont'd)*

Diagnosis	Source	Cell line designation	Originator(s)	Year	Reference
Burkitt's lymphoma	Ascitic fluid	OB-2, OB-3	Osunkoya, B.	1964	Osunkoya, B., and Mottram, F., *Cancer Res. 27*:2500, 1967
	Biopsy	Raji	Pulvertaft, R.	1963	
		EB-1	Epstein, M.	1964	Epstein, M., and Barr, Y., *J. Natl. Cancer Inst. 34*:231, 1965
		EB-3	Epstein, M.	1964	Epstein, M., *et al.*, *Wistar Inst. Monogr. 4*:69, 1965
		Ogun	Pulvertaft, R.	1965	Fahey, J., *et al.*, *Science 152*:1259, 1966
		Awo	Pulvertaft, R.	?	Osunkoya, B., and Mottram, F., *Cancer Res. 27*:2500, 1967
		Jijoyce	Pulvertaft, R.	1965	
		AL-2	O'Conor, G., Rabson, A.	1965	O'Conor, G., and Rabson, A., *J. Natl. Cancer Inst. 35*:899, 1965
		IM-4	Buell, D.	1967	Buell, D., and Fahey, J., *Science 164*:1524, 1969
	Jaw	OB-1, OB-6, OB-7	Osunkoya, B.	1964	Osunkoya, B., and Mottram, F., *Cancer Res. 27*:2500, 1967
		MOB-8, MOB-9, MOB-10	Osunkoya, B., Mottram, F.		
		AL-1	Rabson, A.	1965	Rabson, A., *et al.*, *Int. J. Cancer 1*:89, 1966
	Biopsy	Kudi	Pulvertaft, R.	1965	Osunkoya, B., and Mottram, F., *Cancer Res. 27*:2500, 1967

Burkitt's lymphoma (cont'd)	Lymph node	SL_1	Stewart, S.	1965	Stewart, S., *et al.*, *J. Natl. Cancer Inst. 34*:319, 1965
		EB-5	Epstein, M.	1966	Epstein, M., *et al.*, *Brit. J. Cancer 20*:475, 1966
	Ovary	EB-2	Epstein, M.	1964	Epstein, M., and Barry, Y., *J. Natl. Cancer Inst. 34*:231, 1965
		EB-4	Epstein, M.	1966	Epstein, M., *et al.*, *Brit. J. Cancer 20*:475, 1966
	Pleural fluid	ESP-1	Priori, E.	1970	Priori, E., *et al.*, *Nature New Biol. 232*:61, 1971
	Spinal fluid	Ob-5	Osunkoya, B.	1964	Osunkoya, B., and Mottram, F., *Cancer Res. 27*:2500, 1967
		MOB-11	Osunkoya, B., Mottram, F.		
	Thigh	Ob-4			
	?	B35M	Minowada, J., Kamei, H.,	?	Minowada, J., and Kamei, H., *Proc. Am. Assoc. Cancer Res. 8*:47, 1967
	?	Daudi	Klein, G.	1966	Allderdice, P. W., *et al.*, *J. Cell Sci. 12*:809, 1973
	?	P-2K	Pulvertaft, R.	?	Tanigaki, N., *et al.*, *J. Immunol. 97*:634, 1966
Mycosis fungoides	Lymph node	WI-L1 (HUP-1)	Levy, J.	1966	Levy, J. A., *et al.*, *Cancer 22*:517, 1968

Human Brain Tumor Cells in Matrix Culture 6

TEDDY HOLMSTRÖM

1. Introduction

Organ cultures of various embryonic tissues and of both benign and malignant tumors have been successfully used in various investigations. The basic aim of this technique is to maintain the architecture, differentiation, and growth of the tissue as similar as possible to the *in vivo* situation. One of the best-known methods is the Trowell-type organ culture system, in which tissue explants are grown on small pieces of lens paper placed on a grid of steel mesh (Trowell, 1954). Although this type of organ culture system allows growth of the fragment as a whole, it does not permit outgrowth of the cells at the periphery of the primary explant. This weakness is partly overcome in three-dimensional matrix culture systems, which permit both maintenance of primary explants and replication of cells with reproduction of original tissue structures within the pores of the supporting matrix.

Leighton (1951) was among the first to report growth of tumors in matrix cultures *in vitro*. He used a combined matrix of commercially available cellulose sponge and plasma clot for growing mouse mammary adenocarcinoma, and described the formation of organized aggregates of cells in the lumina of the matrix. The successful growth of eight other transplantable animal tumors in the same system was reported in 1954 (Leighton, 1954). Epithelium, especially, could be recognized in the outgrowth of the tumors *in vitro*. Papillary and glandular patterns could be seen in the newly formed

TEDDY HOLMSTRÖM III Department of Pathology, University of Helsinki, Helsinki, Finland.

cell groups of this mammary tumor. Leighton further improved the system by coating the lacunae of the cellulose sponge with a thin layer of collagen and showed the superiority of this matrix to either cellulose or collagen sponge alone for growing Walker tumor 256 (Leighton *et al.*, 1967). In the collagen-coated sponge, the cells adhered well to the walls of the lacunae and showed good proliferation. The same could be seen in the collagen sponge alone, but the soft sponge progressively deteriorated, the lumina collapsed, and the cells became necrotic. In the untreated cellulose sponge, adhesion of the cells to the walls of the lacunae was poor.

A large number of other sponge materials have now been tested as matrices. Human fibrin foam was introduced by Kalus and Klement (1966), who grew human embryonic tissues on the matrix. The explants remained viable, and specific organotypic structures could be seen in the proliferating zone between the explant and the matrix. In 1968, they reported successful growth of human tumors (Kalus *et al.*, 1968). They used human epithelial tumors predominantly, and showed definite growth and formation of tumor-specific structures within the lacunae of the upper layers of the fibrin foam. A clear difference in growth pattern between benign and malignant tumors could be demonstrated; the benign tumors maintained their histological structure, whereas the malignant tumors grew into the matrix. The growth capacity of the malignant tumors *in vitro* was positively correlated with their level of differentiation *in vivo.*

Another type of matrix culture system was used by Wolff and Wolff (1961) and Wolff (1963). They grew animal and human tumor explants using chick mesonephros both as a supporting matrix and as a nutritional source. Some of these tumors were transferred serially from mesonephros to mesonephros for several years. Direct contact between the tumor tissue and the mesonephric tissue was not needed, but the mesonephric tissue secreted growth-promoting substances that served to feed the malignant cells.

Human brain tumors grow relatively well in monolayer cultures (Kersting, 1968; Pontén and McIntyre, 1968; Wahlström *et al.*, 1969). Similarly, matrix cultures of human brain tumors have been successful (Holmström *et al.*, 1970; Holmström and Saksela, 1971). These and some further results will be discussed in this chapter.

2. General Matrix Culture Techniques

2.1. Sponge Matrix

In the original work by Leighton (1951), commercially available cellulose sponge was used. This was cut into small pieces, about 8.0 by 5.0 by 1.0 mm in size. The sponge was boiled three times in distilled water for a total of 90 min. The pieces were then immersed in acetone, ether, and absolute alcohol successively, for 15 min in each. The triple boiling in distilled water was then repeated.

The properties of the matrix are improved by coating the walls of the lacunae with a thin layer of collagen (Leighton *et al.*, 1967). The fibrillary collagen used is a commercial preparation by Ethicon (Ethicon, Inc., Somerville, N.J.).

A 1% solution of collagen is prepared in a methanol–water base containing 2% cyanoacetic acid. A few drops of this is placed on a slice of dry cellulose sponge with a tissue culture pipette. The mixture is kneaded thoroughly into the sponge with forceps. The sponges are dried overnight at 38°C. The matrices are then washed for 12–24 h in 50% methanol containing 0.5% ammonium hydroxide. One-hour washes are carried out twice in sterile distilled water and once in Hank's solution, and the sponges are then stored at 4°C in fresh Hank's solution. The pieces of sponge can then be used in the same manner as described later for fibrin foam.

2.2. Embryonic Tissues

Various embryonic tissues have been used for investigations on the invasion of normal tissues by malignant cells. Easty and Easty (1963) used rat kidney or liver in a Trowell-type system for investigations on mouse melanoma. Pieces of normal and neoplastic tissue were placed side by side on top of the Trowell grid, and the malignant melanoma cells infiltrated the rat liver or kidney tissue. Wolff (1963) reported good growth of various human surgical tumors explanted on chick mesonephros. This technique is described in detail in Chapter 8.

2.3. Fibrin Foam

Human fibrin foam is a commercial, sterile, disposable product made by lyophilization of human fibrinogen by the Institute of Sera and Vaccines, Prague, Czechoslovakia. The fibrin foam is cut into small pieces about 8 by 6 by 3 mm in size. The pieces are placed in petri dishes with growth medium, e.g., Eagle's basal medium supplemented with serum and antibiotics. The hygroscopic fibrin foam draws growth medium into itself, the pieces sink to the bottom of the dish, and the fluid level is adjusted to the upper surface of the foam. The tumor material is cut into small pieces of about 1 mm^3 and placed on the fibrin foam cubes, one or two pieces on each. The dishes are incubated in humidified air and 5% CO_2 at 37°C. After cultivation, the cultures are fixed in Carnoy's solution and embedded in paraffin by routine methods. Histological sections are cut through the tissue fragment at right angles to the surface and mounted on gelatin-treated slides. The slides are stained with orcein or hematoxylin and eosin. For radioautography of labeled cultures, the preparations are hydrated and covered with Kodak AR 10 film by the stripping film technique. The dried slides are exposed for 7 days in dark, lightproof boxes at 4°C. Developing, fixing, and rinsing are done by routine methods. The slides are dried in air for 3–4 days, dipped in xylene, and covered with Canada balsam and coverslips. Special techniques used are described below.

3. Growth Behavior of Various Tumors

3.1. Meningiomas

Of all the various types of brain tumors cultivated in this system, including eight meningotheliomatous meningiomas, seven neurinomas, and ten gliomas, the seven fibromatous meningiomas investigated grew best (Holmström and Saksela, 1971). They showed a significantly greater ability to grow into the matrix as compared with the other tumors when penetration into the lacunae of the fibrin foam was measured (Fig. 1). The grade was the maximum number of launar layers that the outgrowing cells had penetrated; and for fibromatous meningiomas it was about 3 and for meningotheliomatous meningiomas about 1. The degree of penetration correlated well with the proliferating activity of the tissue, measured by tritiated thymidine uptake (Holmström *et al.*, 1970).

The viability (the percentage of explants that were viable) for fibromatous meningiomas was about 90% and for meningotheliomatous meningiomas about 80% (Fig. 2). Both types of meningiomas retained their original histological structure well in the primary explants, and meningotheliomatous meningiomas, especially, often showed reproduction of concentric, laminated structures in the lacunae of the matrix (Figs. 3 and 4).

3.2. Neurinomas

The seven neurinomas showed good viability in the matrix culture system used, about 80% (Fig. 2). The original histological structure with interlacing cell bundles and nuclear palisading was preserved in the primary explants.

The outgrowth from the explants was of the same order of magnitude as for meningotheliomatous meningiomas; i.e., the cells penetrated the first or second lacunar layer of the foam (Fig. 1). The number of outgrowing cells was small and consisted of single cells lining the walls of the lacunae, and therefore no characteristic structures were formed. In some explants, no outgrowth occurred, although the original structure was well preserved in the primary explant (Fig. 5).

3.3. Gliomas

The nine gliomas grown in this matrix culture system were graded according to Kernohan from II to IV (Kernohan *et al.*, 1949). The viability of the

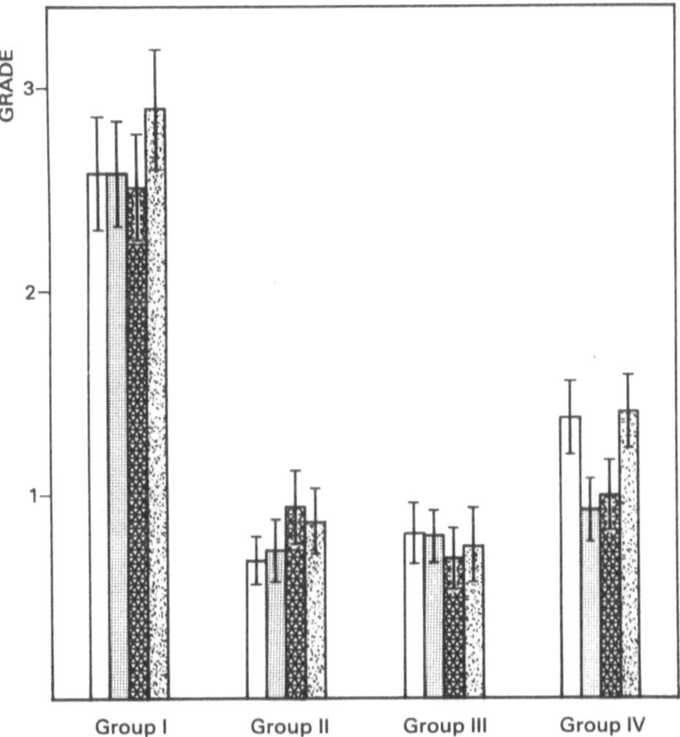

FIG. 1. Penetration into the matrix for the histologically different tumor groups. I, Fibromatous meningiomas; II, meningotheliomatous meningiomas; III, neurinomas; IV, gliomas. Mean values with standard error of the means are shown (Student's t-test). Columns from left to right indicate explants grown in autologous serum, aged serum pool, clumping serum and nonclumping serum. Note the significantly higher growth potential of fibromatous meningiomas in all sera used, and the difference of the growth capacity of gliomas in clumping and nonclumping sera. Copyright by *Acta Pathologica et Microbiologica Scandinavica.*

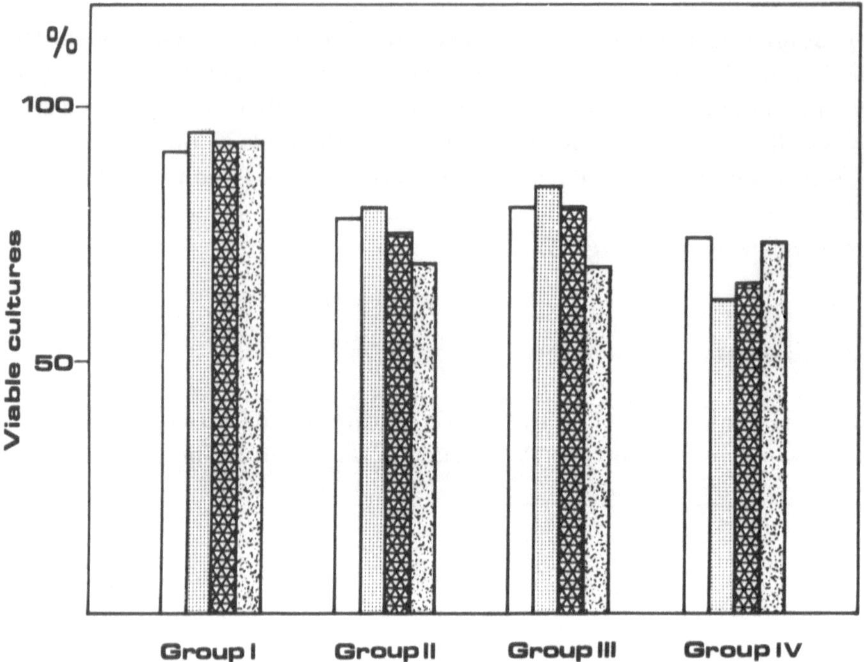

FIG. 2. Viability of tumor explants in the histologically different tumor groups. Columns and groups are analogous to those in Fig. 1. Note the somewhat higher viability for fibromatous meningiomas. Copyright by *Acta Pathologica et Microbiologica Scandinavica.*

primary explants was low, about 60%, and many became necrotic (Fig. 2). On the other hand, the outgrowths from the viable explants extended deep into the matrix; the highest grade recorded was 6 and it was usually on the order of 2 or 3. Because of the low viability, the mean grade was about 1.5. The outgrowing cells had the same cytological characteristics as the mother explants; they were spindle-shaped and pleomorphic, and were single or organized into small groups. They did not form any typical structures (Fig. 6).

FIG. 3. Matrix culture of fibromatous meningioma at 3 days. Note well-preserved histological structure and diffuse border onto the matrix. Bar in the lower right-hand corner indicates 10 μm. Copyright by *Acta Pathologica et Microbiologica Scandinavica.*

FIG. 4. Matrix culture of meningotheliomatous meningioma at 7 days. Reproduction of the concentric laminated structure in the first lacunar layer. Bar in the lower right-hand corner indicates 50 μm. Copyright by *Acta Pathologica et Microbiologica Scandinavica.*

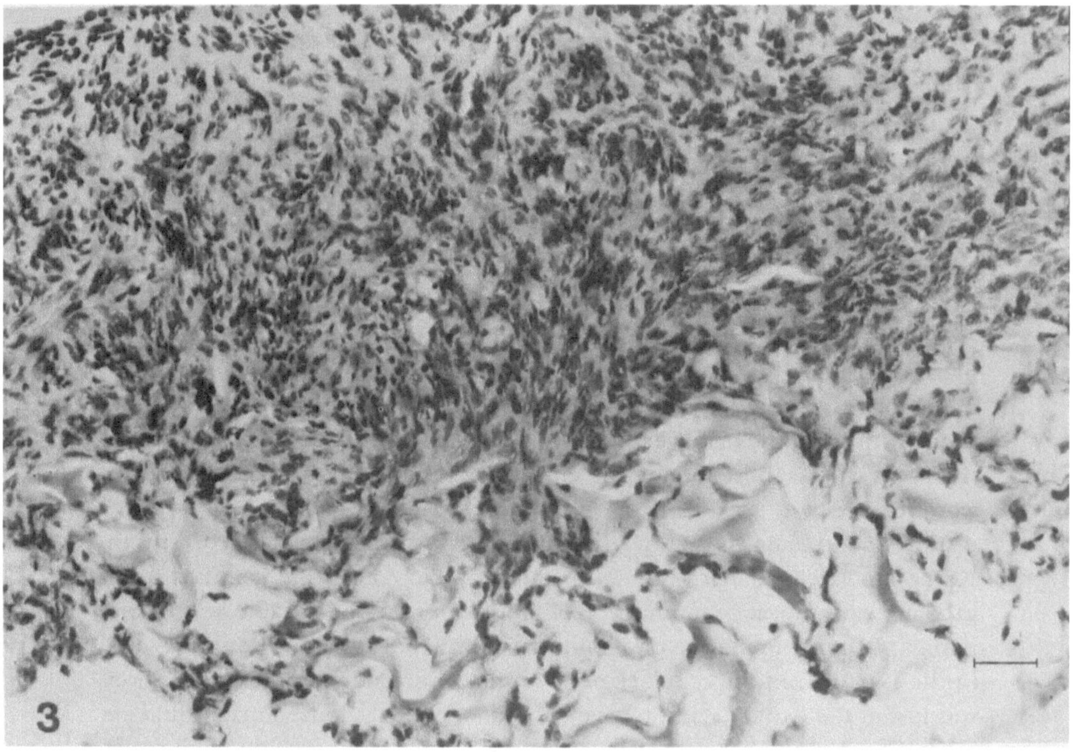

3

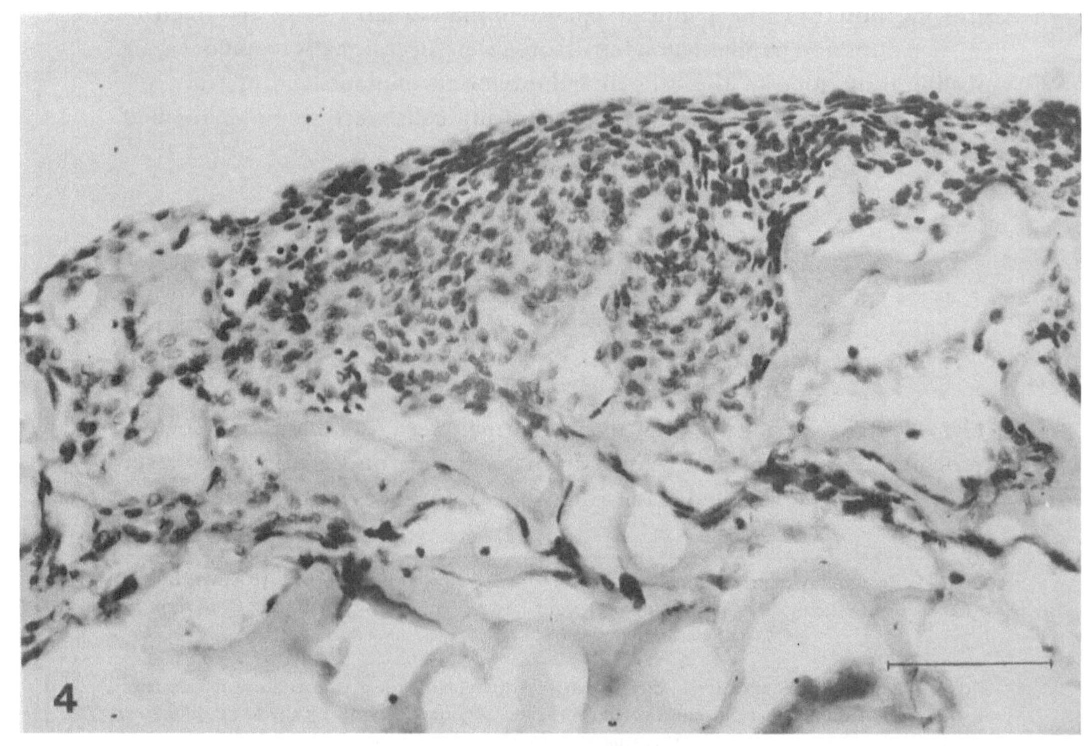

3.4. Others

One specimen of a malignant papilloma of the choroid plexus was grown on the fibrin foam. The explants remained viable and preserved their typical histological structure. Penetration into the lacunae was slight or failed, and at most only a few cells lined the walls of the lacunae of the matrix. Consequently, no characteristic structures were formed.

One case of a chordoma derived from the clivus region was grown on the matrix. Histologically the tumor was a malignant one. However, the growth in the matrix was rather poor; most of the explants became necrotic, and the outgrowth from the viable explants was slight. It consisted of single cells of the same type as those seen in the mother explant and no typical structures were formed.

Two ependymonas, one of grade I and one of grade III, according to Kernohan (Kernohan *et al.*, 1949), one papillary and one cellular, were grown on the fibrin foam matrix. All explants remained viable and in the papillary ependymona the papillomatous epithelial structure could be seen in the explants. In the cellular ependymona, the pseudo-rosette formation was lost in the explants, but typical cuboidal cell with dense nuclei could be seen. The invasiveness was very slight in both cases, only of grade 1. The cells growing out from the papillary ependymona explants were arranged in small groups and papillomatous structures were occasionally formed. In the proliferating zone of the cellular ependymona explants, no organotypic arrangements could be seen; the outgrowing cells were single or formed small groups.

4. Influence of Various Factors on Growth

4.1. Effect of Various Human Sera

The effects of various noninactivated human sera, i.e., clumping serum, nonclumping serum, and pooled human serum, on cells in monolayer cultures have been studied extensively. The differences in these effects have

FIG. 5. Fourteen-day matrix culture of a neurinoma showing well-preserved structure, but no outgrowth into the matrix. Bar in the lower right-hand corner indicates 10 μm. Copyright by *Acta Pathologica et Microbiologica Scandinavica.*

FIG. 6. Oligodendroglioma after 11 days in matrix culture. Note the great variation in the size of nuclei. Bar in the lower right-hand corner indicates 50 μm. Copyright by *Acta Pathologica et Microbiologica Scandinavica.*

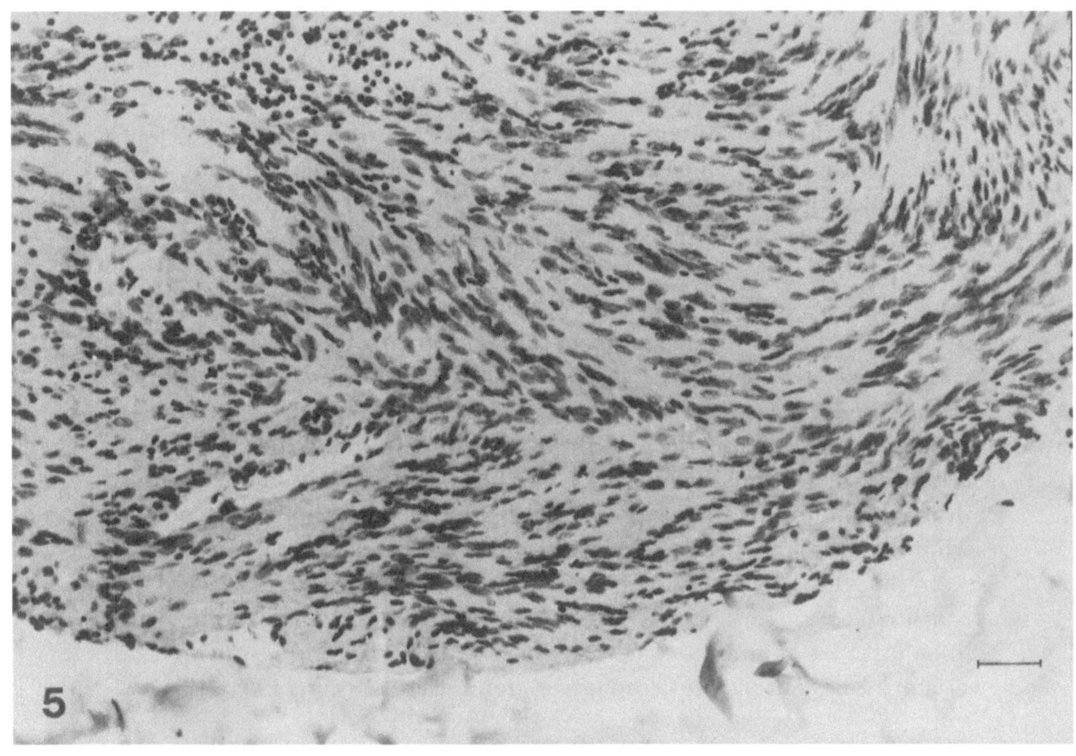
5

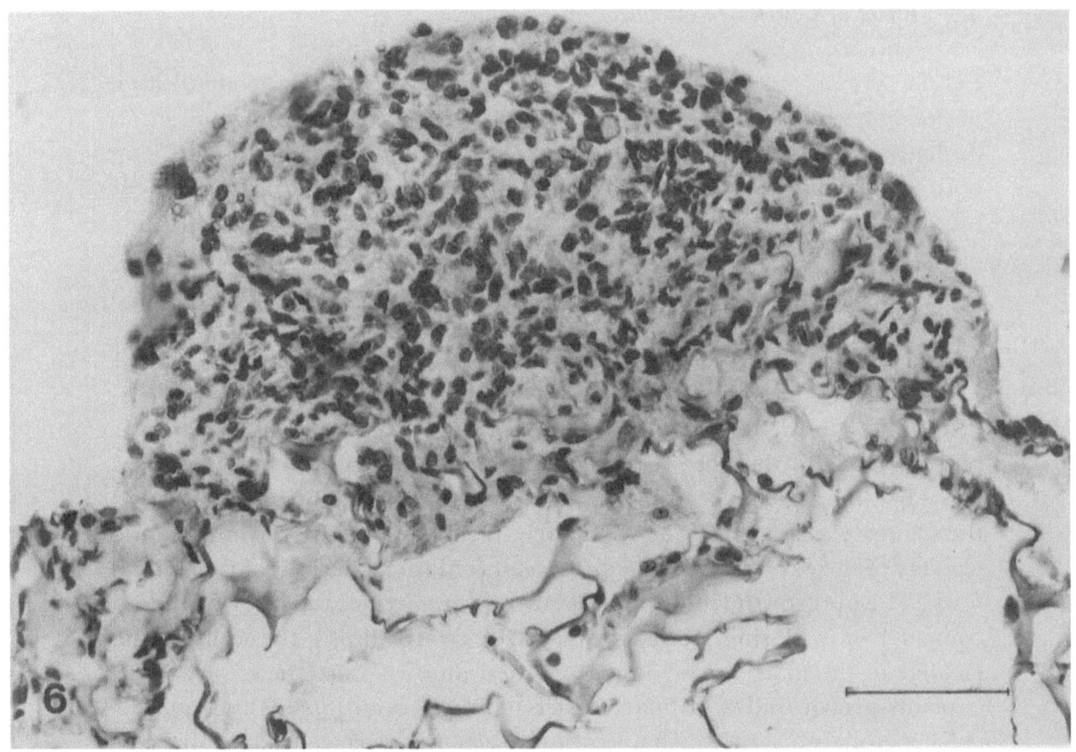
6

been shown to be due to binding of serum components to the growth surface of the cells. The same difference was noted with all tissue culture cell lines studied, both transformed established lines and normal diploid cells. Treatment of the glass surface with these sera generally reduced the number of cells attaching to the surface, the clumping type of serum causing the strongest effect (Nordling, 1967). A certain degree of direct action of these sera on the cells could not be excluded, although the effect was shown to be mostly indirect. This was suggested by data concerning the division behavior of HeLa cells grown in these sera (Saksela, 1962). In the present matrix culture system, these sera were compared with fresh autologous serum. In the benign tumor group, the growth-promoting capacity of the various sera used showed no statistically significant difference. In the glioma group, however, significantly less penetration into the matrix was noted with pooled serum or clumping serum than with autologous serum or nonclumping serum (Fig. 1). The matrix was not pretreated with these sera, as were the growth surfaces in the experiments described above. Therefore, the growth-inhibiting effect of noninactivated serum pool and clumping serum must, at least partly, be a direct one, although no definite conclusions can be drawn.

4.2. *Effect of Chick Mesonephros on Gliomas*

In the organ culture system developed by Wolff and Wolff (1961), mesonephric tissue of chick embryos was used both as nutritional source and as matrix for explants of human tumors, and had a favorable influence on both the viability and the growth of explants. The effect was not dependent on direct contact between tumor explant and mesonephros tissue; the same effect could be seen when a thin membrane was placed between the two tissues and even in explants grown in conditioned medium. A modification of this system was developed to improve the viability and penetration of glioma explants grown in the fibrin foam matrix culture system. A carpet of pieces of chick mesonephros tissue was prepared on the bottom of a petri dish, and a cube of fibrin foam was placed on this. A tumor tissue explant was placed on top of the fibrin foam cube in the usual way. The mesonephros tissue became attached to and grew into the matrix from the bottom up, and the glioma explant grew into the matrix from the top. By this means, the viability of the explants could be preserved for longer periods of time, up to 6 wk. The outgrowth from the explants was not accelerated, however, and consisted only of single cells or small cell groups lining the walls of the lacunae of the matrix. The depth of penetration was also the same as with explants grown under ordinary matrix culture conditions. If the layer of chick mesonephros on which the culture was placed was sealed in a thin layer of gelatin, no effect at all could be noted. A conditioned medium made of chick mesonephros did not have any effect on either the growth capacity or the viability of the explants.

4.3. *Effect of Nerve Growth Factor on Neurinomas*

Nerve growth factor (NGF), MR61 (Wellcome Reagents Ltd., Wellcome Research Laboratories, Beckenham, Kent, England), has been shown to give a good outgrowth of fibers from chick embryo sensory or sympathetic ganglion after 18–24 h incubation at 37°C (Cohen, 1959). One unit of NGF per milliliter of final tissue culture medium has generally been used. To the present matrix cultures of neurinoma explants, NGF was added to the growth medium in two different strengths, 1 unit/ml and 3 units/ml final concentration. Fresh NGF in the same concentrations was added every second day, and the next day, i.e., on days 3 and 5 of cultivation, the cultures were terminated and treated in the usual manner. The penetration and viability were compared with those of explants from the same tumors grown under standard conditions. The viability of the explants and the outgrowth of cells were equally good in all three lines; no significant differences were noted. The penetration into the matrix was grade 1 or 2, and the outgrowing cells lined the walls of the lacunae and did not form any organotypic cell aggregates. The typical histological structure of the primary explants, with interlacing cell bundles and nuclear palisading, was well preserved.

5. *Reaggregation of Cells from Primary Monolayer Cultures*

5.1. *Glioma Cells and Normal Glia Cells*

Normal glia cells were cultivated from brain tissue obtained from a patient undergoing a neurosurgical operation for a meningioma where resection was necessary. The cells of two gliomas (astrocytoma grades III and IV) were used in two different experiments each and the normal glia cells served as controls. The cells were harvested by trypsinization and centrifuged at 1000 rpm so that a cell pellet formed at the bottom of the centrifuge tube. A small piece of the pellet was placed on top of the matrix with a Pasteur pipette. Three cultures of every line were set up and the cultures were terminated at 1-wk intervals. The glioma cells remained viable and lined the walls of the lacunae; they were pleomorphic, with variations in nuclear size and shape. They never filled a whole lacuna, and did not reproduce any structures. The viability of the nonneoplastic glia cells was much lower, and only a few cells stayed viable and lined the walls of the lacunae without forming any structures.

5.2. Meningiomas

Two meningotheliomatous meningiomas were used as a cell source and the primary monolayer cultures were made by routine methods. The matrix cultures were set up in the same manner as described for glioma cells and normal glia cells. The meningioma cells showed good growth in monolayer cultures, and the cells remained viable in the matrix cultures. Penetration into the matrix was of grade 1–3, and the cells were arranged in small groups and the lacunae were sometimes filled. A concentric organization of the cells as in psammoma bodies was occasionally seen.

5.3. Neurinomas

The cells in the pellet from the primary monolayer cultures of two neurinomas did not show any reaggregation or formation of neurinoma-like structures. Penetration into the matrix was chiefly the same as for cells growing out from primary explants; i.e., the cells lined the walls of the lacunae and did not form any typical structures.

6. Conclusions

As compared with monolayer cultures, this fibrin foam organ culture system offers certain advantages. The maintenance of the original morphology of tissue and the cells in the proliferating zone may be due to the microenvironment created within the small lacunae of the foam matrix. Essential nutrients produced by the cells themselves are perhaps not diluted into the medium, and a cross-feeding following the principles demonstrated by Eagle and Piez (1962) can take place. For these reasons, reaggregation of dispersed cells theoretically should take place more easily, and this was shown to be the case for meningioma cells but not for normal glia, glioma, or neurinoma cells.

This type of matrix culture system may, however, be further developed for studies on tumor responses to different exogenous influences. The growth of the tumor explant into the matrix can be graded, and the proliferative activity of the tumor *in vitro* can be measured. The method is rather rough, however, and growth is not always good enough to yield statistically significant differences. The measurement of DNA synthesis by radioautography on histological sections of labeled cultures is more exact, and smaller differences are detected by this method, but it is too laborious and expensive for routine use. The easiest and most exact method seems to be to count the radioactivity in the whole culture with a scintillation counter and then correlate it with the amount of DNA in the culture, the result being expressed as an activity index. However, some technical problems remain unsolved.

The system is generally hampered in long-term cultures by the increasing amount of necrosis of the primary explants. The continuous maintenance of cell proliferation necessary for increased penetration into the matrix has not been achieved even with growth-promoting factors. However, it is hoped that in the future technical difficulties will be resolved and the full potential of the matrix culture methods may be applied, for example, to the analysis of tumor responses to therapeutic substances.

7. *References*

Cohen, S., 1959, Purification and metabolic effects of a nerve growth–promoting protein from snake venom, *J. Biol. Chem.* **234:**1129–1137.

Eagle, H., and Piez, H., 1962, The population-dependent requirement by cultured mammalian cells for metabolites which they can synthesize, *J. Exp. Med.* **116:**29–43.

Easty, G. C., and Easty, D. M., 1963, An organ culture system for the examination of tumor invasion, *Nature (Lond.)* **199:**1104–1105.

Holmström, T., and Saksela, E., 1971, Growth of human brain tumor explants in matrix cultures in different human sera, *Acta Pathol. Microbiol. Scand.* **79:**399–406.

Holmström, T., Saksela, E., Nyström, S., and Saxén, E., 1970, Growth of human brain tumors in matrix cultures in fresh autologous serum, *Acta Pathol. Microbiol. Scand.* **78:**313–322.

Kalus, M., and Klement, V., 1966, Cultivation of organ fragments on fibrin foam, *Folia Biol. Praha* **12:**468–472.

Kalus, M., Ghidoni, J. J., and O'Neil, R. M., 1968, Growth of tumors in matrix cultures, *Cancer* **22:**507–516.

Kernohan, J. W., Mahon, R. F., Svien, H. J., and Adson, A. W., 1949, Simplified classification of gliomas, *Proc. Mayo Clin.* **24:**71–75.

Kersting, G., 1968, Tissue cultures of human gliomas, in: *Progress of Neurological Surgery*, Vol. 2, pp. 165–202, Karger, New York.

Leighton, J., 1951, A sponge matrix method for tissue culture: Formation of organized aggregates of cells *in vitro*, *J. Natl. Cancer Inst.* **12:**545–561.

Leighton, J., 1954, The growth patterns of some transplantable animal tumors in sponge matrix tissue cultures, *J. Natl. Cancer Inst.* **15:**275–293.

Leighton, J., Justh, G., and Esper, M., 1967, Collagen-coated cellulose sponge: Three-dimensional matrix for tissue culture of Walker tumor 256, *Science* **155:**1259–1261.

Nordling, S., 1967, Adhesiveness, growth behaviour and charge density of cultured cells, *Acta Pathol. Microbiol. Scand. Suppl.* **192:**1–100.

Pontén, J., and McIntyre, E. H., 1968, Long term culture of normal and neoplastic human glia, *Acta Pathol. Microbiol. Scand.* **74:**465–486.

Saksela, E., 1962, The effect of different human sera on the karyologic picture of HeLa cells: A contribution to the knowledge of environmental influences on cell populations, *Acta Pathol. Microbiol. Scand.* **153:**1–73.

Trowell, O. A., 1954, A modified technique for organ cultures *in vitro, Exp. Cell Res.* **6:**246–248.

Wahlström, T., Saksela, E., Troupp, H., and Nyström, S., 1969, The growth of normal and neoplastic human glia in association with autologous and homologous lymphocytes *in vitro, Scand. J. Clin. Lab. Invest.* **23:**72 (Suppl. 108).

Wolff, Et., 1963, Long-term organotypic cultures of human surgical tumors at the expense of substances elaborated by the mesonephros of chick embryo, in: Symposium on Organ Cultures *Natl. Cancer Inst. Monogr.* **11:**180–195.

Wolff, Et., and Wolff, Em., 1961, Le rôle du mésonephros de l'embryon de poulet dans la nutrition de cellules cancéreuses. II. Etude par la méthode de la membrane vitelline, *J. Embryol. Exp. Morphol.* **9:**678–690.

Neoplastic Human Glia Cells in Culture

7

Jan Pontén

1. *Introduction*

The panorama of human malignant tumors is by far the best described in nature. Over 100 different histogenetic varieties are known, and their biological traits have been abundantly documented. Their *in vitro* characterization lags far behind, however, mainly because of the considerable technical difficulties involved in establishing cultures from human neoplastic tissue. Primary explants usually yield only necrobiotic neoplastic cells which rapidly die out. Such cultures have found a limited use in connection with certain morphological problems, but have in the main been disappointing. Permanent lines of proven neoplastic origin which would be of much greater general value are still few in number. It would be of immense importance if a method could be invented by which all types of neoplasia could be reproducibly grown in the laboratory in long-term culture.

With appropriate technique, a fairly high proportion of explants of human gliomas develop into permanent lines (Manuelidis, 1969; Pontén and Macintyre, 1968; Westermark *et al.*, 1973). This chapter will stress this aspect rather than morphological studies on early cultures, a subject which has been reviewed elsewhere (Manuelidis, 1965; Lumsden, 1963; Kersting, 1961; Nakai, 1963; Windle, 1958).

Jan Pontén Division of Cell Biology, The Wallenberg Laboratory, University of Uppsala, Uppsala, Sweden

Human cells from normal tissues have a notable experimental advantage over those from most other species in their remarkable stability in tissue culture (Swim and Parker, 1957; Hayflick and Moorhead, 1961). The cells have a uniform morphology resembling that *in vivo*, a diploid karyotype, well-regulated proliferation and locomotion, and a finite life span. The last parameter, manifested by the gradual development of irreversible degenerative alterations after a period of perfect viability, makes it possible to use infinite growth as a simple criterion for neoplastic origin of derived cells (Pontén and Macintyre, 1968). Human lymphoid cells are the only exception to this rule, since permanent lines can be established with ease from apparently normal cells (Moore *et al.*, 1967; Nilsson *et al.*, 1968). This is not the case with mice and other unstable species, where one always (i.e., even in tumors other than malignant lymphomas) has to rule out that stroma cells which have undergone spontaneous infinite growth transformation *in vitro* make up the resulting permanent lines rather than the neoplastic cells themselves (Pontén, 1971).

We have shown that nonneoplastic glia cells behave as other nonlymphoid human cells. They grow as diploid, morphologically simplified astrocytes (Fig. 1) which always die out *in vitro*, usually after some 20 passages (Pontén and Macintyre, 1968). Against this background one can be confident that any line of glial origin—regardless of its morphology, metabolic requirements, chromosome constitution, etc.—can be regarded as being of neoplastic origin as soon as it distinguishes itself by an infinite life span.

2. *Technical Procedures*

Glioma cells are as a group easier to establish in short- and long-term tissue culture than any other human neoplasia (except possibly Burkitt's lymphoma). Carcinomas almost invariably die out very quickly (Moore and Koike, 1964), whereas sarcomas (Pontén and Saksela, 1967; McAllister *et al.*, 1969) and melanomas (Oettgen *et al.*, 1968) seem to have an intermediate position.

Early pioneering work used the plasma clot technique (Lumsden, 1963; Kersting, 1961; Nakai, 1963; Windle, 1958). The method made it possible to study the morphology and growth pattern of different types of intracranial tumors with accuracy. As a rule, all the major histological groups maintained enough of their structural traits to permit classification *in vitro*. Attempts at correlating microscopic grade of malignancy with tissue culture appearance

FIG. 1. Normal human glia cells in culture. Regular monolayers of monomorphic cells.

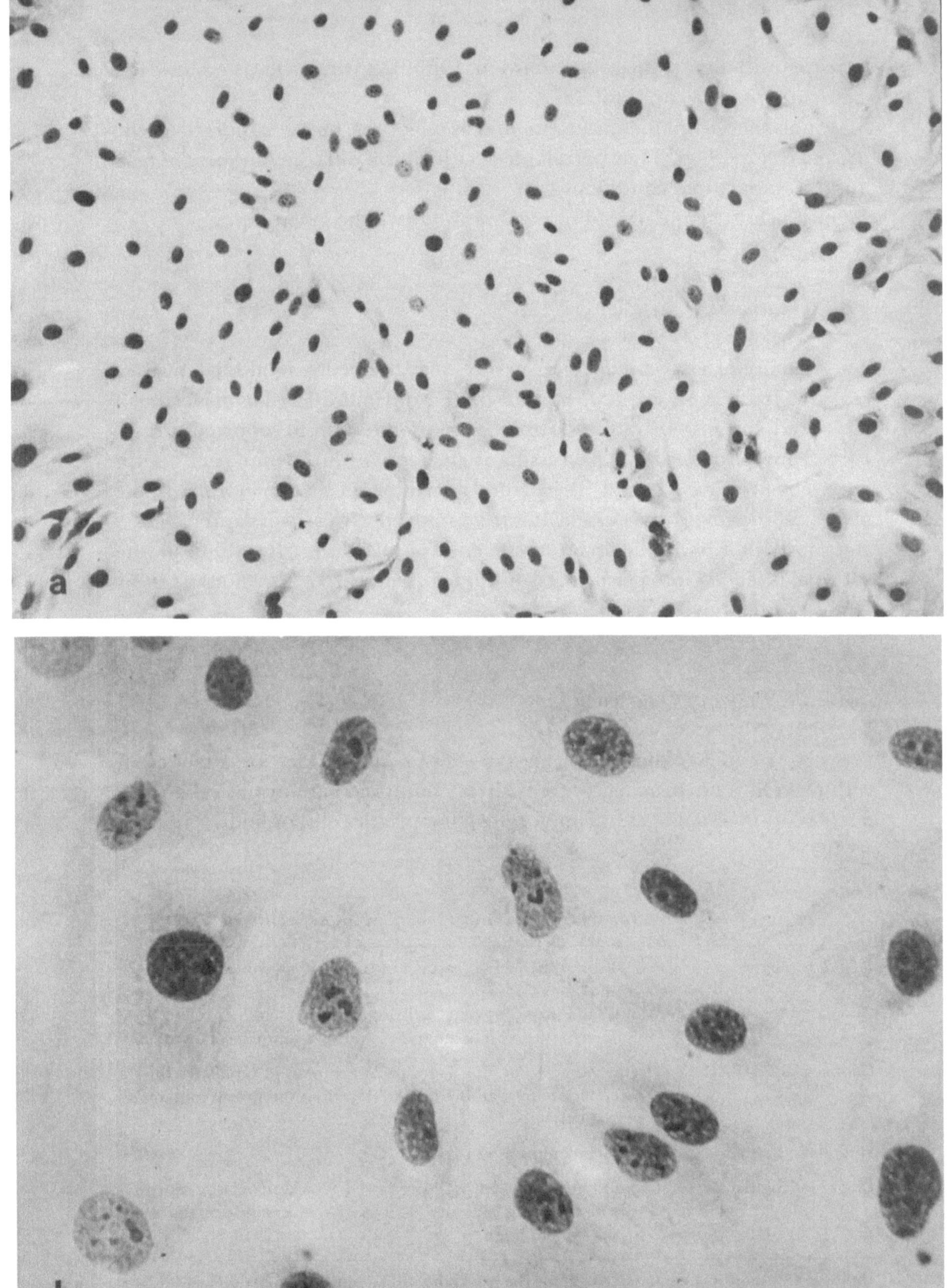

have met with limited success (Lumsden, 1963; Kersting, 1964) and have not led to any practical applications.

Monolayer techniques have, in this as in other fields, superseded the plasma clot method. They permit serial cultivation of large numbers of cells under standardized conditions.

Only a short summary of our own methods will be given here.

2.1. *Treatment of the Biopsy*

The viability of extirpated tumor tissue starts to decline immediately after removal from the patient. The rate of the devitalization has never been measured, but may be rather slow since Manuelidis (1965) reported success even from autopsies. Our processing is started within 30 min after operation. The specimen is first freed from necrotic and grossly normal tissue including meninges and vessels. It is then minced with scissors and pipetted vigorously in a few milliliters of tissue culture medium. After dilution, the material is seeded into plastic petri dishes incubated at 37°C in moist CO_2–air atmosphere to give a pH of 7.2.

2.2. *The Primary Outgrowth*

Properly treated explants will always show some degree of attachment within 24 h. The primary outgrowth is composed of normal cells (glia, fibroblasts, macrophages, meningocytes), neoplastic cells, or both. Its extent

TABLE 1

Character of Primary Outgrowth in Human Malignant Glioma

Histology	Distinctive features of primary outgrowth
Glioma grade I–II	Always dominated by cells indistinguishable from outgrowth from nonneoplastic brain tissue; never transition into permanent lines
Glioma grade III–IV	Highly variable, ranging from no attachment to rapid attachment with efficient migration and proliferation; this group contains all permanent lines
Medulloblastoma[a]	No attachment of tumor cells
Oligodendroglioma[a]	Rapid attachment with well-preserved typical neoplastic morphology in migrating cells; at a later stage irreversible deterioration; no permanent lines

[a] Still too few biopsies examined to exclude the possibility that a minor proportion would show another behavior than that indicated in the table.

and quality differ considerably from case to case. The reasons for this variation are partly obscure, but some guidelines were obtained from a study of 88 specimens in an unselected consecutive series (Westermark *et al.*, 1973). Table 1 shows that glioma grade III–IV and oligodendroglioma have given the most favorable primary cultures.

The malignant gliomas undergo large alterations in their composition during the first few passages. In a proportion of the cases where the malignant elements are virtually unable to attach, the cultures will soon be completely composed of normal glia and fibroblasts. In other instances, the glioma cells attach and migrate well but nevertheless fail to survive subculturing, a development also seen in oligodendroglioma. In a third group, the malignant elements will start to multiply and eventually form established lines as elaborated below.

2.3. Serial Passage

Glioma cultures can be grown in any standard medium for mammalian cells. We have used Eagle's MEM (Eagle, 1959) supplemented with 10% young calf serum and antibiotics. Subcultivation is done by trypsinization. It is important not to seed the cells too sparsely, and 1:2 splits are recommended for routine purposes.

2.4. Storage

Standard procedures with addition of dimethyl sulfoxide, slow freezing, and maintenance in liquid nitrogen preserve human glioma cells with essentially unimpaired viability for many years.

3. Determinants for the Establishment of Permanent Glioma Lines

From previous work with gliomas as well as other malignancies, the impression has been gained that the establishment of lines is a random event (Moore and Koike, 1964). The probability is very low for carcinomas and higher for gliomas. It follows that no predictions about the chances for success can be made at the time when the cultures are started. Westermark *et al.* (1973) investigated gliomas systematically from this point of view. Table 2 summarizes the negative and positive factors found to influence rate of establishment. It reveals an unexpected and totally unexplained fact—that

TABLE 2

Determinants for the Establishment of Permanent Tissue Culture Lines from Human Gliomas

	Influence on establishment of permanent lines	
	Favorable	Unfavorable
Histological type	Glioma grade III–IV	Glioma grade I + II, ependymona, oligodendroglioma
Site of tumor	Temporoparietal region	Other locations
Sex of patient	Male	Female
Age of patient	No systematic influence established	
Cytology of primary outgrowth	Presence of spindle cells (bipolar neuroblasts?)	Well-differentiated astrocytes, immature blast cells

male temporoparietal gliomas are easier to establish than any other sex–location combination. In this group, permanent lines were obtained from 12 of 28 (43%) grade III–IV gliomas. This is the highest success rate published for any series of human neoplasms. In the whole series of 68 grade III–IV gliomas, 13 established lines were from men and only one from a woman in spite of an approximately equal sex distribution in the original material. It may be concluded that establishment of gliomas is not altogether a random event but is governed by partially defined factors intrinsic to the tumor and/or its bearer.

4. *Properties of Neoplastic Human Glia in Vitro*

A probably incomplete survey of the literature indicates that more than 50 glioma lines have been claimed as permanently established lines. Unfortunately, many of these (Manuelidis, 1969) have not been properly identified and some may be extraneous cell contaminants. Nevertheless, Table 3 underlines the fact that gliomas are easier to cultivate than other human malignancies.

4.1. *Morphological Spectrum*

In vivo malignant gliomas are characterized by a multitude of different forms—a fact clearly reflected by a complex nomenclature. In long-term

TABLE 3

Human Glioma Lines Reported in the Literature

Author	Number of permanent lines	Reference
Manuelidis	28	*Ann. N.Y. Acad. Sci. 159*:409, 1969
Wilson *et al.*	7	*Arch. Neurol. 15*:275, 1966
Westermark *et al.*	18[a]	*Acta Pathol. Microbiol. Scand. Sect. A, 81*:791, 1973
Maunoury *et al.*	5	*Neurol. Chir. 18*:8, 1972

[a] Most of these lines have been individually identified by surface antigens, isozymes, and chromosomes to exclude contamination by HeLa cells or cross-contamination within the glioma line collection (Beckman *et al.*, 1971).

cultures *in vitro*, considerable simplification has taken place. Established cell lines tend to become cytologically much more uniform than the multiform picture encountered *in vivo*. Certain permanent alterations have been observed after many passages (Manuelidis, 1969), but most reported glioma lines seem to be remarkably stable even after many years *in vitro*. Table 4 and Figs. 2–6 show five main categories into which established glioma lines may

TABLE 4

A Morphological Grouping of Human Glioma Lines Established at the Wallenberg Laboratory, Uppsala

Characteristic feature	Designation of cell line
Astrocytoid (Fig. 2)	251 MG Cl.*a*[a]; 343 MG; 348 MG; 495 MG Cl.*a*[a]; 539 MG
Pleomorphic (Fig. 3)	373 MG
Epithelioid (Fig. 4)	87 MG; 251 MG Cl.*e*[a]; 343 MG
Bipolar (Fig. 5)	105 MG; 118 MG; 138 MG; 178 MG; 251 MG Cl.*b*[a]; 372 MG; 399 MG; 410 MG; 489 MG; 495 MG Cl.*b*[a]; 563 MG; 692 MG; 716 MG
Bimorphic (Fig. 6)	706 MT[b]

[a] Clones obtained by single cell isolations *in vitro*.
[b] Origin from glia cells never proven. See caption of Fig. 6.

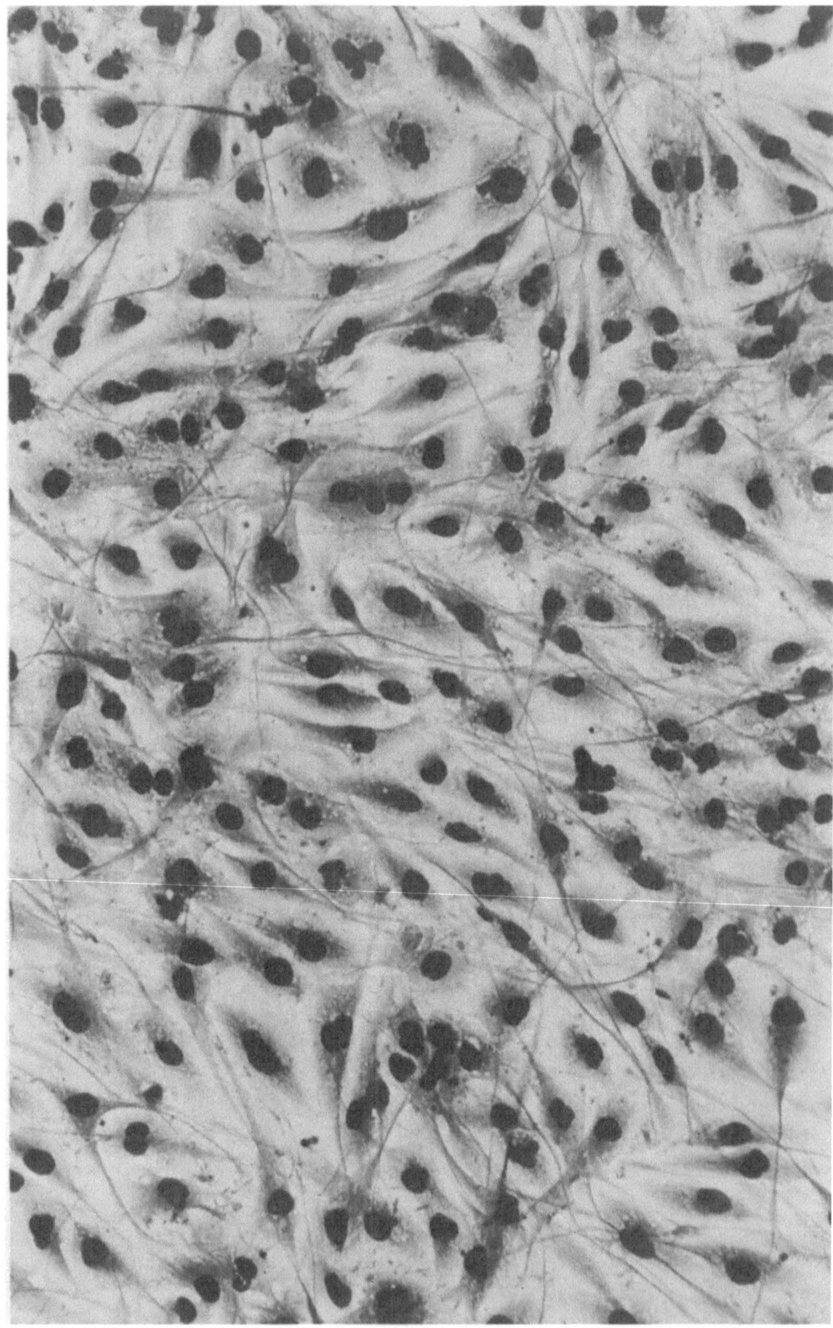

FIG. 2. Clone *a* from line 251 MG displaying typical astrocytoid morphology with well-developed long, branching cytoplasmic extensions.

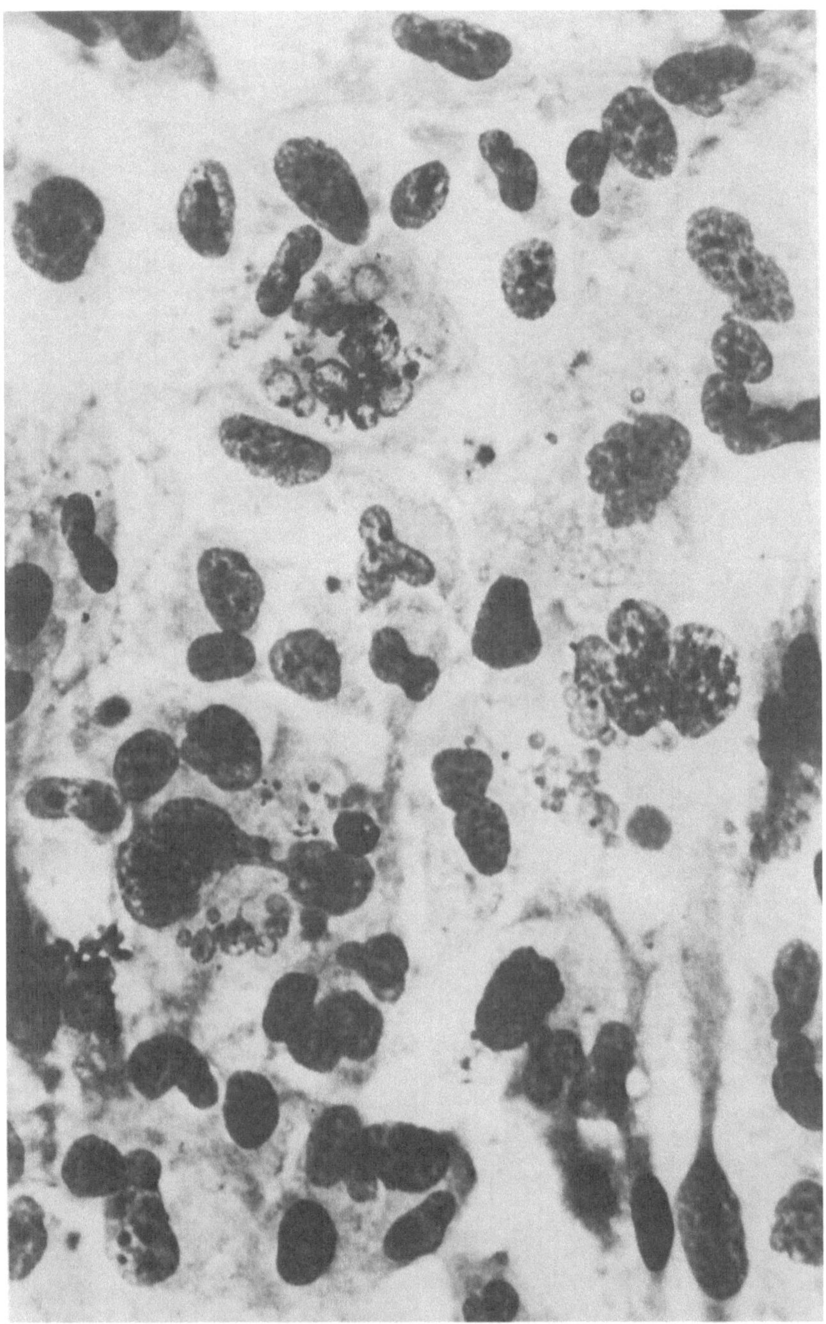

FIG. 3. Pleomorphic glioma line (373 MG) with highly irregular nuclei.

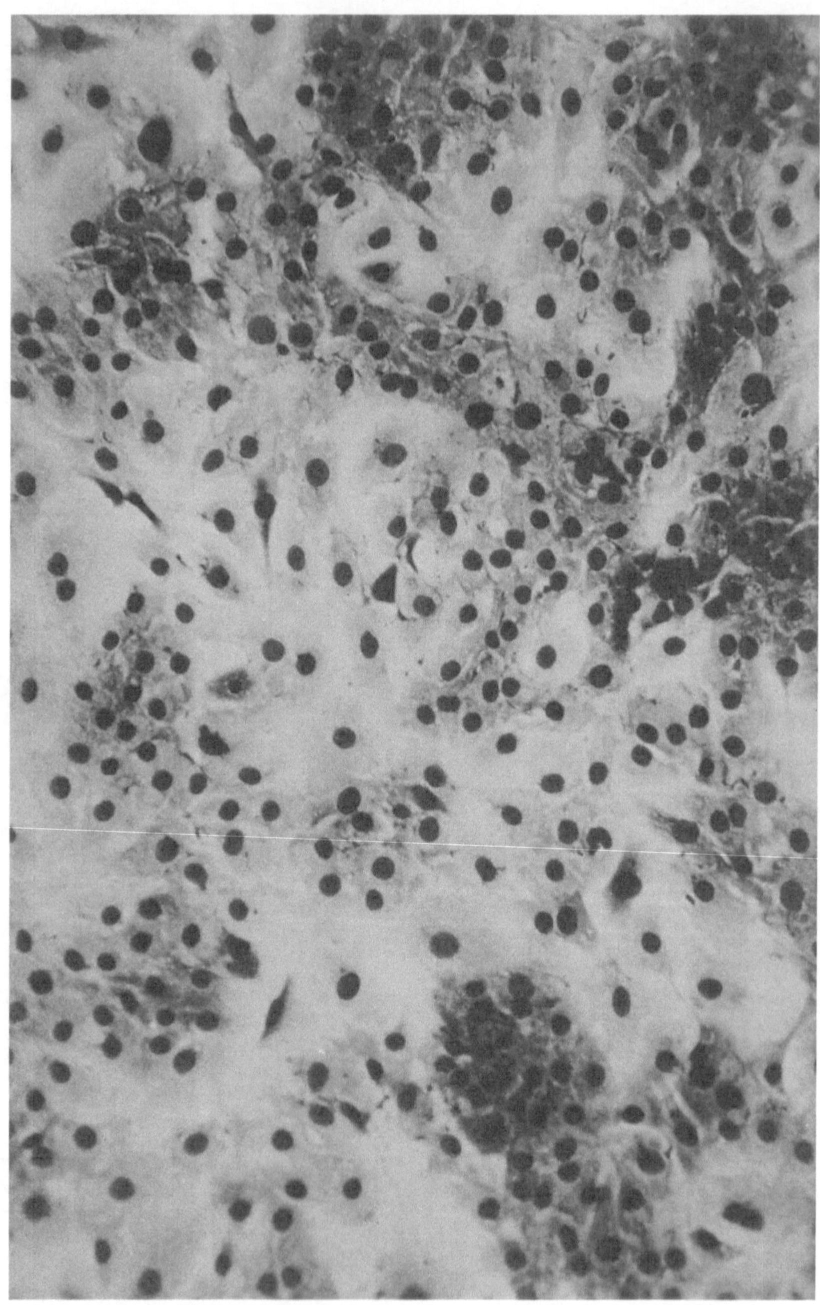

FIG. 4. Example of epithelioid glioma line (87 MG) with polygonal, often well-spaced cells without any definite polarity. Irregular growth pattern with focal heaping up of cells.

be grouped, but the experienced observer may be able to discern subtle individual differences within the groups. In a few instances, clones have been isolated which differ morphologically from the wild cell population (Table 4).

4.2. Medium Requirements

No large systematic studies have been performed on the metabolic needs of neoplastic human glia cells in culture. We have failed to find any difference between Ham's F-10 (Ham, 1963) and Eagle's MEM in the capacity to support growth. Also, adult human serum and fetal and newborn calf serum are equally effective. The optimal serum concentration seems to be around 10%.

4.3. Formation of Permanent Lines

In our unselected material of grade III–IV gliomas, the frequency of permanent lines was about 20%. If, however, only male parietotemporal tumors were considered, this figure rose almost to 50%. In almost all instances, it was possible to predict within 1 month after explantation whether any given line would be established. At this time, atypical cells should multiply well enough to permit repeated subcultivations. Those explants which fail to develop into permanent lines usually lose their tumor cells after a short time in culture, and by 1 month only normal cells will be found. Multiple pieces from the same tumor carried in parallel behave in the same fashion; i.e., either established lines will develop from all primary cultures or there will be neoplastic cell degeneration in all of them roughly simultaneously. This shows that factors intrinsic to the tumor take part in determining whether a given neoplasm will show the property of endless multiplication *in vitro*.

4.4. Density-Dependent Proliferation Control: Topoinhibition

Normal glia cells are characterized by an unusually strict proliferation control which is directly related to the local cell density. Figure 7 shows a typical growth curve. It is seen that virtually no multiplication (monitored by DNA synthesis and cell counting) takes place beyond a terminal density of 70,000 cells/cm^2. This corresponds to a moderately crowded monolayer (Fig. 1) where all cells have established stable and extensive cytoplasmic contact, but no nuclear overlapping. At this stage, the cells are reversibly arrested in the G_1 phase of the cell cycle. If a layer is scored mechanically, the glia adjacent to the wound will enter DNA synthesis after a delay of about 20 h and proliferate until the defect is healed. This behavior is characteristic of cells with well-preserved growth control and is often regarded as a reflection of one of the mechanisms which *in vivo* keeps the cell number constant in "stationary tissues with latent capacity for regeneration" (e.g., glia, connective tissue, liver, kidney epithelium).

Deviations from the stringent density-related multiplication control characteristic of nonneoplastic human glia have been studied in several representatives from the morphological glioma groups of Table 4. *Maximal exponential growth rate* of cells not in contact with each other varied from line to line. The average value was somewhat lower than that of normal glia. Lines were found which multiplied faster or slower than the control cells. Maximal growth rate of sparse cells does thus not constitute a discriminating feature between nonneoplastic and neoplastic glia cells in culture. *Terminal cell density* (TCD) (Fig. 7) also varied within wide limits among the glioma lines. To avoid undue influence of cell shape and size, we have used a crowding index (C.I.) to express one aspect of defunct multiplication control. It is defined as the ratio between cell concentration at terminal density and the concentration of cells necessary to just cover a given growth area (Westermark, 1973*a*). For normal glia grown under standard conditions the C.I. is 1.4. Eight tested glioma lines showed an increased C.I. ranging from 2.0 to 10.2 (Westermark, 1973*b*). This shows that glioma cells are not inhibited at the same low cell concentration as normal glia. In this respect, they resemble animal cells transformed spontaneously or by oncogenic viruses *in vitro* (Pontén, 1971).

Terminal cell density and its corollary, the crowding index, do not *per se* indicate whether the observed absence of a net increase in cell number is caused by inhibited proliferation or a balance between unimpaired multiplication and cell loss. To solve this problem, glioma lines were subjected to radioautography after labeling of DNA with radioactive thymidine. The result was a wide scatter between the individual lines with respect to sensitivity of DNA synthesis to increasing cell density. Some lines (e.g., 87 MG and 118 MG) did not display any density-dependent inhibition of cell multiplication. Other lines showed a moderate response, and a few (i.e., 138 MG and 251 MG) were markedly inhibited at high local cell concentrations

---

FIG. 5. Two examples of glioma lines classified as bipolar, indicating the morphological limits. (a) 105 MG, which is partly polygonal but shows a sufficient degree of cell polarity to justify its inclusion in the bipolar group. (b) 178 MG, with extremely elongated bipolar cells almost resembling fibroblasts.

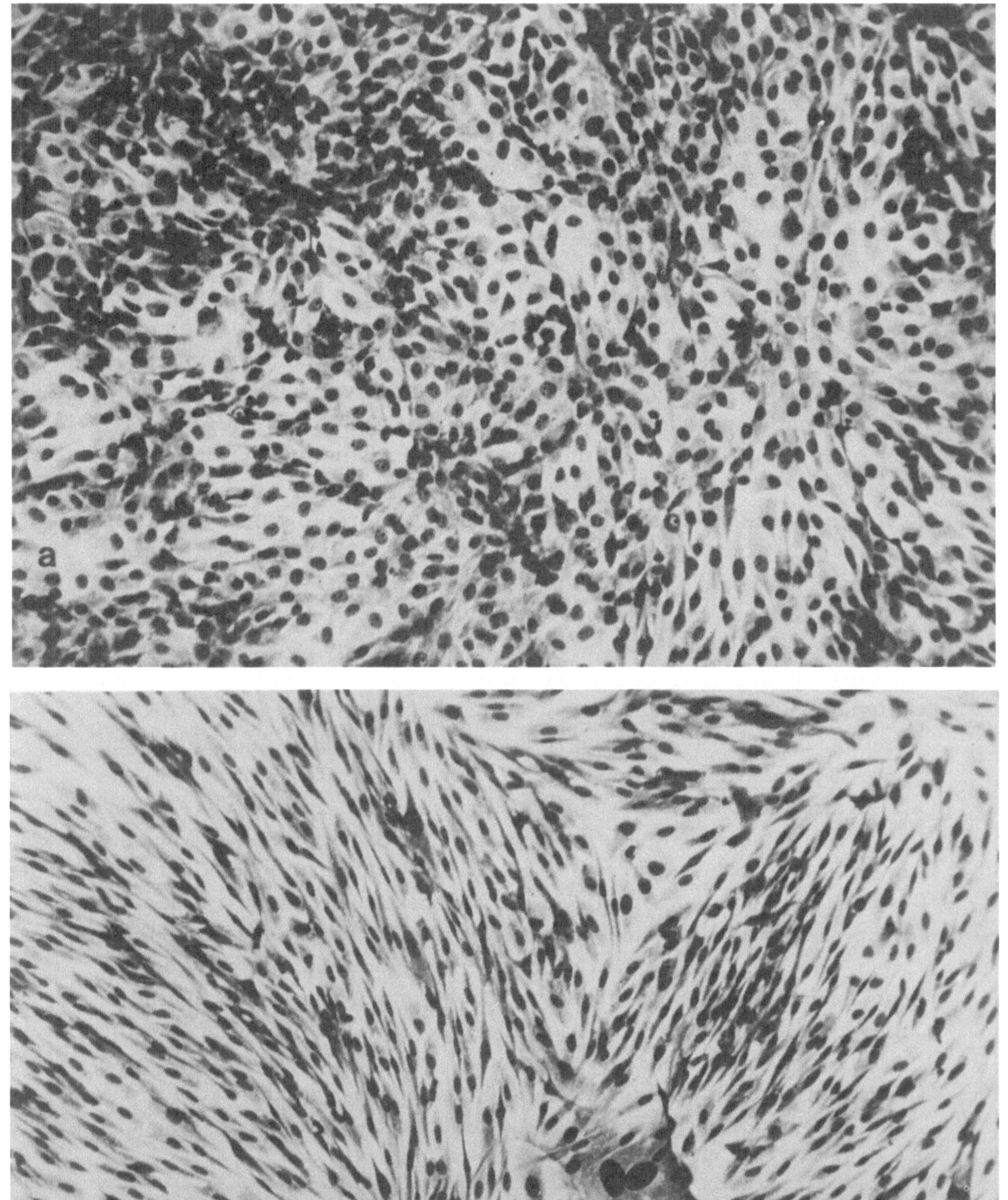
a
b

(Westermark, 1973*b*). Further analysis of these phenomena suggested that most glioma lines responded to increased cell density with a diminished growth rate. However, the response was abnormally sluggish and never complete. All glioma lines analyzed showed a small but significant escape or *residual DNA synthesis* which could not be further depressed by increasing the local glioma cell concentration.

Residual DNA synthesis has been established in all glioma lines and in glia cells transformed by oncogenic viruses. We suggest that the inability of transformed cells to completely shut down proliferation as a response to increased local density may be the most important *in vitro* indication of their deficient growth control. It is presumably a better approximation of *in vivo* growth conditions than, for instance, rapid logarithmic growth of sparse cells. The nature of this malfunction will probably not be elucidated until more is known about normal cell multiplication control.

From experiments with glia which largely conform to similar studies on rodent (Todaro *et al.*, 1965) and chicken (Temin, 1971) cells, we know that terminal-density cells are blocked at a point of the cell cycle which is at least 18 h before the G_1–S transition. Resting glia cells may be triggered into the cell cycle by the addition of fresh serum (Pontén *et al.*, 1969) or by mechanical wounding of the cell sheet (Westermark, 1973*b*,*c*). In both instances, nuclear DNA synthesis can be registered after a delay of 18 h. Preliminary data (A. Lindgren *et al.*, unpublished, 1973) suggest that the "pre-S" period can be divided into two parts: G_0 and G_{1c} in principally the same manner as has been suggested for embryonic chicken cells (Temin, 1971). G_{1c} is defined as the period prior to the DNA synthesis phase when the interphase cell is tooled up with respect to gross content of macromolecules essential for DNA synthesis. In G_0, cells cannot start DNA synthesis because the necessary metabolic steps have not been taken. It is a true resting phase where the cell is committed to other functions than preparations for subsequent division. Since it has to take time to tool up for DNA synthesis, theoretically there must be a period interposed between G_0 and G_{1c} when the cell is still not committed to DNA synthesis but has left the true resting phase and begun preparations for a coming S phase. This hypothetical cell cycle phase, which we may term "G_{1e}" (e stands for "early"), should be reversible,

FIG 6. 706 MT with its two aspects. (a) The surface-attached component with a slight resemblance to certain bipolar lines. (b) Cells spontaneously growing in suspension with no tendency to attach to plastic or glass; rounded, pleomorphic elements characterized by intense bubbling along the outer surface. The original biopsy was from an intracerebral, poorly differentiated tumor, possibly glioblastoma multiforme. However, its origin could never be definitely established histologically and the possibility of metastasis was never excluded, although a careful autopsy failed to reveal any extracranial neoplasia. It is labeled MT (malignant tumor) because of its uncertain nature.

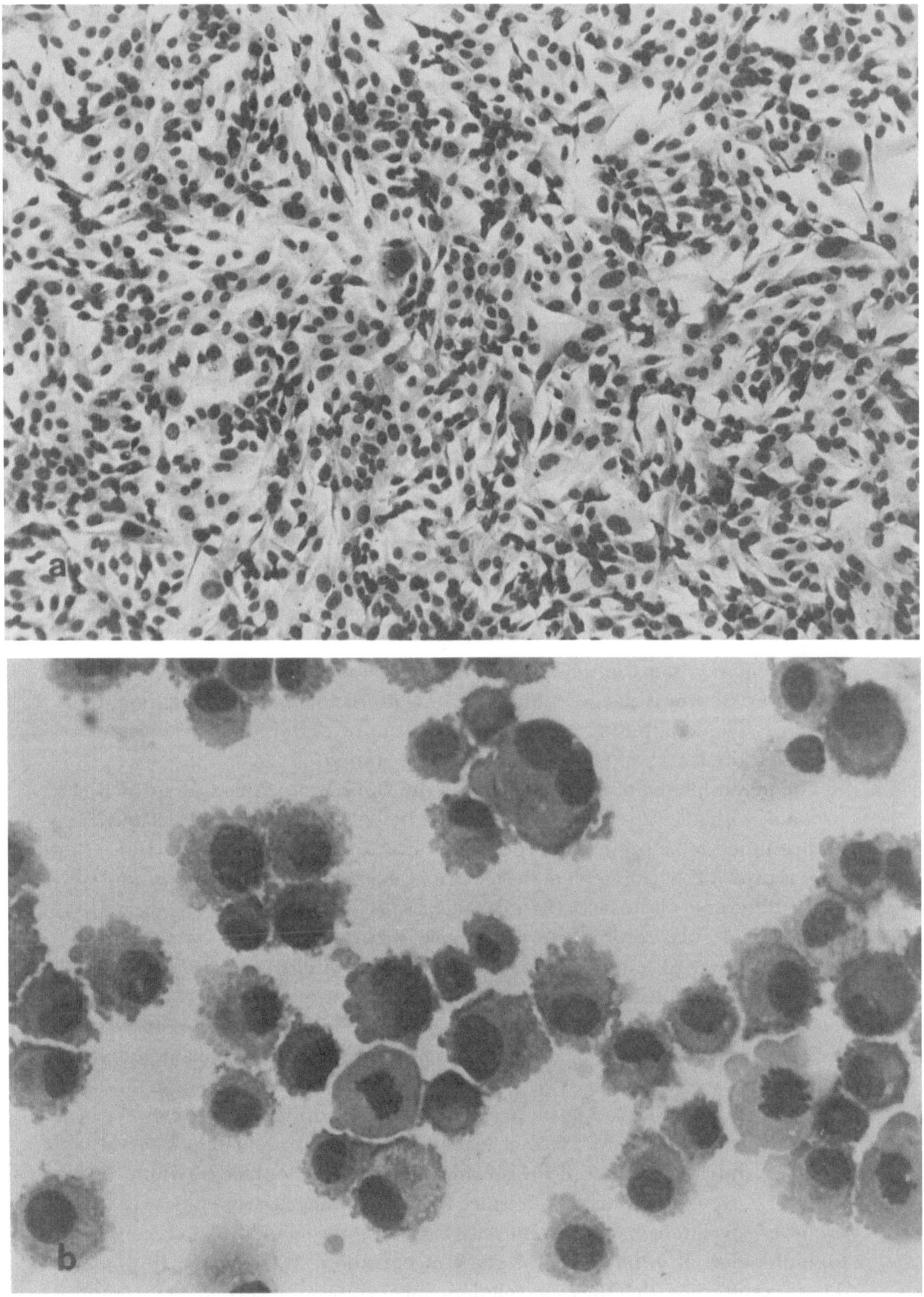

a

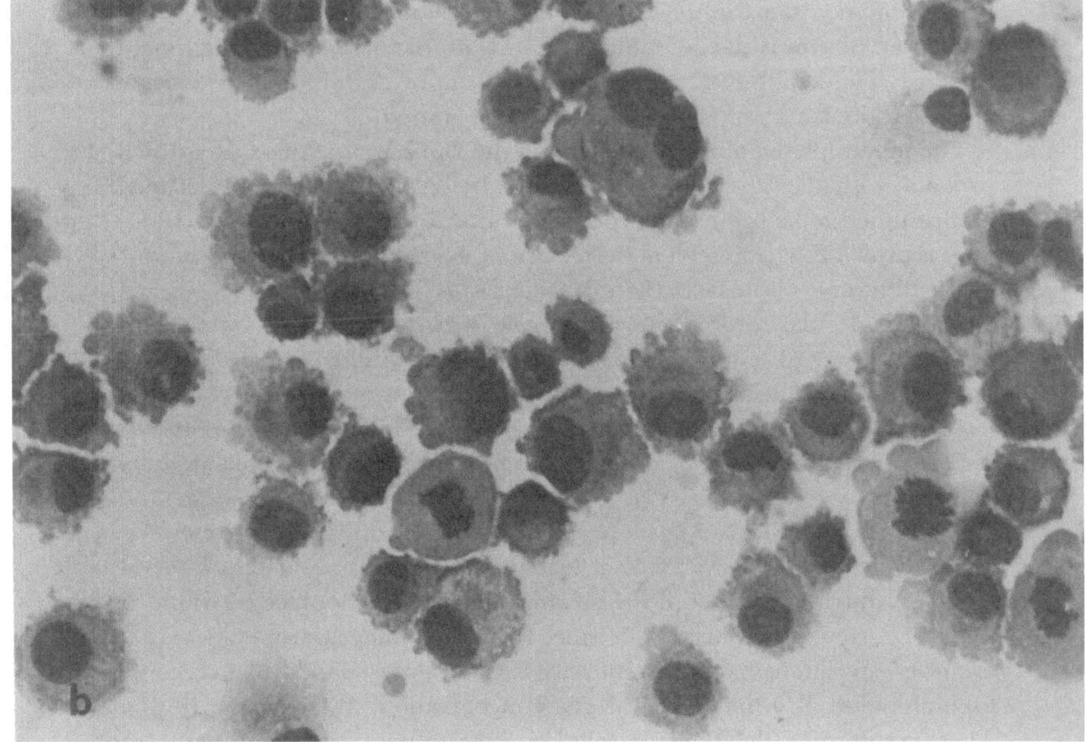

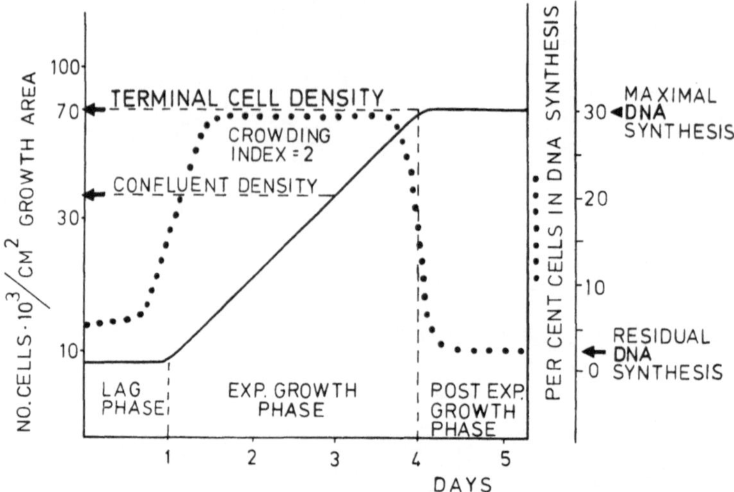

FIG. 7. Schematic representation of the effect of increasing local cell density on the multiplication of normal human glia cells. Note sharp decrease in DNA synthesis at the terminal cell density, where the glia cells remain essentially stationary with insignificant residual DNA synthesis.

permitting reentrance into G_0. The point of no return is located at the G_{1e}–G_{1c} transition. Serum is needed only up to this point for the cell cycle to run forward. The length of G_{1c} is about 4 h; G_0 can by definition be of infinite duration; the length of G_{1e} has not been determined.

The topoinhibited glia cell is resting in the G_0 phase. At this stage, which probably resembles the state of the undisturbed glia cell *in vivo*, the cell may be presumed to be preferentially engaged in its "differentiated" functions. This is probably what is seen in the electron microscope as a "specialization" of the different cell surfaces (Brunk *et al.*, 1971).

Macromolecular serum factors influence the growth state of animal cells profoundly (see review by Temin *et al.*, 1972). One or more components are necessary for survival, attachment, movement, and multiplication (Lipton *et al.*, 1971; Dulbecco, 1970; Temin *et al.*, 1972). The importance of serum factors for multiplication of glia cells has been explored to some extent by our group.

It was first established that there exists a linear relationship between serum concentration and TCD, at least within the concentration interval 5–30%. A fourfold increase of the serum concentration doubled the value of the TCD. Another important inference from the same experiment was that even very frequent medium renewal ("steady state") failed to overcome topoinhibition at a defined local glia concentration (Westermark, 1971). These results show that the extracellular concentrations of certain factors in fresh serum determine the degree of maximal cell packing. Whether this is mediated via permanent alterations in cell shape and/or size or is due to a more direct action of serum on multiplication control has not been determined. The results also show that serum is able to increase the level of TCD but not to prevent topoinhibition from becoming manifest. In general, the findings suggest some sort of antagonism between cellular factors responsible for topoinhibition and serum components which stimulate growth.

Attempts to purify at least one principle involved in the multiplication control have met with partial success. From human plasma, a polypeptide has recently been isolated in highly purified form. It has a molecular weight of about 5000 and may be attached to a larger carrier molecule in native serum. The polypeptide—tentatively named "somatomedin B"—stimulates DNA synthesis in normal glia cells (Westermark and Wasteson, 1974). It is not yet known whether this polypeptide is solely responsible for the serum effect or whether there are additional factors present.

The growth stimulatory serum activity rapidly disappears in the presence of glia cells. The rate of decline and the fate of the presumably degraded molecules remain to be examined.

All glioma lines tested respond pathologically to serum. Rapid growth is sustained by 1% serum or less—concentrations where hardly any multiplication of normal glia will occur. When serum is removed from normal glia, cells beyond the point of no return will complete their cycle to become arrested in G_0. Glioma cells will not show this prompt response but will enter new cell cycles repeatedly even in the absence of serum (B. Westermark *et al.*, unpublished). It will be important to determine whether this apparent relative independence from serum macromolecules can be specifically related to somatomedin B (Uthne, 1973) or other related polypeptides.

This is not the place to go into all the details of the deficient multiplication control of human glioma cells, but the situation may be crudely summarized by the following statements: (1) All glioma lines—regardless of morphology and chromosome constitution—show measurable deviations from the strict topoinhibition of normal glia cells. (2) A superhigh terminal cell density, an increased crowding index, and a capacity to continue proliferation even among stationary normal glia have been obligatory findings in several tested lines. (3) The deficient response to topoinhibition has only occasionally been absolute; in most cases, it seems to be of a quantitative rather than a qualitative nature. (4) All glioma lines need considerably less serum than normal glia to sustain growth and to reach comparable degrees of cell packing. (5) Suggestive evidence exists that glia cells are topoinhibited in a true resting phase (G_0), whereas glioma cells cannot, by topoinhibition alone, be retained in G_0. Instead, there are always cells in G_{1e} or G_{1c} which eventually enter mitosis irrespective of the local cell concentration. (6) Glia cells transformed by simian virus 40 or feline sarcoma virus show the same principal abnormal traits as glioma cells derived from brain tumors (see review by Westermark, 1973*a*).

4.5. Control of Cell Movement

Normal glia cells have been followed by time-lapse cinematography. Their locomotion is governed by a leading lamella equipped with plasma membrane "ruffles" (Abercrombie *et al.*, 1970*a*) traveling backward on the dorsal cell surface (Abercrombie *et al.*, 1970*b*). When the leading lamella encounters the outer surface of another cell, a remarkable series of events will follow. Ruffling is shut off within a few minutes. Instead, an intercellular adhesion is formed. When the leading lamella begins to contract, the cells are pulled together and usually remain affixed to each other. As the cell density increases among a population of multiplying glia, lateral contacts become extensive until the entire growth area is covered at a density of about 35,000 cells/cm^2. Cell division will go on at a reduced rate until the terminal density of about 60,000 cells/cm^2 is reached. Accommodation for this last crop of cells is provided by increased cell packing. This is accomplished by slight thickening and overlapping of the cytoplasm. At their terminal density, the glia cells will form a regular pattern with no overlapping nuclei. The thin outer part of the cytoplasm forms projections which intertwine with each other. In this state, the cells remain in fixed positions having established contacts with each other and with the solid support by means of special attachment devices resembling desmosomes *in vivo* (Brunk *et al.*, 1971).

Glioma lines always show deviations from the pattern above. In extreme cases, ruffling appears to be completely uninfluenced by contact with other cells, in other lines there is almost perfect shutoff of ruffling after contact. All but a few of our lines show "vertical" ruffling. This phenomenon, never seen in normal glia, is characterized by the extrusion of thin ruffles (Fig. 8) directly from the dorsal surface straight up into the fluid medium without the normal origin from the lateral edge. A third abnormal feature is an inability to form normal stable intercellular adhesions. Even in dense cultures, tightly packed cells, with variable frequency between individual lines, will snap back from each other leaving part of the growth area empty.

The effect of the above disturbances is modified by the strength of the adhesions between the ventral cell surface and the solid support. If this force is small, cells will crawl over each other, producing a characteristic criss-cross pattern with much cellular overlapping in dense areas. In cases of strong adhesion to the solid support, cells will remain attached to it in spite of lively

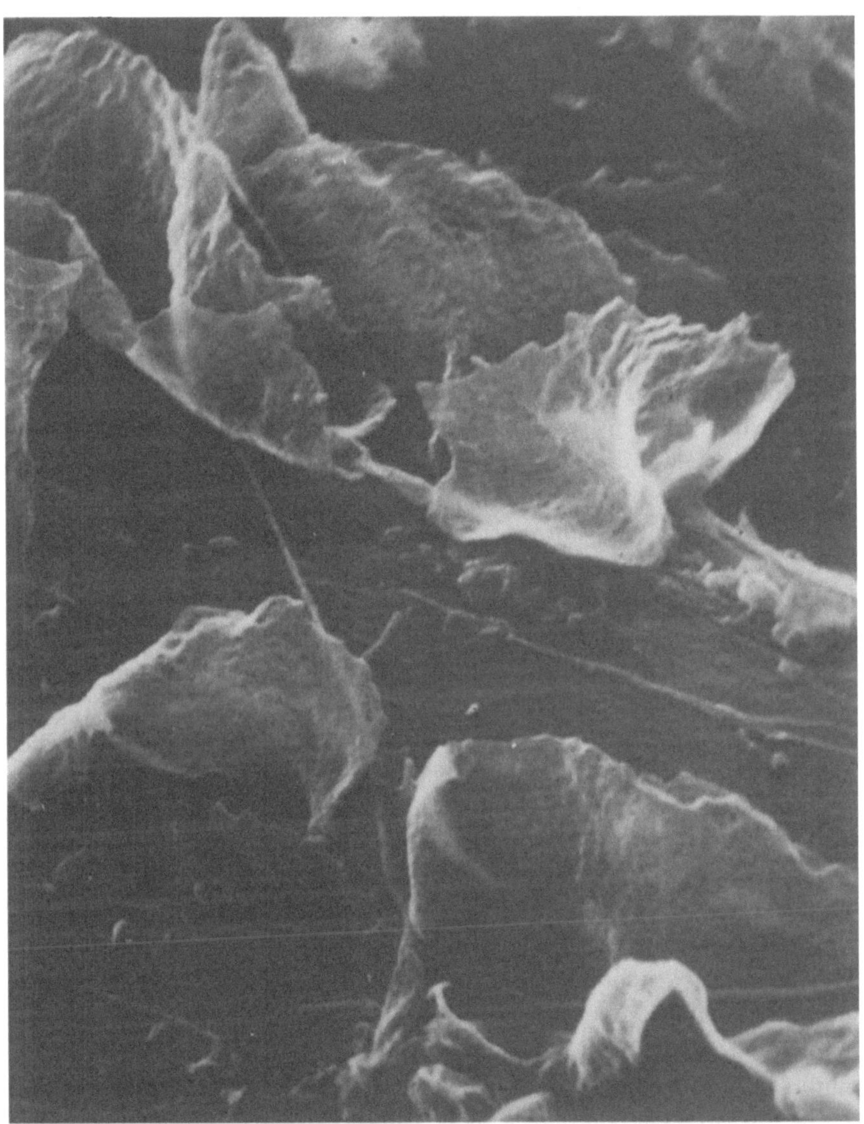

FIG. 8. Scanning electron micrograph of malignant glioma cells. Area with large, slender lamellae, representing "atypical ruffling of the membrane." ×10,000.

plasma membrane movements. No nuclear overlapping will occur and cells will only slowly change their positions. This type of relaxed movement control can only be revealed by time-lapse filming; by ordinary microscopy, glioma cells would appear to be arranged as a regular monolayer.

4.6. *The Glioma Cell Surface*

Electron microscopic studies have revealed besides atypical vertical ruffling, considerable differences between normal and neoplastic glia cells *in vitro*. The normal cells have a smooth dorsal surface (Fig. 9). Immediately under the plasma membrane is a thin but regular and continuous sheet of microfilaments presumed to be the main "muscle tract" of the cell. The ventral surface contains specialized desmosome-like attachment devices in immediate contact with the solid support. Between these, the membrane is shaped into rounded vaults studded with endocytotic vesicles. The morphology suggests that the ventral surface is most active in the uptake of macromolecules and particulate matter.

The glioma surface has varied considerably between the individual lines. In all instances, specialization has been less perfect than among the normal glia cells. For instance, endocytosis may be diffusely distributed over the entire plasma membrane and the microfilaments may show a patchy distribution. The most conspicuous feature, however, has been the occurrence of protrusions, some of which seem to be connected with thin stalks to the main cell body (Fig. 10). Sometimes these connections seem to break spontaneously with the release of bags of cytoplasm containing lysosomes and other organelles.

The overall impression of the structure of the glioma membrane is one of extreme activity. Movement is hyperactive, and large segments of the membranes are lost either in the process of endocytosis or by loss of cytoplasmic extrusions. The importance of the apparent instability is unknown. It may be a sign of deficient regulation of membrane synthesis, assembly, and movement comparable to the "general cellular disorder and malfunction" which accompany a malignant transformation. But it may also, as is often suggested for neoplastic cells in general, reflect the key pathological feature of neoplasia—a disturbed membrane function. According to this theory, the membrane acts as a censor against the outer world, shutting off stimulatory signals once cell division becomes unnecessary. A malfunction disturbs the censor function, permitting constant emittance of stimulatory signals which cause the unphysiological proliferation characteristic of the malignant state. The two hypotheses are variants of the old theme of

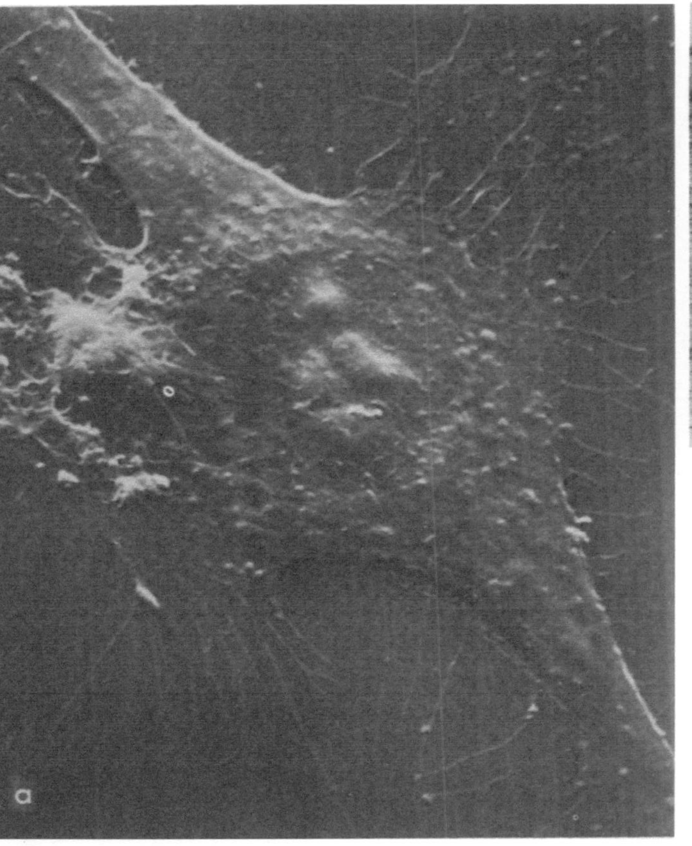

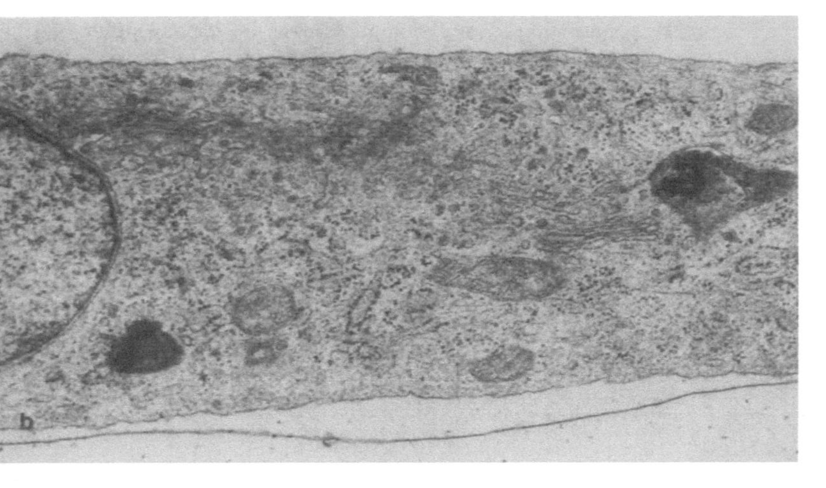

FIG. 9. Scanning (a) and transmission (b) electron micrographs of normal glia cells. Cells are thin and flattened with a smooth upper surface, apart from a small peripheral area with "ruffling of the membrane" in the left-hand photo. Left: ×3200; right ×32,000.

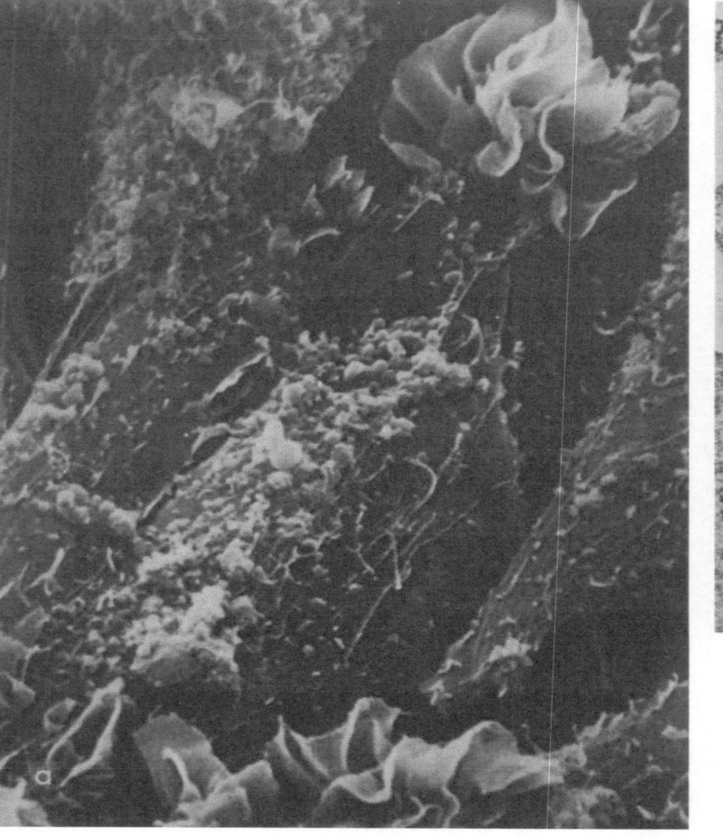

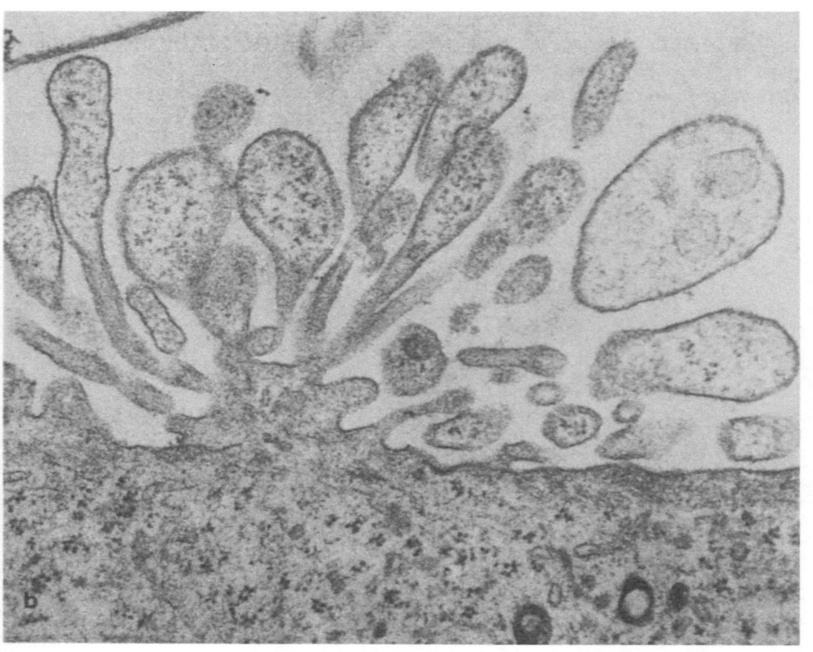

FIG. 10. Scanning (a) and transmission (b) electron micrographs of malignant glioma cells. Cells form numerous protrusions from the upper surface, some of which represent "atypical ruffling." Left: ×3200; right: ×32,000.

whether a certain alteration in a malignant cell is of primary or secondary importance for the neoplastic state.

Several groups have claimed that transformed and normal cell membranes differ with respect to their response against certain lectins, a class of proteins or glycoproteins from plants and lower animals with strong binding affinity for different membrane-bound sugars (see Sharon and Lis, 1972). The most extensive studies have been performed with concanavalin A—a protein which binds to L,D-mannopyranoside, L,D-glucopyranoside and L-*N*-acetyl-D-glucosaminoside groups. Con A binds approximately equally to normal and transformed cells but agglutinates the latter with much greater efficiency. This has been ascribed to clustering of receptors on the outside of neoplastic membranes in contrast to an even distribution on the outer surface of normal cells (Nicolson, 1973). These studies have been based on comparisons between normal and transformed rodent cells.

We have investigated Con A agglutination of human glioma lines (Glimelius *et al.*, 1974), and certain differences were found between individual lines. However, as a group they did not differ significantly from glia and certain other normal human cells. It seems probable that no difference in Con A agglutinability has been demonstrated which distinguishes normal and neoplastic glia cell membranes *in vitro*. This suggests that the findings on rodent cells cannot be generally applied.

Since ATP is involved in important membrane functions such as ionic transport and mobility, we have conducted a limited study of its synthesis. It is known that cells may synthesize ATP in their membranes from precursors added from the outside, a finding that suggests a certain degree of cell membrane autonomy with respect to ATP synthesis (Ågren and Ronquist, 1969). We have compared normal glia and glioma cells in this respect (Ågren *et al.*, 1971*a*). It was found that the neoplastic cells formed 3–6 times more ATP than the corresponding normal cells. The responsible enzymes were apparently located at the cell membrane. Degrading ATPase activity showed the reverse situation; i.e., it was high in normal and very low in neoplastic glia (Ågren *et al.*, 1971*b*).

These findings emphasize that glia and glioma membranes are very different. It is possible that the high formation of ATP is in some way related to the enhanced mobility of the glioma membrane.

4.7. *Interactions with Normal Cells*

Eight different glioma lines (87 MG, 105 MG, 118 MG, 138 MG, 178 MG, 251 MG, 343 MG, 373 MG) have been grown in contact with normal stationary glia (Westermark, 1973*e*). All neoplastic populations multiplied, but the rates of proliferation differed. This was in marked contrast to normal glia cells, which under the same conditions could not initiate their cell cycle (Westermark, 1973*d*).

There has so far been no clear correlation between this sign of an impaired growth control and other parameters mentioned earlier in this review. Weiss *et al.* (1973), working with an inbred rat strain, concluded that the degree of inhibition of locomotion and proliferation that normal cells exert on the neoplastic cells is the most relevant *in vitro* indicator of tumorigenicity *in vivo.* If so, quantitative assessment of the growth of neoplastic cells or stationary normal cells could be developed into a useful *in vitro* tool for determination of the clinical malignancy of human neoplastic cells.

4.8. Immunological Properties

Strong evidence has been presented for the presence of immunity in glioma patients. This is partly nonspecifically directed against glia cell antigens in general (Wahlström *et al.*, 1973*a*).

A study (Wahlström *et al.*, 1973*b*) has been made of our glioma lines with respect to a possible tumor-specific antigen distinct from the general glial antigenicity. Rabbit serum obtained from animals immunized with lyophilized glioblastoma multiforme tissue was extensively absorbed with various normal human organs including brain and also with fresh HeLa cells. The resulting sera reacted only with cell lines cultured from malignant gliomas in indirect immunofluorescence tests. Normal glia was negative, as were skin fibroblasts and three different human sarcoma lines. The morphological pattern could be divided into three types for the 14 glioma lines tested. One was a delicate, often segmentary lining at the cell margin ("fine" in Table 5); the second was a coarse fluorescence which gave the impression of a thick brushlike layer of tiny extensions on the cell membrane ("coarse" in Table 5); and the third, found only in line 251 MG, consisted of a dense fibrillary network in the cellular membrane.

These patterns were consistent characteristics of the individual lines and may depend on stable variations in cell surface topography.

It is, of course, not possible to exclude that the differences between normal and neoplastic glia surface reactivity with antibody are of a quantitative rather than a qualitative nature.

We may, with this reservation, conclude that glia *and* glioma cells share brain-specific antigen(s). In addition, glioma cells contain surface-bound antigen(s) apparently specific for neoplastic cells. Whether these antigens play any role in growth regulation *in vivo* is still unknown. It has been suggested that a systematic response against brain-specific antigens may be

TABLE 5

Identification of Human Glioma Lines

	Basic cytology[a]	Sex	Isozymes G6PD	PGM$_1$	PGM$_3$	Fluorescent antibody	Mixed hemad-sorption	Reference[b]
87 MG	epi	F	B	2–1	2–1	Fine		(d, a, b)
105 MG	bip	M	B	1	1	Coarse		(d, a, b)
118 MG	bip	M	B	2–1	1	Fine		(d, a, b)
138 MG	bip	M	B	2–1	1	Fine	Indiv. distinct	(d, e, a, b)
178 MG	bip	M	B	1	1	Fine	Indiv. distinct	(d, e, b, c)
251 MG	epi	M	B	1	1	Fibrous	Indiv. distinct	(d, e, b, c)
343 MG	astro	M	B	1	2	Fine	Indiv. distinct	(d, e, b, c)
348 MG	astro	M	B	1	1			(b, c)
372 MG	bip	M	B	2–1	1			(b, c)
373 MG	pleo	M	B	1	1	Coarse		(d, b, c)
399 MG	bip	M	B	1	2–1	Fine		(d, b, c)
410 MG	bip	M				Fine		(d, c)
489 MG	bip	M	B	1	2	Coarse		(d, b, c)
495 MG	bip	M	B	2	1	Coarse	Indiv. distinct	(d, e, b, c)
539 MG	astro	F				Fine		(d)
563 MG	bip	M						
692 MG	bip	M				Fine		(f)
706 MT	bimo	F				None		(f)
716 MG	bip	M						

[a] epi, Epithelioid shape; bip, bipolar shape; astro, starlike shape; pleo, strong pleomorphism; bimo, bimorphic, see Fig. 6.

[b] (a) J. Pontén and E. MacIntyre, *Acta Pathol. Microbiol. Scand. 74*:465, 1968. (b) G. Beckman *et al., Hum. Hered. 21*:238, 1971. (c) B. Westermark, J. Pontén, and R. Hugosson, *Acta Pathol. Microbiol. Scand. 81*:791. (d) J. Pontén, this chapter. (e) J. Pontén and E. Saksela, *Int. J. Cancer 2*:434, 1967. (f) T. Wahlström *et al., Cell Immunol.*, submitted. (g) J. Å. Espmark *et al.*, ASM Meeting, Miami, Paper M325, 1973. (h) K. Nilsson *et al., Clin. Exp. Immunol. 7*:477, 1970.

the reason for the peculiar common absence of extracerebral metastases from malignant gliomas (Wahlström *et al.*, 1973*a*).

4.9. Chromosomes

The chromosomes of glioma lines have not yet been systematically investigated. However, crude karyotyping has established that all our lines are heteroploid. Most cells are subtetraploid with highly variable numbers. One line (118 MG) was near diploid and has remained essentially stable during a long sojourn *in vitro*.

4.10. Infection by Oncogenic Viruses

We have studied the effects of the following oncogenic viruses on normal glia cells: simian virus 40 (SV40), feline sarcoma virus (FSV), and Rous sarcoma virus (RSV).

SV40 will induce a transformation in glia cells which manifests itself by strongly reduced topoinhibition. Cells will be little if at all influenced by an increased local cell density (Westermark, 1973*a*). Their movement control also seems impaired since they will form irregular cell piles. Transformation is, particularly initially, accompanied by cell destruction. At a passage level which exceeds the normal by some 50%, transformed populations will enter a crisis with progressively slower growth terminating in complete lysis. We have not been able to establish a permanent SV40-transformed line with an infinite life span. The sequence above is essentially similar to that described from human fibroblasts exposed to SV40, with the exception that a few fibroblast lines have been recovered from "crisis" (Pontén *et al.*, 1963).

FSV is very effective in transforming human glia. After 10 days, cytologically altered cells are already clearly visible. They have all the morphological hallmarks of cells transformed by oncogenic RNA viruses (see Pontén, 1971). Transformed cells have a reduced sensitivity to crowding with respect to proliferation and cell membrane movements. They rapidly become predominant but will also eventually enter irreversible lysis, and no permanent FSV-transformed line has thus been produced. All cultures release FSV.

Glioma cells are also susceptible to FSV and become chronic virus releasers. They undergo the same characteristic cytological alterations as normal glia. Their capacity for endless multiplication is not lost after the virus infection.

RSV will produce slight and rapidly reversible cytological alterations in normal glia populations. This interaction has not been further studied.

Certain glioma lines will react to RSV by cytological alterations, which, however, generally disappear because of overgrowth of uninfected cells. One cell line—118 MG—has been successfully transformed into a permanent line apparently completely composed of RSV-altered cells. The morphology is typical. The state of the RSV genome has been investigated. The transformed cells behave as "virogenic" elements; i.e., they fail to release infectious virus but may be induced to do so by close contact with chicken cells (Macintyre and Pontén, 1967; Macintyre *et al.*, 1969). The line 118 MG-EH (EH stands for strain Engelbreth-Holm of RSV) has been used to assay RD114 virus—an agent of probable feline origin—isolated from a human rhabdomyosarcoma after transplant passage through an RNA virus infected kitten (Nelson-Rees *et al.*, 1973; McAllister *et al.*, 1971).

4.11. *Identification Problems*

Foreign cell contamination is a major danger in work with permanent tissue culture lines. Since 1962 a number of reports (see Gartler, 1967; Peterson *et al.*, 1968) have revealed both inter- and intraspecies cell contamination in human cell lines.

The most common inadvertent admixture seems to be HeLa cells. Lines contaminated by HeLa may be uncovered by the isozyme pattern of glucose-6-phosphodehydrogenase (G6PD) and phosphoglucomutase (PGM). G6PD occurs as two variants, type A being almost exclusively confined to Negros. HeLa cells are type A, and lines stated to be derived from Caucasians that show type A of G6PD are therefore strongly suspect of HeLa contamination.

Espmark *et al.* (1973) applied mixed hemadsorption techniques for the alloantigenic mapping of established human cell lines. A large panel of sera from multiparous women was used and an individual profile of reactivity could thus be constructed for each line under test. All diploid nonestablished lines had individual patterns, in contrast to 14 lines from the American Type Culture Collection which were diagnosed as certainly or probably contaminated with cells.

Glioma lines from other sources than the Wallenberg laboratory (Table 3) have never been tested for their authentic origin. At least in some cases, as judged from the illustrations and verbal descriptions, HeLa contamination seems possible.

The majority of our glioma lines have been analyzed by a number of markers listed in Table 5.

Table 5 contains 18 lines of undisputable glioma origin (the MG lines) as judged from the histology of the biopsy. One line (706 MT) was of probable but never histologically proven glioma origin (see Fig. 6).

The fluorescent antibody marker (Wahlström *et al.*, 1973, 1974) was specific for glioma cells since it did not react with normal glia, normal fibroblasts, or three tested sarcoma lines. In all 14 MG lines tested, specific fluorescence was seen at the cell membrane, indicating that the lines were of human glioma origin. 706 MG was the only negative specimen, presumably reflecting its peculiar histology which suggested either anaplastic glioma, origin from mesenchymal components of the brain, or metastasis (although no other tumor was found at autopsy).

All MG lines tested for G6PD and PGM isozymes showed a non-HeLa pattern. The five lines which were tested for alloantigenic marker with mixed hemadsorption (Espmark *et al.*, 1973) had individual profiles.

These facts in conjuction with a stable cytology with individual major or minor traits for each line make us conclude that no cell contamination has occurred in our lines. The 19 permanent Wallenberg lines from human brain tumors constitute the largest published collection of well-characterized human neoplastic lines obtained from a consecutive series of biopsies.

5. *Glioma Lines as Models for Neoplasia*

For a long time, it was considered futile to study neoplastic cells *in vitro*. This conviction was based on the fact that normal rodent cells almost invariably transformed spontaneously into tumorigenic lines after only a few months in culture. *In vitro* conditions were by themselves considered so artificial that all cells were rendered neoplastic in the absence of addition of any known carcinogens.

The important work by Hayflick (1965) has shown this generalization to be in error. Human cells and later chicken cells were found to retain all hallmarks of normality even after prolonged serial cultivation. It is against this background that neoplastic human cells derived from malignancies *in vivo* are of considerable general biological interest. In the glia–glioma system, it is possible to compare normal and malignant cells isolated and grown under similar conditions. Both partners retain original basic characters during serial cultivation. Any differences would therefore be expected to reflect genuine and important traits in malignant cells.

In the adult brain, the astrocytes are essentially stationary; i.e., they are parked in G_0 but may be stimulated to proliferate, for instance after trauma. Mitotic figures are extremely rare in the undisturbed adult human brain. On the other hand, glioma cells have mitoses, the number of which seems inversely related to the degree of differentiation.

The glia–glioma system recapitulates these features in a remarkable manner *in vitro*, at least at a superficial descriptive level.

Normal glia cells will become parked in an apparent G_0 at a critical local density which cannot be exceeded by any known stimulation from the outside. Under identical conditions, glioma cells are only moderately inhibited and it has been impossible to accomplish a true stationary phase except by such artificial means as a sharp reduction in the exterior serum concentration or total deprivation of serum.

The human glia–glioma system would, briefly summarized, serve as a model in at least the following situations:

Growth control studies: Here it would be important to find out the mechanism behind the apparently deficient multiplication control of glioma cell populations. Is it caused by plasma membrane dysfunction which makes it impossible for the cell to react properly to its neighboring cells by stopping at G_0, even if extensive intercellular contacts have been created? Is the glioma cell reaction to serum growth factors entirely different from that of normal glia? Certain facts such as a substantially lower serum requirement and hyperexcitability by serum suggest that such is the case. Is the intrinsic growth control disturbed to the extent that new cell cycles are initiated even if normally adequate inhibitory signals are generated from the cell periphery? The presence of significant residual DNA synthesis is compatible with such an idea.

Immunological studies: Considerable evidence indicates the presence of tumor-specific immunological responses against most human neoplasia, including brain tumors. So far, the *in vitro* reactions have almost exclusively been carried out between lymphocytes, fresh tumor cells, and serum in various combinations. The use of primary tumor cells has precluded standardized techniques, and the unavailability of proper normal control cells has made it difficult to distinguish between tissue-specific and tumor-specific reactions. The availability of a fairly large collection of established glioma lines and normal glia cells (which may also be cultivated from a tumor-bearing individual) should be a valuable tool for the resolution of problems in human tumor immunology. They may serve as sources for purification of antigens and reference objects in clinical studies. It is interesting to note that all of our tested glioma lines have a membrane-bound antigen which is not demonstrated on normal glia, sarcoma cells, or normal fibroblasts.

Action of carcinogens of human cells: With chemical carcinogens and X-rays, it has been possible to transform only rodent cells *in vitro*. Since these have a high inherent tendency for transformation, it is not known whether the transforming activity should be considered a true induction of neoplasia or an enhancement of an inherent tendency (promotion). Stable human glia cells are sensitive to chemical carcinogens, and our recent finding (Pontén, 1973) that ethylnitrosourea transforms such cells may be useful in approaching the important problem of the activity of putative carcinogens in man.

Since oncogenic viruses transform human glia, it should be possible to compare such cells transformed *in vitro* with those obtained from tumors *in vivo*. Our preliminary data indicate that principally the same type of growth disturbances exist in virally transformed cells as in glioma cells.

More examples such as the search for a viral etiology could be cited as models where glia–glioma cells would be useful. It seems to be a significant step forward that techniques have been developed for the growth of human tumor cells outside of the body. This is necessary for conducting systematic experiments and for applying the vast amount of existing animal data to human cells. Important species differences exist, and solution of the vexing problem of the etiology and nature of cancer in man may perhaps be possible only by study of human cells.

6. References

Abercrombie, M., Heaysman, J. E. M., and Pegrum, S. M., 1970*a*, The locomotion of fibroblasts in culture. I. Movements of the leading edge, *Exp. Cell Res.* **59:**393.

Abercrombie, M., Heaysman, J. E. M., and Pegrum, S. M., 1970*b*, The locomotion of fibroblasts in culture. II. "Ruffling," *Exp. Cell Res.* **60:**437.

Ågren, G., and Ronquist, G., 1969, Formation of extracellular adenosine triphosphate by tumour cells, *Acta Physiol. Scand.* **75:**124.

Ågren, G., Nilsson, K., Pontén, J., Ronquist, G., and Westermark, B., 1971*a*, Formation of extracellular adenosine triphosphate by normal and neoplastic human cells in culture, *J. Cell. Physiol.* **77:**331.

Ågren, G., Pontén, J., Ronquist, G., and Westermark, B., 1971*b*, Demonstration of an ATPase at the cell surface of intact normal and neoplastic human cells in culture, *J. Cell. Physiol.* **78:**171.

Beckman, G., Beckman, L., Pontén, J., and Westermark, B., 1971, G-6-PD and PGM phenocytes of 16 continuous human tumor cell lines, *Hum. Hered.* **21:**238.

Brunk, U., Ericsson, J., Pontén, J., and Westermark, B., 1971, Specialization of cell surfaces in contact-inhibited human glia-like cells *in vitro, Exp. Cell Res.* **67:**407.

Dulbecco, R., 1970, Topoinhibition and serum requirement of transformed and untransformed cells, *Nature (Lond.)* **227:**802.

Eagle, H., 1959, Amino acid metabolism in mammalian cell cultures, *Science* **130:**432.

Espmark, J. Å., Ahlqvist-Roth, L., Chapple, P. J., and Cartwright, L. N., 1973, Alloantigenic characterization of permanent human cell lines, presented at the ASM Meeting, Miami Beach, May 6–11, Paper M325.

Forsby, N., Brunk, U., Ericsson, J., Pontén, J., and Westermark, B., 1972, Ultrastructural features of *in vitro*-cultivated malignant gliomas, *Acta Pathol. Microbiol. Scand. Sect. A* **80:**430.

Gartler, S. M., 1967, Genetic markers as tracers in cell culture, in: Decennial Review Conference on Cell Tissue and Organ Culture, *Natl. Cancer Inst. Monogr.* **26:**167.

Glimelius, B., Westermark, B., and Pontén, J., 1974, Agglutination of normal and neoplastic human cells by concanavalin A and *ricinus communis* agglutinin, *Int. J. Cancer* **14:**314.

Ham, R. G., 1963, An improved nutrient solution for diploid Chinese hamster and human cell lines, *Exp. Cell Res.* **29:**515.

Hayflick, L., 1965, The limited *in vitro* lifetime of human diploid cell strains, *Exp. Cell Res.* **37:**614.

Hayflick, L., and Moorhead, P., 1961, The serial cultivation of human diploid cell strains, *Exp. Cell Res.* **25:**585.

Kersting, G., 1961, *Die Gewebszuchtung menschlicher Hirngeschwulste*, Springer, Berlin, Gottingen, Heidelberg.

Kersting, G., 1964, Tissue culture and the classification of brain tumours, in: Classification of Brain Tumours (K. J. Zülch, and A. L. Woolf, eds.), *Acta Neurochir. Suppl.* **10:**68.

Lipton, A., Klinger, I., Paul, D., and Holley, R. W., 1971, Migration of mouse 3T3 fibroblasts in response to a serum factor, *Proc. Natl. Acad. Sci.* **68:**2799.

Lumsden, C. E., 1963, Tissue culture in relation to tumours of the nervous system, in: *Pathology of Tumours of the Nervous System*, 2nd ed. (D. S. Russell, and L. J. Ruginstein, eds.), p. 281, Edward Arnold (London).

Macintyre, E. H., and Pontén, J., 1967, Interaction between normal and transformed bovine fibroblasts in culture. I. Cells transformed by Rous sarcoma virus, *J. Cell Sci.* **2:**309.

Macintyre, E. H., Grimes, R. A., and Vatter, A. E., 1969, Cytology and growth characteristics of human tumour astrocytes transformed by Rous sarcoma virus, *J. Cell Sci.* **5:**583.

Manuelidis, E. E., 1965, Long-term lines of tissue cultures of intracranial tumors, *J. Neurosurg.* **22:**368.

Manuelidis, E. E., 1969, Experiments with tissue culture and heterologous transplantation of tumors, *Ann. N.Y. Acad. Sci.* **159:**409.

Maunoury, R., Vedrenne, C., Arnoult, J., Constans, J. P., and Febvre, H., 1972, Culture *in vitro* de tissu glial normal et néoplastique. Croissance, cytologie, ultrastructure, *Neuro-chirurgie, Paris* **18:**8.

McAllister, R. M., Melnyk, J., Finklestein, J. Z., Adams, E. C., Jr., and Gardner, M. B., 1969, Cultivation *in vitro* of cells derived from a human rhabdomyosarcoma, *Cancer* **24:**520.

McAllister, R. M., Nelson-Rees, W. A., Johnson, E. Y., Rongey, R. W., and Gardner, M. B., 1971, Disseminated rhabdomyosarcomas formed in kittens by cultured human rhabdomyosarcoma cells, *J. Natl. Cancer Inst.* **47:**603.

Moore, G. E., and Koike, K., 1964, Growth of human tumor cells *in vitro* and *in vivo*, *Cancer* **17:**11.

Moore, G. E., Gerner, R. E., and Franklin, H. A., 1967, Culture of normal human leukocytes, *JAMA* **199:**519.

Nakai, J., 1963, *Morphology of Neuroglia*, Charles C Thomas, Springfield, I.

Nelson-Rees, W. A., Klement, V., Peterson, W. D., Jr., and Weawer, J. F., 1973, Comparative study of two RD 114 virus-indicator cell lines, KC and KB, *J. Natl. Cancer Inst.*, submitted.

Nicolson, G. L., 1973, Temperature-dependent mobility of concanavalin sites on tumour cell surfaces, *Nature (Lond.)* **243:**218.

Nilsson, K., Pontén, J., and Philipson, L., 1968, Development of immunocytes and immunoglobulin production in long term cultures from normal and malignant human lymph nodes, *Int. J. Cancer* **3:**183.

Nilsson, K., Bennich, H., Johansson, S. G. O., and Pontén, J., 1970, Established immunoglobulin producing myeloma (IgE) and lymphoblastoid (IgC) cell lines from an IgE myeloma patient. *Clin. Exp. Immunol.* **7:**477.

Oettgen, H. F., Tadao, A., Old, L. J., Boyse, E. A., de Harven, E., and Mills, G. M., 1968, Suspension culture of pigment-producing cell line derived from a human malignant melanoma, *J. Natl. Cancer Inst.* **41:**827.

Peterson, W. D., Jr., Stulberg, C. S., Swanborg, N. K., and Robinson, A. R., 1968, Glucose-6-phosphate dehydrogenase isoenzymes in human cell cultures determined by sucrose–agar gel and cellulose acetate zymograms, *Proc. Soc. Exp. Biol. Med.* **128:**772.

Pontén, J., 1971, Spontaneous and virus induced transformation in cell culture, in: *Virology Monographs* (S. Gard, C. Hallauer, and K. F. Meyer, eds.), Wien, New York.

Pontén, J., 1973, Transformation of normal human glia cells by a chemical carcinogen. *XVII Scandinavian Congress of Pathology and Microbiology, Stockholm. June 12–14*, Abstract.

Pontén, J., and Macintyre, E. H., 1968, Long term culture of normal and neoplastic human glia, *Acta Pathol. Microbiol. Scand.* **74:**465.

Pontén, J., and Saksela, E., 1967, Two established *in vitro* cell lines from human mesenchymal tumours, *Int. J. Cancer* **2:**434.

Pontén, J., Jensen, F., and Koprowski, H., 1963, Morphological and virological investigation of human tissue cultures transformed with SV40, *J. Cell. Comp. Physiol.* **61:**145.

Pontén, J., Westermark, B., and Hugosson, H., 1969, Regulation of proliferation and movement of human glia-like cells in culture, *Exp. Cell Res.* **58:**343.

Sharon, N., and Lis, H., 1972, Lectins: Cell-agglutinating and sugar-specific proteins, *Science* **177:**949.

Swim, H. E., and Parker, R. F., 1957, Culture characteristics of human fibroblasts propagated serially, *Am. J. Hyg.* **66:**235.

Temin, H. M., 1971, Stimulation by serum of multiplication of stationary chicken cells, *J. Cell. Physiol.* **78:**161.

Temin, H. M., Pierson, R. W., Jr., and Dulak, N. C., 1972, in: *Growth, Nutrition and Metabolism of Cells in Culture*, Vol. 1, (H. Rothblat and V. J. Cristafolo, eds.), p. 49, Academic Press, New York, London.

Todaro, G. J., Lazar, G. K., and Green, H. J., 1965, The initiation of cell division in a contact-inhibited mammalian cell line, *J. Cell. Comp. Physiol.* **66:**325.

Uthne, K., 1973, Human somatomedins: Purification and some studies on their biological actions, *Acta Endocrinol. Suppl.* **175**.

Wahlström, T., Saksela, E., and Troupp, H., 1973*a*, Cell-bound antiglial immunity in patients with malignant tumors of the brain, *Cell. Immul.* **6:**161.

Wahlström, T., Linder, E., Saksela, E., and Westermark, B., 1974, Tumor-specific membrane antigens in established cell lines from gliomas, *Cancer* **34:**274.

Weiss, R. A., Veselý, P., and Siňdelarova, J., 1973, Growth regulation and tumor formation of normal and neoplastic rat cells, *Int. J. Cancer* **11:**77.

Westermark, B., 1971, Proliferation control of cultivated human glia-like cells under "steady state" conditions, *Exp. Cell Res.* **69:**258.

Westermark, B., 1973*a*, Growth control of normal and neoplastic human glia-like cells in culture, *Acta Univ. Uppsal. Abst. Uppsala Diss. Med.* **164.**

Westermark, B., 1973*b*, The deficient density dependent growth control of human malignant glioma cells and virus transformed glia-like cells in culture, *Int. J. Cancer* **12:**438.

Westermark, B., 1973*c*, Induction of a reversible G1 block in human glia-like cells by cytochalasin B, *Exp. Cell Res.* **82:**341.

Westermark, B., 1973*d*, Growth regulatory interactions between stationary human glia-like cells and normal neoplastic human cells in culture. I. Normal cells. *Exp. Cell Res.* **81:**195.

Westermark, B., 1973*e*, Growth regulatory interactions between stationary human glia-like cells and normal and neoplastic human cells in culture. II. Neoplastic cells.

Westermark, B., Forsby, N., Brunk, U., Ericsson, J., and Pontén, J., 1972, Studies on *in vitro* cultivated human glia and glioma cells. I and II, *Acta Pathol. Microbiol. Scand. Sect. A* **80:**694.

Westermark, B., Pontén, J., and Hugosson, R., 1973, Determinants for the establishment of permanent tissue culture lines from human gliomas, *Acta Pathol. Microbiol. Scand. Sect. A, Pathol. Microbiol. Scand.* **81:**791.

Westermark, B., and Wasteson, Å., 1974, The response of cultured human normal glial cells to growth factors, *Adv. Metab. Dis.*, in press.

Windle, W. F., 1958, *Biology of Neuroglia*, Charles C Thomas, Springfield, Ill.

Wilson, C. B., Barker, M., and Slagel, D. E., 1966, Tumors of the central nervous system in monolayer tissue, *Arch. Neurol.* **15:**275.

Current Research with Organ Cultures of Human Tumors 8

ET. WOLFF AND EM. WOLFF

1. Introduction—Historical

It is of considerable interest, from the standpoint of fundamental and applied research, to culture malignant human tumors *in vitro* in the form of massive, organized nodules such as those which exist in the organism. We shall see later that this objective can be attained by a relatively simple technique which produces genuine miniature tumors, some of which can multiply indefinitely. It is easy to imagine the interest that such techniques arouse from the point of view of experimentation on human cancer, for it is very seldom that one can perform direct experiments on such material. Occasionally human tumors can be transplanted into an animal. However, such instances are rare and one is normally obliged to extrapolate from experiments with animal tumors. This is why we have sought to develop media and conditions which permit the *organotypic culture of human tumors.*

The historical treatment will be brief, for the technique is recent and it has been performed in only a few laboratories. One can cite the attempts to culture tumors *in vivo* in various more or less isolated parts of the organism, such as the yolk sac and allantois of the chick embryo, the anterior chamber of the eye and the peritoneal cavity of a variety of animals, or the cheek

ET. WOLFF AND EM. WOLFF Laboratoire d'Embryologie expérimentale, Collège de France, Paris, France pouch of the hamster. To these one can also add transplantations into animals in which immunological reactions have been lessened by X-irradiation. However, in all these experiments, which more often than not have been performed with animal rather than human tumors, the influence of the host can not be disregarded.

Among the first attempts were the experiments of Greene (1957) on transplantation of animal (Shope's rabbit papilloma) or human (glioblastoma, fibrosarcoma, papillary carcinoma of the thyroid) tumors into the anterior chamber of the eye and into the brain of the guinea pig and the mouse.

Important results have been obtained by means of coelomic or intraembryonic grafts in the chick embryo, which has proved to be a suitable subject for the transplantation of some mammalian tumors. Bueker (1948), Levi-Montalcini and Hamburger (1951), Levi-Montalcini (1952), and Kautz (1952) were the first to show that mouse tumors (S-180 and S-37) transplanted into the coelomic cavity preferentially invade different organs, such as the mesonephros, liver, lung, and gonads. The growth of tumors in these organs or in the surrounding spaces is often considerable. The reaction of the host is no less remarkable, being characterized in particular by a considerable hypertrophy of the spinal and sympathetic ganglia and by a massive invasion of nerve fibers into many organs (Bueker, 1957; Levi-Montalcini *et al.*, 1954).

Transplantation of mammalian tumors onto the extraembryonic membranes of birds has often been fruitful. Thus Murphy (1913) and Karnofsky *et al.* (1952) cultured rat and mouse tumors on the chorioallantoic membrane of the chick. Dagg *et al.* (1956) transplanted onto this same membrane, strains of human tumors previously cultured for several years in monolayers. Toolan's human epidermoid carcinoma (HEp-3) multiplied particularly abundantly, developing numerous metastases in all the organs of the chick.

Taylor and his collaborators have used a very simple method for culturing animal tumors. On introducing small fragments of mouse tumors (mammary carcinoma) or rat tumors (Walker tumor 256) into chick embryo yolk sac, they sometimes obtained an enormous development of the explants (Taylor *et al.*, 1942, 1948). However, they do not seem to have obtained many results by this method with human tumors.

Other techniques, such as the injection of tumor cells into the embryonic circulation, have been successfully applied to tumors of small mammals (Humphreys, 1960; Leighton, 1963).

Work involving the organotypic culture *in vitro* of human tumors, apart from that described in the following chapters, is relatively scanty. Leighton (1954*a,b*) and Leighton *et al.* (1968) have described a method of culture in a sponge matrix impregnated with a nutrient medium consisting of embryo extract, horse serum, and Earle's solution. The cells, obtained either from cultured cell lines or from fresh tumors, form more or less organized masses which proliferate and spread in the interstitial liquid in the pores of the sponge.

More recently, various authors have used organ culture techniques as an aid to resolving certain problems concerning differentiation, *in vitro* carcinogenesis, inhibition of tumor growth, and the properties of cancer cell membranes. Particular mention should be made of the work of Lasfargues and Murray (1959, 1968), Lasfargues and Feldman (1963), and Ambrose and his collaborators (Tchao *et al.*, 1968; Ellison *et al.*, 1969; Yarnell and Ambrose, 1969*a,b*) as well as the recent studies on the culture of human glioblastomas by Rubinstein *et al.* (1973).

Most of this work concerns mouse or rat cancer, although some has been carried out with human tumors. However, it is difficult to separate the techniques employed and the problems raised in man from those concerning animals. The cultures obtained by the authors cited above were in general of short duration, although sufficient for the requirements of their experiments.

2. Steps Leading to the Culture of Organized Tumors in Vitro

Current techniques for the culture of organized human tumors derive from those utilized in our laboratory for the culture of embryonic organs (Et. Wolff and Haffen, 1952; Et. Wolff *et al.*, 1953).

2.1. Organ Culture in Vitro

The essential characteristic of organ culture technique is that the embryonic organs are grown on the surface of a semisolid medium. The culture medium comprises the following constituents:

1% agar in Gey's solution	7 vol
Extract of 8- to 10-day chick embryo	3 vol
Gey's or Tyrode's solution plus antibiotics	3 vol

The warm mixture is poured into a watchglass. When it is cool, the organs to be cultured (e.g., gonads, liver, mesonephros, metanephros, intestine, lung, skin and derivatives, eyes, long bones, facial buds) are placed on the flat surface. This technique can be applied equally well to organs of birds and those of mammals. If required, it is possible to substitute nutrients, RNA, hormones, vitamins, or various growth factors for part of the Tyrode's solution. The embryonic organs, taken before differentiation occurs, grow and differentiate *in vitro*. The average duration of their development is at most 10–28 days at 38°C. Thereafter, they may survive but their development does not persist.

2.2 Heterologous Associations of Embryonic Organs in Vitro: Chimeras of Chick and Mouse Organs

Since it is possible to culture avian and mammalian organs on identical media and at the same temperature, it was tempting to associate them. Accordingly, fragments of testicles and ovaries from chick embryos were associated with fragments of the same organs derived from mammals. Associations between different species have been carried out with lung, liver, and kidney (Et. Wolff, 1954; Et. Wolff and Weniger, 1954).

Heterologous organs (e.g., testicle and mesonephros, lung and liver) can be associated (Bermann, 1960) as well as homologous organs from two species. The main result obtained from such heterospecific combinations is that the organs of the two species can collaborate to form common structures—real organ or tissue chimeras. There is no antagonism between the cells of different origin; on the contrary, there are sometimes affinities. The organotypic culture of tumors also demonstrates such a collaboration.

2.3. Associations of Embryonic Organs of the Chick with Mammalian Tumors

The next step was to associate cancerous mammalian organs with chick embryo organs. It is feasible to associate mammalian tumors with normal mammalian tissue, but superior results have generally been obtained from heterologous associations. Early experiments involved the association of mouse sarcoma S-180 with various organs of the chick embryo (Et. Wolff, 1956; Wolff and Schneider, 1956, 1957*a,b*; Schneider, 1958). Other mouse and rat tumors were cultured in a similar fashion. The results can be summarized as follows: Confronted with the embryonic organ, the tumor fragments fuse intimately with it; in particular, the sarcoma cells penetrate deep into the chick tissues. Intimate association between the two tissues is followed by invasion and finally by replacement of the cells of the embryonic organ with sarcoma cells. Different organs have been tested at different embryonic stages, and many have given positive results, e.g., mesonephros, metanephros, gonads, liver, lung, and intestinal layers. However, the 8- to 10-day mesonephros gave the best results and for that reason has been adopted as the "living medium" in virtually all subsequent experiments, in particular those involving human cancer.

Subsequently, human cell lines, maintained for several years in histiotypic culture *in vitro*, were associated with the mesonephros. These associations were carried out using the cell lines HeLa, KB, and FL (Et. Wolff and Em. Wolff, 1958*a,b*, 1959, 1961*a,b*, 1966) and were fully successful. The tissues of the mesonephros were sometimes completely invaded by the tumor cells; although the structure of the urinary tubes was apparently maintained, the walls of the tubes and the intertubular tissues were replaced by sarcoma cells (Fig. 3).

In this way, cell lines long adjusted to *in vitro* culture conditions were shown to be capable of associating with the mesonephros and of reconstituting sizable nodules recalling their epithelial origin. At this point, we undertook the culture of fragments of tumor removed directly from the patient.

3. Techniques

The techniques employed for the culture of human tumors derive from those developed for cultures of mouse and rat tumors. Initially, the mesonephros was used as nutrient substrate, acting as intermediary between the medium and the tumor. In later studies, dialyzing membranes were interposed between the mesonephros and the tumor. Still later, living embryonic organs were replaced, first by dialysates then by active fractions of these dialysates.

It should be pointed out that the basic medium used in all these experiments, as in those concerning organ cultures, is a nutrient medium which contains either embryo extract and serum or serum alone. Living embryonic organs are used as aliments when they are in direct contact with the cancerous tissues; in addition, they provide *growth-promoting substances.* Extracts of normal tissues, dialysates of these extracts, and various fractions prepared from them provide the tumors with substances indispensable for their growth. In their absence, the culture media, although adequate for normal embryonic organs, are insufficient despite their rich nutrient capacity for the survival and development of tumors.

3.1. *Cultures of Human Tumors on Mesonephros*

The following medium has been developed by us (Et. Wolff and Em. Wolff, 1960*b*):

1% agar in Gey's solution	10 vol
Horse serum	4 vol
Embryo extract diluted at 50% in Tyrode's solution	4 vol
Penicillin and various other antibiotics	several drops

Fragments of the tumor are placed on the medium next to fragments of the mesonephros of roughly similar dimensions (0.1- to 0.2-mm cube). They form a mosaic of small polygons which generally fuse with one another (Fig. 1a).

An improvement in the technique consists of spreading a piece of the vitelline membrane of a nonincubated chicken egg over the medium. The mosaic of tumor and mesonephros fragments is deposited on the membrane. The latter is then folded over the explants so as to envelop them in a kind of bag. The vitelline membrane thus serves as an intermediary between the medium and the explants on the one hand and the explants and the atmosphere on the other. It plays no part in the nutrition of the culture, but facilitates exchanges, allows the explants to spread out more thinly over a larger area, and promotes their fusion.

3.2. *Cultures on Mesonephros with Interposition of a Vitelline Membrane or a Dialysis Membrane*

A logical development of the aforementioned technique was to determine whether the living mesonephros was necessary for the culture of tumors. Must the tumors be in direct contact with the embryonic tissue or can they be sustained by the substances produced by the mesonephros which diffuse across the filtering membrane?

The same technique as before was used, but this time only the fragments of mesonephros were placed in the "bag" formed by the folded vitelline membrane. The tumor fragments were placed on top, thus being separated from the mesonephros by the membrane. The latter was then folded a second time over the tumor explants. Thus the two sorts of explants were separated by a fold of membrane (Fig. 1b). Although the pores of the membrane allowed large molecules to pass, no structured elements could cross: only substances in solution or fine suspension could filter through the pores.

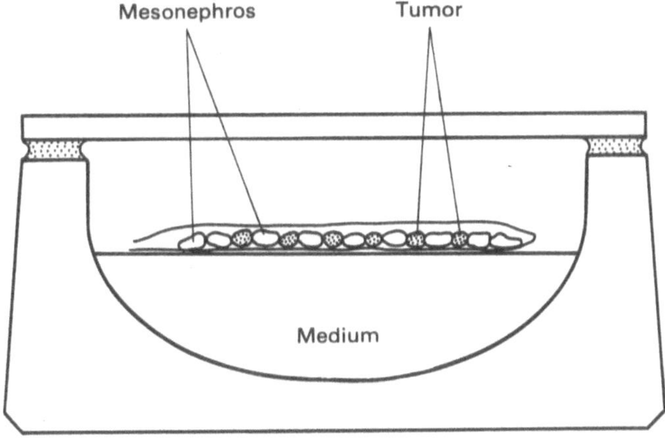

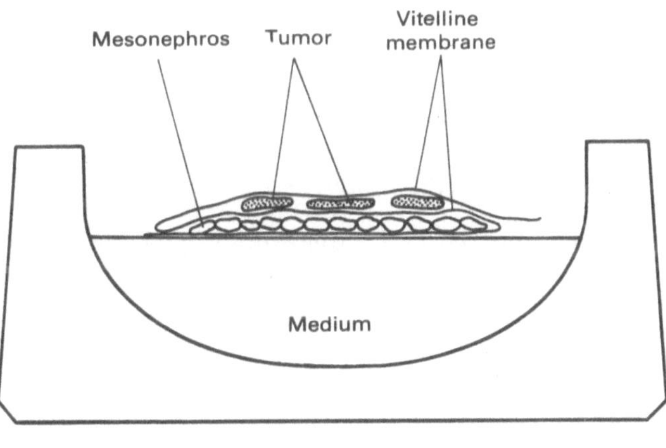

FIG. 1. Diagram of the two tumor culture techniques. (a) Culture of tumor explants in direct contact with fragments on mesonephros. (b) Culture of tumor explants separated from the mesonephros fragments by a vitelline membrane.

Thus the tumor fragments were able to use dissolved substances derived from the culture medium and, equally, diffusable substances exuded from the mesonephros. Both categories of substances have been found to be indispensable for the culture.

In certain experiments, the vitelline membrane was replaced by dialyzing membranes (cellophane, Visking tubing) for which the upper limits of permeability are known (mol wt 15,000).

3.3. Cultures on Nutrient Media Without Embryonic Organs

In subsequent experiments, we replaced the embryonic organs by dialysates of yeast or of liver from young chickens (Wolff *et al.*, 1966). These experiments were suggested by the preceding step, in which tumor explants were nourished by diffusion across a membrane. It should be noted that in such media embryo extract and serum were always present (under certain conditions, however, only the serum was retained).

3.3.1. With Yeast Dialysate

Having found that mesonephros extracts were toxic, we decided to use an extract of an acetone powder of brewer's yeast and, subsequently, the dialysate of this extract (Et. Wolff *et. al.*, 1965).

The composition of the culture medium was as follows:

1% agar in Gey's solution	11 vol
Horse serum	4 vol
Extract of 8½-day chick embryo diluted 50% in Tyrode's solution	4 vol
Yeast extract	1 vol

The yeast extract is prepared in the following way: Yeast (aerobic, Fould-Springer) is treated with 10 vol of acetone at 0°C. The suspension is disrupted in a blender capable of breaking the nuclei and filtered through paper. The residue is left to dry and the fine powder obtained is resuspended in Tyrode's solution and incubated for 3 h at 37°C. After centrifugation at 1000g for 15 min, the supernatant is sterilized by filtration through millipore membranes. It is this preparation which is used in the cultures.

The control media are prepared with the same ingredients minus the yeast extract. The explants used initially were tumor nodules previously cultured for several months on a dialyzing membrane and derived, respectively, from the 107th passage of tumor strain Z200 and the 60th passage of tumor strain Z516.

3.3.2. With Dialysate of Mesonephros from Chick Embryo and of Liver from Young Chicken (Em. Wolff et al., 1966)

a. Dialysate of Mesonephros from Chick Embryo. Cultures grown on a crude extract of 8- to 10-day mesonephros decline rapidly because of the toxicity of the extract. However, the dialysate was found to be favorable for the tumor culture. It is prepared from a homogenate in Tyrode's solution of 8- to 10-day mesonephros. The dialysis is carried out, as for yeast extracts, against distilled water, using Visking tubing. The dialysate is reduced by rotary evaporation to the initial volume of the mesonephros homogenate.

b. Dialysate of Liver from Young Chicken (Croisille et al., 1967). At first, dialysates were prepared in the same manner from homogenates of livers from 8- to 10-day embryos. However, on account of the considerable number of embryos required to prepare these extracts, tests were performed to determine whether dialysates of liver from 3-month-old chickens gave the same results. These were found to be just as active as the extracts of embryonic organs, and for this reason they have been used regularly ever since.

c. Preparation of the Dialysate of Liver Homogenate. Fifty grams of liver from 3-month-old chickens is suspended in 90 ml of a 1:1 dilution of Tyrode's solution with distilled water and homogenized in a blender (type H451, Equipements Industriels, Paris) at 40,000 rpm for 2½ min. The homogenate is dialyzed in tubes of Visking cellulose (Union Carbide, Chicago) at 4°C against a large volume of distilled water. The dialysate is concentrated to 90 ml by rotary evaporation *in vacuo*.

d. Properties of the Dialysates. To determine the approximate size of the pores of the dialysis tubes, we have used solutions of substances of known molecular weight. Cytochrome *c* (mol wt 16,500) does not cross the membrane, lysozyme (mol wt 14,380) is at the limit of retention, whereas ribonuclease (mol wt 12,700) passes easily. Thus we can assert that the dialysates of liver, mesonephros, and brewer's yeast contain only substances with a molecular weight lower than 15,000. All molecules with a molecular weight higher than 15,000, and, in consequence, large protein molecules, are retained in the dialysis bag.

In subsequent experiments, we have fractionated the dialysates and studied the effectiveness of the different fractions. Technical details will be given later, together with a study of the results of these fractionations.

4. *Results*

4.1. *Organotypic Culture of Cells Previously in Cell Culture*

To begin with, we associated *cultures of human cells*, previously grown for a considerable time in monolayers in liquid media. Among those used were the histiotypic cell lines KB, isolated by Eagle from an epithelioma of the buccal floor, HeLa, isolated by Gey from the epithelium of the cervix, and FL, isolated by Fogh and Lund from human amnion cells transformed *in vitro*.

In classical cell culture, the cells of these cancerous lines have an undifferentiated aspect and develop as a monolayer on the glass walls of the culture vessel. For organotypic culture, fragments of this layer are scraped from the walls of the vessel and washed several times. They are associated as a mosaic with fragments of mesonephros from 8½-day chick embryos on the culture medium of Wolff and Wolff. Several hours after the explantation, the organ fragments and the cancer cells have completely fused. The latter migrate into the interior of the mesonephros, which they invade more or less completely (Fig. 2).

In organ culture, each strain has its particularities as regards the shape of the cells, their penetrative ability, and the way in which they form a mass and associate. Each one loses the dedifferentiated aspect it had in cell culture and forms more or less massive nodules, composed of numerous tiers of cells (Fig. 3). These cultures can be transferred to new mesonephros on fresh culture medium every 7–14 days, and some have been maintained in this way for several months. It is likely that they could be kept going indefinitely without any diminution in their capacity for proliferation (Et. Wolff, 1956; Et. Wolff and Em. Wolff, 1958*a,b*, 1959, 1960*a,b*, 1961*a,b*; Em. Wolff, 1962, 1964).

If a filtering membrane such as the vitelline membrane of the hen's egg is put between the mesonephros and the mass of tumor cells, the latter grow, no longer directly on the embryonic tissue, but on substances which are elaborated by the mesonephros and pass across the membrane. Massive nodules, with various degrees of organization, are formed. In certain cases, one obtains stratified epithelial formations (Figs. 4 and 5) which reproduce certain characteristics of the original tumor.

These cell strains have also been successfully grown on liver, gonads, and metanephros, but the mesonephros of the 8- to 10-day chick is the most conducive to the prolonged multiplication of these tumors.

4.2. Short-Term Cultures

A considerable number of short-term cultures have been obtained by means of the two methods employed by Wolff and Wolff, namely parasitic nutrition by contact (Et. Wolff *et al.*, 1962) and nutrition by dialysis across a membrane (Et. Wolff, 1961).

Whereas the media used for the culture of organs do not allow transplanted tumors to survive for more than 2 or 3 days, these two techniques have enabled us to grow, *in vitro*, many human tumors removed directly from the patient during surgical operations or biopsies. Among those which have given positive results are the following:

Glandular gastric epitheliomas
Various types of intestinal adenocarcinomas
Several tumors of the colon
Epidermoid bronchopulmonary tumors
A small-cell anaplastic carcinoma of the lung
A pulmonary adenocarcinoma
Epitheliomas of the bladder
An epidermoid cancer of the tongue
A glandular epithelioma of the corpus of the uterus
A small-cell cervical carcinoma
Breast epitheliomas
Lymphoblastic granulomas and lymphomas
Lymph nodes from patients with Hodgkin's disease

Generally speaking, one can count on a survival time of at least a week when the sample is reasonably rich in healthy tumor cells. Attempts to culture regions where cancer cells are very thinly dispersed and experiments with extremely fibrous tumors are usually unsuccessful.

When directly associated, human tumors and embryonic chick tissues fuse within several hours and form a solid mass which develops in three dimensions. One can often observe active proliferation of the tumor cells, which start from centers of implantation and penetrate the mesonephros; sometimes the mesonephros is completely invaded. Histological sections resemble normal mesonephros in structure, but the walls and interstices of the tubes are replaced by tumor cells (see Fig. 3).

In such chimeras, the cancer cells can be recognized just as easily as if they were labeled. They are readily distinguishable from the embryonic chick cells by their large size and their strongly basophilic nuclei. It would be difficult for even a single tumor cell to escape detection.

Many tumors (principally those of epithelial origin) can be grown for periods of 1–6 wk, which enables certain short-term experiments to be carried out. It is hard to estimate the probability of success in tumor explantation, for many of the tumors which we were given were very deficient in cells, contained large necrotic portions, or were composed mainly of cells in a poor state of preservation. However, as a rough figure, 30–40% of explanted tumors are able to survive for 1–6 wk.

On the other hand, we have noted that tumors of small rodents can be grown more easily than human tumors. This is probably because of the relative ease with which one can obtain perfectly fresh animal tumors and select the most promising parts for culture.

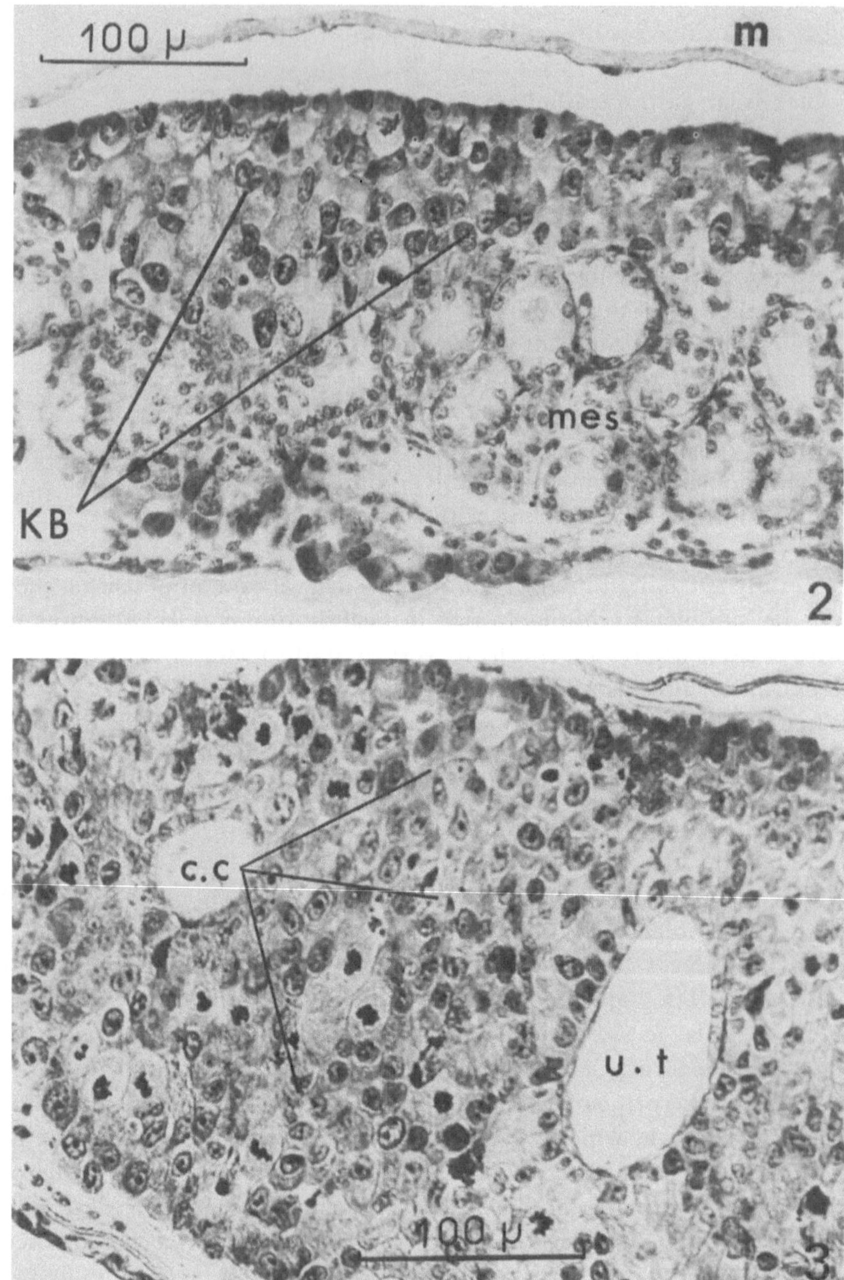

FIG. 2. Section of a nodule of KB cancer cells grown in contact with chick mesonephros. The association is enveloped in a vitelline membrane. KB, Cancer cells; m, vitelline membrane; mes, mesonephros. From Et. Wolff and Em. Wolff (1961). FIG. 3. Complete invasion of a mesonephros explant by HeLa cells. The cells composing the tubes of the embryonic kidney have been lined with or replaced by tumor cells. c.c., Cancer cells; u.t., urinary tubes lined with cancer cells. From Et. Wolff and Em. Wolff (1961*a*,*b*).

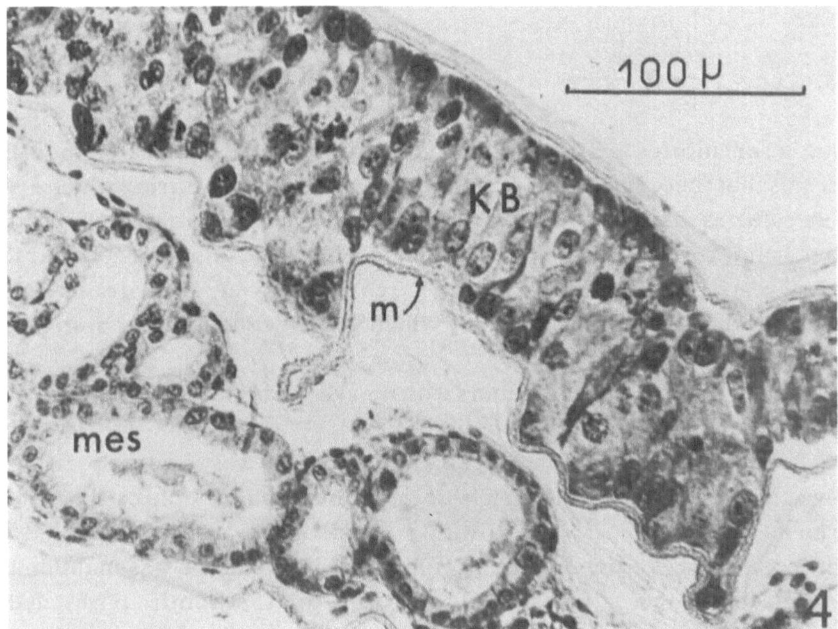

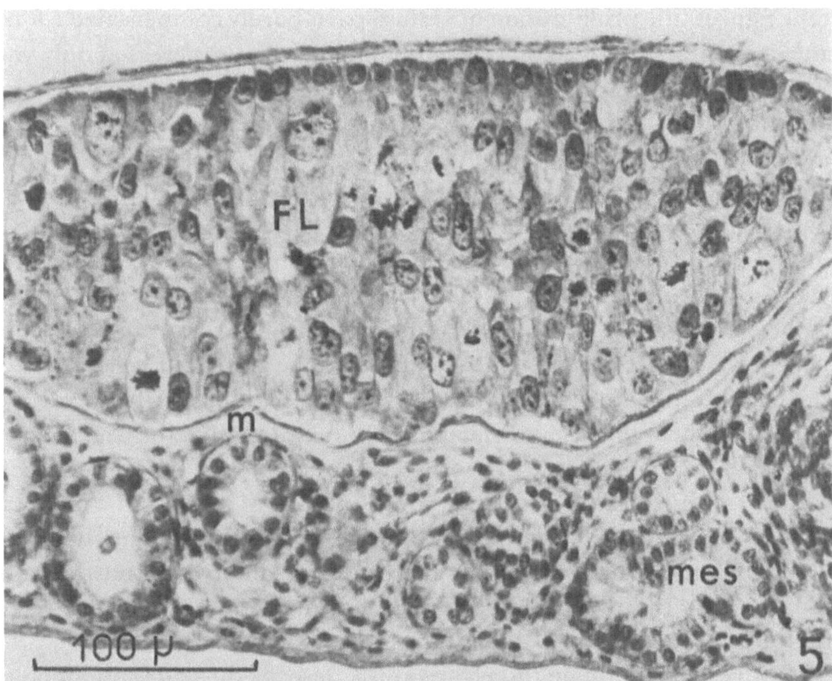

FIG. 4. KB cells cultured in the presence of chick mesonephros, with an interposed vitelline membrane. KB, Cancer cells; m, vitelline membrane; mes, mesonephros. From Et. Wolff and Em. Wolff (1961*a,b*). FIG. 5. Fogh FL cancer cells, transformed *in vitro*, cultured with interposition of a vitelline membrane. Note the palisade-type epithelial arrangement and the numerous mitotic figures. Fl, Cancer cells; m, vitelline membrane; mes. mesonephros. From Et. Wolff and Em. Wolff (1961*a,b*).

4.3. Long-Term Cultures

Long-term cultures are those which have proliferated for at least 6 months. It seems that there is a critical stage around 3 or 4 months during which even those cultures that appear to be prospering have difficulty in passing. On the other hand, certain cultures have exceeded 1 yr, and some have lasted for several years. Two tumors (Z 200 and Z 516) have given rise to strains which persist after more than 10 yr and which have been used for systematic experiments.

Below we give a list of the tumors which have been grown for more than 1 yr, together with their characteristics.

Pulmonary adenocarcinoma Ra 90: This tumor was removed from a 63-yr-old woman and cultured in association with mesonephros. *In vitro*, it formed small, compact clumps with an epithelioid aspect, composed of tightly packed cylindrical or polygonal cells. This culture was maintained through 42 passages (at intervals of 8–12 days) for 15½ months. It was finally abandoned when, despite a generally healthy aspect and the presence of mitotic figures, the proliferation of certain parts barely compensated for the disintegration of others, so that the number of explants increased only very slowly.

Hepatic metastasis of a tumor of the digestive tract (probably of gastric origin), Z 200: The culture was started on January 10, 1962, and the tumor continues to proliferate after 13 yr *in vitro*. It is likely that, accidents excepted, it will be able to multiply indefinitely. The number of explants can be increased *ad libitum*, depending on experimental requirements. There are currently several hundred explants in culture; at certain moments there have been several thousand. The tumor retains approximately its initial structure of an adenocarcinoma composed of epithelioid cells grouped around cavities, or lined up along the vitelline membrane. However, the secretion of mucus into the cavities is less abundant than at the beginning of the culture. Immunological properties are unchanged: the nodules continue to synthesize the carcinoembryonic antigen of Gold and Freedman (Burtin *et al.*, 1970). The number and type of chromosomes have not altered: karyotype analysis reveals the same variability around the same mode as at the beginning of the experiment (deGrouchy and Em. Wolff, 1969).

The two explantation methods previously described—with mesonephros in direct contact (Figs. 6 and 7) or with a vitelline membrane interposed (Fig. 8)—have been used with equal success. The explants cultured in this way tend to exhibit a characteristic morphology—that of smooth, disc-shaped nodules. This external aspect is observed even more clearly in the case of cultures grown on liver or yeast dialysate, as will be mentioned in Section 4.4.

Cylindrical epithelioma of the colon, Z 516: Fragments of a tumor of the descending colon were taken from an 80-yr-old woman and associated with 8½-day mesonephros. The tumor had the aspect of a mucous cylindrical epithelioma of the colon. It was characterized by tubular formations, composed of one or several layers of tall, cylindrical epithelial cells, arranged around wide mucus-containing cavities. This tumor was first cultured on October 29, 1963, and gave rise to more than 700 explants in 1 yr. Only practical considerations have limited this intense proliferation. The results were equally good whatever the culture method employed. With the interposition of the vitelline membrane, the explants take on a characteristic aspect, very different from that of tumor Z 200 (Figs. 9 and 10). They tend to constitute large, mucus-filled vesicles, around which the cellular layers form narrow epithelial bands. These features become more marked when the cultures are grown on dialysates in the absence of mesonephros. Tumor Z 516 multiplied very actively for 10 yr but had eventually to be abandoned following mycoplasma infection.

Tumor AZ 110: This is a tumor of the ascending colon (Et. Wolff and Em. Wolff, 1972; Em. Wolff *et al.*, 1972) taken from a 73-yr-old woman. It was characterized by multiple tubular or adenoid structures. First cultured on February 11, 1970, it continues to flourish 5 yr later. Its histological structure conforms with that of the parent tumor, although the aspect is predominantly adenoid rather than tubular. A certain number of multipolar mitotic figures can be observed in addition to numerous normal ones (Fig. 11).

The rapid growth of this tumor *in vitro* has been demonstrated by measurements of various parameters over defined periods. After 10–13 days of culture following a transplantation on to fresh medium, the dry weight of the explants was found to have increased to 180–575% of the initial value, depending on the series. RNA content increased to 220–660% over the same length of time; the DNA level rose similarly (230–680%).

Tumor AZ 432: This is a hepatic metastasis of rectal origin, removed from a man of 68. The primary culture was started on June 6, 1972 (unpublished work). After biopsy, the metastases had the appearance of a Lieberkühnian adenocarcinoma. The same features are retained in culture, i.e., epithelial structures, forming blind tubes or sinuous ribbons, composed of tall cylindrical cells.

These cultures continue to multiply after more than 2 yr on chick mesonephros. Some have been separated from the mesonephros by a vitelline membrane and have undergone several successive transfers on such media, but their adaptation to this mode of nutrition is apparently not yet perfect.

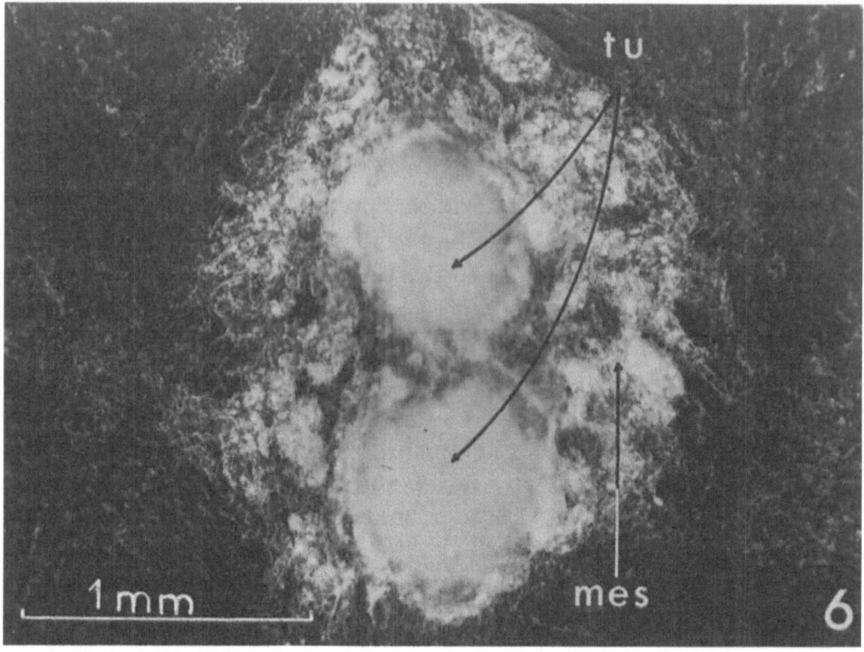

FIG. 6. Appearance of two living tumor nodules of the strain Z 200, cultured on mesonephros. mes, Mesonephros; tu, tumor. From Et. Wolff *et al.* (1965).

4.4. Analysis of Nutritive Requirements of Tumors in in Vitro Cultures

4.4.1. Nutrient Factors and Growth Factors

As already mentioned, none of the explanted tumors can survive in the absence of an embryonic organ or of an extract of an embryonic organ. The basic medium is nevertheless rich in nutrients. Similar to that used for the culture of tissues and organs, it contains embryo extract, horse serum, and a physiological salt solution supplemented with glucose.

However, on the same medium, if the tumor fragments are associated with an embryonic organ, particularly with the mesonephros, they survive and multiply actively. The same result is obtained when filtering membranes, such as the vitelline membrane of the hen's egg, cellophane membranes or Visking cellulose dialyzing membranes, are placed between the organ and the tumor. In subsequent studies, we used media to which extracts or dialysates (crude extract of yeast or the dialysate prepared from it, dialysate of a homogenate of liver from 3-month-old chickens) were added.

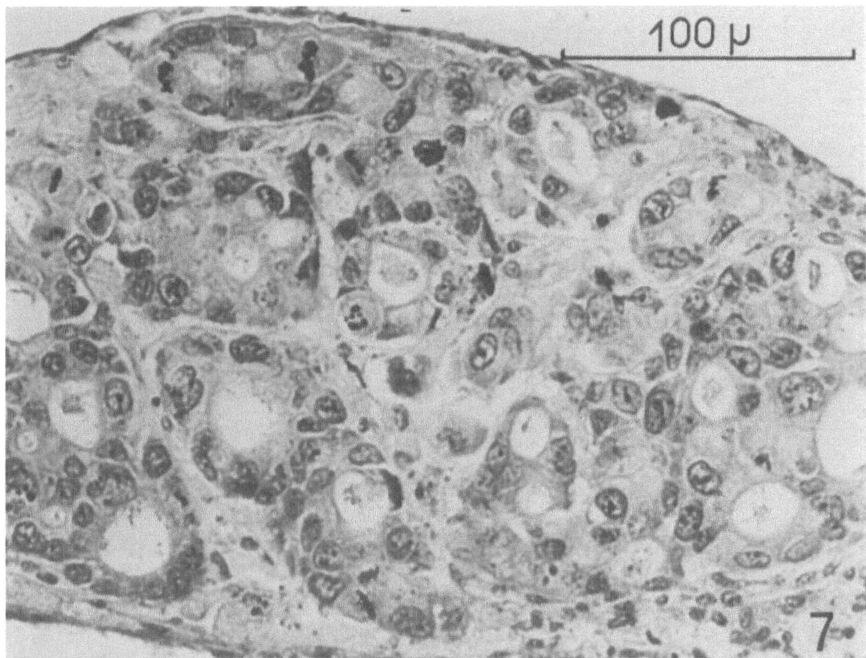

FIG. 7. Histological appearance of a nodule of tumor Z 200 during primary culture on mesonephros. Note the mucus-filled alveoli lined with epithelioid cells. From Et. Wolff and Em. Wolff (1967).

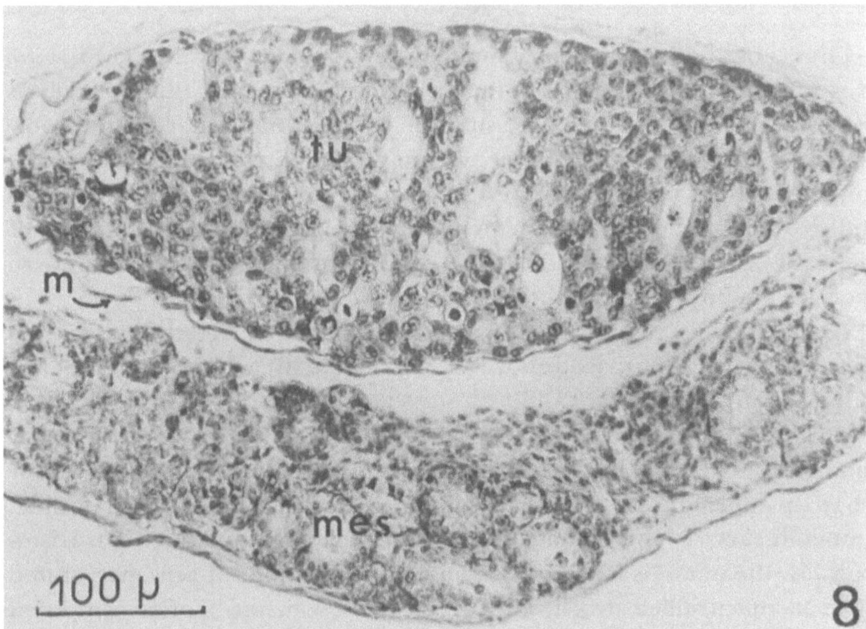

FIG. 8. Transverse section of a nodule of tumor Z 200 cultured on mesonephros with a vitelline membrane interposed. m, Membrane; mes, mesonephros; tu, explant of tumor Z 200. From Et. Wolff and Em. Wolff (1967).

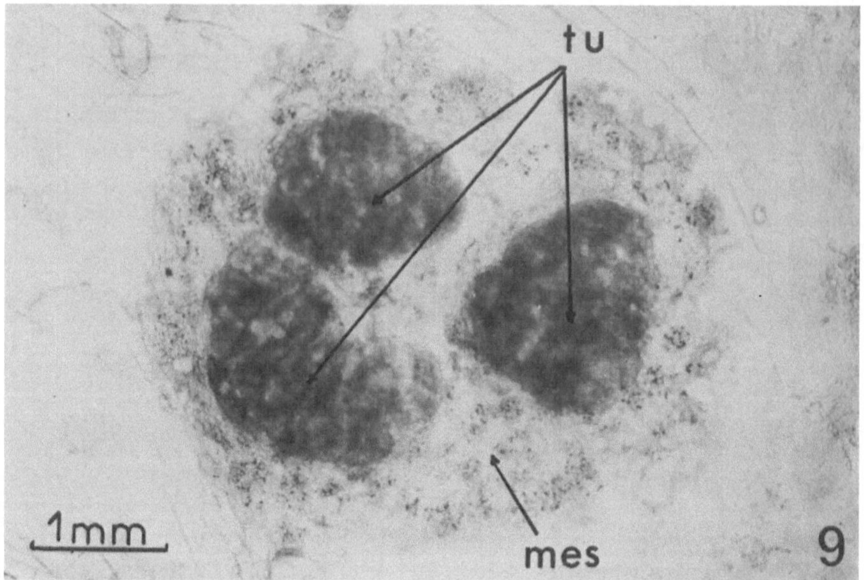

FIG. 9. Explants of tumor of the colon Z 516 cultured on mesonephros. mes, Mesonephros: tu, explants of the tumor Z 516. From Em. Wolff (1964).

Thus substances which enable human tumors to survive and grow *in vitro* exist in embryonic organs or in their extracts. From the results of dialysis experiments, we know that these substances have a molecular weight below 15,000. As a working hypothesis, we may consider that the organotypic culture medium provides the necessary aliments, while the mesonephros and extracts provide growth factors. Only a relatively small proportion of dialysate (one-eleventh of the total volume of medium) is required to produce the growth-promoting effect.

The bulk of our research on nutrient factors has involved the two tumors of intestinal origin described above (Z 200 and Z 516), which have given rise to long-term cultures.

a. Strain Z 200. Explants of Z 200 grown on dialysates acquire a very characteristic morphology which differs considerably from that of tumor Z 516. In appearance they are spheroid or lenticular, with a regular outline, a smooth surface, and homogeneous, translucid contents (Fig. 12). Histologically, the tumor is made up of dense accumulations of cells, perforated by small, mucus-filled alveoli. The surface of these masses is often composed of a cylindrical epithelium with tall cells in which the nuclei are elongated, arranged parallel to the cellular membranes, and situated on the basal side (Figs. 13 and 14).

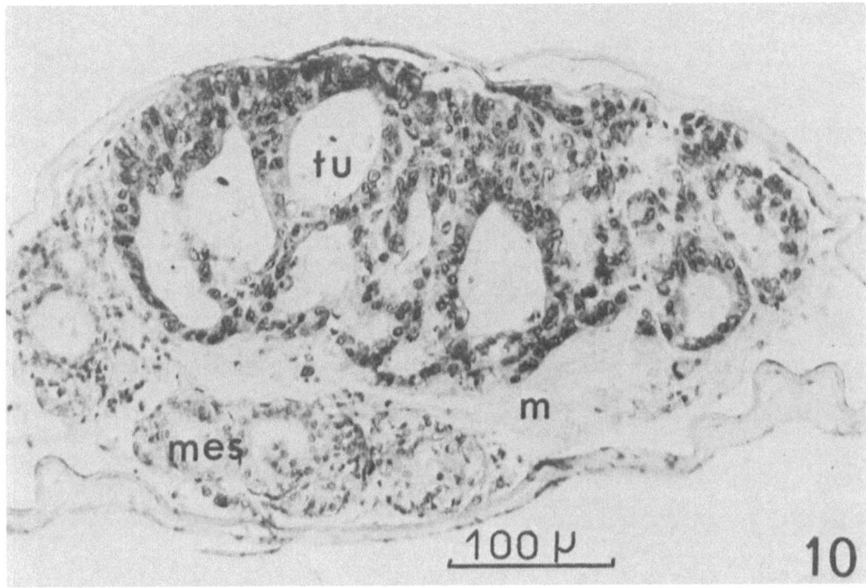

FIG. 10. Histological appearance of the tumor Z 516 cultured on mesonephros with interposed vitelline membrane. m, Membrane; mes, mesonephros; tu, tumor. From Em. Wolff (1964).

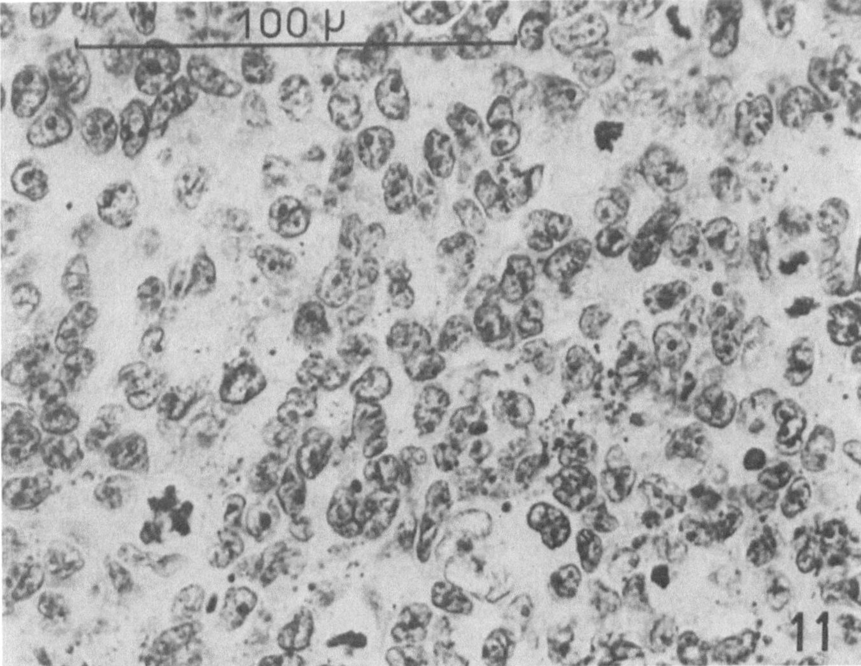

FIG. 11. Section through an explant of the tumor AZ 110 after 2½ yr of organotypic culture *in vitro*. Note the numerous mitotic figures, including a tripolar one (on the left). From Em. Wolff *et al.* (1972).

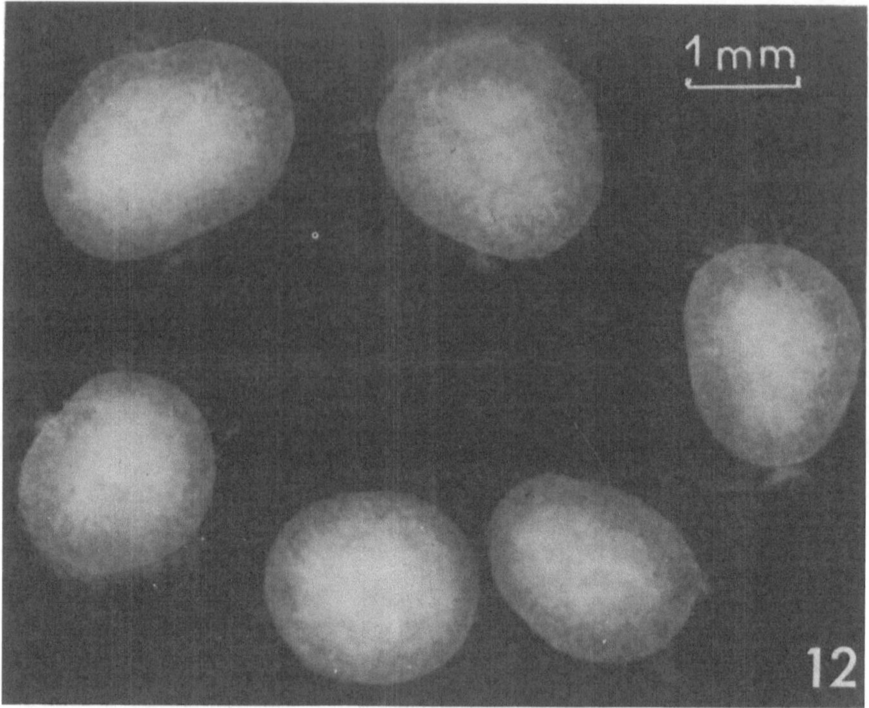

FIG. 12. Nodules of tumor Z 200 cultured on the nutrient medium in the presence of yeast extract. Observed by reflected light, the explants appear as ovoid or discoid nodules with a smooth surface. From Et. Wolff *et al.* (1965).

b. Strain Z 516. The surface of the nodules of strain Z 516 is irregular, folded and carved into numerous furrows and deep clefts. These features confer on it a superficial resemblance to "cerebral cortex" (Figs. 15 and 18). Histological sections show solid masses of tumor cells hollowed out into large, mucus-filled cavities and enveloped in a continuous cortex of plurilayered high cylindrical cells from which thick, sinuous cords ramify toward the interior of the nodule (Figs. 16 and 17).

Thus organotypic human tumors, grown in the absence of any other living tissue, tend to develop an external morphology and a specific structure which are, if anything, more organized than in the parent tumor.

4.4.2. Fractionation of Dialysates

We have sought to determine the nature of the growth-promoting substances contained in the extracts. Studies were carried out in parallel on the dialysates of yeast and liver. In both cases the results were similar, as shown in Figs. 19 and 20 (Croisille *et al.*, 1967).

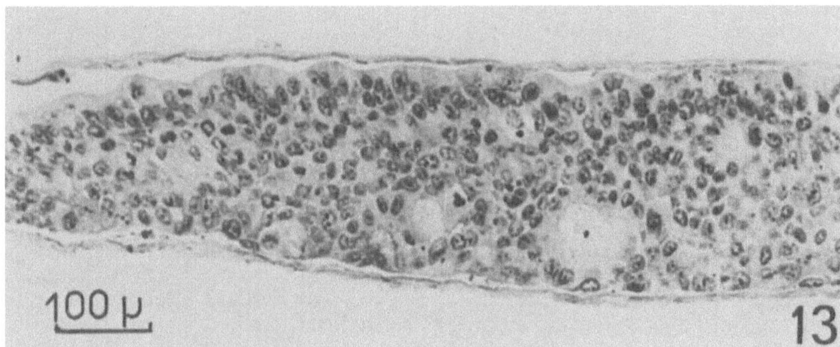

FIG. 13. General view of a transverse section of a nodule. It is dense and massive with several mucus-containing alveoli (below). From Et. Wolff *et al.* (1965).

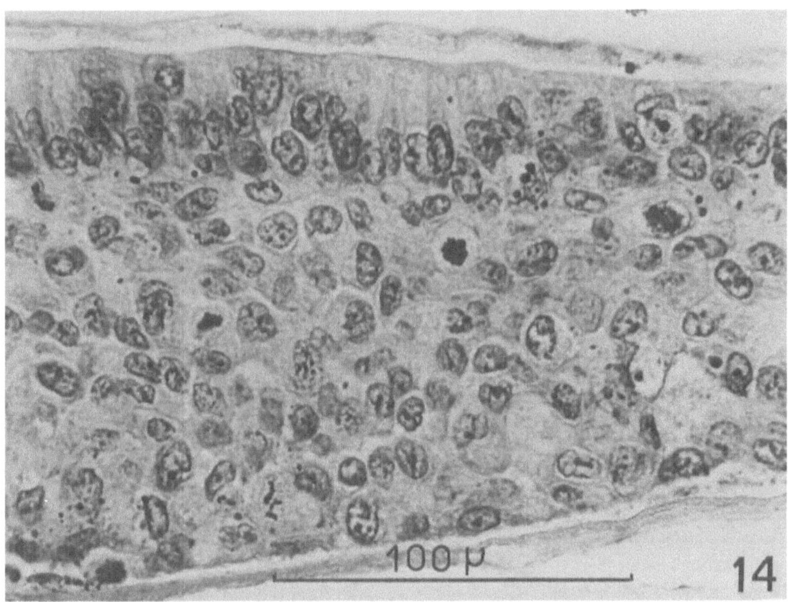

FIG. 14. Section of a massive nodule showing the surface bordered by a single-layered cylindrical epithelium. From Et. Wolff *et al.* (1965).

1. The yeast dialysate was fractionated by gel filtration on Sephadex G 25. Four fractions, Sep A, Sep B, Sep C, and Sep D, were tested in culture. Separately they were inactive, but Sep A and Sep B mixed together (Sep X) gave positive results.

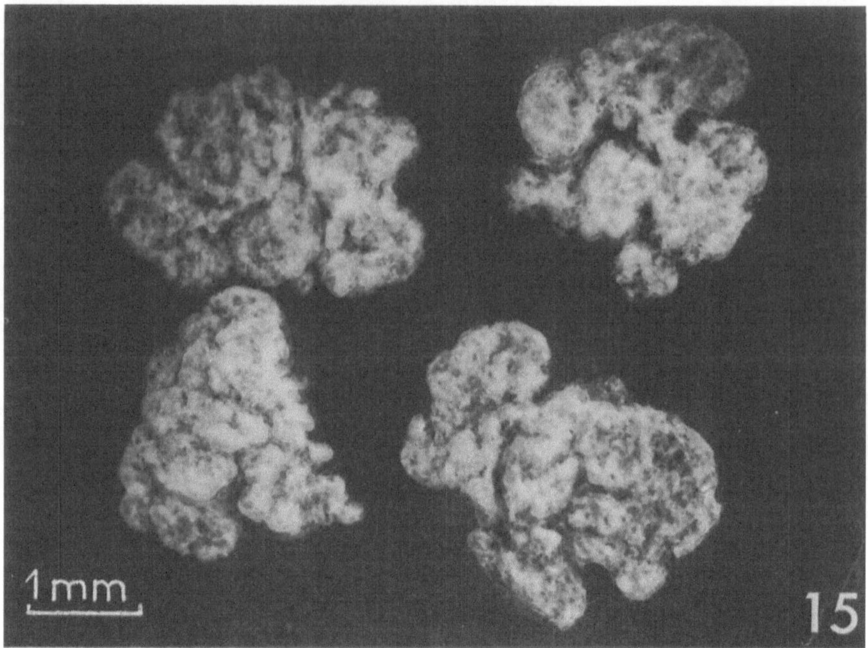

FIG. 15. Tumor Z 516 grown in the absence of mesonephros, but in the presence of yeast extract. Note the corrugated, irregular appearance of the explants, whose surface, viewed by reflected light, recalls the convolutions of the cerebral cortex. From Et. Wolff *et al.* (1965).

In two parallel experiments, Sep X and liver dialysate were fractionated by ion-exchange chromatography. On columns of Amberlite IR 120 (cation exchanger, in the H^+-form), an inactive fraction (Cat A, eluted by water) was separated from a very active one (Cat B, eluted by ammonia). Fractions Cat B and Ano A, whether derived from brewers yeast or 3-month chicken liver, promoted vigorous growth of the two strains of tumor in organotypic culture.

2. In a subsequent step, fractions Cat B and Cat A (from yeast or liver) were further fractionated on columns of Amberlite IRA 400 (anion exchanger, in the OH^--form). Four new fractions were obtained: "neutral" and "acid" from Cat A, "base" and "ampholyte" from Cat B. Only the "ampholyte" fraction was active, whichever the source of the original extract (Figs. 19 and 20). In a subsequent purification step, the "ampholyte" fraction was subjected to chromatography on a column of Sephadex G10. By this means, an active fraction, Dis A, was separated from an inactive one.

Each active fraction was found to be very rich in ninhydrin-positive substances, among which were numerous amino acids. In addition, polypep-

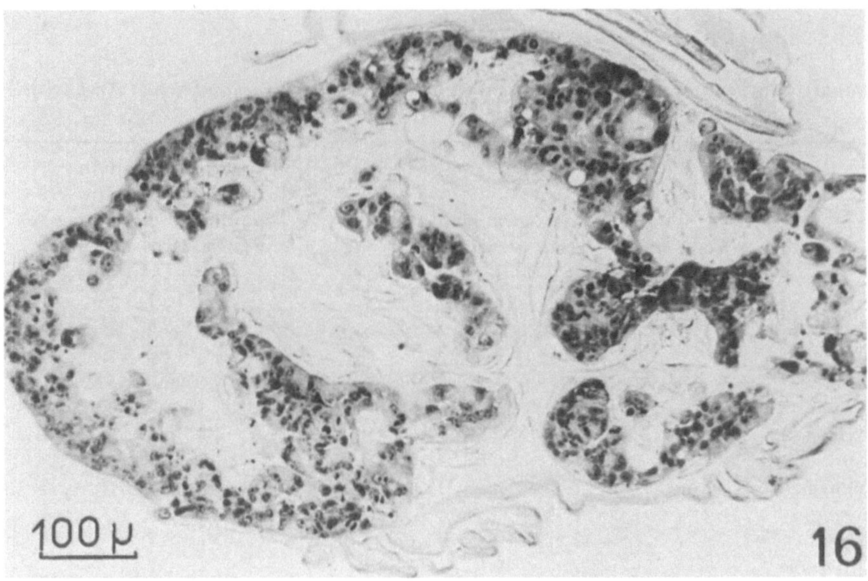

FIG. 16. General view of a section of a nodule of tumor Z 516 grown on yeast extract. Note the superficial cortex giving off cords which ramify toward the center of the nodule. All the spaces are filled with mucus. From Et. Wolff and Em. Wolff (1966).

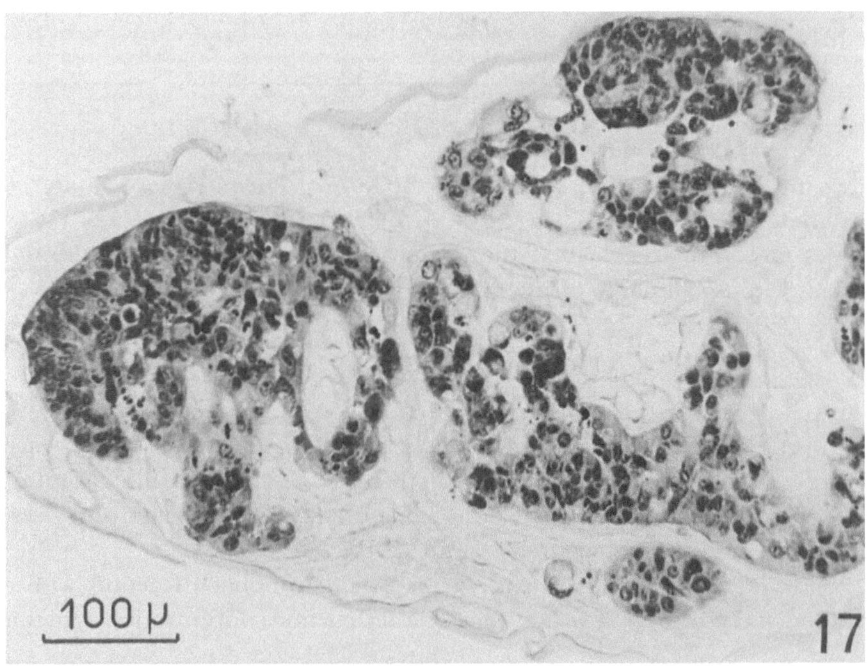

FIG. 17. Another histological section of tumor Z 516. The nodule is carved out into several lobes which are bathed in mucus. From Et. Wolff and Em. Wolff (1966).

TABLE 1

Comparison of Amino Acid Concentrations in Chick Embryo Extract and in the "Ampholyte" Fraction

Amino acids	Concentration in chick embryo extract (mM)	Concentration in the hydrolysate of the "ampholyte" fraction of chick liver dialysate (mM)
Alanine	0.35	16.1
Arginine	0.10	0.5
Aspartic acid	0.22	12.9
Cysteine	—	0.9
Glutamic acid	0.85	18.2
Glycine	0.30	15.0
Histidine	0.08	3.1
Isoleucine	0.10	5.6
Leucine	0.11	11.6
Lysine	0.15	8.7
Methionine	0.01	2.7
Ornithine	0.02	2.1
Phenylalanine	0.07	3.6
Proline	—	8.6
Serine	0.43	10.6
Threonine	0.19	7.6
Tryptophan	+	—
Tyrosine	0.12	2.0
Valine	0.14	12.8

tides, ultraviolet-absorbing substances, and fluorescent and colored material were detected.

It is most remarkable that the same active fraction should be found starting from material so different as brewer's yeast and chicken liver.

4.4.3. Measurement of Amino Acid Concentration (Smith et al., 1971)

The amino acids in the "ampholyte" fraction were determined by means of a Technicon automatic amino acid analyzer. Eighteen amino acids were identified and their concentrations calculated. The amino acid content of the embryo extract, determined at the same time for comparative purposes, was found in general to be much lower (Table 1).

Following these results, we replaced the "ampholyte" fraction with a solution of these 18 amino acids, each one at the same concentration as in this

FIG. 18. Another macroscopic view of a nodule of tumor Z 516 cultured without mesonephros on yeast extract. Note the circumvolutions and the convolutions and furrows, which roughly recall the aspect of a brain.

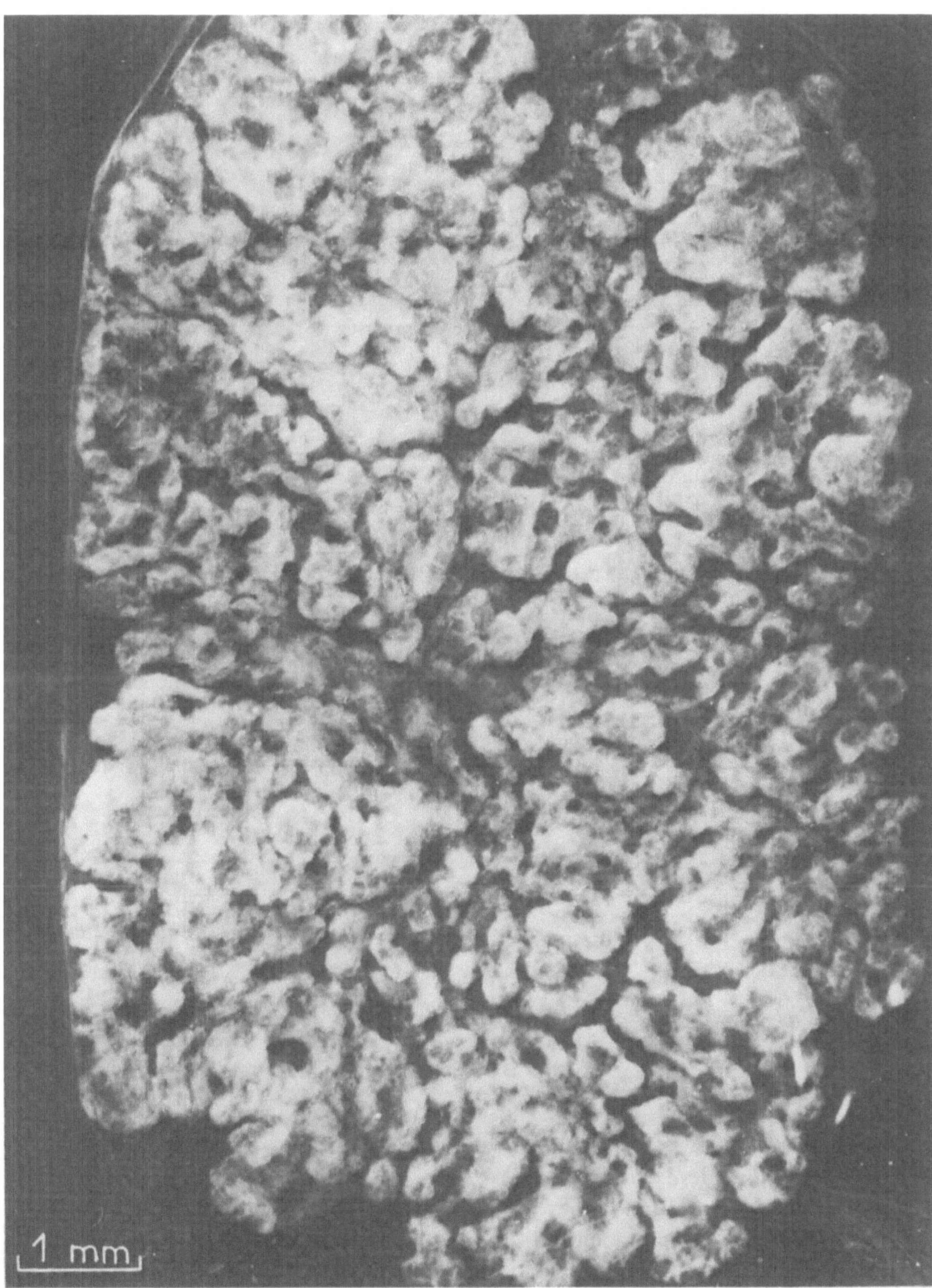
1 mm

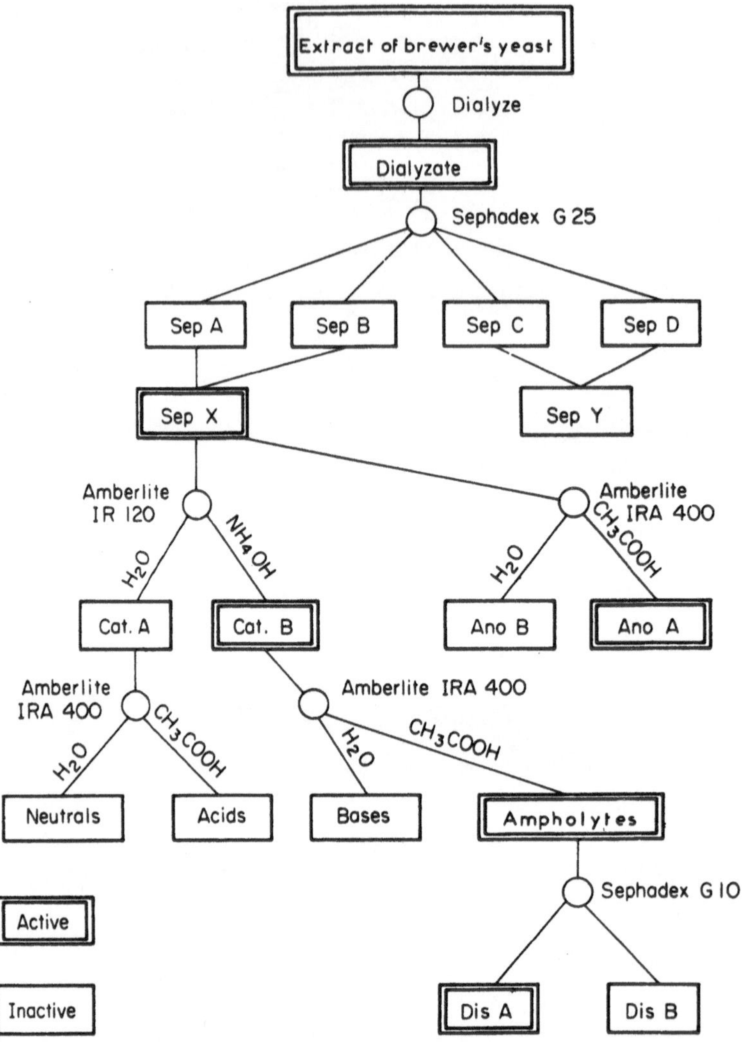

FIG. 19. Fractionation of dialysate of brewer's yeast, leading to results similar to fractionation of dialysate of 3-month chicken liver (Fig. 20). From Em. Wolff *et al.* (1967).

fraction. In this way, we obtained a solution which was very active in the presence of embryo extract.

In order to ascertain whether all 18 amino acids were necessary for tumor growth, we prepared 17 solutions, each with 17 amino acids at the concentrations determined by the previous analysis, but with one (each time different) missing from each solution. By this means, five amino acids have been found

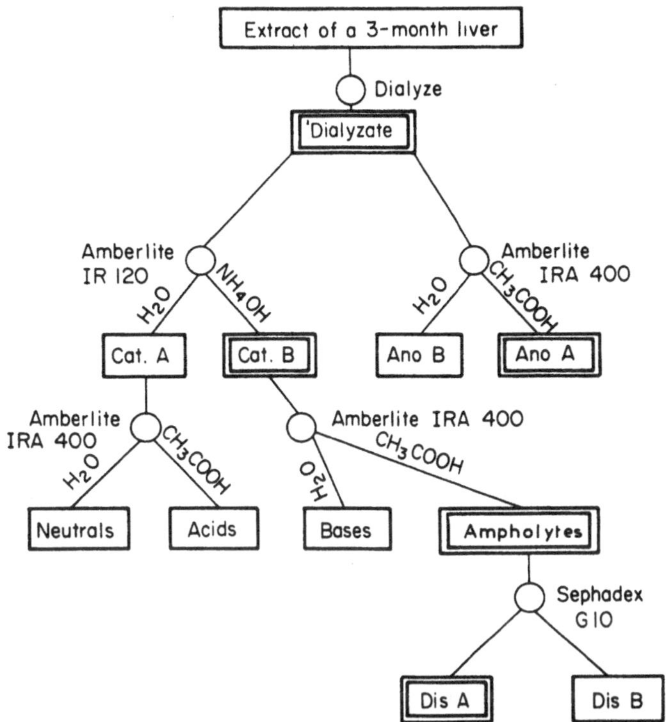

FIG. 20. Fractionation of dialysate of 3-month chicken liver, leading to results similar to fractionation of dialysate of brewer's yeast (Fig. 19). From Em. Wolff *et al.* (1967).

to be indispensable, notably cysteine, methionine, arginine, leucine, and lysine. The concentration of each is 5–200 times that found in the embryo extract. The other amino acids can act as adjuvants but are not indispensable.

4.4.4. *Localization of the Indispensable Growth Factors*

However, do these amino acids represent *all* the factors required for the unlimited growth of the tumors? It should be borne in mind that the five essential amino acids, as well as the 13 others, are already present in the embryo extract and in the serum. Thus it is by virtue of their concentration, i.e., quantitatively rather than qualitatively, that they produce their effect.

To try to clarify this problem, the embryo extract was omitted from the culture medium and the dialysate was replaced with the appropriate amino acid solution (the serum remaining present).

The results were as follows:

1. In the presence of embryo extract, the amino acid solution can replace the dialysate.

2. In the absence of embryo extract, the amino acids cannot stimulate growth.
3. In the presence of boiled embryo extract, the amino acids cannot stimulate growth.

If the embryo extract is left out of the medium and replaced with an equivalent volume of Tyrode's solution, the tumor explants continue to proliferate, provided that one of the dialysates (yeast or liver) is present. Consequently, these two dialysates contain all the growth factors necessary for the multiplication of the tumors. As a result, they are able to assure the unlimited growth of the explants.

The replacement of a dialysate in the culture medium with the corresponding boiled dialysate was without effect on the intensity of proliferation of the explants only if unboiled (fresh) embryo extract was present.

Thus there exists in both the embryo extract and the dialysate one or more factors (F) necessary for growth. This indispensable complement is inactivated by heating the dialysates or the embryo extract at 100°C. In addition, thermostable substances (the amino acids) are present in sufficient amounts only in the two dialysates (Table 2).

In conclusion, at the present time it appears that two categories of factors are indispensable: first, amino acids at concentrations higher than those found in the embryo extract, and, second, substances as yet unidentified

TABLE 2

Combined Action of Certain Constituents of the Culture Medium[a]

	(F) EE	(0) EE replaced by Tyrode's solution	(0) EE boiled
Amino acid solution (AA)	(AA) + (F) +	(AA) + (0) −	(AA) + (0) −
Liver dialysate (AA + F)	(AA + F) + (F) +	(AA + F) + (0) +	(AA + F) + (0) +
Liver dialysate, boiled (AA) + (0)	(AA) + (F) +	(AA) + (0) −	(AA) + (0) −
Yeast dialysate (AA + F)	(AA + F) + (F) +	(AA + F) + (0) +	(AA + F) + (0) −
Yeast dialysate, boiled (AA + 0)	(AA) + (F) +	(AA) + (0) −	(AA) + (0) −

[a] EE, Chick embryo extract; AA, indispensable amino acids; AAS, solution of amino acids; F, thermolabile growth factor; 0, absence of the growth factor F.

which exist in dialysates of yeast or chicken liver and in embryo extract and are destroyed by boiling.

4.5. *Applications of the Organized Culture of Human Tumors*

Several examples will be given here of the research made possible by the technique of organ culture.

4.5.1. *Attempts to Characterize Factors of Maintenance and Growth of Tumors in Vitro*

The topic of the nutritive requirements of cultured tumors has already been treated in detail in Section 4.4. It is of prime interest, for it is probable that the living organism must provide developing malignant tumors with conditions of nitrition (aliments and growth factors) similar to those necessary *in vitro*. These studies can thus contribute to the investigation of a very important problem—that of the development of malignant tumors. It is not enough for a normal cell to undergo a mutation which confers malignant properties on it; this transformation probably occurs in a great number of cells of an organism, at various moments. In addition, the transformed cells must find a favorable environment—in other words, an adequate nutrient medium together with the essential growth factors. Our research with organotypic culture ought to make an important contribution to this area of investigation.

4.5.2. *Attempts to Inhibit Growth*

Of all the experiments which suggest themselves, attempts to inhibit tumor growth are naturally among the most important. Such studies were initiated in our laboratory, particularly by Pageot-Simpson and Et. Wolff (1969) and Simpson (1969), and are being continued at the present time, using substances such as rubidomycin which are employed in the control of cancer and leukemia.

However, the results of such experiments are difficult to interpret, for nothing is more simple than to obtain a cessation of development or to cause the necrosis of an organotypic culture in an environment which provides the explants with no means of defense. Any modification of the medium, the addition of any chemical, any microbial or viral irruption can rapidly result in the necrosis of tumor explants. Obviously, a comparison must be made with normal control cultures. This is what we have tried to do, but it must be emphasized that truly *valid* controls do not exist, since adult organs and tissues cannot be grown in organotypic culture. Thus one must turn to embryonic organs, whose reactions to inhibitors may be different from those of adult organs. Further, embryonic organs can be cultured only for a limited period (generally not more than 1 month), and in any case active growth occurs only during the first few days.

Thus embryonic organs have to be used as controls in experiments which can not be of very long duration. Nevertheless, these studies can provide valuable indications as to the relative resistance of normal and malignant cells in organotypic explants.

4.5.3. Evaluation of the Malignancy of Cell Lines

The degree of malignancy of certain cell lines can be determined by associating them with chick embryo mesonephros in organotypic culture. These experiments have been carried out with various mouse cell lines (Et. Wolff *et al.*, 1960; Barski and Em. Wolff, 1965), but it is reasonable to suppose that the method is applicable to human tumor cells.

As an example, we may consider three cell lines derived from normal fibroblasts of C3H mice. Cell line N1 (derived from clone NCTC 2472 of Sanford and Earle) was highly malignant; line N2 (derived from clone NCTC 2555) was malignant in only 2–3% of the cases in which it was inoculated into C3H mice. Barski's clone M1, a somatic hybrid of N1 and N2, with a karyotype which shows chromosomal markers of both lines, was highly malignant.

Fragments of monolayers of these different cell lines were removed from the culture vessels and associated with chick embryo mesonephros. The capacity of these lines to multiply and penetrate the embryonic tissue provides as good a measure of malignancy as experiments in which the cells are inoculated into animals, and has none of the disadvantages produced by immune response in the latter system. Thus the highly malignant lines N1 and M1 penetrated deeply into the mesonephros from the beginning of the association and could be transplanted to fresh mesonephros for a period of 300 days without losing the capacity to invade and proliferate. Cells from the weakly malignant line N2 penetrated the mesonephros very superficially or not at all and died after the second or third transfer. These results have been reproduced with other cell lines.

4.5.4. Existence in Certain Tumors of Carcinoembryonic Antigens

Certain antigens have been found to exist both in some tumors and in embryonic organs. The antigen of Gold and Freedman (1965), which has been detected in tumors of the human digestive system, is an example. It is absent from the normal digestive tract and from other adult organs, but exists in the digestive apparatus of the human embryo (hence the term "carcinoembryonic antigen," CEA). We have shown (Burtin *et al.*, 1970) that small amounts of this antigen are present in organotypic explants of several tumors of the digestive tract (AZ 110, Z 200, Z 516) after a number of years in culture. Revelation by immunofluorescent techniques has enabled us to determine its localization in the nodules.

Considering these results as well as the fact that the karyotype of the tumor cells has not altered—in terms of both number and structure of the chromosomes—it can be concluded that organotypic cultures of tumors demonstrate a great stability of characters after several years and numerous transfers.

ACKNOWLEDGMENT

We should like to express our best thanks to Dr. Julian Smith for his most valuable collaboration in translating this article.

5. *References*

Barski, G., and Wolff, Em., 1965, Malignancy evaluation of *in vitro* transformation of mouse cell lines in chick mesonephros organ cultures, *J. Natl. Cancer Inst.* **34:**495.

Bermann, F., 1960, Associations xénoplastiques d'organes embryonnaires: Etude de quelques structures mixtes *in vitro* et *in vivo, C. R. Soc. Biol.* **154:**911.

Bueker, E. D., 1948, Implantation of tumors in the hind-limb field of the embryonic chick and the developmental response of the lumbo-sacral system, *Anat. Rec.* **102:**369.

Bueker, E. D., 1957, Screening tumors (*in vivo*) for their effects on the growth of spinal and sympathetic ganglia of the embryonic chick, *Cancer Res.* **17:**190.

Burtin, P., Buffe, D., Von Kleist, S., Wolff, Em., and Wolff, Et., 1970, Mise en évidence de l'antigène carcinoembryonnaire spécifique des cancers digestifs dans des tumeurs humaines entretenues en culture organotypique, *Int. J. Cancer* **5:**88.

Croisille, Y., Mason, J., Wolff, Em., and Wolff, Et., 1967, Analyse biochimique des facteurs déterminant la croissance de tumeurs cancéreuses humaines en culture d'organes *in vitro, Eur. J. Cancer* **3:**371.

Dagg, C. P., Karnofsky, D. A., and Roddy, J., 1956, Growth of transplantable human tumors in the chick embryo and hatched chick, *Cancer Res.* **16:**589.

deGrouchy, J., and Wolff, Em., 1969, Analyse chromosomique d'une tumeur cancéreuse humaine en culture organotypique, *Eur. J. Cancer* **5:**159.

Ellison, M. L., Ambrose, E. J., and Easty, G. C., 1969, Differentiation in a transplantable rat tumour maintained in organ culture, *Exp. Cell Res.* **55:**198.

Gold, P., and Freedman, O., 1965, Specific carcinoembryonic antigens of the human digestive system, *J. Exp. Med.* **122:**467.

Greene, H. S. N., 1957, The significance of transplantability, *Trans. Stud. Coll. Physicians Philadelphia* **24(3):**101.

Humphreys, T., 1960, The fate of Ehrlich ascites cells injected intravenously into chick embryos, *Transpl. Bull.* **26:**118.

Karnofsky, D. A., Ridgway, L. P., and Patterson, P. A., 1952, Tumor transplantation to the chick embryo, *Ann. N.Y. Acad. Sci.* **55:**313.

Kautz, J., 1952, Differential invasion of embryonic chick tissues by sarcomas 180 and 37, *Cancer Res.* **12:**180.

Lasfargues, E. Y., and Feldman, D. G., 1963, Hormonal and physiological background in the production of B particles by the mouse mammary epithelium in organ cultures, *Cancer Res.* **23:**191.

Lasfargues, E. Y., and Murray, M. R., 1959, Hormonal influences on the differentiation and growth of embryonic mouse mammary glands in organ culture, *Develop. Biol.* **1:**413.

Lasfargues, E. Y., and Murray, M. R., 1968, Mouse mammary carcinogenesis *in vitro*, in: *Cancer Cells in Culture* (H. Katsuta, ed.), pp. 231–240, University of Tokyo Press, Tokyo.

Leighton, J., 1954*a*, Studies on human cancer using sponge matrix tissue culture. I. The growth patterns of a malignant melanoma, adenocarcinoma of the parotid gland, papillary adenocarcinoma of the pancreas and epidermoid carcinoma of the uterine cervix (Gey's HeLa strain), *Texas Rep. Biol. Med.* **12:**847.

Leighton, J., 1954*b*, The growth patterns of some transplantable animal tumors in sponge matrix tissue culture, *J. Natl. Cancer Inst.* **15:**275.

Leighton, J., 1963, The appearance of disseminated minute tumor nodules in the chorioallantoic membrane of the chick following intravenous inoculation of ascites tumor cells, *Cancer Res.* **23:**148.

Leighton, J., Mark, R., and Justh, G., 1968, Patterns of three-dimensional growth *in vitro* in collagen-coated cellulose sponge: Carcinomas and embryonic tissues, *Cancer Res.* **28:**286.

Levi-Montalcini, R., 1952, Effects of mouse tumor transplantation on the nervous system, *Ann. N.Y. Acad. Sci.* **55:**330.

Levi-Montalcini, R., and Hamburger, V., 1951, Selective growth stimulating effects of mouse sarcoma on the sensory and sympathetic nervous system of the chick embryo, *J. Exp. Zool.* 116:321.

Levi-Montalcini, R., Meyer, H., and Hamburger, V., 1954, *In vitro* experiments on the effects of mouse sarcomas 180 and 37 on the spinal and sympathetic ganglia of the chick embryo, *Cancer Res.* **14:**49.

Murphy, J. B., 1913, Transplantability of tissues to the embryo of foreign species, *J. Exp. Med.* **17:**482.

Pageot-Simpson, P., and Wolff, Et., 1969, La sensibilité différentielle d'une tumeur maligne humaine et des gonades embryonnaires, en culture organotypique *in vitro*, à une substance alkylante, le Melphalan, *C. R. Acad. Sci.* **268:**2997.

Rubinstein, L. J., Herman, M. M., and Foley, V. L., 1973, *In vitro* characteristics of human glioblastomas maintained in organ culture systems, *Am. J. Pathol.* **71:**61.

Schneider, N., 1958, Sur les possibilités de propagation d'un sarcome de Souris sur des organes embryonnaires de Poulet à différents stades du développement, *Arch. Anat. Microsc. Morphol. Exp.* **245:**48.

Simpson, P., 1969, La sensibilité différentielle d'une tumeur humaine et des tissus somatiques et germinaux des gonades embryonnaires en culture organotypique *in vitro*, *Eur. J. Cancer* **5:**331.

Smith, J., Wolff, Em., and Wolff, Et., 1971, Nouvelles recherches sur les facteurs permettant la croissance de trois tumeurs cancéreuses humaines cultivées organotypiquement *in vitro* pendant de longues durées, *C. R. Acad. Sci.* **272:**1465.

Taylor, A., Thacker, J., and Pennington, D., 1942, Growth of cancer tissue in the yolk-sac of the chick embryo, *Science* **96:**342.

Taylor, A., Carmichael, N., and Norris, T., 1948, A further report on yolk sac cultivation of tumor tissue, *Cancer Res.* **8:**264.

Tchao, R., Easty, G. C., Ambrose, E. J., Raven, R. W., and Bloom, H. J. G., 1968, Effect of chemotherapeutic agents and hormones on organ cultures of human tumours, *Eur. J. Cancer* **4:**39.

Wolff, Em., 1962, Adaptation de quatre nouvelles souches cancéreuses humaines à la culture organotypique *in vitro*, *C. R. Soc. Biol.* **156:**1217.

Wolff, Em., 1964, Chimères d'organes et cultures organotypiques de tumeurs cancéreuses, in: *Exposés Actuels de Biologie Cellulaire: Les Cultures Organotypiques* (A. Thomas, ed.), pp. 337–376, Masson, Paris.

Wolff, Em., Croisille, Y., Mason, J., and Wolff, Et., 1966, Sur la stimulation de cultures organotypiques de deux épithéliomas humains par des dialysats d'extrait de levure, de mésonéphros et de foie d'embryon de Poulet, *C. R. Acad. Sci.* **262:**2120.

Wolff, Em., Croisille, Y., Mason, J., and Wolff, Et., 1967, Sur le fractionnement des substances favourables à la croissance de nodules cancéreux humains cultivés *in vitro, C. R. Acad. Sci.* **265:**2157.

Wolff, Em., Smith, J., and Wolff, Et., 1972, Etude expérimentale d'une nouvelle tumeur maligne humaine du côlon ascendant en culture organotypique de longue durée, *C. R. Acad. Sci.* **274:**341.

Wolff, Et., 1954, Potentialités et affinités des tissus révélées par la culture *in vitro* d'organes en associations hétérogènes et xénoplastiques, *Bull. Soc. Zool. Fr.* **79:**357.

Wolff, Et., 1956, La culture de tumeurs sur les organes embryonnaires explantés *in vitro, Bruxelles Med.* **36:**2235.

Wolff, Et., 1961, Utilisation de la membrane vitelline de l'oeuf de Poule en culture organotypique. I. Technique et possibilités, *Develop. Biol.* **3:**767.

Wolff, Et., and Haffen, K., 1952, Sur une méthode de culture d'organes embryonnaires *in vitro, Texas Rep. Biol. Med.* **10:**463.

Wolff, Et., and Schneider, N., 1956, Sur l'association d'une tumeur de Souris et d'organes embryonnaires de Poulet en culture *in vitro, C. R. Soc. Biol.* **150:**845.

Wolff, Et., and Schneider, N., 1957*a*, La culture d'une sarcome de Souris sur des organes de Poulet explantés *in vitro, Arch. Anat. Microsc. Morphol. Exp.* **46:**173.

Wolff, Et., and Schneider, N., 1957*b*, La transplantation prolongée d'un sarcome de Souris sur des organes embryonnaires de Poulet cultivés *in vitro, C. R. Soc. Biol.* **151:**1291.

Wolff, Et., and Weniger, J.-P., 1954, Recherches préliminaires sur les chimères d'organes embryonnaires d'Oiseaux et de Mammifères en culture *in vitro, J. Embryol. Exp. Morphol.* **2:**161.

Wolff, Et., and Wolff, Em., 1958*a*, La propagation d'une souche de cancer humain sur des organes embryonnaires de Poulet cultivés *in vitro, C. R. Acad. Sci.* **246:**1116.

Wolff, Et., and Wolff, Em., 1958*b*, Les résultats d'une nouvelle méthode de culture de cellules cancéreuses *in vitro, Rev. Fr. Etudes Clin. Biol.* **3:**945.

Wolff, Et., and Wolff, Em., 1959, Sur le comportement de souches cancéreuses humaines en association avec des organes embryonnaires de Poulet cultivés *in vitro, C. R. Soc. Biol.* **153:** 1898.

Wolff, Et., and Wolff, Em., 1960a, Comment un sarcome de Souris se nourrit-il des tissus du rein embryonnaire de Poulet? *C. R. Soc. Biol.* **154:**2182.

Wolff, Et., and Wolff, Em., 1960*b*, Mise en évidence de substances favorables à la prolifération de cellules cancéreuses dans le rein embryonnaire du Poulet, *C. R. Acad. Sci.* **250:**4076.

Wolff, Et., and Wolff, Em., 1961*a*, Le rôle du mésonéphros de l'embryon de Poulet dans la nutrition de cellules cancéreuses. II. Etude par la méthode de la membrane vitelline, *J. Embryol. Exp. Morphol.* **9:**678.

Wolff, Et., and Wolff, Em., 1961*b*, Cultures de cellules cancéreuses humaines sur des organes embryonnaires de Poulet explantés *in vitro*, in: *Colloque International Nogent 1960, "La Culture Organotypique,"* Editions du C.N.R.S., Paris.

Wolff, Et., and Wolff, Em., 1966, Cultures organotypiques de longue durée de deux tumeurs humaines du tube digestif, *Eur. J. Cancer* **2:**93.

Wolff, Et., and Wolff, Em., 1967, Factors of growth and maintenance of tumours as organized structures *in vitro*, in: *Ciba Foundation Symposium on Cell Differentiation* (A. V. S. de Reuck and J. Knight, ed.), pp. 208–215, J. and A. Churchill Ltd., London.

Wolff, Et., and Wolff, Em., 1972, Caractères d'une nouvelle tumeur maligne de l'intestin humain en culture organotypique de longue durée, *Rev. Suisse Zool. (Fasc. Suppl.)* **79:**343.

Wolff, Et., Haffen, K., and Wolff, Em., 1953, Les besoins nutritifs des organes sexués embryonnaires en culture *in vitro, Ann. Alim. Nutr.* **7:**5.

Wolff, Et., Barski, G., and Wolff, Em., 1960, Mise en évidence de différents degrés de malignité de souches cellulaires de Souris en culture d'organes embryonnaires de Poulet, *C. R. Acad. Sci.* **251**:479.

Wolff, Et., Wolff, Em., and Renault, P., 1962, Sur la culture organotypique de carcinomes humains très proliférants, en présence de mésonéphros d'embryons de Poulet, *Pathol. Biol.* **10**:116.

Wolff, Et., Wolff, Em., and Croisille, Y., 1965, Culture organotypique de deux épithéliomas humains en l'absence de substratum vivant, *C. R. Acad. Sci.* **260**:2359.

Yarnell, M. M., and Ambrose, E. J., 1969*a*, Studies of tumour invasion in organ culture. I. Effects of basic polymers and dyes on invasion and dissemination, *Eur. J. Cancer* **5**:255.

Yarnell, M. M., and Ambrose, E. J., 1969*b*, Studies of tumour invasion in organ culture. II. Effects of enzyme treatment, *Eur. J. Cancer* **5**:265.

Metabolic Gradients in Tissue Culture Studies of Human Cancer Cells* 9

JOSEPH LEIGHTON AND RUY TCHAO

1. Introduction

When cancer is first identified in a person, we find on histopathological evaluation that the new growth appears as a tissue organized in characteristic multilayered arrangements of cells. Inevitably, those tumor cells in immediate intimate association with the circulation of the host, as represented by the blood vessels in the tumor, are in a different metabolic status than are tumor cells many cell diameters away from the blood vessels. As a specific expression of this gradient, the observations of Tannock (1968) are appropriate. He found in a transplantable mammary carcinoma that tumor cells in close proximity to blood vessels had a high index of tritiated thymidine incorporation, whereas a few cell diameters away from the vessels labeling was much less. A common observation of diagnostic histopathology is that tumor cells close to vessels are clearly viable while in the same microscopic field the tumor cells most distant from the same vessels are necrotic. Several factors contribute to these conditions, including pO_2, pCO_2, pH, and the concentrations of essential metabolites and cell products. The situation is

*This work was supported by NIH-NCI Research Grants CA 13219 and CA 14137 and Contract G-72-3858.

JOSEPH LEIGHTON AND RUY TCHAO Cancer Bioassay Laboratory, Department of Pathology, The Medical College of Pennsylvania, Philadelphia, Pennsylvania extremely complex; these factors are interrelated and yet each may have unique effects on the system.

Gradients of metabolites are regularly observed in tissue culture studies oriented toward organotypic growth. The goal of many investigators has been to modify conditions so that a small organotypic fragment shall be composed of a maximal thickness of viable cells. In our work, we are probing the nature of the gradient itself since metabolic gradients are the usual setting in intact tissues, whether normal or cancerous. We have directed our interest to the role of oxygen tension since this component is readily manipulated *in vitro* and is of great importance in all metazoan forms. We take our orientation from many sources. One point of departure is work on invertebrate marine hydroids, which was initiated more than a generation ago.

2. *Examples of Metabolic Gradients in Multicellular Organisms*

2.1. *Invertebrates*

Various invertebrates of the hydra type are essentially of cylindrical appearance, with specialized distinctive structures at both ends. At one end, a thickened base is adapted for attachment to available supporting structures. At the other end, a motile "head" with a feeding stoma is surrounded by tentacles that bring food to the oral opening. When such organisms are modified by amputation of both specialized polar structures, either end may become the new feeding head depending on the conditions of "cultivation." The role of gradients of oxygen tension in regeneration has been studied in the marine hydroid *Tubularia* since the beginning of this century. T. H. Morgan (1903) reported that when the cut end of a *Tubularia* stem was placed in sand, regeneration was inhibited at that end. Barth (1940) found that the rate of regeneration was dependent on the oxygen tension in the seawater. Miller (1937) observed that when segments with cut ends at each pole were exposed to seawater with differing oxygen tensions the pole exposed to the higher tension became the feeding end. These observations were made even more interesting by Goldin's work (1942) indicating that acid metabolites of *Tubularia* inhibit regeneration, even in the presence of high oxygen tensions. Spiegelman and Goldin (1944) observed a parallel inhibitory effect of progressively lowered pH on aerobic respiration and on regeneration even in the presence of high oxygen tensions. They concluded that the effect of low pH on *Tubularia* regeneration is not a direct specific effect, but is mediated through its action on enzyme systems involved in aerobic respiration.

This description of *Tubularia* is relevant to the present chapter since it places experimental consideration of metabolic gradients, particularly of oxygen, in a historical perspective. Furthermore, since acid products of metabolism modify regenerative growth and respiration in some metazoan forms the situation may have partial parallels when we evaluate the role of metabolic gradients of human cells *in vitro* and *in vivo*.

2.2. Normal Mammalian Organs

Gradients of oxygen tension are clearly in operation in some forms of hepatic regeneration. In the liver with normal vascular anatomy, proliferating liver cells after hepatic injury are found in largest numbers around the portal zones, where the concentration of oxygen provided by branches of the hepatic artery is greatest. This association of arterial blood and hepatic cell proliferation was examined directly by Sigel *et al.* (1968). They studied "the role of the direction of intrahepatic blood flow upon the location of hepatocyte formation in regenerating liver" by a series of transplantation experiments. Autotransplants of liver lobes with arterial blood perfusing the hepatic lobules in the normal direction, i.e., from portal vein to central vein, were accompanied by the normal pattern of localized proliferation of hepatocytes in the portal area. Where the circulation was reversed in the transplantation procedure, arterial blood entering the lobule through the central vein and leaving through the portal vein, hepatocyte proliferation in the region of the central veins exceeded that found near the portal veins.

2.3. Solid Neoplasms

On routine examination of tumor specimens in diagnostic clinical histopathology, the presence of metabolic gradients is abundantly evident. Figures 1 through 4 are illustrative. Transitional cell carcinoma of the urinary bladder, grade I, appears grossly as several small cauliflower-shaped lesions protruding from the bladder wall into the bladder cavity. In many parts of such tumors, distinct polypoid structural units are seen with central vascular cores surrounded by stratified neoplastic transitional cells. A portion of such a unit is seen in Fig. 1. The blood supply is identified as the elongated tubular structure on the left. The open channel on the right is between adjacent "polyps" of tumor, and is continuous with the cavity of the urinary bladder. The metabolic gradient, which must be supported by the blood vessel, is composed of an uninterrupted stratified neoplastic epithelium approximately 20 cells thick.

Figure 2 is from the edge of a primary carcinoma of the breast. The hard scirrhous bulk of the tumor is seen above as densely fibrous tissue almost devoid of cells. The margin of the tumor mass, in three-dimensional terms the surface zone of an expanding sphere, is in contrast densely cellular. Many elongated irregular branching aggregates of carcinoma are seen. At the periphery of this cellular zone, in the lowest part of the photograph, is adipose tissue. The nutrition for the growing tumor mass may be derived from two sources, blood vessels passing through the adipose tissue to the tumor and the adipose tissue itself. A morphological gradient is depicted by the three zones in the figure, and this arrangement suggests that a metabolic gradient is almost inevitable. Goldacre and Sylvén (1962) have indeed demonstrated such a gradient in studies on experimental tumors in animals. Following the intravenous injection of dyes, staining was abundant in the growing margin of the tumor and not in the large central bulk of the tumor.

Figure 3 is a section of lung in which metastatic mammary carcinoma is seen in a distended lymphatic vessel. This focus of tumor resembles in great detail a fragment of carcinoma in "organotypic" culture. There is no blood supply within the substance of the tumor fragment. All nutrients enter and leave from its surface. The fragment has a discrete oval configuration and can be divided into two recognizable zones. The outer zone is composed of viable, easily recognized adenocarcinoma. The center consists of necrotic tumor cells without distinctive histopathology. Obviously a gradient of metabolites is present extending from the surface of the tumor nodule to its necrotic core.

FIGS. 1–4. Four illustrations of the histological appearance of cancer in man. Each photograph depicts the morphological expression of a metabolic gradient. All four are stained with hematoxylin and eosin. ×120. (1) Transitional cell carcinoma of the urinary bladder, grade 1. Tubular structures on the left are blood vessels. Surrounding the vessels, and seen in the center of the field, is a stratified neoplastic epithelium about 20 cell diameters thick. The cleft on the right is the space between two adjacent tumor structures and is presumably continuous with the cavity of the urinary bladder. (2) Carcinoma of the breast observed at the periphery of a hard tumor mass infiltrating adipose tissue. The bulk of the tumor is represented by the tissue in the upper part of the field which consists of dense collagen bundles and occasional small cells. The cellular margin of the tumor mass is seen in the center of the figure and consists of many prominent nests of tumor cells. Perhaps this is analogous to the zone of piling up in the aerobic portion of a meniscus-gradient culture. Adipose tissue in the lowest part of the figure would be expected to be the target for further infiltrative spread of the tumor. (3) A focus of carcinoma of the breast that has spread to the lung, as seen within a dilated lymphatic vessel. The fragment of carcinoma, devoid of an internal vascular supply, recalls an organotypic culture. Two zones are evident, a periphery of viable cells arranged as stratified neoplastic glands and a center of necrosis. These two zones are evidence of a metabolic gradient. Viable cells in the deeper aspects of the cortex must exchange metabolites by diffusion through overlying cells. (4) Malignant melanoma. Three nutritive vessels are surrounded by multilayers of viable tumor cells. In areas most distant from the vessels, necrotic cells appear as thin irregular bands separating "lobules" of viable tumor cells. These necrotic bands are too remote from the vessels for the tumor cells to be sustained.

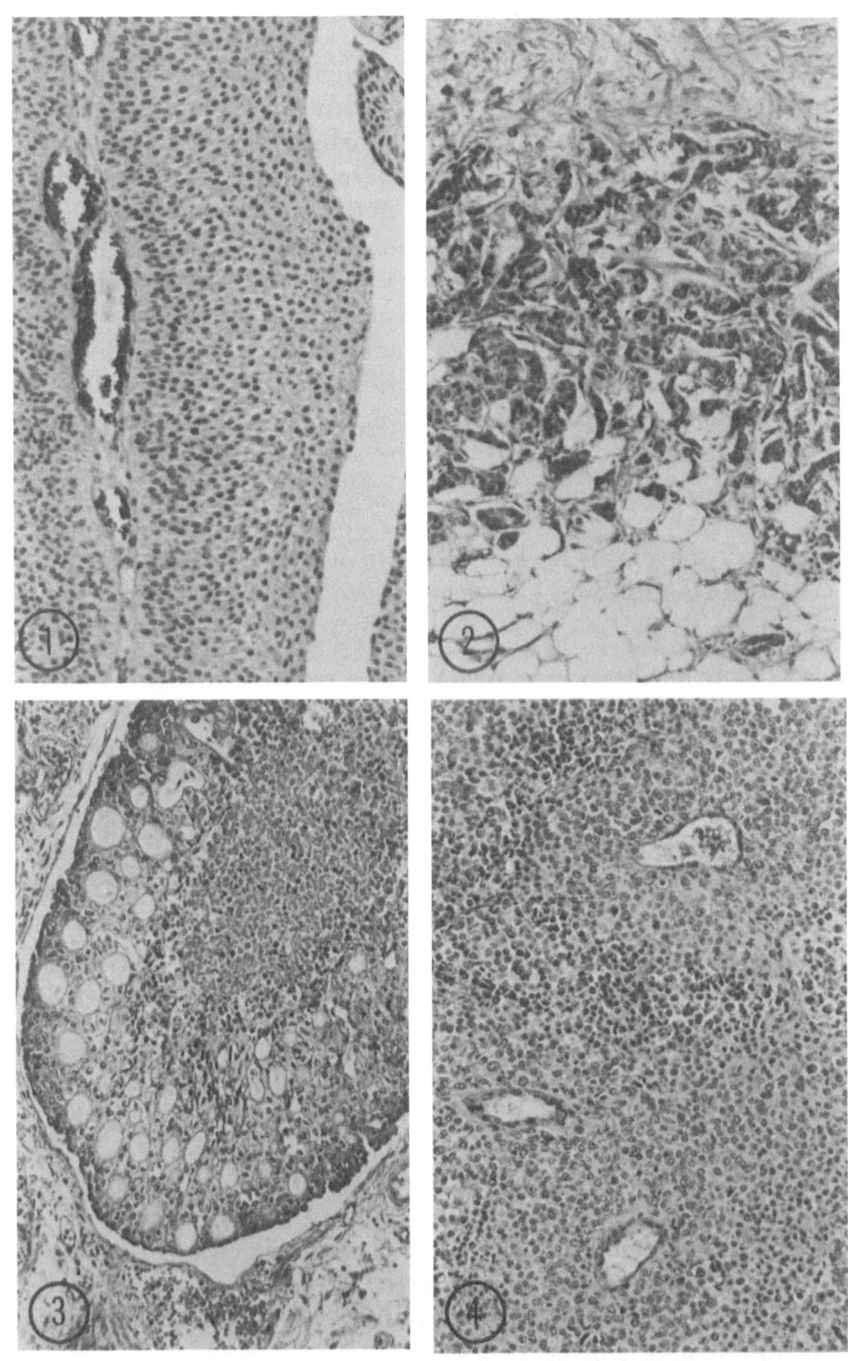
1
2
3
4

The morphological expression of metabolic gradients in tumors can be recognized equally well in vascularized solid tumors. Figure 4 is such an instance in a malignant melanoma. Three vessels are identifiable. The one in the upper half of the figure is surrounded by viable tumor cells, as are the two near each other in the lower part of the figure. The viable tumor cells surrounding all vessels are not continuous. Instead, the populations of viable cells are separated by irregular bands of hyperchromatic necrotic and dying tumor cells. Diffusion of metabolites from vessels into the surrounding substance of the tumor can support only a limited thickness of viable tumor parenchyma. From Tannock's studies (1968), we can presume that the percentage of cells in G_0 increases as the distance from the supporting blood vessels increases. For a therapeutic modality to act effectively on the cells of a solid tumor, the activity of the agent must express itself on a population of tumor cells in a spectrum of metabolic states, including a relatively aerobic setting adjacent to vessels and a continuous gradient of increasingly anaerobic conditions at progressive distances from the vessels.

3. *Metabolic Gradients in Three-Dimensional Organotypic or Histotypic Cultures on Collagen-Coated Cellulose Sponge*

The techniques for preparing collagen-coated cellulose sponges have been described in detail (Leighton, 1973) and will not be repeated here. Instead, procedures will be described for studying gradients in three-dimensional matrix culture.

Gradients can be provided for study in the growth resulting from inocula of suspensions of cells or in the growth from discrete explants. Explants of carcinomas that are placed gently on the surface of collagen-coated sponges often remain discrete after 5–7 days of culture or longer, growing in an organotypic manner. The orientation of the sponge culture for paraffin embedding is a crucial feature if gradients are to be evaluated. The culture must be trimmed for embedding and oriented in paraffin so that the 6-μm thick histological section encompasses the gradient from the surface to the depths of the culture.

3.1. *Organotypic Culture of Tumor Explants*

Four examples of organotypic culture are presented in Figs. 5–8 to illustrate the patterns of gradient expression observed in explants of tumors cultured in matrix. These illustrations should be considered in close comparison with the first four figures, especially Fig. 3.

The gradients seen in Fig. 1–4 from intact clinical tumors have their histopathological counterpart in organotypic culture. In Fig. 5 we see a fragment of tumor after a few days in organotypic culture. The donor tumor was the malignant melanoma illustrated in Fig. 4. Tumor fragments were placed on the surface of collagen-coated sponge. After 5–7 days, the explants had spread laterally, but were organotypically distinctive. In Fig. 5 we see, on the left, the surface of the explant bathed by the gas–medium interface and contiguous with it a broad zone of viable cells. The undersurface of the explant in contact with collagen-coated sponge is also contiguous with a viable zone of cells, but this layer is more irregular and thinner than the upper zone near the gas phase. Both surfaces were bathed by the same liquid medium, but one was "enriched" by the oxygen in the air above the culture. Within the fragment itself, sandwiched between the wide and the narrow zones of viability, is a necrotic zone. Its status is comparable to that of the zones of necrosis seen previously in intact tissues in Figs. 3 and 4.

Two carcinomas growing as organotypic fragments provide further illustration of this common pattern, a viable cortex and a necrotic center. Figure 6 is a fragment of mammary cancer, Fig. 7 of papillary adenocarcinoma of the thyroid. The explants considered thus far, Figs. 5–7, all had been placed on the surface of the matrix, in contact with the air–medium interface to their left. Viability is oxygen oriented in all three cases and away from the underlying matrix, which is to the right of the field. In occasional experiments, explants have been placed on the sponge sandwiched between sponge and the glass wall of the culture tube. In such circumstances, growth and migration of viable cells also take place toward the medium–air interface, but in this case toward and into the matrix. One such culture is illustrated in Figure 8, a human fibrous mesothelioma.

3.2. *Experimental Combinations of Cells*

When collagen-coated sponge is inoculated with suspensions of cells, proliferation may be accompanied by the formation of tissue. For example, a suspension of the mouse fibroblast cell line 3T6 forms a connective tissue (Leighton *et al.*, 1970) in which a distinctive gradient of structure is seen from the free surface of the sponge to its depths. Combinations of chick embryonic tissues and human tumor cells form tissues in which a segregation or sorting out is seen when the cultures are examined from the gradient point of view. Figures 9 and 10 are two such combinations. Figure 9 is a combination of chick embryo lung and fibrosarcoma of human lung. Note that the fibrosarcoma cells grow as a covering over irregularly necrotic, organized components of the embryonic lung. Most of the sponge is infiltrated by a sparse connective tissue that does not appear to be neoplastic. Figure 10 is a combination of chick embryonic tissue from the general region of the mesonephros and cells from a peritoneal effusion of a patient with ovarian cancer. Dark-staining viable tumor cells appear both as aggregates and singly, covered by a thin layer of connective tissue of chick embryonic origin.

Figures 11 and 12 illustrate a second simple approach to examining the interaction of mammalian and chick embryonic cells. A suspension of mammalian cells is injected into a chorioallantoic vein of the 11- or 12-day-old chick embryo (Leighton, 1967). Within minutes to hours, the embryo is removed and an appropriate organ is selected for studying "metastatic growth" *in vitro* in the context of organotypic culture. Figure 11 shows a fragment of liver, injected 1 wk earlier with the human mammary cancer cell line BT-20 and promptly cultivated on matrix. Viable liver appears as a thin outer zone. Necrotic liver makes up most of the field. Proliferating cancer cells appear between necrotic and viable liver. This is in contrast to the location of growth of a rat ascites hepatoma, which grew preferentially on the outer surface of viable liver (Leighton, 1968). Figure 12 is a fragment of embryonic heart with a cultivation history similar to that of the culture depicted in Fig. 11, except that the human cells were strain HeLa. A few HeLa cells are seen, primarily as small collections just below the outer surface of viable chick cells.

We have yet to initiate a systematic exploration of the comparative biological qualities of clinical tumors or human cell lines in the context of their morphological expressions when grown in three-dimensional gra-

FIGS. 5–8. Four illustrations of organotypic cultures of human tumors on a matrix of cellulose sponge. The cultures were embedded so that histological sections depict the gradients of metabolites from the gas–medium interface on the left into the depths of the cultures on the right. All sections are stained with hematoxylin and eosin. ×120. (5) A fragment of the malignant melanoma seen as a surgical specimen in Fig. 4. The aspect of the fragment at the gas–medium interface, seen on the left, is composed of viable cells many cell diameters deep. The opposite surface rests on the matrix. Its supporting medium permeating the sponge is remote from the gaseous atmosphere in the culture and the depth of viable cells is less. A substantial zone of necrosis is seen between the thick and the thin viable areas of tumor. (6) An explant of mammary carcinoma. The thin viable cortex is composed of carcinoma cells, supporting stroma, and lymphocytes. The deeper aspects of the fragment are necrotic. (7) An explant of papillary carcinoma of the thyroid gland. Viable carcinoma in histotypic papillary arrangement is seen on the periphery of the explant. The center is necrotic. (8) Growth from an explant of fibrous mesothelioma in an unusual experimental setting. The explant was sandwiched between the glass surface and the 1-mm-thick slice of collagen-coated cellulose sponge. The gas–medium interface is to the left of the field, on the medium-bathed surface of the sponge. Tumor cells have migrated into the matrix toward the gas–medium interface, forming the "cortex" of the culture. The remainder of the explant, on the right of the field, consists of necrotic tumor cells. In all of these figures, 5 through 8, proliferating or viable cells are found consistently in relation to the gas–medium interface.

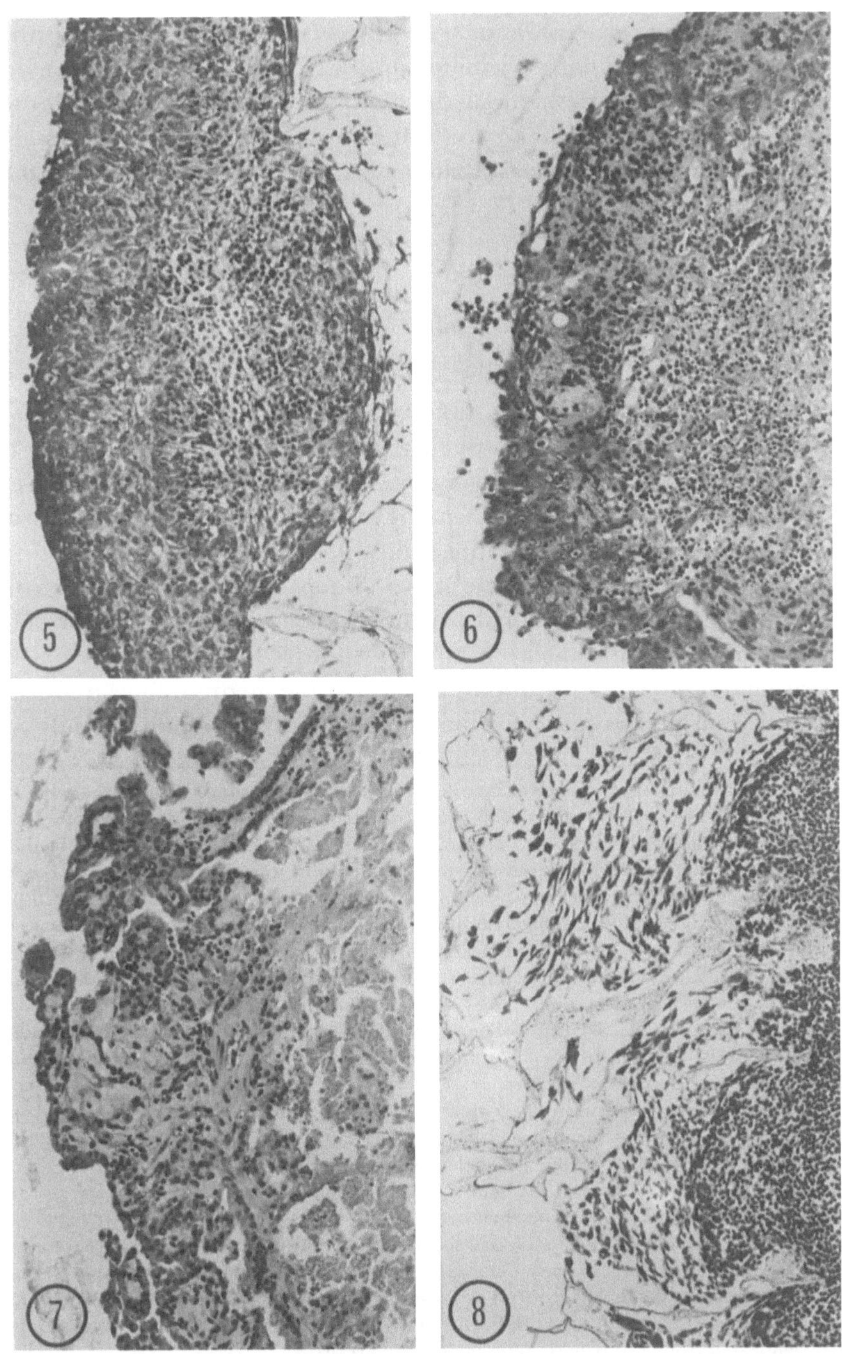
5
6
7
8

dients or organotypic culture. We think that such studies might best be initiated in the model in which human cells are injected intravenously in the embryo, followed by the cultivation of a heavily seeded organ such as the liver in an organotypic preparation. From bits of experience, we suspect that all human cell lines will not grow in the same way, with the same patterns, or in the same zone. Instead, we think, they will express themselves in different ways, allowing such cell lines to be studied and compared in a new, more meaningful context as neoplasia than is now possible in other accepted *in vitro* models.

4. *Gradients in Monolayer Growth: Meniscus-Gradient Culture*

Edwin Osgood demonstrated in the 1950s that the effects of gradients of metabolites on cells *in vitro*, especially gradients of oxygen tension, can be studied very well in several ways using two-dimensional monolayer cultures. Meniscus-gradient culture is our variant of Osgood's first gradient tissue culture method (Osgood and Krippaehne, 1955).

The study of metabolic gradients in two-dimensional culture differs from the models of three-dimensional organotypic or histotypic growth. The metabolic gradient in monolayer cultures appears to be primarily one of decreasing oxygen tension from the surface of the medium to its depths, a direct relationship between cells and medium. On the other hand, the

---

FIGS. 9–12. Four illustrations of sponge matrix cultures of combinations of human cancer cells and chick embryo cells. All are stained with hematoxylin and eosin. ×120. (9) A combination of fibrosarcoma of the lung and chick embryonic lung. Tumor cells have reached the most superficial aspect of the culture, closest to the gas–medium interface. Irregularly necrotic organoid remnants of embryonic lung are immediately beneath the fibrosarcoma cells. Most of the matrix is filled with a loose, sparsely cellular connective tissue that does not appear to be neoplastic. (10) A combination of ovarian carcinoma cells obtained from a peritoneal effusion and embryonic tissue from the mesonephric region. The most superficial aspect of the culture consists of a thin layer of embryonic tissue covering carcinoma cells that appear singly and as aggregates in a loose connective tissue. The substance of the matrix is devoid of any organoid tissue. (11 and 12) Growth of human tumor cell emboli in organotypic cultures of chick embryonic organs. Suspensions of tumor cells were injected intravenously in 11-day-old embryos. The embryos were promptly removed, and organs for cultivation were selected and then prepared as explants on the sponge. In Fig. 11 is a fragment of embryonic liver seeded with the mammary cancer cell line BT-20. The field consists of a narrow band of dark-staining viable cells on the left. The remainder of the field consists of necrotic liver. The viable cortex of the culture is made of two zones. Its outer half is composed almost exclusively of viable liver cells. The inner half has a combination of liver cells and a substantial number of the larger carcinoma cells. In Fig. 12 is a fragment of chick embryonic heart seeded with HeLa cells. A thin layer of embryonic connective tissue cells covers the explant. A few groups of HeLa cells lie immediately below, on the outer surface of the broad band of myocardium. Below the viable myocardium, clearly delineated from it, is pale-staining necrotic heart tissue.

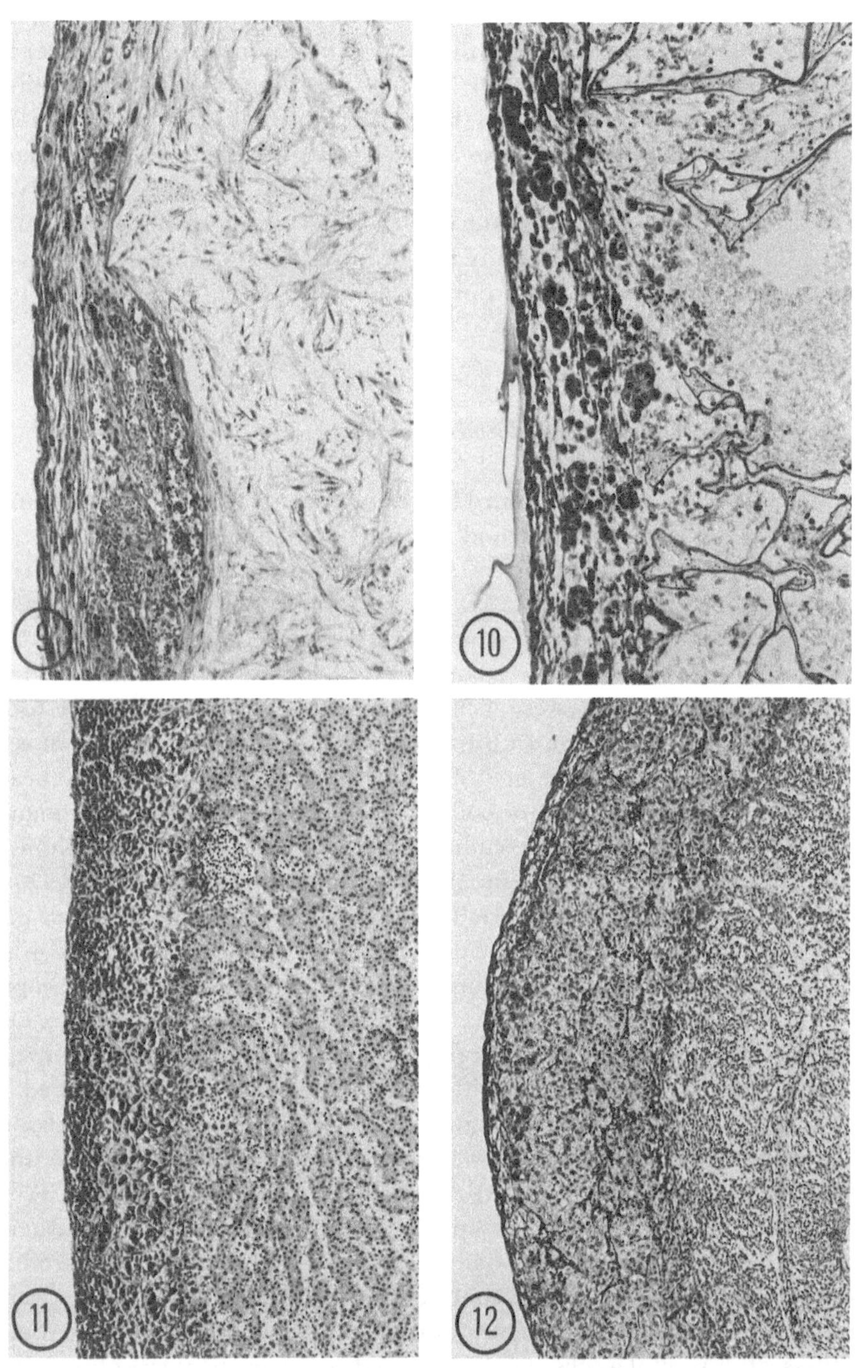
9
10
11
12

gradient in three-dimensional organotypic or histotypic culture is more complex since all diffusible metabolites, of which oxygen is only one, must diffuse through successive layers of cells to support those cells that retain viability within the explant. While the three-dimensional context is closer to the situation *in vivo* (see Fig. 3), the use of three-dimensional culture requires costly technical resources, primarily a histology laboratory. When, however, two-dimensional cultures are to be terminated, fixed, and stained for further microscopic evaluation, the cost is almost negligible. If observations are to be made on living cultures, monolayers are distinctly advantageous. The patterns of growth can easily be monitored at various positions in the oxygen gradient and appropriate fields of living cells selected for time-lapse observations.

4.1. Origins of the Meniscus-Gradient Method

Osgood and his associates introduced several gradient tissue culture methods in the mid-1950s (Osgood, 1955; Osgood and Krippaehne, 1955; Osgood and Brooke, 1955). Their investigations were concerned primarily with hematopoietic cells.

Our active interest in using monolayers to study gradients followed an accidental observation in our laboratory in 1970. Stock cultures of dog kidney cell line MDCK were being maintained with the bead-in-tube technique (Leighton, 1958). In this procedure, continuous cultures of cell lines are maintained in tubes incubated in a vertical position. The glass bead in the tube serves as a scraper or policeman. When growth is overabundant, brief vigorous agitation of the culture, applied just before the medium is replaced, releases surplus cells into the medium. At one time early in 1970 it was evident that this routine dislodgement of cells with the bead had not been performed for some time. On macroscopic examination, a pale gray opaque ring of growth was seen just below the meniscus. On microscopic examination, this proved to be a massive piling up of cells in highly organoid papillary cystic structures. Another population of cells, derived from human ovarian cancer and maintained with the same technique, was examined at once. It had the same gross appearance as the first group. On microscopic examination, the pattern was also highly organoid, but uniquely so and different from MDCK. This experience was repeated using MDCK in Leighton tubes containing coverslips. The tubes were seeded with suspensions of cells in medium and maintained initially in the near-horizontal position. After attachment and confluency were attained, some tubes were incubated in a vertical position, while others were kept at a 45° angle. In both settings, after several weeks of cultivation a distinct gradient was observed.

The role of oxygen in the phenomenon of piling up and organization of MDCK cells at the aerobic end of the gradient was demonstrated by a colleague, Dr. Robert K. Prince. He prepared gradient cultures on microscope slides in large Leighton tubes. (These tubes were developed in conjunction with the Bellco Glass Co., Vineland, N.J.) Two series, each cultured in the near-vertical position for 23 days, are illustrated in Fig. 14. On the left is the control, fed with fresh medium two or three times weekly and restoppered each time. On the right is a tube fed in the same manner, but kept open in a gaseous environment of 95% O_2 and 5% CO_2. Compare the zones of dense growth just below the meniscus. This area of the control on the left averages 3 mm in width. On the right, in the culture receiving an atmosphere enriched with oxygen, it is about 8 mm wide. Microscopically we see the control in Fig. 15 and the enriched culture in Fig. 16. Organization and transport function (cyst formation) are much greater in the zone of piling up in the presence of an increased oxygen tension. These results suggest that for the papillary adenocarcinoma MDCK the maximal expressions of function and elaborate cell-to-cell organization are achieved in an environment favoring aerobic respiration.

As this study of MDCK progressed, the senior author was comparing several epithelial cell lines in meniscus-gradient culture in collaboration with Professor Hajim Katsuta in the latter's laboratory at the University of Tokyo. In particular, two urinary bladder carcinoma cell lines of rat origin were compared (Leighton and Katsuta, 1973). A preliminary standardization of meniscus-gradient technique evolved as we compared monolayer cultures of various established cell lines.

4.2. *Current Techniques for Epithelial Cell Lines*

Preparation of meniscus-gradient cultures is conducted in two stages.

Stage 1: Tubes with a flat surface, containing an 11- by 35-mm coverslip, are inoculated with a suspension of cells in 1 ml of fresh medium at a concentration of cells known to provide confluent growth in a few days. The tubes are incubated in the conventional horizontal position. Medium is replaced as indicated by changes in pH and the cultures remain in a horizontal position until near-confluency is attained.

Stage 2: As confluent growth on the coverslip becomes imminent, the medium in the culture is replaced with 2 ml of fresh medium and the tubes are subsequently incubated in a vertical position. Tubes are fed twice weekly, or, if absolutely necessary because of the rapid fall in pH, three times weekly. One should avoid disturbing the cultures by microscopy and the attendant inevitable agitation of the medium until shortly before a replenishment of the medium.

Many cell lines drop the pH of the medium markedly overnight. Our current practice in dealing with this situation is to feed such cultures with a medium of high pH, 8.0 or 8.2. This provides the cells with an environment of wide sweeps in pH, changing in a few days from 8.2 to 6.8 or lower and then on feeding abruptly reverting to 8.2. Such oscillations in pH are an important additional factor operating on the cells in the presence of the continuous gradient of decreasing oxygen tension, a gradient which itself is established and disrupted every few days with each new feeding.

The following general features characterize the growth after several weeks of cultivation, based on our experience with six carcinoma cell lines. Four distinct contiguous strata of cells are seen. Just at the meniscus, there is a 0.5- to 1.0-mm-wide band of cells in a monolayer. A second zone follows, the one with piling up of cells, consisting of a collar 2–4 mm wide. The cells are densely packed in this region, often arranged in highly organoid multicellular structures. This is the portion of the gradient that is recognized easily in the living culture and that after fixation and staining has a very dark color. Proceeding down the gradient, the third zone is a wide monolayer of viable cells that are obviously larger than those of the first two zones, and among which enormous mononucleated tumor giant cells are frequently found. For some cell lines, the third zone is itself composed of two distinct strata of viable cells of very different cytological appearance. The width of the third zone is highly variable from one cell line to the next, being influenced, for any one cell line, by the frequency of media replacement and the final low pH of the depleted medium. The fourth and last zone is one of

---

FIGS. 13–16. (13) Two views of a meniscus-gradient culture tube, with a ruler numbered in centimeters. The tube resembles the familiar Leighton tube, except that the closed end is flat rather than a hemisphere. This modification provides a secure footing for the rectangular coverslip, which is also held in place by capillary forces between the flat surface of the tube and the underside of the coverslip. (14) Meniscus-gradient cultures of MDCK grown on standard microscope slides in large Leighton tubes and fixed after 23 days in a near-vertical position. The slide on the left was cultured in the usual manner; that is, the tube was stoppered except for brief periods of feeding three times weekly. The slide on the right was in a tube that was not stoppered, but was fed as the control and kept in a saturated atmosphere of 95% O_2 and 5% CO_2. The cultures have been stained with hematoxylin and eosin after fixation. An artifact is seen in the center of each slide where two coverslips, placed on the slide after staining and mounting, are in contact. In the upper part of each slide is the curved border reflecting the meniscus. In the control slide, on the left, a band of dense opacity is seen about 4 mm below the meniscus. The band of opacity itself is approximately 3 mm wide. Contrast the zone of dense opacity of the control with the experimental slide on the right. The opaque zone on the right is broader, 7 or 8 mm wide. (15) Details of a representative area from the narrow dense zone, the zone of piling up, of the control slide seen in Fig. 14. The MDCK cells consist of a monolayer on which are superimposed many compact connected and isolated aggregates of papillary adenocarcinoma. Occasional cysts are found, one of which is seen in the lower left corner of the figure. ×120. (16) Details of a representative area from the broad dense zone of the culture exposed to 95% O_2 and 5% CO_2 for 23 days. Superimposed on the monolayer are myriads of functional cystic papillary aggregates in complex organoid arrangements. ×120.

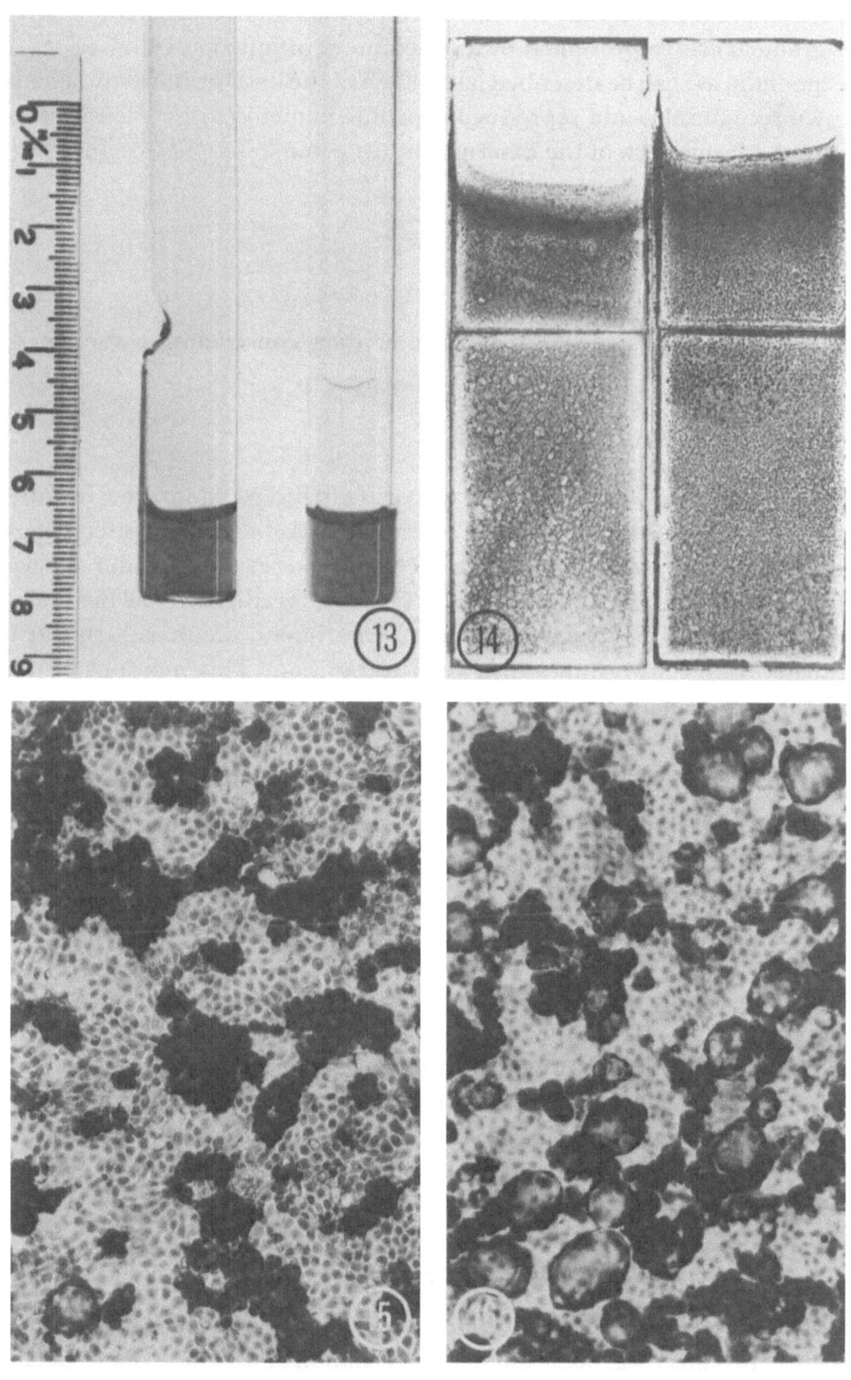
13
14

cell degeneration, necrosis, and sloughing. The third and fourth zones share a 10-mm-wide or more span of the gradient below the zone of piling up, to the bottom of the coverslip. The early development of necrosis in the span of the gradient can be prevented by a supplement of mucopolysaccharides in the medium, as shall be described later. Each of the lines we have studied has its own recognizable and reproducible profile in meniscus-gradient culture within the framework of the description just given.

4.3. *Standardization of Technique*

Standardization must depend on further data concerning a number of factors.

4.3.1. *Orientation of the Tube*

As mentioned previously, our first experiments were conducted in tubes held in two positions, vertical and at an angle of 45°. Gradient effects were observed in each, and the zones at 45° were wider than in the vertical cultures. It should be mentioned that in Osgood's gradient model the slide is also at an angle. Ever since our first experiment, we have arbitrarily incubated our culture tubes in a vertical position. This may not be the optimal arrangement.

4.3.2 *Shape of the Culture Tube*

Our current technique employs a tube modified for meniscus-gradient culture as illustrated in Fig. 13. It is similar to the widely used Leighton tube except that the closed end of the tube is flat rather than hemispherical. This modification (provided by the Bellco Co., Vineland, N.J.), together with the capillary seal between the coverslip and the flat wall of the tube, keeps the coverslip in a stable position. Another type of tube, used in earlier investigations (Leighton and Katsuta, 1973), has two wide parallel glass surfaces permitting phase optics study. This tube has been used by Katsuta in many investigations, including his work on transformation of liver cells in the NAGISA zone (Katsuta *et al.*, 1965). Current studies in our laboratory involve a direct comparison of the tube illustrated in Fig. 13 and the Katsuta tube.

4.3.3. *Restoration of the Gradient After Feeding*

The feeding schedule has been arbitrarily set at two or at most three times weekly. This choice was made out of a combination of habit and of no specific information. If data yet to be obtained were to demonstrate that the oxygen gradient is completely restored within an hour after it has been disturbed, feeding intervals of 1 or 2 days might be satisfactory, and wide sweeps in pH might not be a necessary variable in the system. We plan to explore this question using methylene blue and other oxidation–reduction dyes. Such data may be confirmed with a sequence of oxygen electrodes set at different depths in the tube.

4.3.4. *Composition of the Culture Environment*

The topic of the composition of the culture environment encompasses all of the complexities of cell nutrition, complicated by a continuous gradient of decreasing oxygen tension and of wide oscillation in the environmental pH. It also includes the composition of the gas phase and the total pressure of the gaseous atmosphere over the culture medium.

4.3.5. *Duration of Cultivation in the Gradient*

Cells immersed in medium for only 2 or 3 days are quite different in appearance from those seen after 3 or 4 wk of cultivation. The sorting of cells by both appearance and arrangement is a response to prolonged maintenance of the culture in the gradient. From the point of view of therapeutics, very different data may be obtained depending on when in the time sequence of cultivation a pulse of therapy is applied and when the cultures are terminated for detailed microscopic study.

4.3.6. *Indices of Observation*

Indices of observation are now at the technically simplest, most economical level. Cultures are examined with the light microscope just before medium is replenished. At the end of the period of cultivation, cultures are fixed and stained with hematoxylin and eosin, and prepared as permanent mounts for light microscopy. It remains to be determined how valuable will be the data derived by more sophisticated means of observation. Among the reasonable possibilities for examining various levels in the gradient are stains of enzyme histochemistry such as alkaline phosphatase, cytogenetic techniques, and electron microscopy. A more dynamic view of events in the living culture requires time-lapse cinephotography. It may be desirable to compare cells at various levels of the gradient in subsequent biological experiments. Such isolates can be obtained from cultures on plastic coverslips or Gelfilm (Upjohn) by cutting these substrates into segments transverse to the axis of the original gradient. Aerobic and anaerobic segments from gradient cultures of human cell lines can be studied in an intact host by topical inoculation of the segments on the chorioallantoic membrane of the chick. Techniques for such inoculation are simple (Leighton, 1967).

5. *Application of the Meniscus-Gradient Method*

In this discussion, we will concentrate on applications of the meniscus-gradient model that are currently under investigation in our laboratory, and merely mention a few other directions in which the model may be useful.

5.1. *Characterization of Cell Lines*

Catalogs of available tissue culture cell lines, human or animal, are particularly inadequate as to descriptions of growth pattern and cell morphology. Our recent experience with conventional monolayer cultures of six carcinoma cell lines provided renewed recognition of this inadequacy. Each of these six epithelial cell lines proved to be characteristically distinctive when examined in meniscus-gradient culture. Four of them were derived from the urinary bladder, two of rat (Toyoshima *et al.*, 1971) and two of human origin RT4 (Rigby and Franks, 1971) and T24 (Bubenik *et al.*, 1960). Figures 17 through 20 illustrate the appearance of the human bladder cancer lines at two positions in the gradient. Figures 17 and 18 are of RT4 and Figs. 19 and 20 of T24. Figures 17 and 19 are from the aerobic zone of piling up, just below the meniscus. Figures 18 and 20 show an anaerobic region 7 mm below the meniscus. All photographs were made at a magnification of 120. Note the difference in cell size in the two zones for each of the cell lines, and compare the morphology of the two lines at both levels.

These lines derived from human malignant urothelium, as well as the two from rat bladder cancer, all have a unique pattern of morphology in meniscus-gradient culture. This suggests that the model system may serve as a means of general characterization of many cell lines. Furthermore, if one were seeking an epithelial cell line with a particular capacity for giant cell

---

FIGS. 17–20. Illustrations of two human bladder cancer cell lines, RT4 and T24, in meniscus-gradient culture, showing aerobic and anaerobic parts of the culture. All are stained with hematoxylin and eosin. ×120. (17) RT4, a field from the zone of piling up just beneath the air–medium interface. (18) RT4, a field from the anaerobic part of the culture, 7 mm below the air–medium interface. Compare the size of the cells in Figs. 17 and 18. (19) T24, a field from the zone of piling up just beneath the air–medium interface. (20) T24, a field from the anaerobic part of the culture, 7 mm below the air–medium interface. Note cells in mitosis including several grossly abnormal forms. Compare the size of the cells in Figs. 19 and 20.

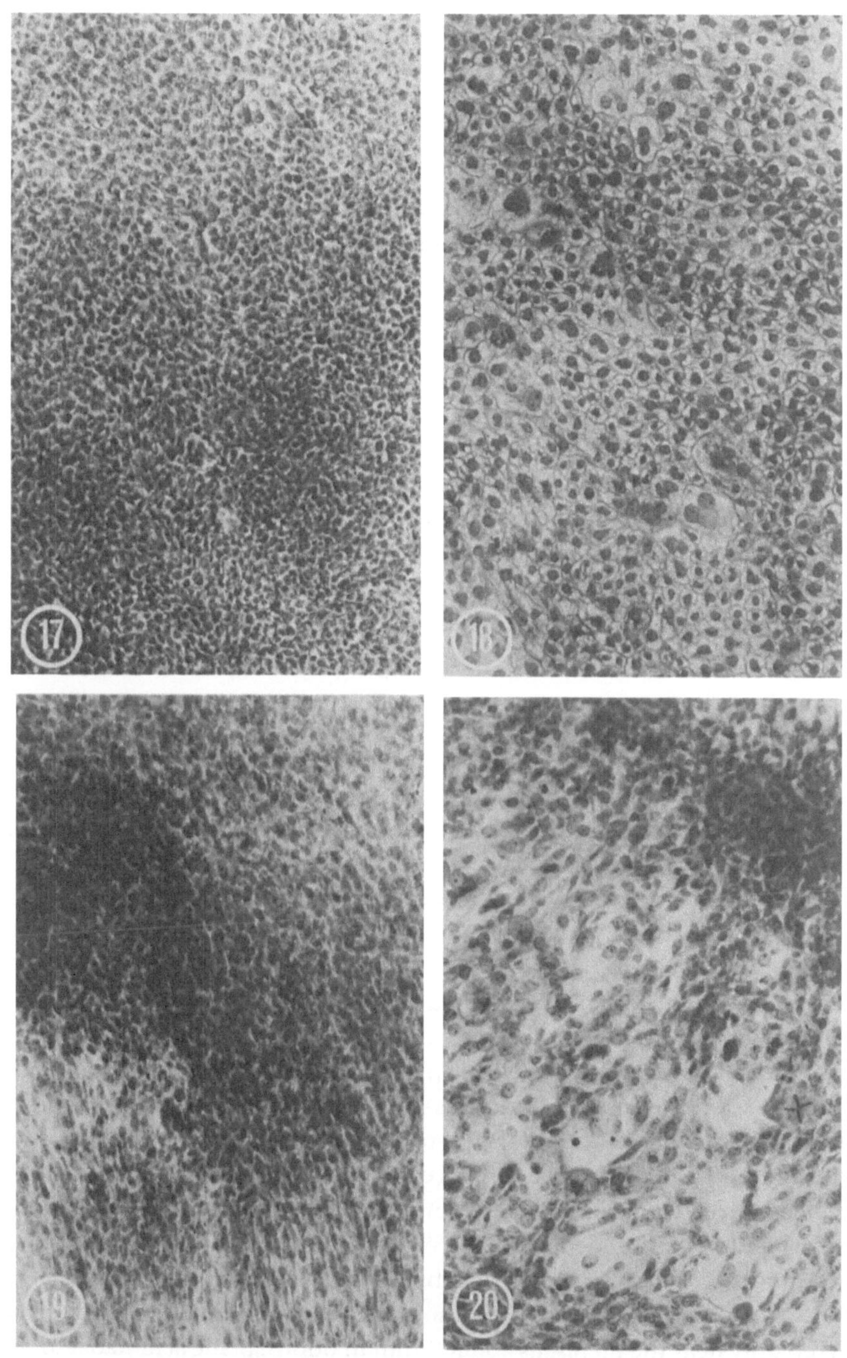
17
18
19
20

formation, Nara bladder tumor II is immediately identified as an excellent candidate. This line, derived from a chemically induced bladder cancer in the rat, produced enormous numbers of mononucleated tumor giant cells in the zone about 6 mm below the gas phase (Leighton and Katsuta, 1973). This fact is not evident without cultivation in the gradient model.

5.2. *Diagnostic Evaluation of Clinical Tumors*

Certain clinical tumors of apparent similar type, as evaluated by diagnostic histopathology, express different biological behavior in the host. Carcinoma of the urinary bladder grade I (Fig. 1) is one example. Eighty percent of patients with these tumors can be managed conservatively, requiring cystoscopy and local destruction of new tumor growths at long intervals. On the other hand, 20% of patients so treated have, in 4 or 5 yr, invasive carcinoma of the urinary bladder usually of a more malignant histopathological grade, and require extensive surgery. We are currently studying cancer of the human urinary bladder in meniscus-gradient culture, and plan to compare a series of patients with grade I and II carcinomas. As one aspect of this investigation, recurrent growths in the same patient's bladder will be cultured. Here we will be looking for changes in characteristics that may foretell significant changes in the neoplastic process in the patient.

5.3. *Experimental Therapeutics*

Carcinoma cells growing *in vitro* in a continuous gradient of decreasing oxygen tension provide a particularly appropriate setting for evaluating therapeutic agents, since their clinical counterparts exist in a gradient setting as illustrated in Figs. 1–4. We have observed that two carcinoma cell lines are modified substantially by supplementation of the medium with mucopolysaccharides.

The human mammary carcinoma cell line BT-20 is responsive to a supplement of mucopolysaccharides in the medium. In control medium, on a schedule of feeding twice weekly, a prominent multilayering of viable cells is seen in the zone just below the gas–medium interface. However, after 3 wk, from 3 mm below the surface to the bottom of the tube there are extensive necrosis and exfoliation of cells. Hyaluronic acid had no influence on the cultures. Heparin prevented some cells from detaching and the viable zone was about 6 mm deep. Chondroitin sulfate prevented the cells from detaching and the cells remained viable to the bottom of the culture, about 10–12 mm below the meniscus, although the piling up phenomenon occurred only near the meniscus about 2 mm in depth. Sialic acid had a totally different effect. It not only prevented the cells from detaching but also induced the appearance of pleomorphic cells. The piling up of cells at the meniscus became less pronounced. Figures 21 through 24 illustrate the effect of chondroitin sulfate.

Figures 21 and 22 are from a control culture and present two patterns, the viable zone of piling up and the necrotic sloughing off zone 10 mm below the surface. In experimental cultures, where the medium was supplemented with 0.05% chondroitin sulfate, the cells in the deep anaerobic part of the culture were protected. Figures 23 and 24 show the zone of piling up and the growth 10 mm below the surface, respectively, in a treated experimental culture. Figures 21 and 23, control and treated, both near the surface, are very much alike. Figures 22 and 24, from a zone 10 mm below the surface, show entirely different pictures.

The mechanisms responsible for the protective phenomenon illustrated in the contrasting Figs. 22 and 24 have not been identified. Since we have observed a similar result with another carcinoma cell line, MDCK, the phenomenon is probably one of some importance (Takeuchi *et al.*, 1974). For example, it may provide a clue to the role of mucopolysaccharides in clinical carcinomas. These substances are prominent constituents of many solid tumors, and conceivably play a protective role for carcinoma cells in metabolic adversity, including the action of cytotoxic agents administered as therapy. In our current investigation of this possibility, we are examining the effects of Bleomycin and Thiotepa on carcinoma cell lines in meniscus-gradient culture. After the effects of the chemotherapeutic agents alone have been clearly characterized, we will determine whether a supplement of mucopolysaccharides modifies the effect of the cytotoxic chemicals on the carcinoma cells. These investigations constitute preliminary probes in therapy with an emphasis on differential effects determined by oxygen gradients. Since metabolic gradients are an integral part of solid tumors, therapy may be improved by actively considering such spectra of metabolic states.

Subsequent work in experimental therapeutics will involve two meniscus-gradient settings of parallel series of cultures. In the first, agents will be evaluated shortly after the gradient has been established. In the second, they will be administered to parallel series of cultures several weeks after the tubes have been placed in a vertical position, after the sorting out of cells in response to selective pressures has taken place. The responses of tumor cells in these two temporal gradient settings may be quite different. They may have clinical analogies. The acute gradient may correspond to rapidly growing transplantable solid tumors of animals. The cultures of greater duration, after selective pressures of the gradient have acted, may have a counterpart in the slow-growing solid tumors of man.

In either of the experimental gradients, combinations of therapeutic agents may provide useful information. If certain chemicals act primarily in the aerobic part of the cultures and others act selectively on the anaerobic portions, some combinations may produce broad-spectrum effects. In addition, drugs which individually have marginal or doubtful effectiveness may in appropriate combinations have useful synergistic effects on selected segments of the gradient.

5.4. *Carcinogenesis and Other Problems*

A variety of other applications of the method might be considered including problems of carcinogenesis, tumor progression, immunology, and virology. Since we have no data in these areas, it is inappropriate to discuss these matters at length here. A few words are in order on the matter of carcinogenesis *in vitro*. In three separate institutions, Goldblatt, Katsuta, and Sanford have examined the effects of oxygen tension on transformations *in vitro* (Goldblatt and Cameron, 1953; Goldblatt *et al.*, 1973; Katsuta *et al.*, 1965; Katsuta and Takaoka, 1968; Sanford, 1965*a, b*; Sanford and Parshad, 1968; Parshad and Sanford, 1971). The results of these excellent investigators are not concordant. We suggest that the meniscus-gradient model may be useful in resolving apparently differing observations.

6. *Perspectives*

We believe that we have made a reasonable case for considering gradients of metabolites in tissue culture studies that aim at understanding cancer in man. The meniscus-gradient model is one appropriate means of probing phenomena of cancer cell biology related to gradients. As the essential qualities of the model are better understood through future investigation, we will have some picture of the way in which cells at various positions relate

FIGS. 21–24. Four illustrations depicting the protective effect of a mucopolysaccharide, chondroitin sulfate, on the anaerobic portion of meniscus-gradient cultures of human mammary cancer cell line BT-20. Hematoxylin and eosin. ×120. (21) A field from the zone of piling up in a control culture. (22) A field from the anaerobic part of the gradient, 10 mm below the gas–medium interface, in a control culture. (23) A field from the zone of piling up in a culture supplemented with 0.05% chondroitin sulfate. Note that Figs. 21 and 23 are interchangeable in appearance. (24) A field from the anaerobic part of the gradient, 10 mm below the gas–medium interface, in a culture treated with a supplement of 0.05% chondroitin sulfate. Compare this figure with the untreated culture illustrated in Fig. 22.

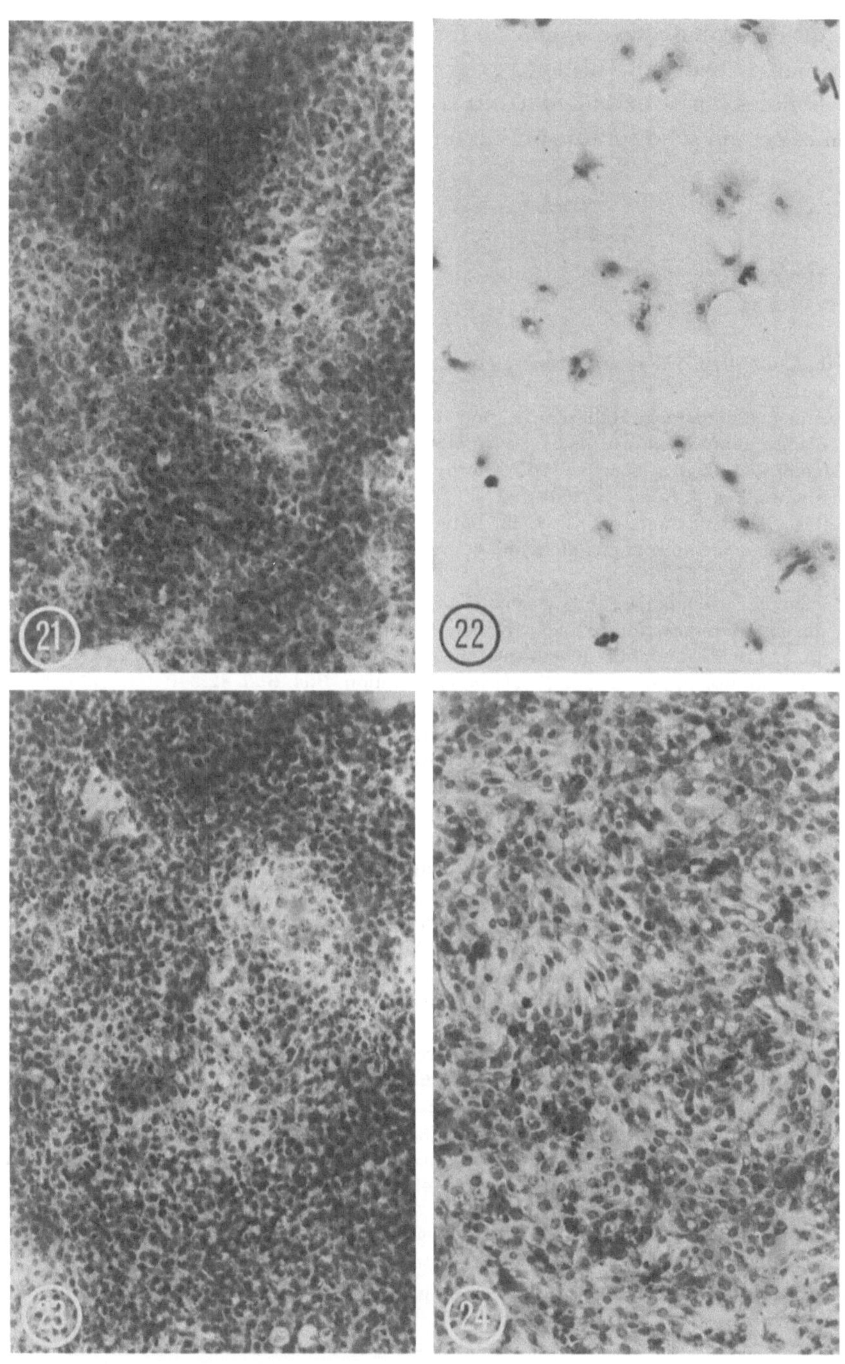
21
22
23
24

to one another, the extent to which they interact, integrate, and respond as an ecological unity. It is within the realm of possibility that their total pattern and their polarization and the development of highly organoid complexes near the gas phase have significant features in common with the response of the marine hydroid *Tubularia* to gradients of oxygen tension. The same possibilities can be extended to our real concern, the coordinated interrelation of cells in solid tumors in the context of their metabolic gradients.

7. References

Barth, L. G., 1940, The relation between oxygen consumption and rate of regeneration, *Biol. Bull.* **78:**366.

Bubenik, J., Perlmann, P., Helmstein, K., and Moberger, G., 1970, Immune response to urinary bladder tumours in man, *Int. J. Cancer* **5:**39.

Goldacre, R. J., and Sylvén, B., 1962, On the access of blood-borne dyes to various tumor regions, *Brit. J. Cancer* **16:**306.

Goldblatt, H., and Cameron, G., 1953, Induced malignancy in cells from rat myocardium subjected to intermittent anaerobiosis during long propagation *in vitro, J. Exp. Med.* **97:**525.

Goldblatt, H., Friedman, L., and Cencher, R. L., 1973, On the malignant transformation of cells during prolonged culture under hypoxic conditions *in vitro, Biochem. Med.* **7:**241.

Goldin, A., 1942, A quantitative study of the interrelationship of oxygen and hydrogen ion concentration in influencing *Tubularia* regeneration, *Biol. Bull.* **82:**340

Katsuta, H., and Takaoka, T., 1968, Cytobiological transformation of normal rat liver cells by treatment with 4-dimethylaminoazobenzene after NAGISA culture, in: *Cancer Cells in Culture* (H. Katsuta, ed.), pp. 321–334, University of Tokyo Press, Tokyo, Japan.

Katsuta, H., Takaoka, T., Doida, Y., and Kuroki, T., 1965, Carcinogenesis in tissue culture. VI. Morphological transformation of rat liver cells in NAGISA culture, *Jap. J. Exp. Med.* **35:**513.

Leighton, J., 1958, Economic maintenance of continuous lines of human cells with bead-in-tube cultures, *Lab. Invest.* **7:**513.

Leighton, J., 1967, The spread of cancer explored in the embryonated egg, in: *The Spread of Cancer*, pp. 115–192, Academic Press, New York.

Leighton, J., 1968, Neoplastic blockade, a new concept in the destruction of normal tissue by cancer, in: *Cancer Cells in Culture* (H. Katsuta, ed.), pp. 143–156, University of Tokyo Press, Tokyo, Japan.

Leighton, J., 1973, Cell propagation on miscellaneous culture supports: Collagen-coated cellulose sponge, in: *Tissue Culture: Methods and Applications* (P. F. Kruse, Jr., and M. K. Patterson, Jr., eds.), pp. 367–371, Academic Press, New York and London.

Leighton, J., and Katsuta, H., 1973, Meniscus-gradient culture of carcinomatous epithelial cell lines of bladder and kidney origin, in: *Chemotherapy of Cancer Dissemination and Metastasis* (S. Garattini and G. Franchi, eds.), pp. 31–43, Raven Press, New York.

Leighton, J., Estes, L. W., Goldblatt, P. J., and Brada, Z., 1970, The formation of histotypic fibrous collagen in matrix tissue culture by 3T6 mouse fibroblasts: A response to ascorbic acid, *In Vitro* **6:**153.

Miller, J. A., 1937, Some effects of oxygen on polarity in *Tubularia crocea, Biol. Bull.* **73:**369 (abstr.).

Morgan, T. H., 1903, Some factors in the regeneration of *Tubularia, Arch. Entw.-Mech.* **16:**125.

Osgood, E. E., 1955, Tissue culture in the study of leucocytic functions, *Ann. N.Y. Acad. Sci.* **59:**806.

Osgood, E. E., and Brooke, J. H., 1955, Continuous tissue culture of Leucocytes from human leukemic bloods by application of "gradient" principles, *Blood* **10:**1010.

Osgood, E. E., and Krippaehne, M. L., 1955, The gradient tissue culture method, *Exp. Cell Res.* **9:**116.

Parshad, R., and Sanford, K. K., 1971, Oxygen supply and stability of chromosomes in mouse embryo cells *in vitro, J. Natl. Cancer Inst.* **47:**1033.

Rigby, C. C., and Franks, L. M., 1971, A human tissue culture cell line from a transitional cell tumour of the urinary bladder: Growth, chromosome pattern and ultra-structure, *Brit. J. Cancer* **24:**746.

Sanford, K. K., 1965*a*, An attempt to induce malignant transformation of cells *in vitro* by intermittent anaerobiosis, *J. Natl. Cancer Inst.* **35:**719.

Sanford, K. K., 1965*b*, Malignant transformations of cells *in vitro*, in: *International Review of Cytology*, Vol. 18 (G. H. Bourne and J. F. Danielli, eds.), pp. 249–311, Academic Press, New York.

Sanford, K. K., and Parshad, R., 1968, Oxygen supply and neoplastic conversion of mouse embryo cells *in vitro, J. Natl. Cancer Inst.* **41:**1389.

Sigel, B., Baldia, L. B., Brightman, S. A., Dunn, M. R., and Price, R. I. M., 1968, Effect of blood flow reversal in liver autotransplants upon the site of hepatocyte regeneration, *J. Clin. Invest.* **47:**1231.

Spiegelman, S., and Goldin, A., 1944, A comparison of regeneration and respiration rates of *Tubularia, Proc. Soc. Exp. Biol. Med.* **55:**252.

Takeuchi, J., Tchao, R., and Leighton, J., 1974, Protective action of mucopolysaccharides on dog kidney cell line MDCK in meniscus-gradient culture, *Cancer Res.* **34:**161.

Tannock, I. F., 1968, The relation between cell proliferation and the vascular system in a transplanted mouse mammary tumour, *Brit. J. Cancer* **22:**258.

Toyoshima, K., Ito, N., Hiasa, Y., Kamamoto, Y., and Makiura, S., 1971, Tissue culture of urinary bladder tumor induced in a rat by *N*-Butyl-*N*-(4-hydroxybutyl) nitrosamine, *J. Natl. Cancer Inst.* **47:**979.

Human Lung Cancer in Tissue Culture

10

RUSSELL P. SHERWIN AND ARNIS RICHTERS

1. Introduction

1.1. The Varieties of Pneumothelial Cancers

Most epithelial lung cancers are believed to originate from the bronchial mucosa, and these "bronchogenic carcinomas" have been subdivided into three major entities, epidermoid cancer, adenocarcinoma, and undifferentiated carcinoma. While more elaborate classifications have been proposed, in particular that by the World Health Organization (Kreyberg *et al.*, 1967), criteria for distinguishing the subtypes have not been universally accepted or uniformly applied. As a consequence, there has been a tendency to overlook the great diversity of cancer cell types within the lung. At the root of the problem is the little attention being given to the numerous and distinctive normal cells of the "pneumothelium," i.e., the respiratory tract lining from the bronchus into the alveolus. Some progress has been made with the advent of electron microscopic studies of both nonneoplastic and neoplastic tissues of the lung. Of special interest is the discovery that the "oat-cell" cancer is derived from the Kultschitsky cell of the bronchial mucosal lining and submucosal glands (Bensch *et al.*, 1968). Also, it now appears that one type of "bronchioloalveolar" cancer originates from type 2 pneumocytes of the alveolus (Adamson *et al.*, 1969; Coalson *et al.*, 1970).

RUSSELL P. SHERWIN AND ARNIS RICHTERS University of Southern California, School of Medicine, Department of Pathology, Los Angeles, California

However, these two types of lung cells are the *only* ones that have been identified as "parent cells" for human lung cancers.

1.2. The Concept of the Parent Cell

This deficit in cell identification has two particularly serious implications: (1) The inability to recognize the parent cell of a lung cancer greatly impairs the documentation of primary origin; i.e., for the *majority* of lung cancers, autopsy exclusion of metastatic disease is, at the present time, mandatory. This poorly appreciated problem has been presented earlier in greater detail (Sherwin, 1966). (2) Correlative studies of the cancer cell and its nonneoplastic counterpart are impossible when the parent cell giving rise to the cancer is unknown. (3) Comparisons of lung cancer tissue culture experiences are only as valid as the level of parent cell identification. For example, data from two adenocarcinomas cannot be strictly compared when one is derived from a type 1 pneumocyte and the other from either a type 2 pneumocyte or one of many different mucosal lining cells. With these aspects in mind, and with the added information that our own experience with human lung cancers in tissue culture (Sherwin *et al.*, 1967) indicates a great variety of neoplastic lung cell types, the concept of the "parent cell" should receive high priority for future tissue culture studies.

Another important consideration when culturing human lung cancer is the documentation of the cancer cells in the tissue culture preparations. These aspects have been covered in our earlier reports (Sherwin *et al.*, 1968) and will be discussed in the text that follows.

2. Methodology and Summary of Results

2.1. The Tissue Culture Preparations

A correlated *in vivo–in vitro* study of human lung cancer was carried out. Serial sections of the whole lung (Gillette and Sherwin, 1965) afforded a more precise interpretation of the pathology. Histological sections of the explants after varying periods of *in vitro* life not only provided support for documentation of monolayers but also gave data on semiorgan culture cancer properties. Phase contrast microscopy, supplemented by time-lapse cinephotomicrography, allowed direct observation of histocultures as they underwent transitions into monolayers. Cytological stains of the monolayers gave an additional large-volume dimension to the study. Full details of the tissue culture methodology have been reported earlier (Sherwin *et al.*, 1967). In brief, the most viable-appearing cancer tissue was selected for explantation, and generally 58 explants from each cancer were cultured in Leighton tubes and Rose chambers. A parallel study was carried out for nonneoplastic lung tissues. For all studies, the tubeslip preparations were fixed at 4 h, 24 h, 48 h, 96 h, 7 days, and weekly up to 6 wk. The explants were processed for histological examination, and the cellular outgrowths were stained with the May–Giemsa–Grünwald technique. Eagle's double-strength amino acid medium was used exclusively and to this were added 20% calf serum, 5% beef embryo extract ultrafiltrate, 100 u/100 ml of penicillin, 100 μg/ml of streptomycin, 500 mg/100 ml of glucose, 0.25 mg/ml L-glutamine, and phenol red indicator (0.0025% final concentration). There were four explants per tube and six per Rose chamber, with the latter including a cellophane strip.

2.2. *Cancer Yield in Primary Cultures*

The findings to be presented were based on observations and data derived from 113 human lung cancers, the majority of which were received as resected lungs or lobes of the lung. Definitive studies included the following: (1) Lung cancer was documented in short-term tissue culture (Sherwin *et al.*, 1968) involving 46 human lung cancers. This report covered the principles of documentation of the cancer in tissue culture. A parallel study (Sherwin *et al.*, 1967) of the same material covered aspects of the dynamic behavior of these cancers. In the series, 75% of the cancers explanted yielded tissues or cells identifiable as cancer through either phase contrast observations or stained culture preparations. (2) An expanded study, involving a total of 68 human lung cancers, emphasized the interactions of lymphocytes with neoplastic and nonneoplastic cells (Richters *et al.*, 1971). The overall yield of identifiable cancer in culture was again similar (74%). The most consistent outgrowth was obtained with epidermoid cancer (90%), adenocarcinoma was the least productive (53%), and undifferentiated carcinoma was intermediate (72%). (3) A study of 20 consecutively received lung cancers was particularly directed toward determining the frequency of viable cancer in the explants, the occurrence of a cancer rim around the explants, and the emergence of a cancer monolayer from the explants (Table 1). It was particularly noteworthy that the explants of three of seven adenocarcinomas were characterized by a one-cell-thick cancer rim whereas those from five of six epidermoid cancers showed multilayered cancer cells (Figs. 7 and 8). The special aspects of cytostructure (Table 2) and dynamic behavior for the combined study are discussed in the text that follows.

TABLE 1

Survival and Proliferation of Explanted Cancer in Vitro[a]

Lung No.	Pathological diagnosis[b]	4 h	24 h	48 h	96 h	7 days	14 days	21 days	28 days	35 days	42 days	≥43 days
		R B O	R B O	R B O	R B O	R B O	R B O	R B O	R B O	R B O	R B O	R B O
1 (L1)	Adenocarcinoma	N	N	N	N	− − −	− − −	− − −	− + −	− − −	N	N
2 (L2)	Adenocarcinoma	N	N	N	N	N	− ± +	N	N	N	N	N
3 (L3)	Squamous cell carcinoma	N	N	− + +	N	N	− − +	− + ±	− + +	− − −	N	N
4 (L8)	Adenocarcinoma, bronchiolar type	− + +	− + +	− + +	− − −	− − −	− − −	N	− − −	− + −	N	− − −
5 (L9)	Mixed epidermoid and adenocarcinoma	− + −	− + +	+ + +	− + −	+ + −	+ + −	+ + −	− ± −	− − −	N	− − −
6 (L11)	Adenocarcinoma	− + +	+ + +	+ + −	+ + +	+ + +	+ + +	+ + +	+ + +	+ + +	N	N
7 (L12)	Squamous carcinoma	− + +	+ + −	+ + −	− − −	+ + +	+ + +	+ + +	N	− + −	− − −	N
8 (L13)	Adenocarcinoma	− + +	− + +	− + +	+ + +	+ + +	+ + −	+ + ±	+ + ±	− + ±	+ + ±	N
9 (L14)	Squamous cell carcinoma, exophytic	− + −	+ + +	+ + +	+ + −	− − −	+ + +	+ + +	+ + +	+ + +	− + +	+ + +

10 (L15) Epidermoid carcinoma	− + −	− + −	+ + −	+ + −	+ + −	+ + +	+ + ±	N	+ + ±	− − ±	+ + ±
11 (L17) Squamous cell carcinoma	− + −	+ + −	N	+ + −	+ + −	+ + +	+ + +	− ± ±	+ + ±	− − −	N
12 (L18) Adenocarcinoma	N	N	− + +	− + −	− + +	− − +	− + +	− + +	N	N	N
13 (L20) Adenocarcinoma	N	− + +	− − +	− − +	− − −	− + +	− − −	N	− − ±	N	− − −
14 (L21) Adenocarcinoma	N	− + +	+ + +	− + +	+ + +	+ + +	− + +	− + +	− − −	N	N
15 (L22) Undifferentiated, small cell type	N	− + +	N	+ + +	+ + +	+ + +	+ + +	+ + +	+ + +	− + +	− + +
16 (L23) Squamous carcinoma and adenocarcinoma	N	+ + +	+ + +	N	+ + +	+ + +	+ + +	− − ±	N	− − +	+ + −
17 (L24) Adenocarcinoma	− + +	− + +	− + +	− + ±	− − −	− − −	− + −	− + ±	N	− − −	N
18 (L26) Undifferentiated carcinoma	− + +	+ + +	+ + +	+ + +	N	+ + +	N	− − −	N	N	N
19 (L27) Undifferentiated carcinoma	N	+ + +	N	− + +	− + +	− + ±	N	N	N	N	N
20 (L28) Epidermoid carcinoma	N	N	+ + +	N	+ + +	+ + +	N	N	N	N	N

[a] R. Rim (outgrowth present in histological section); B. button (histological section of explant); O. outgrowth; N. no cancer in outgrowth or explant.
[b] From Department of Pathology records.

TABLE 2

Organs, Tissues, and Cells in Vitro[a]

I. Organ and semiorgan culture
   A. Structurally intact
   B. Major structural alteration

II. Histoculture or organoid culture (primary tissue architecture)
   A. Multilayer
   B. Unilayer–bilayer

III. Tissue culture, monolayer (secondary tissue architecture)
   A. With primary cell shape in tissue form
   B. With secondary cell shape in tissue form

IV. Tissue culture, multilayer and aggregates (secondary architecture)
   A. Cell proliferation (e.g., matrix cultures)
   B. Nonproliferative (passive tissue conversion)

V. Cell culture (individual cells)
   A. Primary cell shape
   B. Secondary cell shape

[a] Original (or primary) structure is characterized by intact *tissue-to-tissue* and *cell-to-cell* relationships, plus cell *shapes* equivalent to those *in vivo*. In histoculture, tissue-to-tissue relationships are minimal or lost but the two other characteristics remain. Cell culture can have cells with either original shape or a shape influenced by the new environment, and the cells may be in tissue (i.e., monolayer) form or individual, as in nonaggregate suspension preparations.

3. Cytostructural Expressions of Lung Cancer in Culture

3.1. Semiorgan (Organotypic) Cultures

A true organ culture of a lung cancer requires perfusion of an entire lung or lobe of a lung. There are no reports concerning such preparations, and serious technical difficulties can be expected with such approaches. Cultures which involve a portion of the cancer mass are more properly designated "semiorgan cultures," or as Maximow (1925) suggested, "organotypic cultures." This form of culture has the extremely important attribute of providing structurally intact tissue for study. Specifically, the tissue-to-tissue relationships, e.g., connective tissue, epithelium, cancer, lymphatic channels, and blood vessels, have been maintained in a state essentially the equivalent of the *in vivo* situation (Fig. 6). The disadvantage of this preparation is that nutrition and metabolic activities are seriously compromised, particularly in the central portions of the explants, and major changes in the tissue and cell relationships ultimately occur. Special perfusion methods to overcome this deficiency have yet to be worked out satisfactorily for the study of human lung cancers, but a number of advances have been made (Gullino *et al.*, 1970; Easty, 1970) which should lead to progress in this area. However, even with optimal perfusion of semiorgan cultures there is still the substantial disadvantage that direct observations of the cancer cells cannot be made; i.e., data must be gained through histopathological processing. The histological sections can of course provide very useful data. For example, Figs. 7 and 8 illustrate the so far consistent differences between semiorgan cultures of epidermoid and adenocarcinoma of the lung.

3.2. Histocultures (Organoid Cultures)

In the histoculture, *structural* integrity is minimal or absent; i.e., we are dealing with an essentially two-dimensional structure, approximately three cells deep. The true relationships of connective tissue, vessels, and other elements to each other and to the cancer are partially or completely lost. However, the *cell-to-cell* relationships of the cancer tissue itself are still maintained (Figs. 1–5), and this *architectural* integrity is identical to or very close to that found in the *in vivo* state. To obtain such preparations, semitransparent slices of cancer tissue are cut either freehand or by the use of special devices. Observations can readily be made immediately after explantation through the use of optically appropriate culture chambers and phase contrast microscopy. These attributes are also found with the small masses of organoid tissue that occur spontaneously (Figs. 2, 9, and 11), a phenomenon referred to as cancer cell "spilling out" (Lasfargues and Ozzello, 1958). When the spilled-out masses of cancer tissue are present in rounded forms, i.e., each cell is rounded rather than flattened, they are highly refractile with phase contrast microscopy and their cytostructural definition is relatively poor (Fig. 10). However, useful information is available from such observations. Some of these masses have been seen to move actively and to change shape, an outstanding behavioral characteristic that should have biological meaning. The rounded masses may spontaneously become flattened, or they can sometimes be pressed flat through the use of cellophane tape. In either case, the result with phase contrast microscopy is excellent cytostructural detail of architecturally intact tissue. The architectural pattern of the histocultures very faithfully reflects that of the histological sections, including epidermoid whorls (Fig. 11) and glands of adenocarcinoma (Figs. 12 and 13).

The two major attributes of histoculture are (1) provision for direct observations of living cancer *tissue* as well as stained preparations after variable periods of *in vitro* life, and (2) a foundation for the documentation of cancer in culture, including monolayers and suspension cultures derived

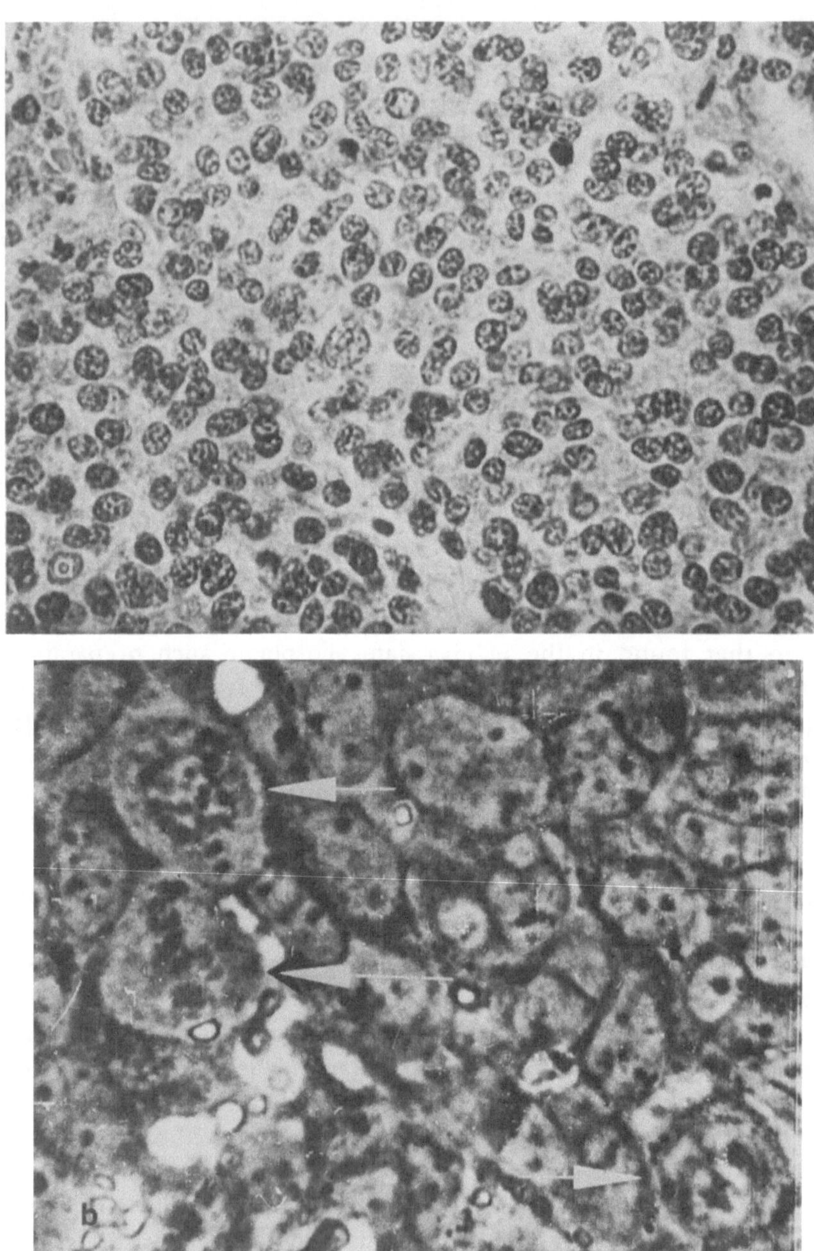

FIG. 1. (a) Undifferentiated carcinoma, histological section. This routinely stained (hematoxylin and eosin) section shows round to elliptical nuclei, multiple nucleoli, and relatively little cytoplasm. (b) Same carcinoma, but histoculture of thin, semitransparent mass recorded by time lapse, phase contrast filming less than an hour after explantation. This is a 16 mm film extract. The oval to elliptical nuclei with multiple small nucleoli correspond to those seen in (a). Three cells (arrows) are in division, but the film records show that only the one in metaphase completes division. ×240 on 16-mm film.

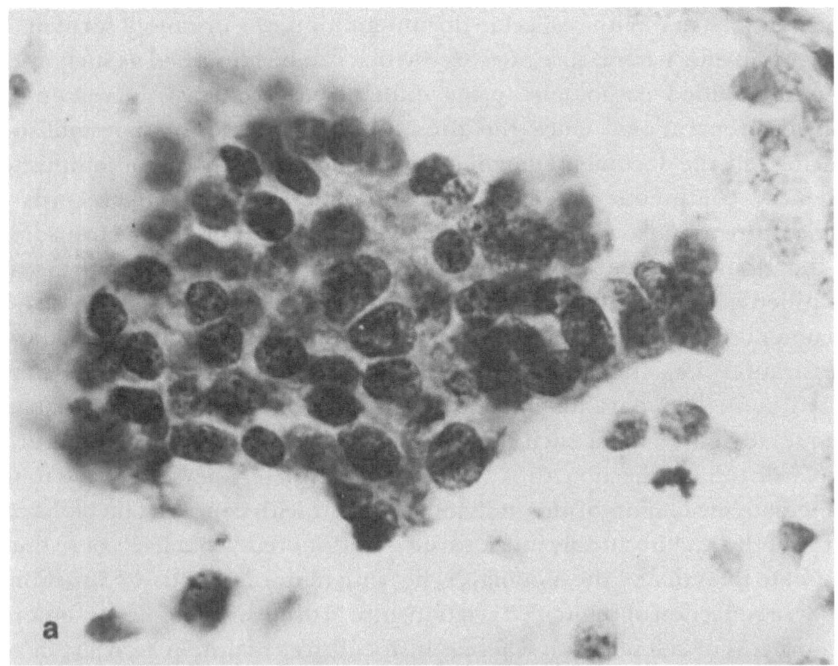

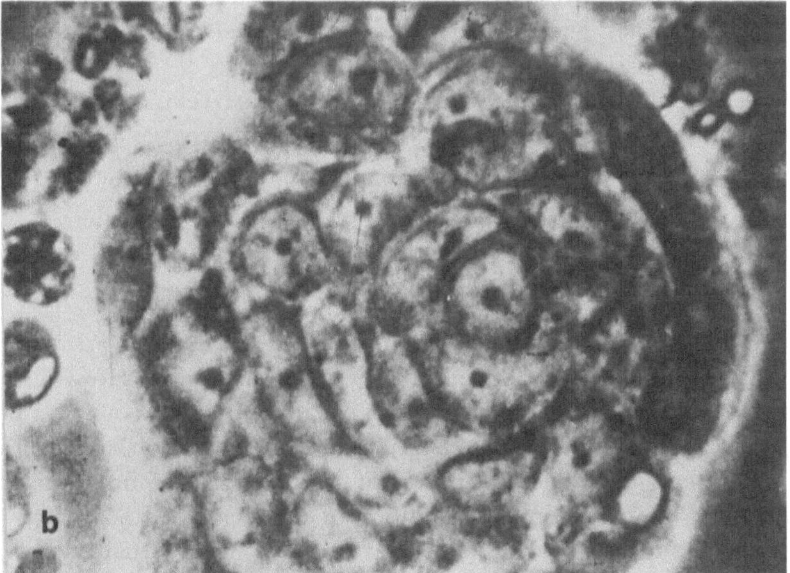

FIG. 2. (a) Undifferentiated carcinoma, histological section. A portion of *in vivo* cancer appears to be isolated, probably within a lymphatic channel. These "islands" of cancer often "spill out" when the tissue is explanted. (b) Undifferentiated carcinoma, phase contrast observation of "spilled-out island" in culture. This island corresponds to that of (a). Note that a "whorl" pattern is evident here which was poorly defined in the hematoxylin and eosin section.

from monolayers. With respect to documentation, the organoid form of the cancer is in effect a thin slice of cancer which can be identified as such by the specially trained pathologist, using either phase contrast microscopy or stained preparations. Once the presence of cancer *tissue* is established conclusively the documentation of cancer *monolayers* is readily accomplished either by continuous time-lapse cinephotomicrographic film records of histoculture monolayer transitions (Figs. 3 and 9) or by observing transitions in the stained preparations (Figs. 4 and 5). Once the monolayers are identified in this manner, cell suspensions derived from them can in turn be documented. It is important to emphasize that the tissue form of culture preparation, i.e., the histoculture, has many advantages over the fixed, dehydrated, and paraffin-embedded histological section. A particularly unique attribute is that such tissues can be observed within minutes after biopsy or tumor resection, thus affording a completely new approach to the immediate evaluation of the individual patient with cancer. The biological status of the architecturally intact tissue is undoubtedly much closer to the *in vivo* state than that of the monolayer, bearing in mind that tissue function is in part a reflection of cell-to-cell relationship. Moreover, monolayers emerge as a process of cell selection whereas histocultures maintain a variety of cell types including primitive cells as well as differentiated cancer cells, stromal cells, and leukocytes. Such preparations lend themselves to a great number of challenges in basic and clinical research (Richters *et al.*, 1971; Sherwin *et al.*, 1969; Sherwin, 1975). One final point: the cell interrelationships and cell surfaces have not been disturbed by proteolytic enzymes employed in culture procedures.

3.3. Monolayers (Sheets and Individual Cells)

As mentioned earlier, the identification of cancer cell monolayers is readily achieved when they are derived from the histocultures. However, the explant may give rise to monolayers without affording observable histoculture-monolayer transitions. In such instances, documentation is difficult and essentially dependent on the finding of residual foci of intact primary architecture, as, for example, the whorls of epidermoid cancer (Fig. 11). When the monolayer is completely devoid of primary architecture, the potential exists for documentation through chromosomal markers, but such

FIG. 3. (a) Undifferentiated carcinoma, tissue culture sheet, phase contrast. In this second example of an undifferentiated cancer, three mitoses are present and one of them is tripolar. At the right margin, the cells are spreading as they convert to a monolayer. (b) A monolayer area of the same cancer shows only a small residium, extreme left, of organoid tissue. ×180, 35 mm.

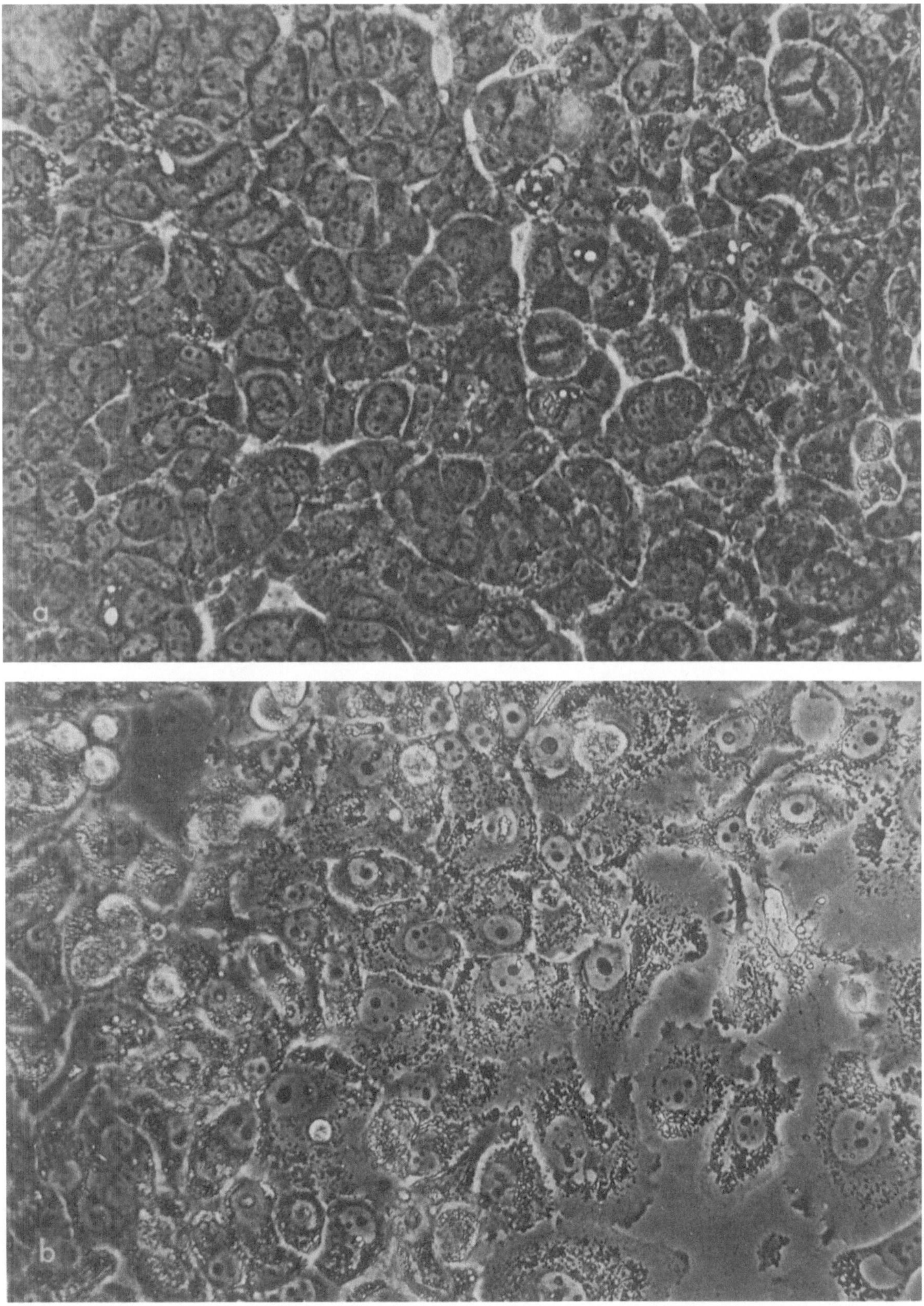

a

b

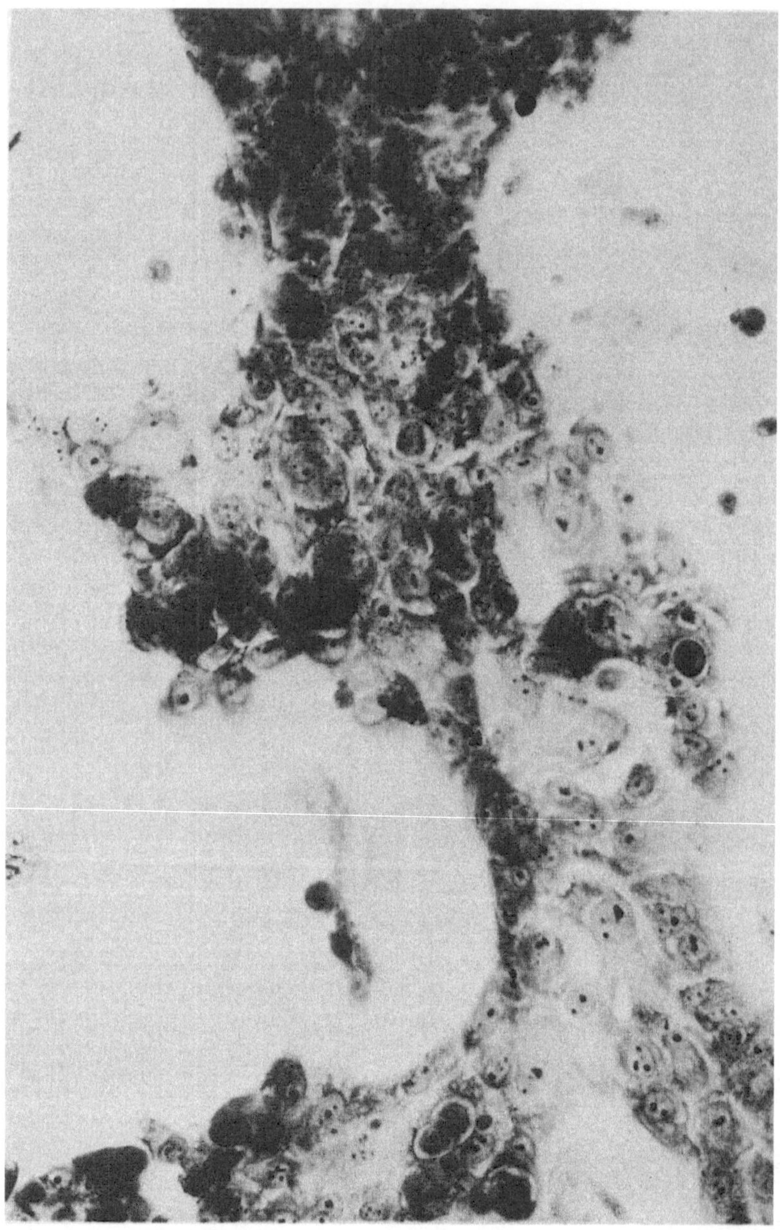

FIG. 4. Transition of cancer from organoid tissues to monolayer. An organoid cancer outgrowth, top half, is in the process of converting to a monolayer, bottom half, May–Grünwald–Giemsa stain. ×160, 35 mm.

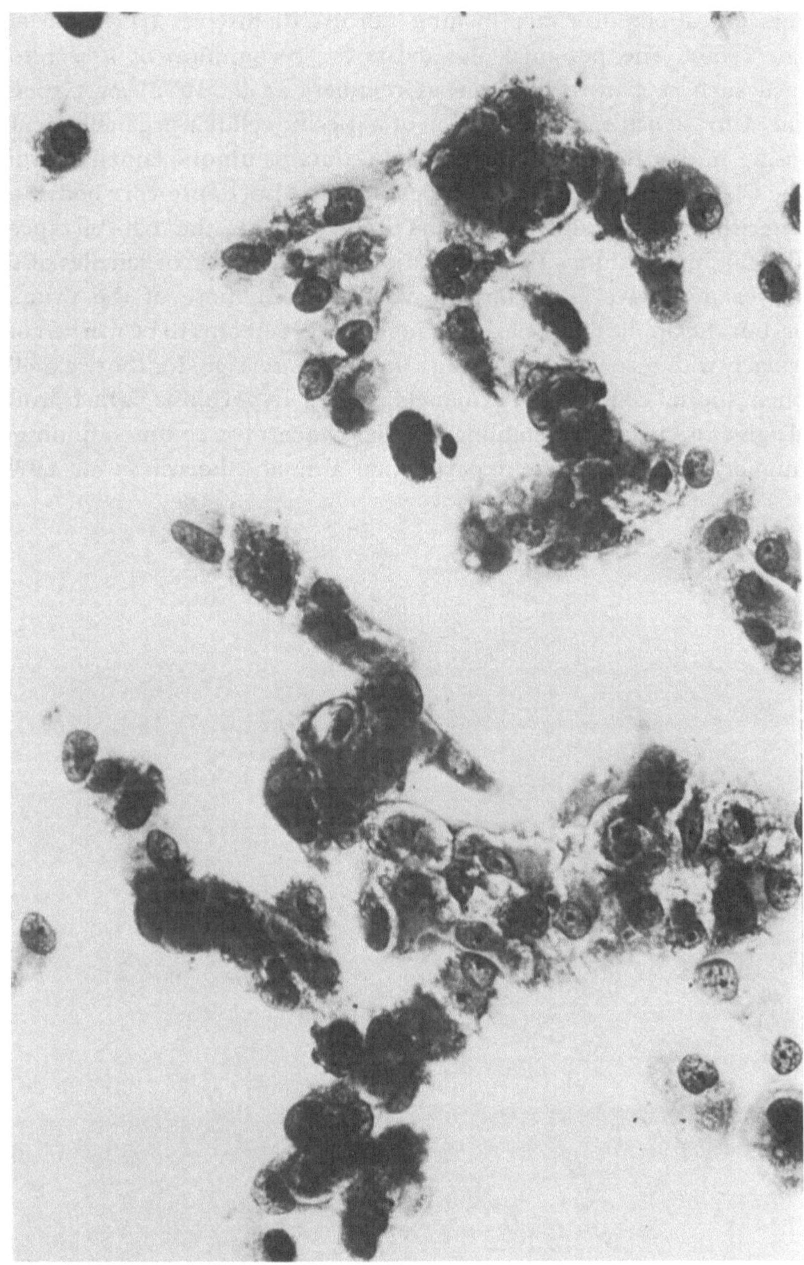

FIG. 5. Cords of cancer. The organoid tissue has partly converted to a monolayer but has retained some features of original architecture, including whorls. May–Grünwald–Giemsa stain.

markers are apparently rare in lung cancers themselves (Davidson and Bulkin, 1966). The potential also exists for recognition of a secretory product, such as growth hormone (Greenberg *et al.*, 1972), or a special enzyme. Ultrastructural identification of a specific cellular organelle is most promising in that the type 2 pneumocyte contains unique lamellar bodies and the Clara cell has distinctive mitochondria. Also, dense-core bodies are characteristic of argentaffin cell tumors of the lung, i.e., the "oat-cell cancer" and the carcinoid tumor. The implication is that specific organelles of the monolayer may have characteristics which match those of the primary tumor, but the applicability of this matching still remains to be worked out, particularly with respect to excluding a *nonneoplastic origin* for the organelles and their special cell types. Germanely, type 2 hyperplasia, which would readily give rise to cells resembling alveolar cancer, is a common finding in the human lung and in the experimental animal (Sherwin *et al.*, 1973).

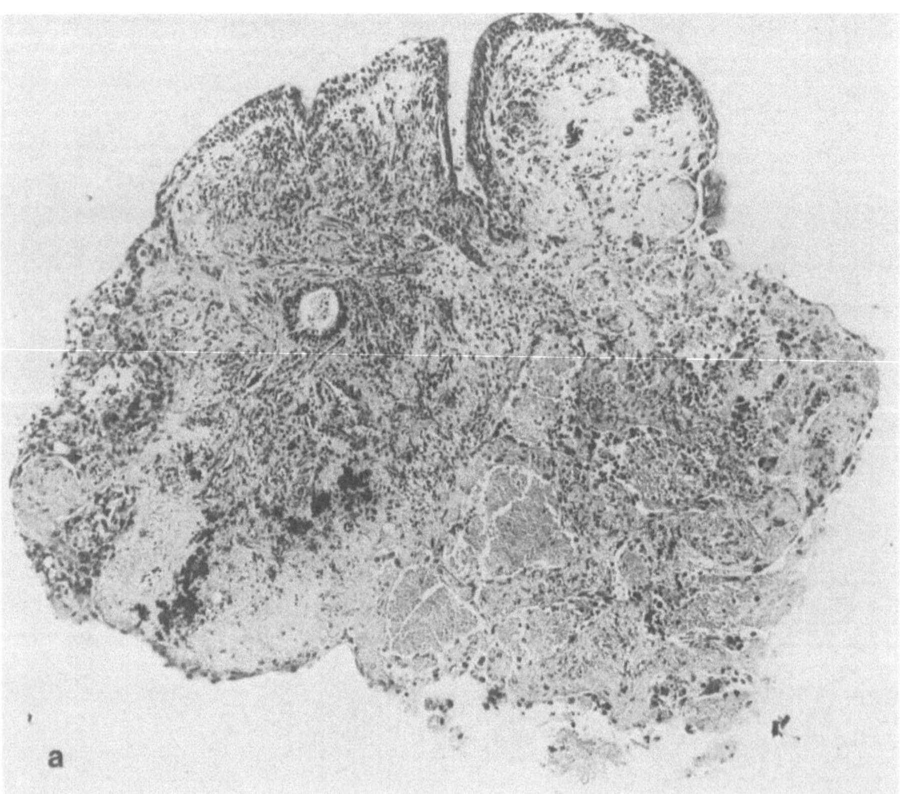

FIG. 6. Squamous carcinoma of the lung, histological section of explant. (a) One-third of the surface epithelium, right margin, is normal, but the central portion shows some atypism, chronic inflammation, and a deep-lying glandular structure representing a tangential cut of the infolding mucosal lining (c). The left one-third of the mucosa is replaced by *in situ* cancer (b).

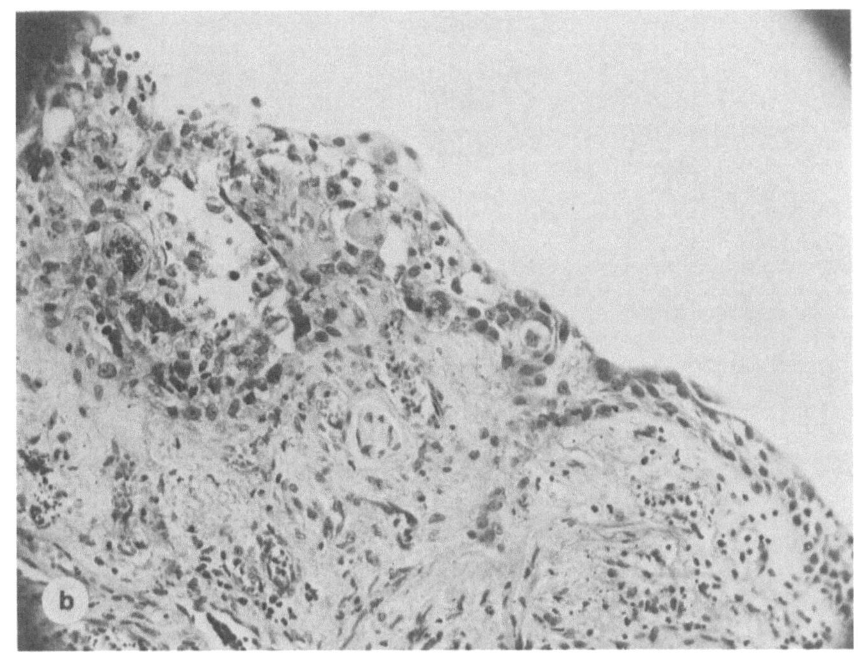
b

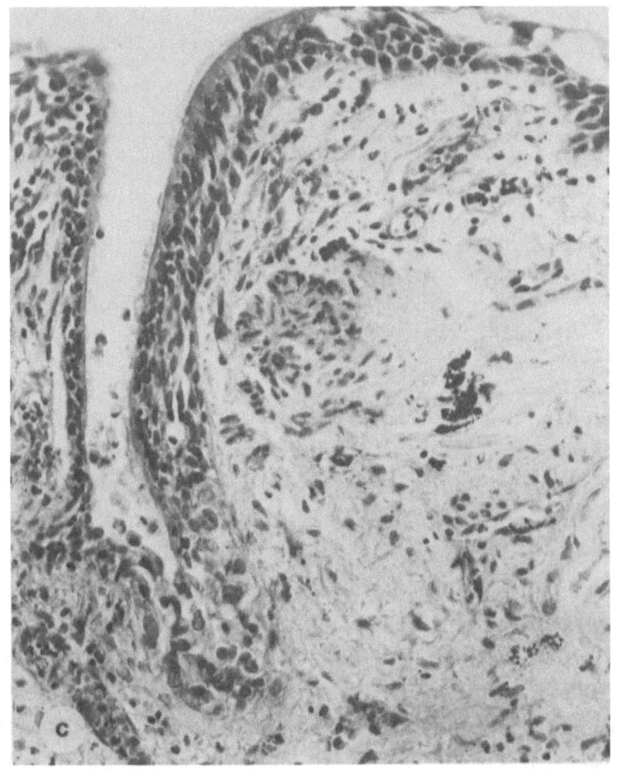
c

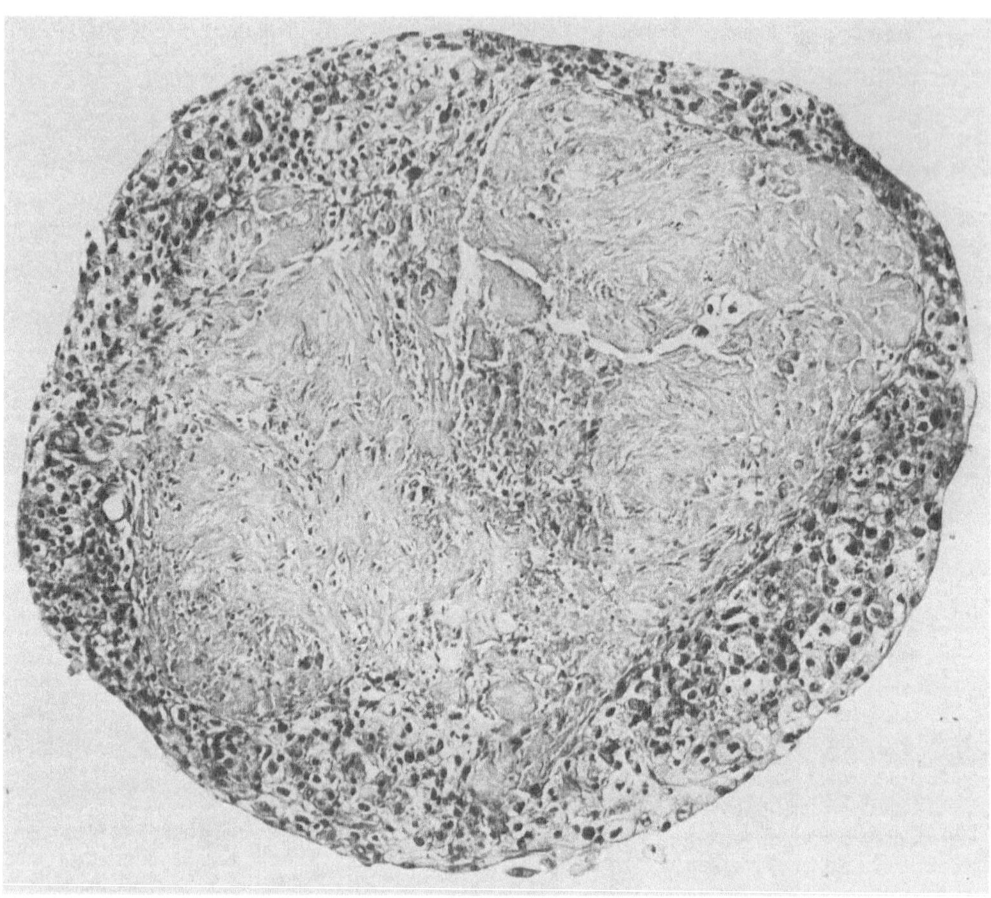

FIG. 7. Squamous carcinoma, histological section of explant after 48 h in tissue culture. The complete outer rim of cancer, with radial orientation of the cells, and the central relatively acellular connective tissue area are the result of tissue culture reorganization. Only the epidermoid cancers showed this.

Another pitfall is that some organelles may be of a specific type but not unique for lung cells, a factor particularly important when dealing with argentaffin cell cancers and the dense-core vesicles (Sherwin, 1968). Weak support for cell identification can be obtained by demonstrating continuity between cancer cells in the explant and cells of a monolayer emerging from the same explant. So far, this has not been accomplished with human lung cancer, but the principle has been applied in studies of nonneoplastic thyroid tissue (Sherwin *et al.*, 1965). Continuity between human prostatic cancer cells in an explant and an outgrowth of cells around the explant rim, evidence supporting monolayer identity, has also been reported (Stonington and Hemmingsen, 1971). However, all conclusions based on continuity

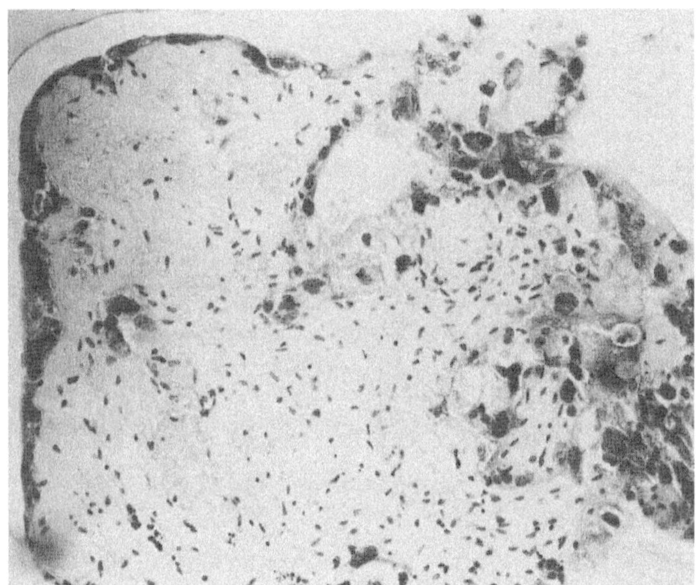

FIG. 8. Adenocarcinoma in explant, histological section after 72 h in culture. Only a single cell layer of cancer surrounds the explant, and it appears to be in continuity with acinar structures and a residual cancer mass.

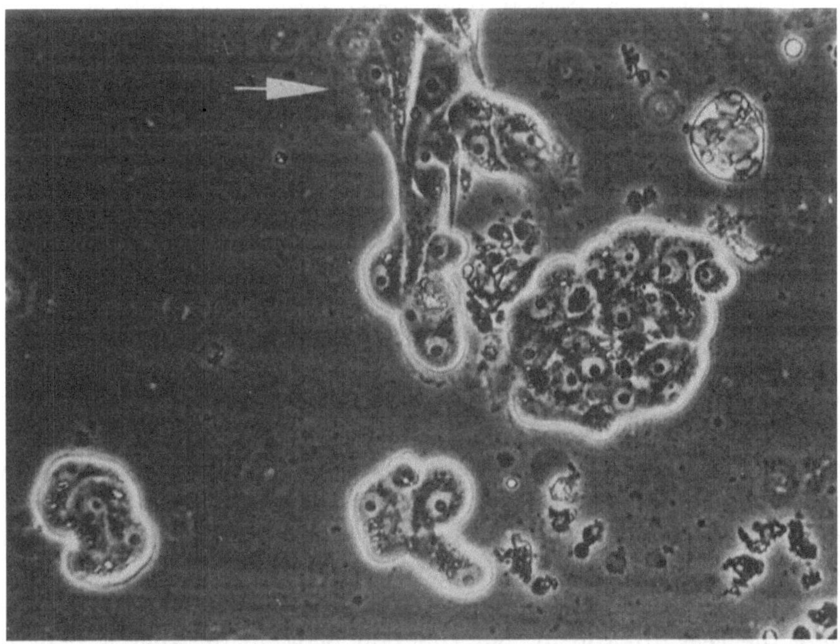

FIG. 9. Adenocarcinoma, spilled-out semiorganoid islands, in culture for 4 days. The original architecture is mainly intact except for a few spread cells (arrow).

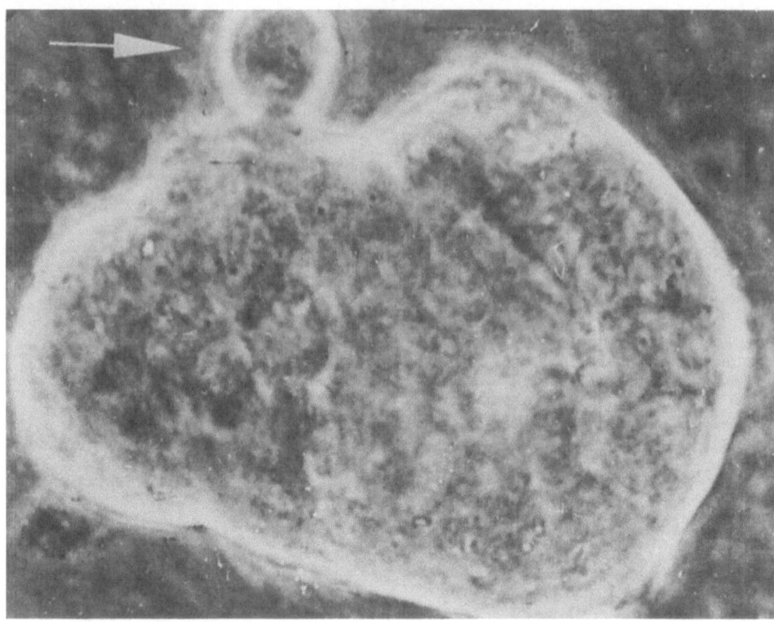

FIG. 10. Spilled-out island of semiorganoid adenocarcinoma. Cancer tissue has emerged from the explant in this isolated, rounded, and refractile form (IIA; *cf.* Table 2). Frequent change of shape and active movements occur. When spreading occurs, the islands resemble those shown in Figs. 12 and 13. Division often occurs by emergence of a single cell (arrow), reproduction totally outside the mass, and reentry of the two daughter cells.

findings must be reconciled with the present lack of a uniform definition of continuity and a uniform application of criteria for such documentation. We have tentatively accepted some lung cancer monolayers on a more liberal basis, for example, an undifferentiated lung cancer where almost every explant yielded an early and prolific outgrowth of cells having a unique type of membrane activity. Moreover, myriads of spilled-out, solid cancer tissue islands appeared to be converted directly into monolayers composed of identical cell types. Occasionally, a flagrant pleomorphism of cells within a monolayer can be strong support for cancer cell identity, and this interpretation is further strengthened by animal transplantation studies (Reed and Gey, 1962) where the three-dimensional tumor masses produced show properties resembling those of the original cancer tissue. For details concerning human lung cell lines reported to be derived from lung cancer, see the listing of lung cell lines in Chapter 5 of this book.

A variant of the monolayer is individual cell growth, in effect a situation where the cells are spread, but cohesion between the cells is poor or completely lost. With respect to lung cancer, a most outstanding *in vivo* and *in vitro* example is the so-called giant cell carcinoma. We have recently demonstrated the origin of this type of cancer from an epidermoid carcinoma. The study was a correlative one involving histological sections of cancer and explant, cytological staining of various tissue culture presentations, and time-lapse cinephotomicrographic recordings (Fig. 14).

3.4. Multilayers (Active and Passive)

Cancer explants may give rise to multilayers by either one of two processes, a vertical and active proliferation of cancer cells or a passive "settling down" of multiple layers of cancer cells within the explant (Sherwin *et al.*, 1967). There are two subtypes of vertical proliferation, one a piling up of cells of the monolayer as part of "loss of contact inhibition" and the other a three-dimensional proliferation effected by the use of special culture procedures (e.g., sponge matrix) or transplantation of tumor into animals (e.g., subcutaneous tissues and hamster cheek pouch).

4. Benign Neoplasia, Atypical Cellular Proliferation, and Normal Cell Populations of the Lung

Attention to nonneoplastic cellular populations is important since cancer explants usually contain a great variety of both normal and atypical cells (Fig. 6) and cellular outgrowths of the atypical cells can readily mimic the cytostructure of cancer monolayers.

4.1. Epithelial Cells

Much work remains to be done in the area of nonneoplastic epithelial cell identification (Figs. 16 and 17), particularly since the only normal lung cell in a monolayer that can be identified with certainty is the ciliated cell with attached tuft of cilia (Fig. 16). Criteria for distinguishing human lung cell types through histochemical tests have yet to be uniformly defined and applied. It should also be noted that a positive mucous reaction does not tell whether the cell is from the bronchial lining or the submucosal gland. Time-lapse recordings of histocultures of mucus-secreting glands (Sherwin and Richters, 1967) have the potential of identifying the cells when they change over to a monolayer since continuous observations are made of the conversion.

4.2. Mesenchymal Cells

There are a variety of "spindle cells" in the lung. In addition to the "fibrocytes" associated with collagen, reticulum, and elastica, there are "septal" cells, pericytes, smooth muscle cells, and endothelial cells. Very limited information is available concerning tissue cultures of the normal and neoplastic "spindle cell" entities of the human lung.

4.3. Leukocytic–Histiocytic Cells

From our own studies, there appears to be a large number of different kinds of histiocytes, distinguished from each other by size, shape, membrane characteristics, and locomotor and presumably functional properties. Although their presence in lung cancer is no doubt quite variable, histiocytes

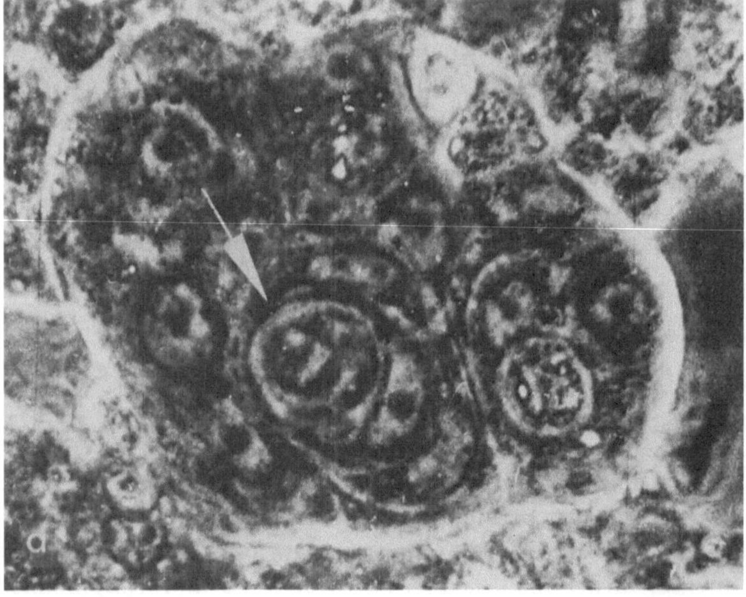

FIG. 11. Epidermoid cancer. (a) Semiorganoid culture (IIB) of epidermoid carcinoma. The cancer tissue is the same one shown in Fig. 6, including whorl formation (arrow) where a cell on the periphery of another appears to surround or engulf it. (b) Histological section of explant, 24 h *in vitro*. In this area, a single whorl can be found among the basal cells (arrow). Most of the tissue is of the well-differentiated squamous type. (c) Explant 24 h *in vitro* of epidermoid cancer (same as in b), histological section. The whorled pattern of this cancer is evident in a number of foci. Hematoxylin and eosin.

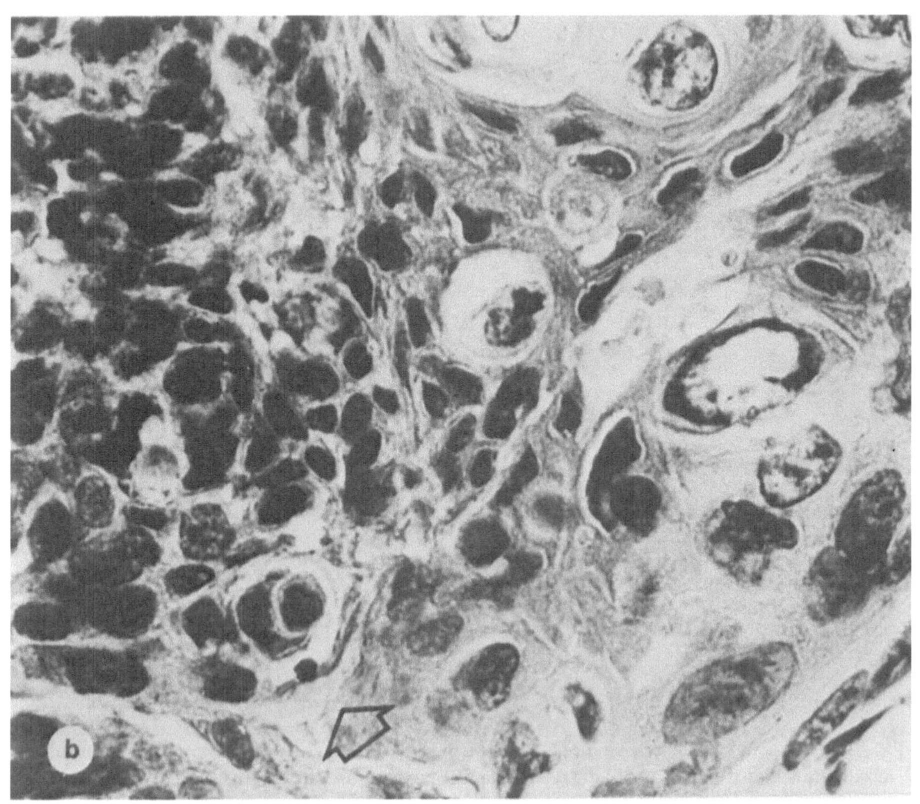
b

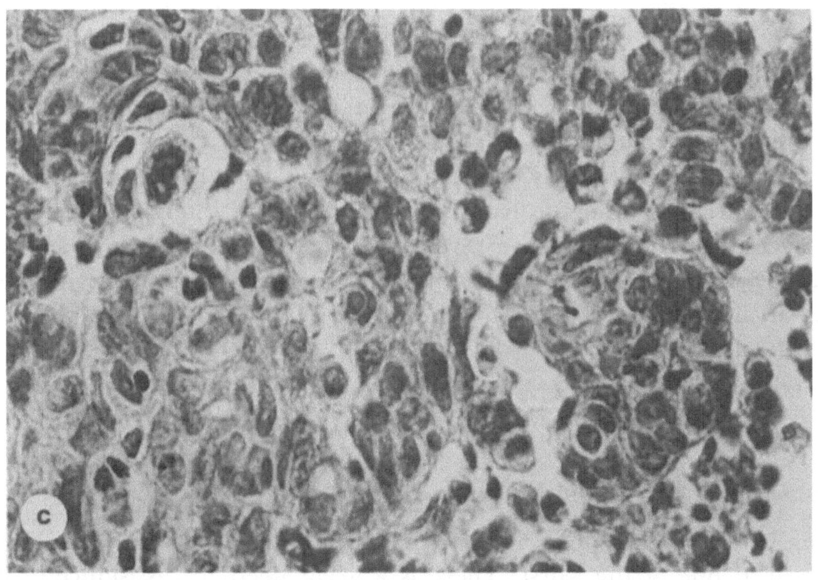
c

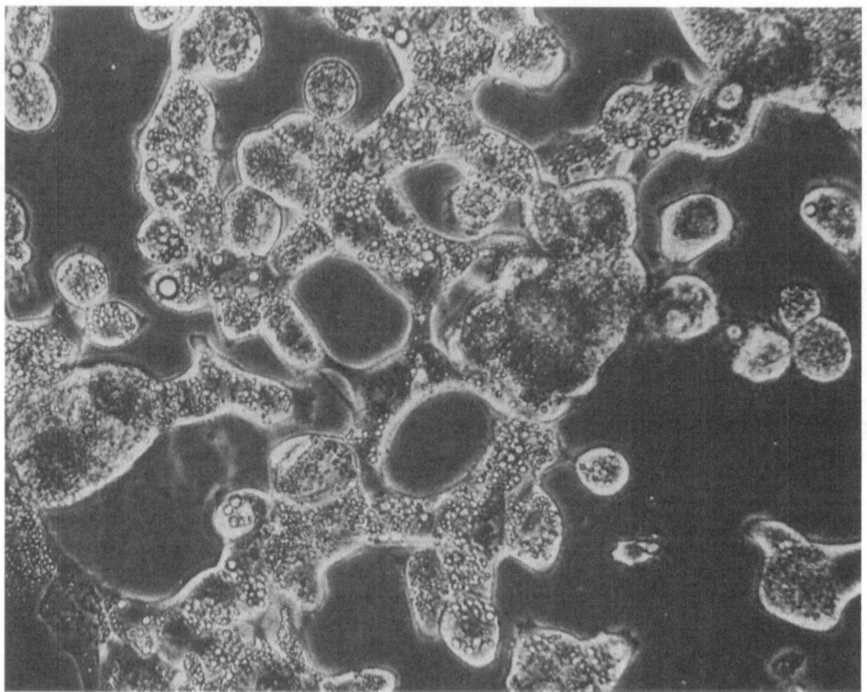

FIG. 12. Glandular adenocarcinoma of the lung in tissue culture. There is a glandular arrangement of the cells and a suggestion that their cytoplasm contains secretory droplets.

appear to be an important part of the host response to cancer. Rarely do they give rise to neoplasia. A group of usually benign histiocytic proliferations is derived from the "epithelioid cell," a histiocyte variant. In addition to the eosinophilic and plasmacytic histiocytomas of the lung, we have reported one that involved the mast cell (Sherwin *et al.*, 1965*b*), including tissue culture findings.

In regard to lymphocytes, we have carried out some preliminary studies dealing with autochthonous lymphocyte–lung cancer interrelationships in tissue culture, and these have revealed a defective relationship between lymphocytes and cancer cells, particularly with respect to quantitative comparisons between random and special lymphocyte interactions (Richters *et al.*, 1971).

5. Future Direction and Goals

5.1. Clinical Applications

Lung cancer is the single most common cancer in man, and its clinical outlook is one of the worst. There is a great need for assistance to the

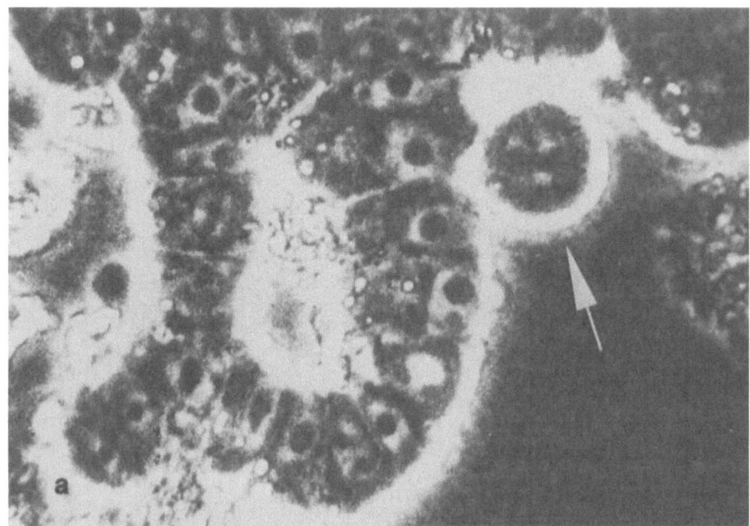

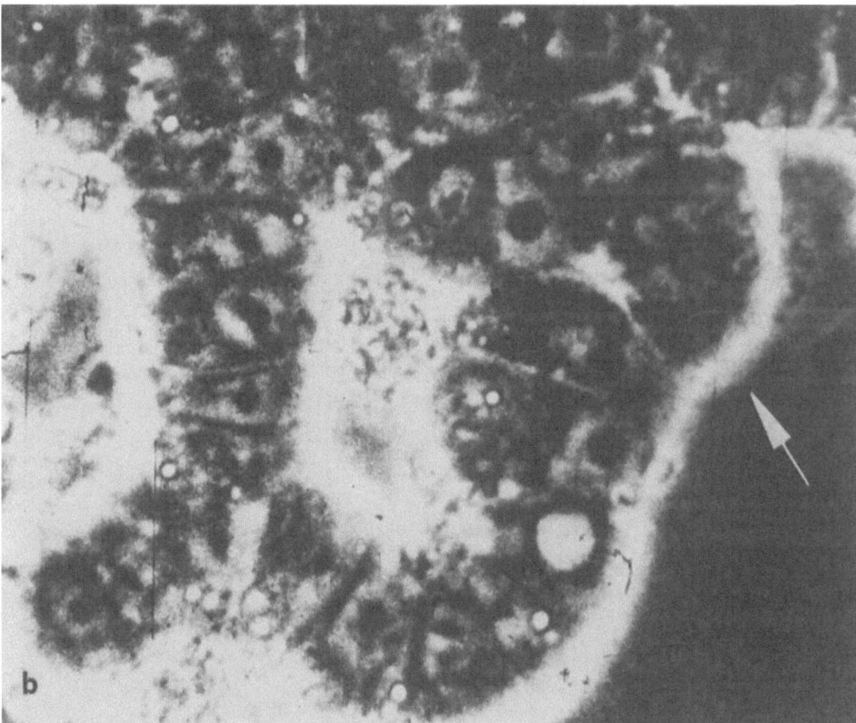

FIG. 13. Glandular adenocarcinoma of lung. This tumor had been interpreted as a poorly differentiated epidermoid carcinoma from the histological sections but in culture presented and maintained a glandular pattern for several weeks. When the tumor cells divided, they generally did so outside of the "acinus" (Fig. 13a) and on completing division reentered the acinus to maintain a perfect alignment (Fig. 13b, arrow indicating beginning alignment).

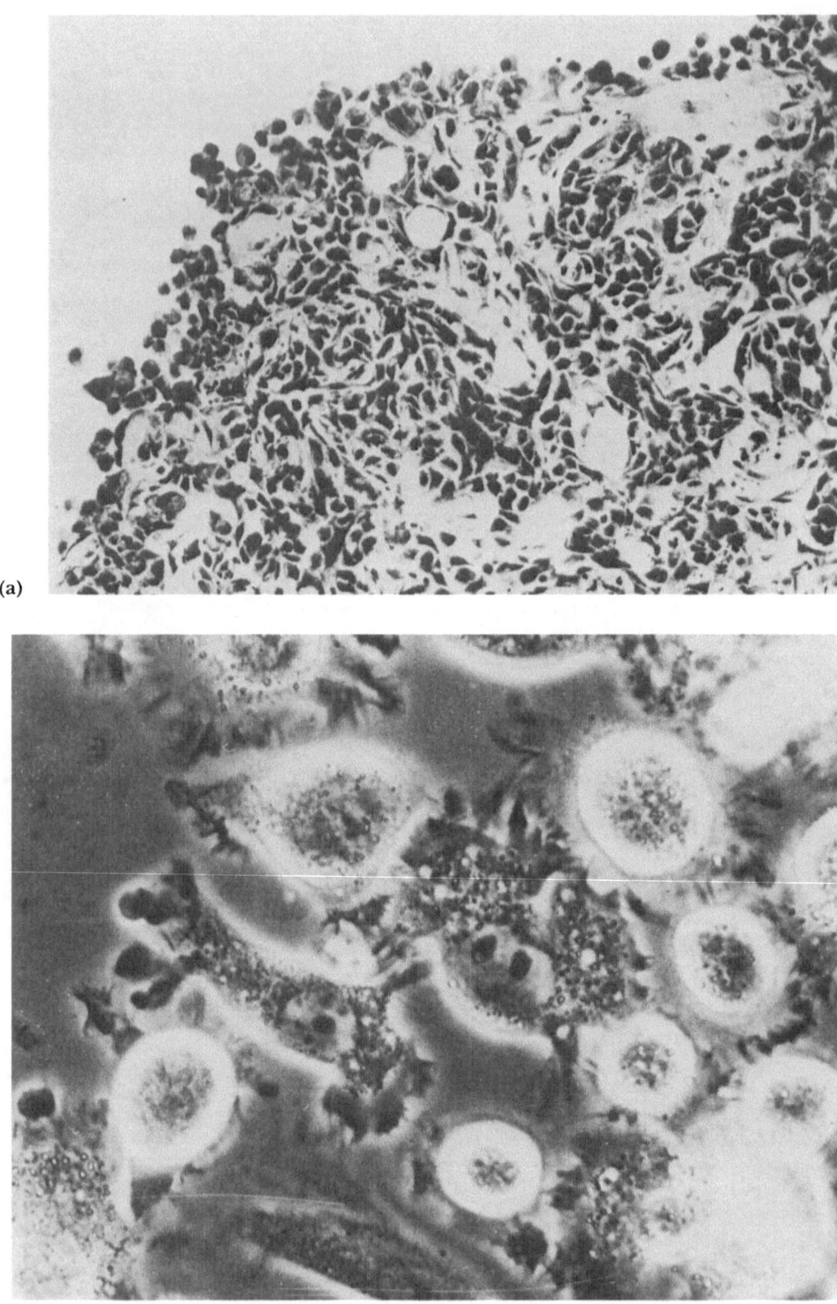

FIG. 14. Explant, 4 days *in vitro*, of epidermoid carcinoma and transition to giant cell carcinoma. (a) The squamous cells are degenerating while the viable basal cells round up and desquamate at the explant margin. (b) When the rounded basal cells spread, they show pronounced membrane activity and great mobility. Phase contrast 4 days *in vitro*.

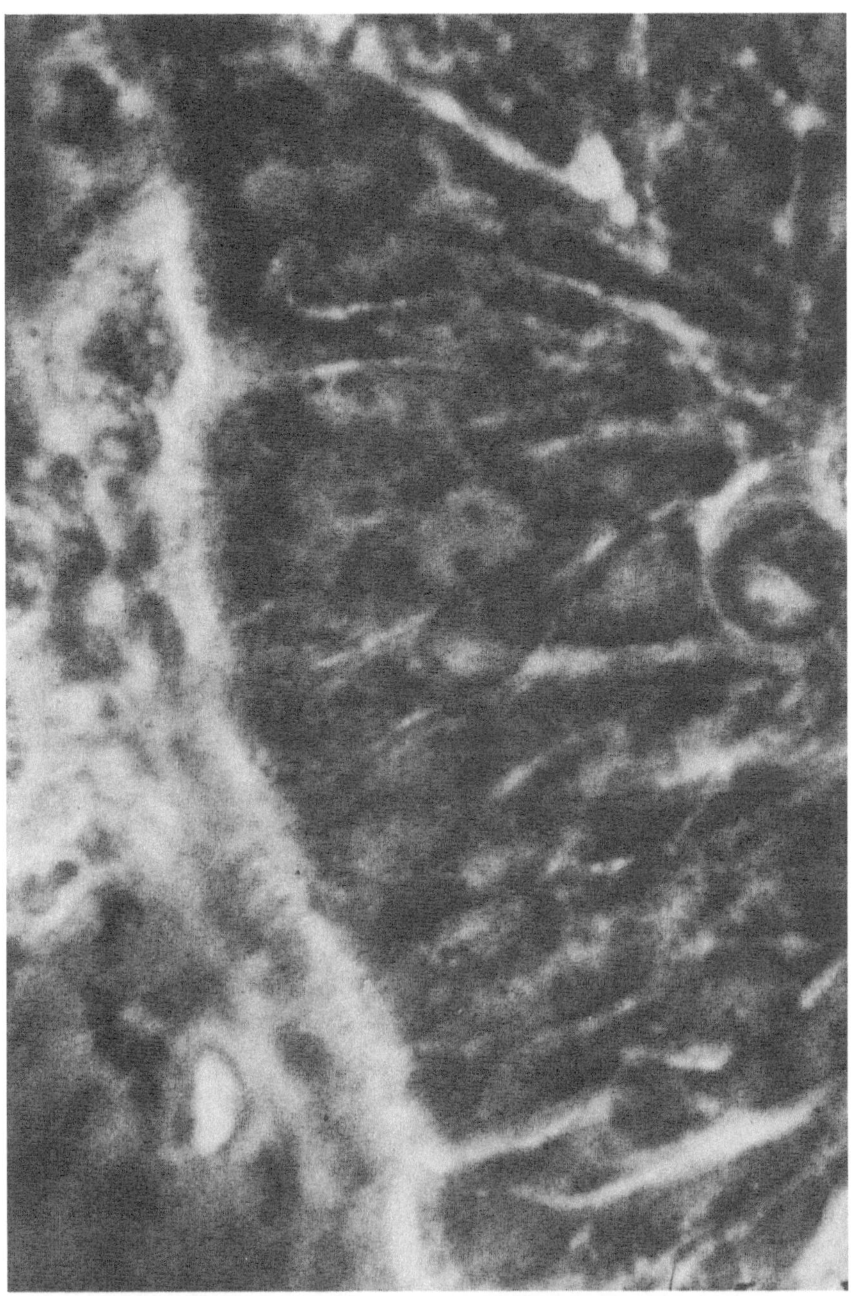

FIG. 15. Normal epithelium of the bronchial mucosa, semi-organoid culture. A thin slice of the mucosa was explanted immediately after operative removal and cinephotomicrographic records were taken at scanning speed. The pseudostratified structure of the lining is apparent. At the free edge of the lining, a continuous row of beating cilia can be seen, with the faster motion of the tips producing a blurred image.

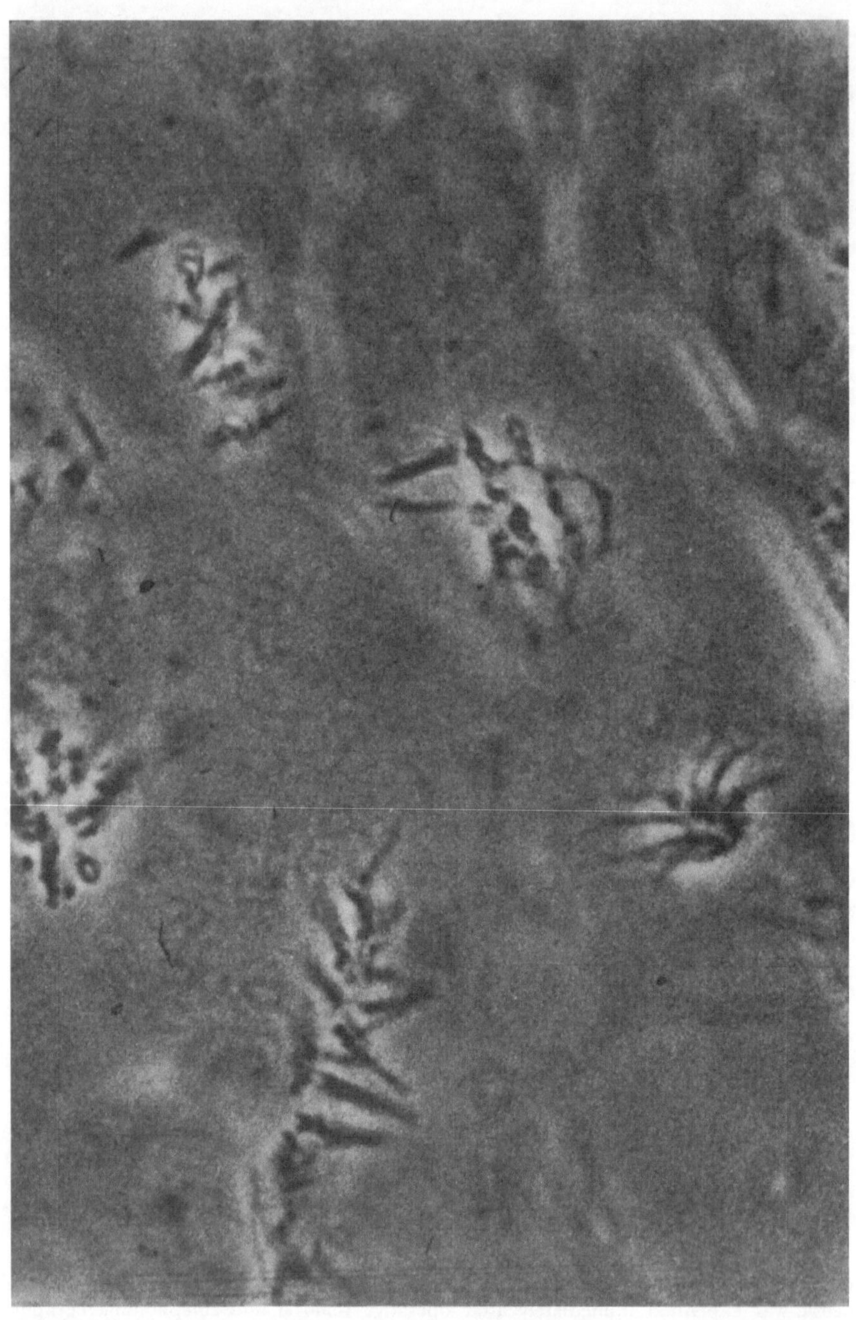

FIG. 16. Ciliated cell monolayer. A monolayer of epithelial cells has emerged from the explant, with each cell exhibiting a central tuft of cilia, seen only when the plane of focus is above the cell.

clinician and also for new information at the cellular and molecular levels. Tissue culture studies can be of substantial help in meeting this need; however, certain critical problems concerning the culturing of human lung cancers must first be resolved. A successful culture must not only provide an appropriate yield but must also be supported by conclusive cell identification. As described in this presentation, histoculture can clearly contribute to the solution of this particular problem. The intact cytostructure is a valid basis for achieving documentation of the *in vitro* cancer cells, and the relative ease with which the histoculture form can be obtained in primary culture affords a foundation for attempts to establish cancer cells in long-term culture.

5.1.1. The Problem of Primary Origin

Once documented lung cancer cells, in their various culture presentations, are available for study, a number of pressing problems can be attacked. Foremost among the problems is the question of the cancer's cell of origin. With the exception of the type 2 pneumocyte, which gives rise to one of the relatively infrequent alveolar cancers, no lung cell has been identified as the "parent cell" of a human lung cancer. Thus it is currently impossible for the clinical oncologist in most cases to distinguish conclusively between a primary and a metastatic lung cancer during the lifetime of the patient. A multidisciplinary approach to this problem has yet to be carried out, and the potential applications of histoculture are essentially unexplored. The problem is further complicated in that the common type of lung cancer, squamous carcinoma, is composed of a type of cell not normally present in the lung. Also, the argentaffin cell does not strictly qualify as a "parent cell" of either oat-cell cancer or the carcinoid tumor, since its full identity cannot yet be established. The dense-core vesicles by which it is characterized do not have the specificity of the lamellar bodies of type 2 pneumocytes. Significantly, a number of metastatic lung tumors show essentially identical dense-core vesicles, in particular islet cell cancers of the pancreas, malignant or ectopic pheochromocytomas (Sherwin, 1968), and malignant carcinoid tumors arising from the small bowel. Moreover, there is the consideration that the argentaffin cell of the bronchial mucosa may be different from that found in the submucosal gland, a factor that can be of clinical significance.

5.1.2. The Evaluation of Prognosis and Therapy Decisions

No two human lung cancers, or cancers in general, will be found to be exactly alike. The unique presentation and clinical course for each cancer result from extreme variability of two major factors, intrinsic aggressiveness of the cancer and the response of the host to the neoplastic process. The availability

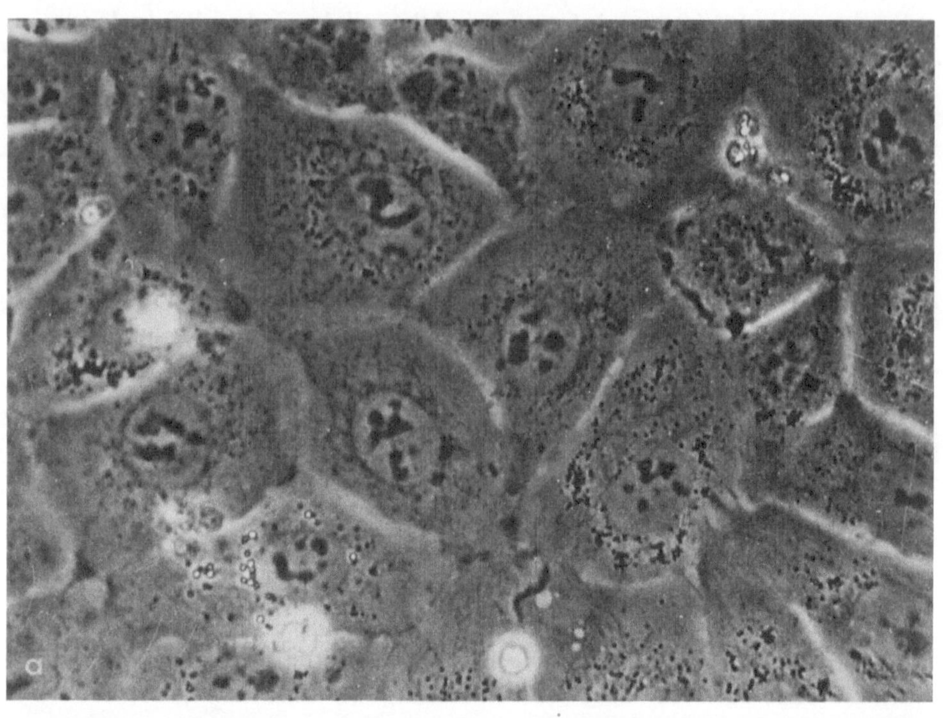
a

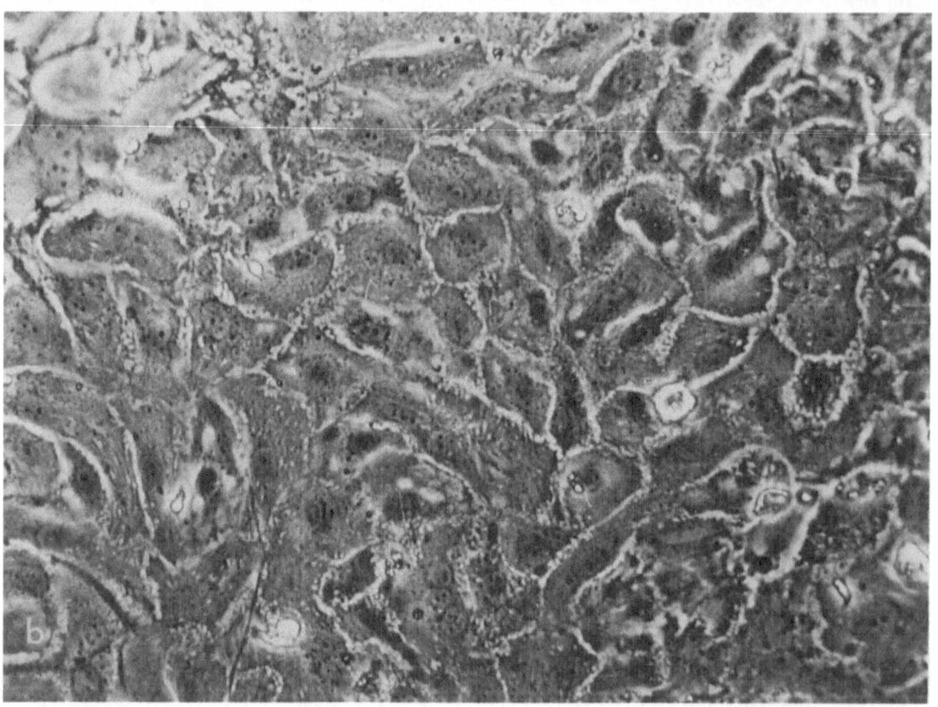
b

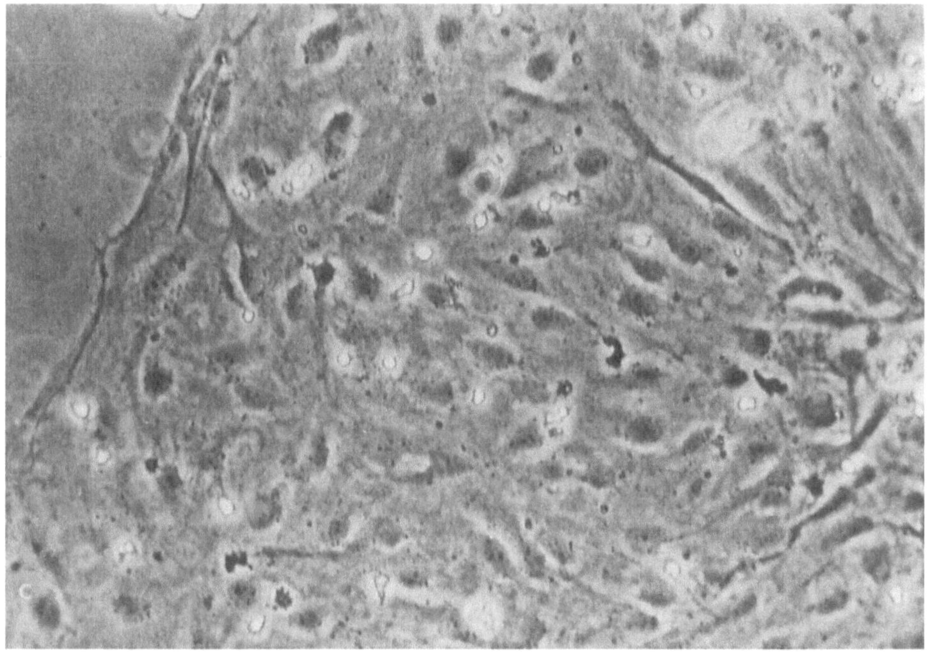

FIG. 17. Nonneoplastic epithelial cells. (a) Both ciliated and nonciliated epithelial cells have a polygonal appearance. (b) The polygonal cells typically develop a "prickle cell" appearance after 2 wk in culture. (c) This monolayer shows a different type of epithelial cell, one usually associated with explants of small bronchi or bronchioles.

of histoculture preparations of the cancer should now make it possible to obtain much new information concerning both factors. New aspects of aggressiveness can be studied, especially such properties as cohesion, adhesion, mitotic cycle events, locomotion, and specific biochemical and ultrastructural changes. The histoculture should be particularly advantageous for assistance with the identification of cancer cell type as well as the recognition of favorable variants of the cancer (Sherwin, 1966). With respect to host resistance, a beginning has already been made in evaluating autochthonous cell systems in the study of lymphocyte and other leukocyte interactions with cancer cells and tissue (Richters *et al.*, 1971; Sherwin *et al.*, 1973). With respect to decisions concerning therapy, one great advantage of histoculture is the presence in each preparation of cells other than the cancer, thus affording a variety of baselines for evaluating the effects of chemotherapeutic drugs or radiation challenge. In a pilot study of a human lung cancer under continuous irradiation, time-lapse cinephotomicrography was especially useful, affording recorded measurements of mitotic cycle events. Quantitative data were obtained on "metaphase plate time," i.e., the time between formation of the metaphase and the first evidence of separation of the metaphase plate. Also, the film recordings revealed numerous instances of mitotic arrest, emphasizing the need to consider completion of mitosis as well as the number of mitotic cells (Sherwin *et al.*, 1969) when evaluating growth rate.

5.2. Basic Science Applications

5.2.1. Cell Characterization

Without going into detail, it is apparent that the histoculture preparation lends itself to many disciplines of cell characterization. Particularly useful approaches should be searches for chemotherapeutic and hormonal surface receptor sites, and membrane properties in general. Clearly, many biochemical and structural research methods can be applied to such preparations.

5.2.2. Cell Interactions and Extrinsic Factors

Although much has been learned about different kinds of lymphocytes and their lymphokines, very little is known about dynamic properties of lymphocytes involving cell-to-cell contacts. Recently, a rather remarkable number of distinctive and unique activities on the part of the lymphocyte have been recognized (Sherwin *et al.*, 1973). It is our belief that the contrasting behaviors of tail attachments and surface membrane appositions of lymphocytes to target cells have equally diverse functional meanings. Other lymphocyte phenomena also appear to subserve special functions.

ACKNOWLEDGMENTS

The authors thank Drs. Weldon K. Bullock and William H. Kern for their cooperation during the study. Valda Richters, our coinvestigator for most of the studies, gave valuable advice and assistance, and Doritz Kreimer provided excellent assistance in the preparation of the manuscript. The work was supported by American Cancer Society Grants No. 312 and 339, NIH Grants CA 06946-01, 2, 3, and the Hastings Foundation.

6. References

Adamson, J. S., Senior, R. N., and Merrill, T., 1969, Alveolar cell carcinoma: An electron microscopic study, *Am. Rev. Resp. Dis.* **100:**550–558.

Bensch, K. G., Corrin, B., Pariente, R., and Spencer, H., 1968, Oat-cell carcinoma of the lung (its origin and relationship to bronchial carcinoid), *Cancer* **22:**1163–1172.

Coalson, J. J., Mohr, J. A., Pirtle, J. K., Dee, A. L., and Rhoades, E. R., 1970, Electron microscopy of neoplasms in the lung with special emphasis on the alveolar cell carcinoma, *Am. Rev. Resp. Dis.* **101:**181–197.

Davidson, E., and Bulkin, W., 1966, Long marker chromosome in bronchogenic carcinoma, *Lancet* **2:**227.

Easty, G. C., 1970, Organ culture methods, in: *Methods in Cancer Research*, Vol. V, (H. Busçh, ed.), p. 1, Academic Press, New York and London.

Gillette, L. V., and Sherwin, R. P., 1965, A Mylar and Aclar plastic method for giant histologic sections of the lung, *Am. Rev. Resp. Dis.* **92:**238–244.

Greenberg, P. B., Beck, C., Martin, T. J., and Burger, H. G., 1972, Synthesis and release of human growth hormone from lung carcinoma in cell culture, *Lancet* **1:**350–352.

Gullino, P. M., 1970, Techniques for the study of tumor physiopathology, in: *Methods in Cancer Research* (H. Busch, ed.), pp. 45–91, Academic Press, New York and London.

Kreyberg, L., Liebow, A. A., and Uehlinger, 1967, Histological typing of lung tumors, in: *International Histological Classification of Tumours*, No. 1, World Health Organization, Geneva.

Lasfargues, E. Y., and Ozzello, L., 1958, Cultivation of human breast carcinomas, *Natl. Cancer Inst. J.* **21:**1131–1147.

Maximow, A., 1925, as quoted by Easty, G. C., 1970, Organ culture methods, in: *Methods in Cancer Research*, Vol. V, (H. Busch, ed.), p. 2, Academic Press, New York and London.

Reed, M. V., and Gey, G. O., 1962, Cultivation of normal and malignant human lung tissue. 1. The establishment of three adenocarcinoma cell strains, *Lab. Invest.* **11:**638–652.

Richters, A., Sherwin, R. P., and Richters, V., 1971, The lymphocyte and human lung cancers, *Cancer Res.* **31:**214–222.

Sherwin, R. P., 1966, The identification of lung cancer and the recognition of favorable variants, in: *Pathology Annual 1966* (S. C. Sommers, ed.), pp. 257–312, Appleton-Century-Crofts, New York.

Sherwin, R. P., 1968, The adrenal medulla, paraganglia and related tissues, in: *Endocrine Pathology* (J. M. B. Bloodworth, Jr., ed.), pp. 256–315, Williams and Wilkins, Baltimore.

Sherwin, R. P., 1975, *The Compleat Oncologic Pathologist, Progress in Experimental Tumor Research*, S. Karger Publ., in press.

Sherwin, R. P., and Richters, A., 1967, *The Embattled Cell* (film), distributed by American Cancer Society, New York, N.Y.

Sherwin, R. P., and Richters, A., 1972, Pathobiologic nature of lymphocyte interactions with human breast cancer, *J. Natl. Cancer Inst.* **48:**1111–1115.

Sherwin, R. P., and Richters, A., 1973, Pathobiology of lymphocyte interactions, in: *Pathology Annual 1973* (S. C. Sommers, ed.), pp. 379–406, Appleton-Century-Crofts, New York.

Sherwin, R. P., Gardner, M., and Richters, V., 1965*a*, The use of autopsy tissue (thyroid gland) for *in vitro* studies, *Am. J. Clin. Pathol.* **43:**114–121.

Sherwin, R. P., Kern, W. H., and Jones, J. C., 1965*b*, Solitary mast cell granuloma (histiocytoma) of the lung, *Cancer* **18:**634–641.

Sherwin, R. P., Richters, V., and Richters, A., 1967, Behavior of cancers of the human lung in short-term tissue cultures, *Cancer* **20:**1–22.

Sherwin, R. P., Richters, V., and Richters, A., 1968, The documentation and behavior of human lung cancer in short term tissue culture, in: *Cancer Cells in Culture* (H. Katsuta, ed.), pp. 3–18, University of Tokyo Press, Tokyo.

Sherwin, R. P., Sondhaus, C. A., Eisenman, J. I., and Richters, A., 1969, Effects of continuous irradiation on human and animal semiorganoid tissues: *In-vitro* time-lapse cinephotomicrographic studies, presented May 10, 1969, Association of University Radiologists, San Francisco.

Sherwin, R. P., Margolick, J. B., and Azen, S. P., 1973, Hypertrophy of alveolar wall cells secondary to an air pollutant (2 ppm NO_2): A semiautomated quantitation, *Arch. Environ. Health* **25:**297–299.

Stonington, O. G., and Hemmingsen, H., 1971, Culture of cells as a monolayer derived from the epithelium of the human prostate: A new cell growth technique, *J. Urol.* **106:**393–400.

Cell Lines from Humans with Hematopoietic Malignancies

11

GEORGE E. MOORE

1. Introduction

Temporary cultures of hematopoietic cells have been studied by cell biologists since 1913. Unfortunately, most cultures were eventually overgrown by fibroblasts. Several investigators claimed that they had established permanent hematopoietic cell lines, but, in retrospect, the data used to support such claims were unacceptable. Several epithelioid cell lines derived from bone marrow cultures probably represented malignant cells that had metastasized from primary carcinomas. Epstein and Barr (1964) and Pulvertaft (1964) reported the successful culture of lymphoid cells from biopsies of Burkitt's lymphoma. Shortly thereafter, Iwakata and Grace (1964) established a lymphoil cell line from the blood of a patient with chronic myelogenous leukemia. In July 1966, we (Moore *et al.*, 1967) established lymphoid cell lines from the blood of two normal persons.

In recent years, there has been a blizzard of publications about human hematopoietic cell lines. This chapter will be concerned primarily with cell lines derived from patients with hematopoietic malignancies including the lymphomas. It is important to observe that seemingly normal hematopoietic cell lines also can be derived from leukemia patients, and one must be very

GEORGE E. MOORE Head, Surgical Oncology, Denver General Hospital, and Professor of Surgery, University of Colorado Medical Center, Denver, Colorado careful that the cell lines labeled as "leukemic" have characteristics of malignancy.

2. Establishment of Hematopoietic Cell Lines

The peripheral blood has been a most convenient source of cells for culture because of the freedom from fibroblasts and the ease of obtaining cell samples. Apparently there is at least one immature lymphoid cell in every 25,000 cells that has the capability of surviving, adapting itself to culture conditions, and multiplying at a rate that eventually produces a self-sustaining cell line. Nonmalignant clinical conditions that provoke a release of immature cells into the blood, such as virus infections, raise the efficiency of establishing cell lines. It is just as easy to establish cell lines from elderly persons as from children. As will be mentioned later, it is difficult to establish cell lines from the blood of newborns without the addition of the Epstein–Barr virus.

It is relatively simple to establish both normal lymphoid and malignant hematopoietic cells from patients with myelogenous leukemia but very difficult to establish them from patients with lymphatic leukemia and lymphomas other than Burkitt's lymphoma. As will be discussed later, leukemias derived from "B" or bone marrow-derived lymphocytes are much easier to cultivate than those from "T" or thymus-dependent lymphocytes.

Investigators failed to establish hematopoietic cell lines before 1964 because the cultures were discarded before there was evidence of growth. Fresh cultures contain many metabolically active cells, and indeed after 3 days in culture there is usually an increase in the number and activity of mononuclear cells. Yet by 7–10 days, there are often only a few scattered macrophage-like cells attached to the glass and the viability of the suspended cells is usually less than 25%. The gradual acceleration of growth of these residual cells has been described (deGrouchy *et al.*, 1970); after an average lapse period of 40–60 days, there is a rapid and sustained growth rate. Table 1 illustrates the range of the lapse period. Two disease states that may be associated with a brief lapse period are infectious mononcleosis and, less frequently, acute leukemia. These exceptions probably result from the sustained growth of many progenitor cells in contrast to the clonar origin of most cell lines.

The explanatory theories for the prolonged lapse period include (1) a mutation of a surviving cell followed by rapid growth, (2) a malignant transformation of a surviving cell, (3) viral transformation by the Epstein–Barr virus (EB virus), either to a dedifferentiated state or to a

TABLE 1

All Lines Established (RPMI Numbers)

Days after initiation											
1-10	11-20	21-30	31-40	41-50	51-60	61-70	71-80	81-90	91-100	101-110	>111
	1777 7177	3367 7610	1048 7369	1006 6028	1017 5866	1016 3177	1027 2247	1028 3196	1058 3048	1119 4766	1026 2967
	1787 7187	7008 7620	1867 7401	1066 6048	1047 6018	1038 3187	1068 3028	1067 3967	1108 4107	1128 6167	1096 3038
	6277 7667	7018 9048	1968 7439	1120 6088	1056 6107	1077 3197	1078 3217	1088 5287	1228 7161	1868 6197	1126 4078
	7157	7127 9126	2367 7469	1122 6467	1057 6267	1097 3227	1178 4207	1106 5307	1238 7169	1938 7271	1218 5018
		7339 9156	1467 7479	1137 7028	1098 7038	1117 4177	1198 4667	1116 7129	1248 7181	2048 7359	1348 6038
		7360 9966	2567 7580	1166 7048	1107 7058	1148 5257	1276 5567	1158 7141	1286 7201	2078 7467	1358 6068
			2667 7590	1186 7070	1130 7068	1156 5277	1318 6078	1208 7209	1288 7259	3567 7520	1657 7251
			3078 7670	1196 7098	1157 7088	1296 6098	1388 6217	1478 7239	1717 7420		1837 7507
			3137 7680	1216 7117	1168 7119	1338 6207	1418 6257	1488 7249	1737 7910		1857 7870
			3287 7690	1247 7121	1257 7147	1378 6666	1578 6567	1498 7261	1978 9146		2127 8286
			5088 7820	1258 7159	1268 7171	1398 7111	1647 7109	1517 7309			9116
			5146 8008	1279 7199	1278 7191	1438 7139	1668 7151	1577 7310			
			6008 8038	1528 7269	1328 7219	1468 7211	1677 7179	1628 7320			
			6237 8068	1548 7276	1458 7231	1518 7241	1687 7189	1658 7340			
			7131 8098	1607 7349	1527 7321	1627 7311	1708 7206	1747 7390			
			7137 8126	1718 7350	1538 7322	1637 7330	1727 7216	1798 7550			
			7217 8466	1728 7351	1568 7331	1648 7450	1757 7221	1858 7860			
			7281 8766	1738 7370	1588 7389	1688 7459	1812 7307	1878 8057			
			7289 9058	1767 7371	1598 7399	1697 7461	1828 7329	1888 9068			
			7291 9246	1827 7380	1618 7409	1698 7517	1838 7379	1898 9106			
			7301 9256	1957 7381	1638 7410	1699 7640	1887 7440	2157 9217			
			7341 9287	1977 7391	1678 7419	1758 7666	1897 7560	9766			
			7347 9297	2058 7421	1707 7441	1788 7766	1948 8296				
			7361 9357	2107 7429	1710 7466	1807 7810	1958 9286				
				2187 7430	1748 7480	1808 7850	2088 9487				
				2237 7431	1768 7489	1847 8097	2098 9587				
				3107 7460	1778 7540	1907 8106	2177				
				3186 7471	1817 7627	1917 8127					
				3667 7510	1848 7630	1988 8167					
				3767 7530	1877 7657	1997 8226					
				4018 7650	1908 7710	2018 8337					
				4058 7660	1928 7720	2137 9018					
				4117 7740	1937 7730	2167 9078					
				4267 7750	1947 7760	2217 9166					
				5008 7830	2038 7767	2257 9247					
				5028 8018	2068 7770	3008 9497					
				5068 8116	2197 7780	3068 9557					
				5156 8966	2287 7790	9577					
				5207 9347	3058 7840						
				5266 9507	3157 7880						
				5366 9537	3867 7890						
				5466 9597	4048 8028						
					4068 8047						
					4088 8058						
					4098 8078						
					4170 8088						
					4217 8107						
					4467 8117						
					4567 8187						
					4967 8207						
					5038 8497						
					5058 9028						
					5078 9098						
					5098 9227						
					5106 9377						
					5197 9527						
					5286 9627						
					9897						

malignant form, (4) nongenetic stimulation of one or several cells by antigens, chemicals, or cell injury, and (5) slow clonal growth of a single cell or several cells until they attain a population that will support rapid growth by the release of unidentified cell products.

A review of malignant cell lines provides no indication that they became established in a shorter time than normal cells. In most instances, there is good evidence that a cell line has developed from a single cell, but some of the cell lines that become established in 2 or 3 wk probably represent multiple clones.

3. Practical Methods of Preparing Initial Cultures from the Blood

Samples of from 5 to 40 ml peripheral blood provide a sufficient number of leukocytes (for duplicate cultures) if the leukocyte count is 8,000/mm^3 or more. Disposable 50-ml plastic syringes with 1–8 ml of ACD solution (NIH formula A, Travenol Laboratories) are inverted several times and placed upright in an incubator at 37°C. The syringes are kept in this vertical position for 1–4 h to achieve erythrocyte sedimentation. If sedimentation is excessively slow, 6% dextran (6% Gentran, Travenol Laboratories) in a ratio of 1 part dextran to 10 parts blood is used to facilitate separation. The attached needle is bent into a semicircle and the plasma layer is ejected into a 12-ml conical centrifuge tube (screw-capped), and centrifuged at 100 *g* for 5 min. The supernatant is aspirated and the cell pellet suspended in RPMI-1640 (Moore *et al.*, 1967) medium supplemented with 20% heat-inactivated fetal calf serum (FCS). As will be explained later, the addition of EB virus or irradiated cells (3000 R) containing the virus is helpful for stimulating cultures from the blood of newborns and children.

Macrocultures for initial chromosome analyses using 1.0–2.5 × 10^6 leukocytes per milliliter are set up in 4-oz flint gem oval screw-capped bottles (Brockway) with 10 ml gassed (10% CO_2 in air) GEM 1717 plus 20% FCS supplemented with 20 units of preservative-free heparin and 1.25 ml of a 10:1 dilution of a stock solution of phytohemagglutinin (PHA-M, Difco). Following 3–5 days of incubation at 37°C, chromosome preparations are made according to a modification of Moorhead's method (Moorhead *et al.*, 1960).

Cultures intended for long-term establishment are initiated in the same manner as the PHA cultures, but without the addition of PHA. The leukocyte concentrations are adjusted to between 2 × 10^6 and 10 × 10^6 leukocytes per milliliter whenever possible. At 3- to 7-day intervals, each culture receives 5–10 ml fresh GEM 1717 plus 20% FCS medium depending on evidence of cell metabolism. After three or four feedings, one-half of the cell-free medium is decanted to allow subsequent additions of medium at weekly intervals. A favorable sign of future establishment of lymphoid cells with B-cell characteristics is early adherence of macrophage-like cells to the glass and the formation of pseudoclones.

Favorable signs of T-type lymphoid cells are difficult to detect because the cells are small, remain in suspension, and grow very slowly. Exceptional cells will multiply rapidly without delay. In both instances, patience is required because after 4 wk of culture there are often only a few scattered residual viable cells. The cultures must not be given large amounts of fresh medium. If one has duplicate cultures, it is advantageous to harvest the cells from one or several flasks and add them to the culture with the highest surviving population of cells.

The dramatic onset of the establishment of most lymphoid cell lines is signaled by the appearance of large clumps and wafers of cells in the medium and signs of rapid increase in metabolic activity. The subsequent loss of such a culture through failure of sustained growth should be less than 5%. One must be careful not to add too much fresh medium (over 20% of the volume) and not to subculture the cell line until a high population density has been achieved.

As might be expected, substances and conditions that produce short-term blastoid transformation of lymphocytes have been applied to fresh cell cultures in the hope that more cell lines could be established more quickly, more consistently, and from smaller blood samples. Various authors have reported the use of phytohemagglutinins (Broder *et al.*, 1970), antigens (Baumal *et al.*, 1971), recombinations of cultures (Moore *et al.*, 1968*a*), lysates of established cell lines (Choi and Bloom, 1970*a*), conditioned media (Choi and Bloom, 1970*b*), the Epstein–Barr virus (Gerber *et al.*, 1969; Henle *et al.*, 1967; Pope *et al.*, 1968; Possnerova *et al.*, 1970), and feeder cells (Benyesh-Melnick *et al.*, 1963, 1971; Miller *et al.*, 1969; Pulvertaft, 1964). The study published by Benyesh-Melnick *et al.* (1963) was remarkable because many of their observations about bone marrow cultures are pertinent to cultures of peripheral blood. Of 123 marrow cultures from 71 children, all cultures contained fibroblasts, and four showed lymphoblastoid transformations.These researchers emphasized emperipolesis activity of the lymphocytes and apparently felt that the fibroblasts had a trophic effect. They stated that the lymphoblastoid cells failed to multiply when the accompanying fibroblasts died out. By 1968, Benyesh-Melnick's group reported that, of 757 fibroblast marrow cultures, 59 showed lymphoblastoid transformations after 40–61 days. This group maintained that only fibroblasts derived from human bone marrow were competent feeder cells. Subsequently these investigators established lymphoid cell lines.

Ioachim (1965) studied the emperipolesis of lymphocytes in fibroblasts and epithelial cells. He also concluded that cells of mesenchymal origin supported the growth of lymphocytes but that epithelial cells destroyed them.

Nilsson *et al.* (1970) established a myeloma cell line with the aid of a feeder layer of fibroblasts. Subsequent studies confirmed the continuous dependence of this cell line on the presence of allogeneic cells.

It is my personal opinion that fastidious cells such as those in most patients with lymphatic leukemia and Hodgkin's disease will require feeder cells or modified "organ cultures" until their exact nutritional requirements can be determined.

4. *Growth Stimulants*

There are conflicting reports as to the efficacy of most additives. PHA causes formation of many cell clumps and stimulates cell division and metabolism for the first few days, but does not increase the frequency of establishment. Some investigators such as Gerber and Monroe (1968) feel that the presence of the EB virus is essential for establishment. Henle *et al.* (1967) reported the growth-promoting effect of irradiated Burkitt lymphoma cells containing EB virus on cultures of fresh lymphocytes. Virus-free cells with differing transplantation antigens are also stimulatory but do not necessarily increase the number of cell lines. The stimulatory activity of other viruses has not been reported, but virus infections that release more immature cells into the blood can be helpful. The role of EB virus is difficult to prove or disprove because detection of the virus by electron microscopy (Moore *et al.*, 1970) or virus "footprints"—immunological staining (Minowada *et al.*, 1968; Klein *et al.*, 1968)—is obtained in a majority (some investigators say *all* cell lines) of the human lymphoid cell lines. Critical studies by Chang (1972) demonstrated cell lines which were established from the cord blood of newborns only if EB virus was added; these will be described later. From a practical standpoint, additives—particularly EB virus and feeder cells—are helpful for establishing new cell lines, but they add uncertainties that may affect the subsequent value of the new cell lines.

The influence of carcinogens and irradiation on establishment has not been reported. Such studies would provide indirect evidence that establishment is or is not the result of a genetic transformation, as has been suggested by Gerber and Hoyer (1971) and Henle *et al.* (1967).

Hersh (1971) has reported that the addition of the enzyme L-glutaminase inhibits blastogenic responses to PHA, allogeneic leukocytes, and streptolysin O. This is an important observation. Bain *et al.* (1964) and subsequently Wilson (1966) noted that a mixture of lymphocytes from two individuals stimulated blastoid transformation and proliferation. Calf serum, in contrast to human serum, stimulated the cells. Even the presence of nonlymphoid cells in the original cultures may aid in inducing dedifferentiation and multiplication. Ling and Holt (1967) noted that lymphocyte populations that had been recently stimulated with a pulse exposure to PHA retained their ability to react to stimulants again. It seems reasonable to conclude that continuous stimulation of cultured lymphocytes should be helpful in attaining establishment, but there is no documented evidence to prove this point.

Table 2 indicates the approximate ratios of cultures initiated to the number that became permanent cell lines, reflecting the relative ease, in our experience, of establishing lymphoid cell lines from patients with various diseases.

French investigators have studied the lapse period and concluded that a mutation-like event occurs (Belpomme *et al.*, 1969). Rosenfeld *et al.* (1969) support the hypothesis that the cell clones originate after an unpredictable event—but not a mutation—that results in a gradual increase in the population of the cultured cells. They noted that a large initial population of leukocytes favors successful establishment. They did not agree with us (Moore and Glick, 1967) that the lapse period may represent the time required for a single primitive cell or only a few cells to multiply and form a discernible self-sustaining population.

Other observers have emphasized the importance of the presence of EB virus in the cells and concluded that cells free of Eb virus do not become established (Gerber and Monroe, 1968). Baumel *et al.* (1971) reported that a combination of EB virus with an antigen (tuberculin) to which the donor was

TABLE 2

Approximate Ease of Establishment of Cell Lines from 30-ml Samples of Peripheral Blood with a Minimum Leukocyte Count of 8000/mm³

Infectious mononucleosis	2/3
Other virus diseases	1/2
Acute myelogenous leukemia	2/5
Advanced malignant melanoma	2/5
Chronic myelogenous leukemia	1/3
Other malignancies	1/3
Normal persons	1/5
Lymphomas	1/20
Hodgkin's disease	1/40
Lymphatic leukemia (adult)	1/80

sensitized induced growth of lymphoid cells. Neither antigen nor EB virus alone was sufficient for transformation. The rapid establishment of cell lines from patients with infectious mononucleosis (Pope, 1967; Diehl *et al.*, 1968) supports the view that EB virus transforms the lymphocytes. We have argued that the release of large numbers of immature lymphoid cells into the bloodstream, rather than a qualitative change in the cells, is the critical condition. In our experience, one of the best times to establish cell lines from a normal person is during the recovery period after influenza or a severe head cold, when there is a lymphocytosis. Indeed, Glade *et al.* (1968, 1969*b*) have established many lymphoid cell lines from patients with various viral diseases.

Stevens *et al.* (1969) established 21 lymphoid cell lines from patients with acute infectious hepatitis and noted relatively less success in establishing cell lines from normal individuals. These investigators found, through use of immunofluorescent sera and electron microscopy, that eight of 13 cell lines had EB virus. They concluded that probably all of the donors were previously infected with EB virus and that the infectious hepatitis increased the stimulation necessary for establishment.

It is also relatively easy to establish cell lines from patients with leukemoid reactions associated with lymphocytosis (Moore and Pickren, 1967).

It is difficult to prove that any human lymphocytes are free of the EB virus or its genome. As mentioned, Gerber and Monroe (1968) have stated that the EB virus or its genome is necessary for establishment. We have held a contrary view because of the evidence that other factors stimulate proliferation, such as allogeneic serum, antigens, and other cells present in the culture (Miller *et al.*, 1969). Furthermore, some scientists have noted that the titers of EB virus antibodies do not correlate with frequency of cell line establishment, and establishment may be inversely related to titers of herpes simplex virus (Moore, 1972). This controversy is difficult to resolve since, according to Gerber *et al.* (1969), EB virus antigens detectable by microcomplement fixation tests are present in all cell lines. Gerber and Hoyer (1971) have stressed similarities between oncogenic DNA viruses and the EB virus on the basis of evidence that EB virus stimulates DNA synthesis. Even so, PHA and similar stimulants also provoke the synthesis of DNA in lymphocytes, and there is no evidence for the reproduction of EB virus as an intermediate step.

Gerber *et al.* (1969) reported that whereas a cell line could not be established from the blood of a normal adult with no antibodies to EB virus, the addition of EB virus to buffy coat cultures was followed by the establishment of a cell line in 24 days. On the other hand, Glade *et al.* (1969*b*) reported establishing cell lines from "EB virus–negative" donors, but the virus was detected in the cultured cells. They also established several cell lines without evidence of EB virus from "EB virus–negative" donors.

Zur Hausen *et al.* (1970) and Zur Hausen and Schulte-Holthausen (1970) demonstrated the presence of an average of six EB virus genome equivalents in a Burkitt's lymphoma cell line ("Raji") in which no virus had been detected and two to 20 EB virus genome equivalents per cell in *fresh* Burkitt's lymphoma and nasopharyngeal carcinoma. Since more than 85% of adults have detectable EB virus antibodies, it might reasonably be asked whether the lymphocytes of any normal person are free of EB virus itself or its genome.

The stimulatory effect of the addition of EB virus is understandable, since other viruses transform cells, but the critical issue remains: does the EB virus provoke normal and abnormal (oncogenic) transformation of normal lymphocytes?

It is our opinion that an increase in primitive lymphoid cells in the peripheral blood of patients with advanced malignancies explains the relative ease of establishing cell lines from them. Many investigators have noted these primitive cells during morphological studies of tumor cells in the blood (Sandberg *et al.*, 1959).

The establishment of hematopoietic cell lines from newborns and small children poses two problems: a low blood volume and a lesser infestation with the EB virus. Chang (1970) has reported the establishment of cell lines from 2×10^6 lymphocytes cultured in test tubes. Relatively small blood samples were used, and 10% of 796 cultures provided cell lines. The only successful cultures of cord blood were those to which filtrate of an established cell line with EB virus had been added. Subsequently, Chang (1972) described a filtrable and ether-stable factor from the saliva of patients with infectious mononucleosis that supported the growth of lymphocytes from cord blood. It is possible that this factor was actually EB virus that was ether stable.

From a biological viewpoint, the postulated symbiotic relationship of EB virus and lymphocytes and the stimulation of growth and multiplication of lymphocytes by this are very interesting. It is puzzling that newborns do not have EB virus from exposure during pregnancy. Last, the probable dangers of mutant EB viruses causing leukemia must be considered. No EB virus has been described in any hematopoietic cells except lymphoid forms. It would be important to determine whether the EB virus genome is detectable in granulocytic leukemia.

5. *Cultures of Bone Marrow, Lymph Nodes, and Biopsies*

The culture of bone marrow biopsies can be handled by the same techniques used for leukocytes of the peripheral blood. It is our impression that excessive red cells are inhibitory; therefore, the white cells are resuspended in distilled water for 30 s and *immediately* recovered by the addition of a 2× concentration of culture medium and removed by centrifugation. Most bone marrow cultures will be overwhelmed with fibroblasts before the hematopoietic cells establish themselves. About 25% of a confluent layer of the adherent cells and all of the cells in the medium can be subcultured so that a more favorable balance of cells is maintained. Again, Benyesh-Melnick *et al.* (1968) and Nilsson (1971*a*) have demonstrated the desirable "feeder" influence of such fibroblasts.

Nilsson (1971*b,c*) described a modified organ culture for establishing lymphoid cells from bone marrow and lymph nodes. The tissue fragment was placed on a 3- by 4-mm slide of gelatin sponge supported on a stainless steel grid covered with a sheet of lens paper. The level of the medium was adjusted so that the sponge was wet. The efficiency of lymphoid cell line establishment was nearly 100%. The author added 1×10^6 allogeneic adult normal fibroblasts as feeder cells to cultures of leukocytes from peripheral blood. He used either F-10 medium (Ham, 1963) or RPMI-1640. The cell lines that developed were all lymphoid in nature plus two myeloma cell lines; no myeloid cell lines were reported (Nilsson *et al.*, 1968).

It is notable that such diverse liquid culture techniques favored the growth of lymphoid cells, whereas cloning techniques with soft agar selectively supported the temporary growth of myeloid cells. Lymphoid cell lines have been established incidental to the culture of tumor biopsies and cultures of effusions (Moore, 1972).

The cell lines described by Giraldo *et al.* (1972) in cultures of Kaposi's sarcoma probably represent lymphoid cells that evolved from the mixed cell cultures. The cultures, after a period of 2–3 months, contained many round cells that grew in suspension and contained herpes-like viruses. Unfortunately, studies of immunoglobulin production were not done.

6. *Representative Malignant Cell Lines*

An unfortunate tendency to label lymphoid cell lines according to the clinical diagnosis of the donor has caused much confusion. For example, some "leukemia" cell lines actually represent lymphoid cell lines derived from normal cells in the blood. This is particularly true of cell lines derived from patients with myelogenous leukemia. Even morphological information can be misleading as there are various similar cell forms in almost all cell lines, malignant or normal. The following *indirect* criteria of malignancy should be present before a cell line is labeled malignant: (1) abnormal morphology (a rare example is the abnormal development of the endoplasmic reticulum in myeloma cell lines), (2) abnormal chromosome constitution, (3) abnormal protein synthesis such as production only of light chains, (4) comparatively high cloning efficiency in soft agar, and (5) aggressive growth in immunosuppressed heterologous hosts. Personal conversation with B. C. Giovanella indicates that there is preliminary evidence that the growth or lack of growth of lymphoid cells in nude (athymic) mice may be an excellent discriminatory test. On the basis of our experience, alteration in isoantigen patterns is not an adequate criterion. The reports (Egan and Todd, 1972) of possible tumor antigens of malignant cultured cells may be helpful in the future.

Diehl *et al.* (1971) reported that even normal lymphoid cell lines had aggressive biological growth in immunosuppressed animals and should be considered malignant. We have rejected this interpretation on the grounds that adaptable normal cells can be cultured in totally immunosuppressed newborn animals (and humans). No leukemia in patients injected intravenously with many billions of autochthonous cultured cells (Moore and Gerner, 1970) provides good evidence that the cells were not malignant.

7. Lymphomas

The lymphoid cell lines derived from youngsters with Burkitt's lymphoma by Epstein and Barr (1964) and by Pulvertaft (1964) undoubtedly represent malignant cells. All of these cell lines have either pseudodiploid cells or cells with abnormal chromosome markers (Miles and O'Neill, 1967; Kohn *et al.*, 1967). No common chromosome pattern was found, although certain chromosomes were abnormal more frequently than others.

Any culture of most Burkitt cell lines contains cells with a spectrum of morphological forms: (1) immature lymphoblasts, (2) a few huge 15-μm cells with one to three nuclei, (3) lymphoblasts with double nuclei, (4) deep-staining cells with a plasmablast (or immunoblast) appearance, (5) macrophage-like cells that often adhere to surfaces and contain debris and phagocytized dead cells, and (6) a few medium-sized lymphocytes. The proportion of the different forms varies according to the cell line and the culture conditions.

Those Burkitt cell lines that we (Minowada *et al.*, 1972) and others (Southam *et al.*, 1969) have studied have high cloning efficiencies, and small inocula of cells produce tumorous masses in immunosuppressed mice and rats.

All of these cell lines form clumps, and although most of them grow as suspensions of cells, a few adhere lightly to glass surfaces. The cell lines are easily adaptable to spinner cultures without loss of their doubling time (20–100 h) and viability.

All of the cell lines contain cells that can produce immunoglobulin, but the percentage of Ig-producing cells in some lines may be less than 5%. A majority of the cell lines produce IgM and/or IgM and IgG (Fahey *et al.*, 1966; Takahashi *et al.*, 1969; Minowada *et al.*, 1967, 1968). Cell lines derived from normal persons are much less likely to continue the synthesis of IgM *than the synthesis of IgG* even if *the former* was detectable after establishment.

Cell lines from Burkitt's lymphoma all contain the herpes-like virus designated the Epstein–Barr virus (Epstein and Barr, 1964) or in a few instances (Raji) the genome of the virus (zur Hausen *et al.*, 1970; zur Hausen and Schulte-Holthausen, 1970). The greatest production of the virus occurs during the first few months after establishment. The highest level of EB virus infection can be achieved by rapid growth of the cells under optimal conditions followed by a culture period of 5–10 days at 35°C and reexposure of the cells to optimal conditions for several days before harvesting (Horoszewicz *et al.*, 1970). Some investigators have reported increasing the EB virus infection by exposure of the cells to 5-bromodeoxyuridine (Hampar *et al.*, 1971). The best cells to scan for virus particles with the electron microscope are cells that appear "injured" or degenerating. Often there is a rim of attached proteinaceous debris surrounding those cells with mature virus particles attached to the membrane.

In summary, it is relatively easy to establish cell lines from Burkitt's lymphoma. The lymphoid cells are abnormal and biologically aggressive, contain EB virus, and produce immunoglobulins, especially IgM. The cells have the characteristics of B-cells.

In contrast, it is very difficult to establish *abnormal* cell lines from other kinds of lymphomas. Trujillo *et al.* (1972) cultured minced fragments of lymph nodes under perforated cellophane in Ham's F-10 medium. They reported the establishment of two lymphoid cell lines from patients with lymphomas but temporary growth in cultures from 14 of 19 patients. However, only one of eight cultures from patients with Hodgkin's disease grew temporarily and none established. One cell line, derived from a lymphatic lymphoma has an abnormal karyotype, produces immunoglobulin, and has C-type particles.

Suárez *et al.* (1969) reported the establishment of a lymphoid cell line from a lymphoblastoma. The cell line had an abnormal chromosome constitution.

Pontén (1967) used a modified organ culture to grow fragments of lymph nodes. Three of six cultures from patients with lymphoma underwent "transformation" from fibroblastoid forms to lymphoid cells after 6–12 wk. One cell line had an abnormal karyotype.

Our experience with culture of leukocytes from the peripheral blood of patients with lymphomas and Hodgkin's disease has been discouraging. Of several hundred cultures, only 13 cell lines became established and none of these had characteristics of malignancy. Eisinger *et al.* (1971) reported the emergence of lymphoid cells from organ cultures of lymph nodes from patients with Hodgkin's disease. The cell lines had few characteristics of malignancy, and further studies will be required to confirm the origin of these cell lines from a unique cell associated with the disease. There were sedimentation peaks characteristic of both DNA and RNA viruses. The DNA virus of the herpes group will have to be distinguished from the EB virus before its significance can be judged.

In brief, there is a need for cell lines with characteristics of lymphomas, but new selective methods of retaining the viability of the malignant cells will have to be discovered.

8. Cell Lines from Patients with Leukemia and Myeloma

Benyesh-Melnick *et al.* (1963, 1968) propagated bone marrow samples from children with leukemia and reported the establishment of 11 cell lines from 114 patients. (In contrast, 27 of 48 similar samples from children with infectious mononucleosis became established.) A subsequent study (Benyesh-Melnick *et al.*, 1971) of the chromosome constitution of three "leukemia" cell lines revealed that two cell lines contained 75% cells with a diploid chromosome number and one had a mode of 48 chromosomes. Regrettably, any reliance on chromosome studies alone as a criterion of malignancy was dispelled by the finding that a cell line from a normal person was equally abnormal and that all seven cell lines from children with infectious mononucleosis were very abnormal after many months in culture.

The cell lines that we have established from patients with infectious mononucleosis have not been abnormal and the differing selective survival of cells in the two laboratories requires clarification.

Iwakata and Grace in 1963 cultured the leukocytes of a patient with chronic myelogenous leukemia in a flask with WI-38 cells as a feeder layer. After a lapse period of 46 days, the culture could be subdivided. Personal examination of an early passage of this cell line (RPMI-6410) revealed myeloblastoid cells with a variety of granules in the cytoplasm, but no evidence of maturation into mature granulocytes. Subsequent studies revealed typical lymphoid cells with B-cell characteristics (large size—10–20 μm—formation of large clumps, rapid growth with a doubling time of 20–200 h, and production of immunoglobulins). The cell line contained the herpes-like virus particles that were indistinguishable from EB virus. The cell line had a relatively low cloning efficiency but produced tumors in immunosuppressed hosts, and had a relatively normal karyotype without the Ph or "Philadelphia" chromosome. In such instances, it is difficult to say whether the cell line was still "leukemic" or whether the surviving cells represented normal elements that overgrew the malignant ones. A pertinent paper by Zur Hausen (1967) provided data on seven cell lines from patients with leukemia; all of them had diploid chromosome constitutions.

Armstrong (1966) established two cell lines from patients with acute myelogenous leukemia and one from a girl with "acute" lymphoblastic leukemia of 4 yr duration. The author noted simultaneous establishment in several flasks of each cell sample after a lapse period of 4–10 wk. These cell lines consisted of lymphoid cells with B-cell characteristics and a diploid set of chromosomes. There was no evidence that the cells had leukemic characteristics.

Lucas *et al.* (1966) established a "lymphoid" cell line from a patient with myelogenous leukemia, but 23% of the cells contained the Ph chromosome. This was good evidence that the "lymphoid" cells were actually derived from a myeloid stem cell, but unfortunately when we examined the cell lines several months later there were no Ph-containing cells. Pauly (personal communication) has described a similar cell line. In both instances, the lymphoid cells that survived or replaced the Ph cells had an abnormal karyotype and may still have represented immature myeloid cells. In other words, it is possible that the Ph phenomenon develops only in a more mature stage.

deGrouchy *et al.* (1970) established a cell line from myelogenous leukemia cells with the Ph chromosome after 46 days in culture. Just 5 days after the establishment, no cells with the Ph chromosome were seen, and by 8 months the cell line consisted mostly of tetraploid cells. The authors concluded that the cell line probably arose from a normal lymphoid cell and overgrew the myeloid cells that had a slow division rate.

One cell line, RPMI-4265, was derived from the blood of a patient with chronic myelogenous leukemia after 40 days in culture. A few weeks later, no Ph chromosomes could be detected even though the cells resembled myeloblasts. The predominant mode was 48 chromosomes with several markers; thus the cell line was possibly derived from an abnormal cell. On the other hand, the cells formed clumps, produced immunoglobulin, and were indistinguishable from normal cultured lymphoid cells. Nevertheless, Huang *et al.* (1969) reported that this cell line had a high cloning efficiency in soft agar and Imamura *et al.* (1970) found that it produced tumor masses in immunosuppressed mice. Both of these findings are consistent with abnormal cell lines having malignant characteristics.

We have no firm opinion whether these lymphoid cell lines with abnormal chromosome constitutions, but without the Ph chromosome, represent a replacement of the myeloid cells with abnormal lymphoid cells or a dedifferentiation of the myeloid cells to a more primitive stage in which the Ph chromosomes or any myeloid characteristics are suppressed.

An independent and important observation about RPMI-4265 that may support our thesis of its origin from a myelogenous cell has been provided by Mann *et al.* (1971). They produced antisera to this cell line and claimed that there was a specific reaction with *both* acute lymphatic and myelogenous leukemia cells.

9. *Unique Cell Lines with T-Cell-Like Characteristics*

In contrast to the hundreds of lymphoid cell lines with B-cell characteristics established from normal persons and from patients with various hematopoietic malignancies, only a few cell lines have T-cell characteristics.

Minowada *et al.* (1972) described a unique cell line derived from a child with acute lymphatic leukemia. The cells (MOLT) grew slowly without evidence of an abrupt establishment phase, did not form clumps, were smaller and had a more mature morphology, had no evidence of immunoglobulin production, and formed rosettes with sheep red blood cells. This cell line grew rapidly in immunosuppressed mice as an ascites tumor and had an abnormal chromosome constitution. We have established a similar cell line, RPMI-8402, with T-cell characteristics from another child with acute lymphatic leukemia. Four other cell lines derived from the leukocytes of this patient had B-cell characteristics and originated from normal lymphoid cells. No EB virus has been found in these T-cells.

Foley *et al.* (1965) established a lymphoid cell line from a baby with acute leukemia by the use of a suspension culture. There was no lapse phase before vigorous growth began and the cells were smaller and more mature in appearance than those seen in most cell lines. The chromosome constitution was described as pseudodiploid and the cells did not produce immunoglobulin.

10. *Myeloma Cell Lines*

There have been no difficulties in confirming the derivation of cell lines from patients with malignant myeloma because of the atypical morphology of the cells and the production of abnormal cell products. A cell line, RPMI-8226, produces only Bence-Jones protein (λ light chains) (Matsuoka *et al.*, 1969) and has malignant characteristics (Moore and Kitamura, 1968). The cells are also unique because they adhere to glass surfaces, have no mature EB virus, and do not form clumps.

Nilsson *et al.* (1968, 1970) established myeloma cell lines that produced IgE molecules. The cells resembled plasmablasts. The modal chromosome number was 44, and there were several abnormal chromosomes. No EB virus particles were detected in the cells, as was true of the myeloma cell line RPMI-8226. It is interesting that these cell lines were dependent on the presence of feeder cells for continuous growth even after establishment.

In brief, there seems to be little doubt that both malignant and normal cell lines can be established from the bone marrow, lymph nodes, and blood of patients with leukemia. Scientists must characterize each cell line before labeling it as "malignant" or "benign" or representative of a particular type of leukemia.

11. Morphology

It is difficult to provide exact morphological descriptions of lymphoid cell lines. As mentioned previously, every culture with the exception of the unique myeloma cell lines and the T-like cell lines has a varying spectrum of morphological forms according to the individual cell line and conditions of culture. A number of authors (Moore *et al.*, 1967; Clarkson *et al.*, 1967) have published descriptions and photographs of the microscopic and ultramicroscopic features of cultured lymphoid cells. The predominant form is the immature lymphoblast. Most cell lines contain very few mature lymphocytes. Other cell types include monocytoid cells, macrophage-like cells with phagocytized cells and cell fragments, plasmablast-like cells, and multinucleated cells. The peculiar absence of fibroblast-like cells from established lymphoid cell lines is unexplainable but probably reflects an unfavorable environment.

It is important to remember that *any* of these morphological forms can be cloned and the new cultures will have the same spectrum of cell types.

In brief, it is not possible to distinguish among most cell lines, with or without characteristics of malignancy, on the basis of morphological characteristics. Even the ultrastructures of most cell lines are similar (Chandra *et al.*, 1968).

Morphological features of cultured lymphoid cells that have been given special attention include nuclear inclusions and protrusions (Gough *et al.*,

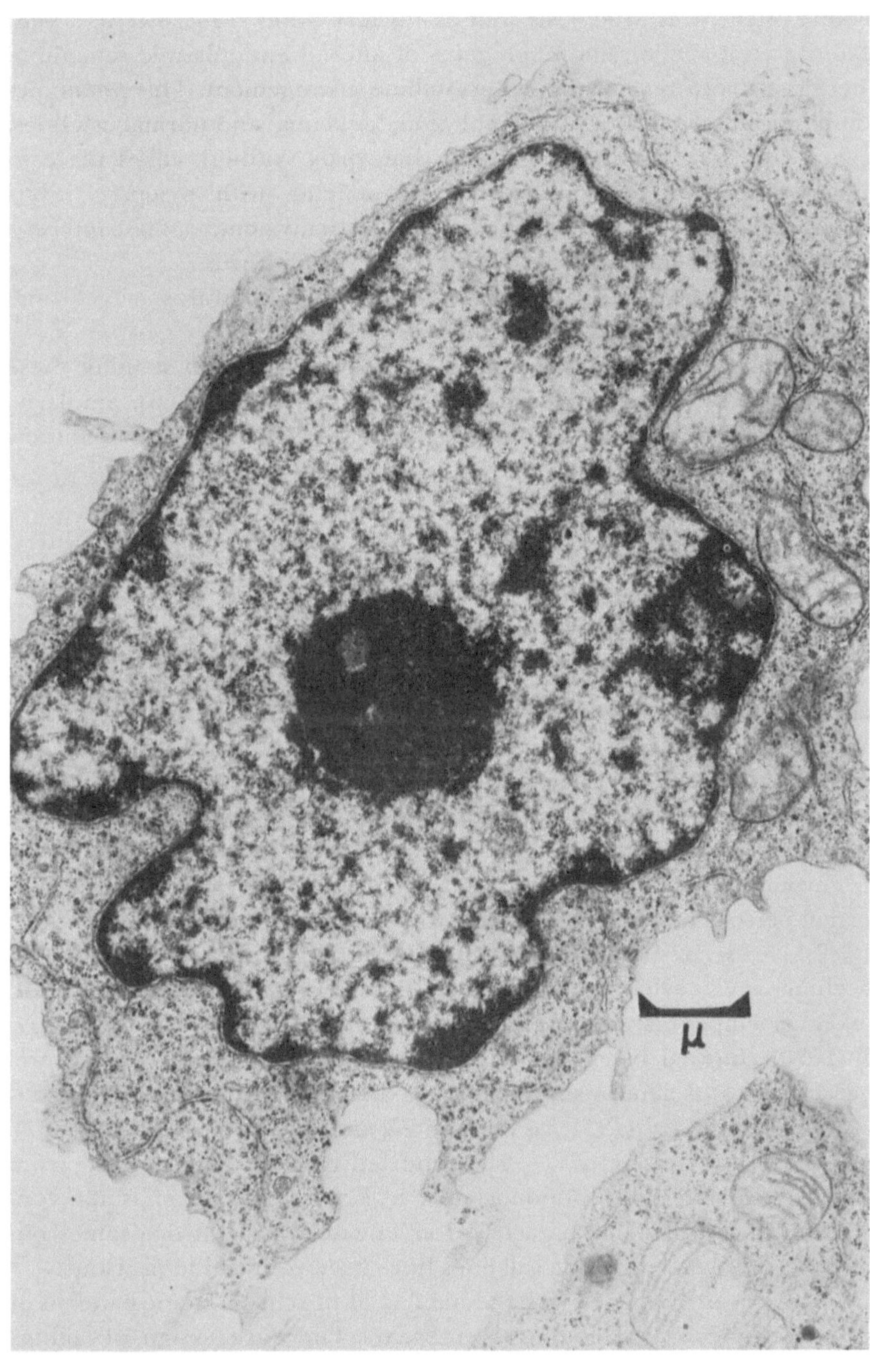

FIG. 1. B-cell RPMI-8866 derived from a patient with acute myelogenous leukemia.

1965; Epstein *et al.*, 1965), as well as nuclear pores (Moore *et al.*, 1968; Chandra *et al.*, 1968), and aggregates of altered endoplasmic reticulum. These last structures may have a crystalline arrangement. This phenomenon has been seen in Burkitt's lymphoma, leukemia, and normal cell lines. Several investigators have suggested that virus synthesis takes place in similar structures in lymphocytes of patients with systemic lupus erythematosus (Gyorkey and Sinkovics, 1971). In my opinion, these interesting structures will not be associated with any specific virus.

Figures 1, 2, and 3 illustrate representative ultrastructural aspects of some of our cultured lymphoid cell lines.

The procedures for making smear preparations of and staining these large, delicate cells have been published (Moore *et al.*, 1968). Similarly, detailed directions for preparing and staining the cells for electron microscopy can be found in a paper by Anderson (1965).

12. Chromosome Studies

The rapid multiplication of human lymphoid cells in culture (20–100 h per generation) makes it easy to obtain cells in the metaphase stage for chromosome studies. It is not necessary to add PHA or similar stimulants; approximately 0.1 μg of colcemid is added to 5 ml of medium and cells, and incubated for 1–6 h. The proportion of mitotic figures present can be determined by smear preparation before fixing the cells. The normality of the chromosome constitution of almost all lymphoid cell lines derived from normal persons parallels that of 3-day cultures of lymphocytes.

Cell lines derived from Burkitt's lymphoma have abnormal karyotypes (Toshima *et al.*, 1967), as do a *few* cell lines derived from patients with leukemia, lymphoma, and myeloma. For example, the cell line that Adams *et al.* (1970) cultured from a patient with lymphatic leukemia had several characteristics of abnormality, including an abnormal chromosome constitution. Adams *et al.* (1971), as well as Steel and Hardy (1970), Pope (1967), and Benyesh-Melnick *et al.* (1971), reported that cell lines derived from patients with infectious mononucleosis had abnormal chromosome constitutions and malignant characteristics. The abnormal chromosome constitutions of several myeloma cell lines have been referred to previously.

We have been impressed with the stability of the chromosome patterns of normal cell lines over periods of several years. There are no signs of "aging" as are described for diploid fibroblast cultures. A few normal cell lines develop aberrant chromosomes, but the causes are unknown. On the other hand, "malignant" cell lines from leukemia patients are very unstable and

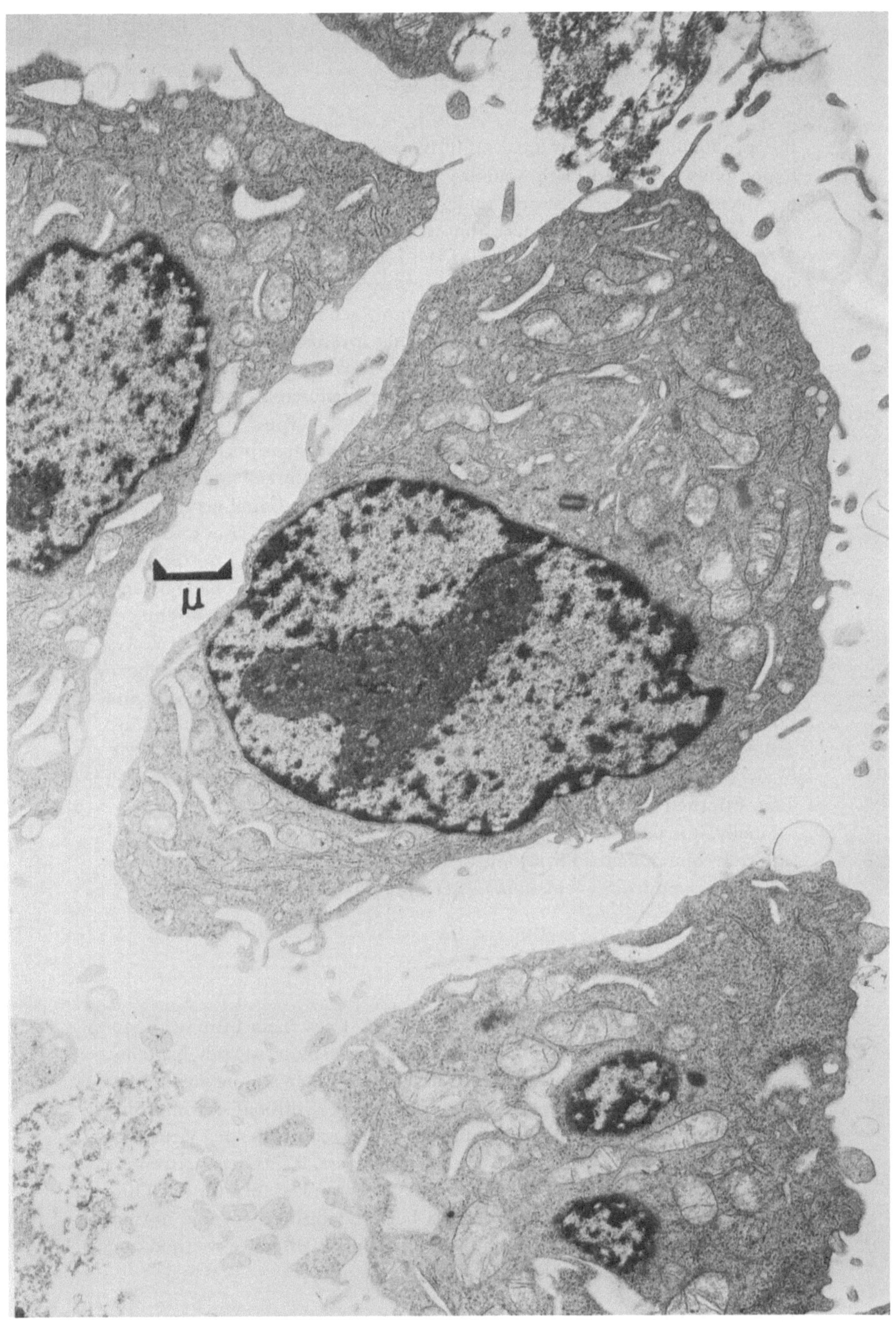

FIG. 2. RPMI-8226 derived from a patient with myeloma.

the predominant pattern may shift from a pseudodiploid mode to a hypodiploid one and then stabilize with a mode ranging as high as tetraploidy. No characteristic or "malignant karyotype" has been described, although some chromosomes are abnormal more frequently than others.

A very puzzling problem concerns the kind of cells that become established from the peripheral blood of patients with myelogenous leukemia. In 1966, Lucas *et al.* reported that a cell line from such a patient had cells with a Ph chromosome. This finding suggested that myeloid as well as lymphoid cells might become established as cell lines. We have several similar cell lines in which the cells had become granulation and questionable Auer bodies. No Ph chromosomes were detected in these cells. deGrouchy *et al.* (1970) observed the presence of Ph-positive cells during the lapse period, followed by their disappearance 5 days after establishment of the cell line. The most acceptable explanation is that the cultures contained residual myeloid cells that were replaced by the faster-growing lymphoid cells. It is not possible to say whether the myeloid cells survived but dedifferentiated into the more primitive lymphoblastoid stage and in doing so "lost" the Ph chromosome. Many hematologists have insisted that the lymphoblast is the progenitor cell for both myeloid and lymphoid cells (Maximow, 1963; Bloom, 1938; Yoffey *et al.*, 1961; Cudkowicz *et al.*, 1964). Further, the Ph chromosome has been reported in patients with myelofibrosis and metaplasia (Forrester and Louro, 1966; Kiossoglou *et al.*, 1966), polycythemia (Kiossoglou *et al.*, 1966), and eosinophilic leukemia and erythroleukemias (Elves and Israels, 1967). In any event, it has not been possible to develop long-term stable myeloid cell lines with the Ph chromosome.

Finally, it is perplexing that the lymphoid cell lines that were associated with cells containing the Ph chromosome are often abnormal, as though they were developed from a leukemia rather than normal cells.

13. Biological Studies

The successful establishment of lymphoid cell lines from humans is not unique. Similar cell lines have been derived from the blood of apes, baboons, and the rhesus monkey (Dunkel and Myers, 1972). It is noteworthy that these cell lines establish after a lapse phase, have a diploid chromosome constitution, produce immunoglobulins, and contain a herpes virus that cannot be distinguished from EB virus. In contrast, it has been extremely difficult to establish normal lymphoid cell lines from rodents. One cell line with characteristics of lymphocytes has been established from a normal mouse (T. Burke, personal communication), but an effective method and growth medium have not been discovered.

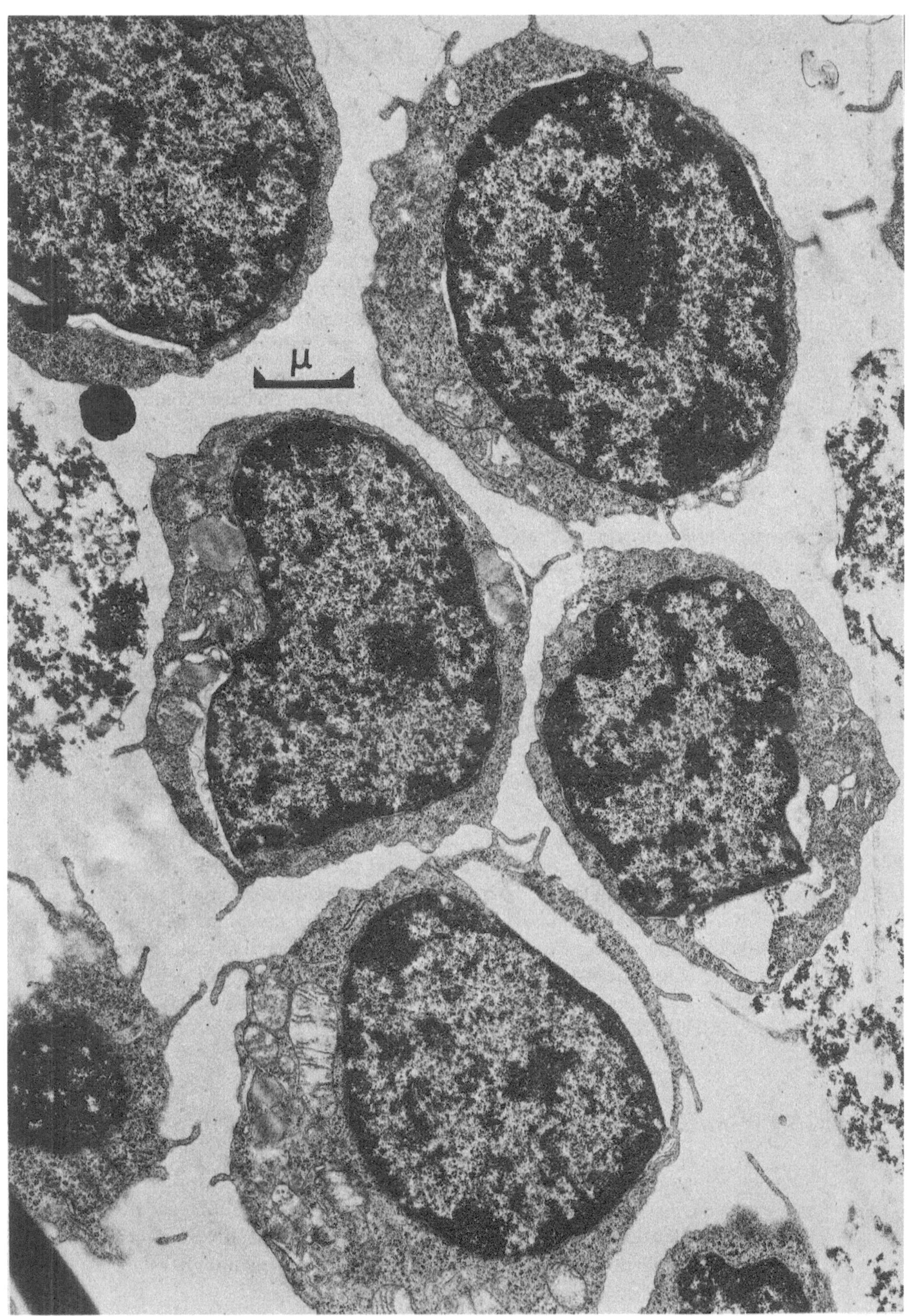

FIG. 3. T-cell MOLT derived from a patient with acute lymphatic leukemia.

14. The Culture of Lymphoid Cells

A number of investigators (Metcalf *et al.*, 1969; Pike and Robinson, 1970; Paran *et al.*, 1970; Iscove *et al.*, 1971; Brown and Carbone, 1971; Harris and Freireich, 1970) have reported the growth of colonies of human hematopoietic cells by culturing the white cells from blood or bone marrow in soft agar with and without feeder layers. The cells forming the colonies are granulocytes. An increased number of colonies develop from the blood of patients with chronic myelogenous leukemia, but only a few small colonies develop from blood of patients with acute myelogenous leukemia. The colony-forming cells from both normal and myelogenous leukemia blood are dependent on a colony-stimulating factor (CSF) found in plasma or urine or provided by feeder cells such as normal peripheral blood cells.

No lymphoid cell colonies evolve from these cultures of fresh leukocytes in agar cultures, and the myeloid cells have not been sustained as long-term cultures. The selective growth of lymphoid cells by this technique and the selective growth of lymphoid cells by the methods using liquid media have biological importance. A search should be made for the proper environment and medium to extend the growth of myelogenous cells as continuous self-replicating clones. A two-phase culture system will probably be required to provide a proper environment for maintenance of some immature cells and for the maturation of other cells. Such a system may be required for successful culture of lymphoma cells and the pathological cells of Hodgkin's disease.

The cloning of established lymphoid cell lines was thought by some scientists to differentiate between "normal" and "abnormal" cell lines. For example, lymphoid cell lines derived from Burkitt's lymphoma have a relatively high cloning efficiency (20–80%) as does the myeloma cell line RPMI-8226 (60%). In contrast, cell lines derived from normal persons have low cloning efficiencies—less than 6% (Huang *et al.*, 1969). This relative assay of biological aggressiveness is helpful and quite well correlated with the presence or absence of abnormal karyotype.

15. Transplantation of Leukemia Cells in Vivo

The heterologous transplantation of both fresh and cultured leukemia cells was achieved by Adams *et al.* (1966), who transplanted a human acute lymphoblastic leukemia in newborn hamsters. A number of investigators (Adams *et al.*, 1966; Southam *et al.*, 1969) have established cell lines in other immunosuppressed heterologous hosts.

Some investigators reported that only those cell lines with malignant characteristics such as an abnormal karyotype could be successfully transplanted. Adams *et al.* (1971) reported that a cell line derived from a child with infectious mononucleosis produced tumorous growths in immunosuppressed neonatal hamsters. Southam *et al.* (1969) noted that a cell line from an individual with infectious mononucleosis had the ability to produce tumors in newborn rats. Deal and Gerber (1971) reported tumor formation in immunosuppressed mice injected with cultured lymphoid cells from normal persons.

This assay may distinguish between normal and abnormal lymphoid cell lines, but is not an absolute test of malignancy. Severely immunosuppressed animals may be merely living culture flasks, and under such conditions both normal and malignant tumors may form.

16. Human Studies

Moore and Gerner (1970) infused volunteer patients having advanced malignancy with $1–236 \times 10^9$ allogeneic cultured lymphoid cells derived from normal persons—none of the patients supported the growth of the infused cells. Of even more significance, autologous cultured cells failed to produce malignant changes. This study therefore provided evidence that lymphoid cell lines had no malignant characteristics, since otherwise the patients would have developed leukemia.

17. Origin of Lymphoid Cell Lines from T- and B-Cells

As noted previously, all normal lymphoid cell lines and a majority of malignant lymphoid cell lines have characteristics of B-cells. We (Minowada *et al.*, 1972, Moore and Minowada, 1973) have reported the establishment of several cell lines from patients with acute lymphatic leukemia that have T-cell characteristics. The myeloma cell line RPMI-8226 has characteristics of both T- and B-cells. No observations have been made of the alteration of T- and B-cell characteristics in a cell line.

Adams *et al.* (1973) have observed that the transplantable human leukemia cells that produce a leukemic state in hamsters are probably T-cells. All of the other leukemia cell lines, including some from patients during remissions of acute lymphatic leukemia, had characteristics of B-cells and did not produce leukemia in the animals.

The derivation of leukemic cells—with evidence of clonal origin—from T- or B-cells may aid in etiological and therapeutic studies. Chronic lymphatic leukemia often consists of B-cells, in contrast to the T-cells of acute lymphatic leukemia. Haran-Ghera and Peled (1973) have provided evidence that leukemias induced in mice with carcinogens seemed to be derived from B-cells, in contrast to the thymic origin of most mouse leukemias that have been induced with radiation and/or virus.

The exacting nutritional requirements of T-cells are evident from the necessity of maintaining high population densities and the adverse effect of replacements with as little as 20% v/v of fresh medium. It would be very desirable to maintain normal lymphoid cells with characteristics of T-cells, macrophages, and plasma cells, but their specific nutritional and environmental requirements are not known.

18. Lymphocyte Destruction of Tumor Cells

The significance of lymphocyte–tumor cell interaction has been known by pathologists for many decades. The amount of lymphoid reaction surrounding tumors has been used to estimate the prognosis of cancers (Black *et al.*, 1955). The culture of normal and malignant lymphocytes has provided new opportunities for studying the mechanisms of tumor cell recognition and destruction by lymphocytes. The relative specificity of these cellular actions between autochthonous cells is indirect evidence that a tumor-specific antigen may exist.

Several clinicians have initiated studies based on the theory that stimulation of the patient's lymphocytes might provide a therapeutic effect on the patient's own tumor cells. Frenster and Rogoway (1970) and Svet-Moldavsky and Kadaghidze (1968) stimulated freshly isolated lymphocytes with PHA or other agents and then reinfused the cells into the cancer patients; a therapeutic effect was reported.

Mitchen *et al.* (1973) compared the effect of unstimulated fresh lymphocytes and cultured lymphoid cells on autochthonous tumor cells. Only a few lymphocytes (one out of 300) were capable of recognition, attachment, and destruction of the tumor cells. Lymphoid cell lines maintained in contact with tumor cells for over a month developed an increased number of "killer" cells. A "blocking" effect of the patient's serum was noted, as has been reported by Hellström and Hellström (1971). The practical limitations of lymphocytotherapy are manyfold, but the most critical need is a method of increasing the proportion of killer cells from less than 1% to nearly 100%.

Despite this and other complexities, Moore and Gerner (1970) infused several patients with 100 g or more of their own cultured lymphocytes.

There was evidence of significant tumor destruction, but no proof that the reactions were specific. Infiltration of the tumor nodules with lymphoid cells and peripheral necrosis provided a histological appearance that might be expected from an immune reaction.

The practical applications of lymphocytotherapy of malignancy will also require culture of the cells in compatible serum or protein-free medium and assessment in patients with a minimal number of tumor cells. An excellent model would be a patient with acute leukemia who is resistant to further chemotherapy and in whom there is a minimal amount of residual leukemia cells.

19. Biochemical Studies

The usefulness of normal lymphocyte cell lines for studies of transplantation or isoantigens has been established. Large quantities of cultured cells have been used for the chemical isolation of individual isoantigens (Reisfeld *et al.*, 1970, 1971; Miyakawa *et al.*, 1971) and for qualitation of genetic expression of the isoantigens (Tanagaki *et al.*, 1972).

Studies of isoantigen patterns of abnormal cultured lymphocytes are still in preliminary development. The probable close association of tumor antigens and transplantation antigens on the cell membrane will make it mandatory to completely identify the isoantigen patterns of both normal and cancerous cells from each patient before interpreting lymphocytic–cancerous target cell reactions. The few isolated instances of "suppression" or undetectability of the major isoantigens on the lymphocytes from patients with advanced malignancy are puzzling and unsolved (personal observation). The HL-A antigens or their expression may vary with other alterations of cultured malignant cells, and thus it is difficult to use them as a criterion of cell identity.

20. Immunoglobulin Production

As noted previously, the vast majority of lymphoid cell lines derived from hematopoietic malignancies, and so far all cell lines from normal persons, are B-cells that synthesize immunoglobulins. The original lymphoid cell lines established from Burkitt's lymphoma were found to synthesize immunoglobulin, particularly IgM (Fahey *et al.*, 1966; Takahashi *et al.*, 1969; Minowada *et al.*, 1967, 1968). About 0.1% to as high as 20% of the cells may have detectable immunoglobulin, but the average involvement of the cultured cells is about 5%. Nevertheless, cloning experiments have shown that all of the cells are capable of producing Ig.

The cells of a cell line often secrete more than one kind of Ig, and a single cell may produce two different heavy chains. The historical thesis that these immunoglobulins of a single cell are directed against a single antigen will probably be proved wrong, but to date the critical experiments have not been accomplished.

Cell lines derived from leukemic cells produce immunoglobulins, with the exception of those from T-cells, as described earlier. Also discussed previously was faulty or incomplete synthesis of Ig by myeloma cell lines.

Various products have been reported to be synthesized by lymphoid cell lines. Aside from immunoglobulins, such products include blastogenic factors, lymphotoxin (Granger and Kolb, 1968), macrophage migration inhibiting factor (Lamelin and Vassalli, 1971), the transfer factor (Lawrence, 1970), and interferon (Green *et al.*, 1969). Apparently interferon production by lymphoblastoid cell lines is less than by fresh or temporarily stimulated lymphocytes. Both "malignant" and "normal" cell lines (Deinhardt and Burnside, 1967) retain the capability to synthesize interferon. Swart and Young (1969) found an inverse relationship between interferon production and the EB virus content of lymphoid cell lines. A reduction in the growth rate of cells in the presence of interferon was observed by Cantell (personal communication). Such a reduction was reported earlier by Paucker *et al.* (1962) for a mouse cell culture (L-cells).

Fresh lymphocytes stimulated by PHA produce large quantities of cyclic adenosine-3′,5′-monophosphate (cyclic AMP) (Smith *et al.*, 1971). Lymphoid cell lines probably synthesize comparable amounts, but no assays have been reported.

Imrie and Mueller (1968) have described a factor released by human lymphocytes in culture that is necessary for the PHA growth response of lymphocytes. This factor is apparently supplementary to the lymphocyte growth factor (LGF) isolated from normal serum. According to Imrie and Mueller, these factors differ from the mitogenic principle found in mixed leukocyte cultures by Kasakura and Lowenstein (1965) and Gordon and Maclean (1965).

Glade and Chessin (1968) found that eight lymphoid cell lines synthesized the C′3 component of the complement system. Bullough and Laurence (1970) have reported the isolation of a lymphocytic chalone that may have clinical usefulness.

The synthesis of tumor-specific products by cultured leukemia cells has not been described, but the aggressive biological behavior of these cells must be reflected by changes in their metabolic patterns. Leukemic lymphocyte cell lines should be very useful in future studies of the coding and mechanisms of immunoglobulin synthesis. Comparative studies of myeloma cell lines with the limited synthesis of light or heavy chains should be helpful.

21. *Summary*

The successful culture of normal and malignant lymphoid cell lines has been of value to the hematologist, the geneticist, the biochemist, and the oncologist. Examples of investigative areas utilizing hematological cell culture include discovery of nutritional requirements of T- and B-cells and effective methods of establishing lymphatic leukemia cells and malignant cells from patients with Hodgkin's disease. Tumor antigens have been reported to be recoverable from cultured leukemia and myeloma cells, and therefore the possibility of developing diagnostic and therapeutic agents may be realized. It may also be possible to use autochthonous cultured lymphocytes for lymphocytotherapy in patients with leukemia. The destruction of the malignant cells by "killer" lymphocytes *in vitro* has been demonstrated, but the nature and degree of reaction in patients have not been clarified.

The availability of both leukemic and normal cell lines from the same patient should be useful in screening chemotherapeutic agents for a specific patient. Similarly, the carcinogenic effect of chemical and physical agents may be detected. The importance of these parallel cell lines for studies of the identification and isolation of tumor-specific antigens and/or other qualitative alterations of the malignant cells is self-evident.

Last, the fundamental question of the normality of lymphoid cell lines from healthy persons in contrast to the malignant characteristics of cell lines derived from patients with leukemia has great biological significance for the dogma that normal mammalian cells have an infinite life span.

It may become possible to establish and culture cells derived from other hematopoietic elements such as the megakaryocyte, the neutrophil, or even the erythroblast. Two- or three-phase cultures with different environmental conditions and different nutritional media will be required for the maintenance of the cells at different levels of maturation.

22. *References*

Adams, R. A., Farber, S., Foley, G. E., Uzman, B. G., Lazarus, H., and Watrouse, P., 1966, Heterotransplantation of human leukemic cells and cell cultures in the lethally X-irradiated syrian hamster, *Cancer Res.* **26:**190.

Adams, R. A., Pothier, L., Flowers, A., Lazarus, H., Farber, S., and Foley, G. E., 1970, The question of stemlines in acute leukemia, *Exp. Cell Res.* **62:**5.

Adams, R. A., Hellerstein, E. E., Pothier, L., Foley, G. E., Lazarus, H., and Stuart, A. B., 1971, Malignant potential of a cell line isolated from the peripheral blood in infectious mononucleosis, *Cancer* **27:**651.

Adams, R. A., Pothier, L., Hellerstein, E. E., and Boileau, G., 1973, Immunoglobulin synthesis and the progression to leukemia in heterotransplanted ALL, CLL, lymphona, and infectious mononucleosis, *Cancer* **31:**1397.

Anderson, D. R., 1965, A method for preparing peripheral leukocytes for electron microscopy, *J. Ultrastruct. Res.* **13:**263.

Armstrong, D., 1966, Serial cultivation of human leukemic cells, *Proc. Soc. Exp. Biol. Med.* **122:**475.

Bain, B., Vas, M. R., and Lowenstein, L., 1964, The development of large immature mononuclear cells in mixed leukocyte cultures, *Blood* **23:**108.

Baumal, R., Bloom, B., and Scharff, M. D., 1971, Induction of long term lymphocyte lines from delayed hypersensitive human donors using specific antigen plus Epstein Barr virus, *Nature New Biol.* **230:**20.

Belpomme, D., Le Borgne de Kaouel, C., Paintrand, M., Grandjon, D., Venuat, A., De Nava, C., Thoyer, C., de Grouchy, J., De The, G., and Mathe, G., 1969, Aspects morphologiques de plusieurs lignees permanentes (I.C.I.) Etablies a partir de sang leucemique humain: Etude a ultrastructurale et chromosomique des cellules avant et apres passage en lignee continue, *Rev. Fr. Etud. Clin. Biol.* **XIV:**848–860.

Belpomme, D., Minowanda, J., and Moore, G. E., 1972, Are some human lymphoblastoid cell lines established from leukemic tissues actually derived from normal leukocytes?, *Cancer* **30:**282.

Benyesh-Melnick, M., Fernbach, D. J., and Lewis, R. T., 1963, Studies on human leukemia. I. Spontaneous lymphoblastoid transformation of fibroblastic bone marrow cultures derived from leukemic and non-leukemic children, *J. Natl. Cancer Inst.* **31:**1311.

Benyesh-Melnick, M., Fernbach, D. J., Dessy, S., and Lewis, R. T., 1968, Studies on acute leukemia and infectious mononucleosis of childhood. III. Incidence of spontaneous lymphoblastoid transformation in bone marrow cultures, *J. Natl. Cancer Inst.* **40:**111.

Benyesh-Melnick, M., Macek, M., Seidel, E. H., and Mackova, V., 1971, Chromosomal analysis of lymphoblastoid cell lines after heterosexual cocultivation with bone marrow fibroblasts, *J. Natl. Cancer Inst.* **46:**369.

Black, M. M., Opler, S. R., and Speer, F. D., 1955, Survival in breast cancer cases in relation to the structure of the primary tumor and regional lymph nodes, *Surg. Gynecol. Obstet.* **100:**543.

Bloom, W., 1938, in: *Handbook of Hematology* Vol. 1 (H. Downey, ed.), p. 373, Hoeber, New York.

Broder, S. W., Glade, P. R., and Hirschhorn, K., 1970, Establishment of long-term lines from small aliquots of normal lymphocytes, *Blood* **35:**539.

Brown, D. H., and Carbone, P. P., 1971, *In vitro* growth of normal and leukemic human bone marrow, *J. Natl. Cancer Inst.* **46:**989.

Bullough, W. S., and Laurence, E. B., 1970, The lymphocytic chalone and its antimitotic action on a mouse lymphoma *in vitro, Eur. J. Cancer* **6:**525.

Chandra, S., 1968, Undulating tubules associated with endoplastic reticulum in pathologic tissues, *Lab. Invest.* **18:**422.

Chandra, S., Moore, G. E., and Brandt, P. M., 1968, Similarly between leukocyte cultures from cancerous and noncancerous human subjects: An electron microscopic study, *Cancer Res.* **10:**1982.

Chang, R. S., 1970, The loss of growth vitality of human lymphoid cell lines derived from healthy adults, *Proc. Soc. Exp. Biol. Med.* **135:**212.

Chang, R. S., 1972, Leukocyte-transforming agent from mononucleosis is ether-stable, *Nature New Biol.* **237:**273.

Choi, K. W., and Bloom, A. D., 1970*a*, Biochemically marked lymphocytoid lines: Establishment of Lesch–Nyhan cells, *Science* **170:**89.

Choi, K. W., and Bloom, A. D., 1970*b*, Cloning human lymphocytes *in vitro, Nature (Lond.)* **227:**171.

Clarkson, B., Strife, A., and DeHarven, E., 1967, Continuous cultures of seven new cell lines (SK-L1 to 7) from patients with acute leukemia, *Cancer* **20:**926.

Cudkowicz, G., Bennett, M., and Shearer, G. M., 1964, Pluripotent stem cell function of the mouse marrow "lymphocyte," *Science* **144:**866.

Deal, D. R., Gerber, P., and Chisori, F. V., 1971, Heterotransplantation of two human lymphoid cell lines transformed *in vitro* by EBV, *J. Natl. Cancer Inst.* **47:**771.

deGrouchy, J., Thoyer, C., Marchan, J. D., Fretault, J., and Paintrand, M., 1970, Etudes cytogenetique, biochimique et morphologique d'une lignee cellulaire continue (Cy-LMC-1), *Ann. Genet.* **13:**157.

Deinhardt, P., and Burnside, J., 1967, Spontaneous interferon production in cultures of a cell line from a human myeloblastic leukemia, *J. Natl. Cancer Inst.* **39:**681.

Diehl, V., Henle, G., Henle, W., and Kohn, G., 1968, Demonstration of a herpes group virus in cultures of peripheral leukocytes from patients with infectious mononucleosis, *J. Virol.* **2:**663.

Dunkel, V. C., and Myers, S. L., 1972, Continuous lymphoblastoid cell line from a rhesus monkey with myelogenous leukemia, *J. Natl. Cancer Inst.* **48:**777.

Egan, M. L., and Todd, C. W., 1972, Carcinoembryonic antigen: Synthesis by a continuous line of adenocarcinoma cells, *J. Natl. Cancer Inst.* **49:**887.

Eisinger, M., Fox, S. M., De Harven, E., Biedler, J. L., and Sanders, F. K., 1971, Virus-like agents from patients with Hodgkin's disease, *Nature (Lond.)* **233:**104.

Elves, M. W., and Israels, M. C. G., 1967, Cytogenetic studies in unusual forms of chronic myeloid leukemia, *Acta Haematol. (Basel)* **38:**129.

Epstein, M. A., and Barr, Y. M., 1964, Cultivation *in vitro* of human lymphoblasts from Burkitt's malignant lymphoma, *Lancet* **1:**252.

Epstein, M. A., Barr, Y. M., and Achong, B. G., 1965, The behaviour and morphology of a second tissue culture strain (EB2) of lymphoblasts from Burkitt's lymphoma, *Brit. J. Cancer* **19:**108.

Fahey, J. L., Finegold, I., Rabson, A. S., and Manaker, R. A., 1966, Immunoglobulin synthesis *in vitro* by established human cell lines, *Science* **152:**1259.

Foley, G. E., Lazarus, H., Farber, S., Uzman, B. G., Boone, B. A., and McCarthy, R. E., 1965, Continuous culture of human lymphoblasts from peripheral blood of a child with acute leukemia, *Cancer* **18:**522.

Forrester, R. H., and Louro, J. M., 1966, Philadelphia chromosome abnormality in agnogenic myeloid metaplasia, *Ann. Int. Med.* **64:**622.

Frenster, J. H., and Rogoway, W. M., 1970, Early clinical trials of activated autologous lymphocytes for human cancer immunotherapy, *Proc. Am. Assoc. Cancer Res.* **11:**28 (abst.).

Gerber, P., and Hoyer, B. H., 1971, Induction of cellular DNA synthesis in human leukocytes by Epstein–Barr virus, *Nature (Lond.)* **231:**46.

Gerber, P., and Monroe, J. H., 1968, Studies on leukocytes growing in continuous culture derived from normal human donors, *J. Natl. Cancer Inst.* **40:**855.

Gerber, P., Whang-Peng, J., and Monroe, J. H., 1969, Transformation and chromosome changes induced by Epstein–Barr virus in normal human leukocyte cultures, *Proc. Natl. Acad. Sci.* **63:**740.

Giraldo, G., Beth, E., Coeur, P., Vogel, C. L., and Dhru, D. S., 1972, Kaposi's sarcoma: A new model in the search for viruses associated with human malignancies, *J. Natl. Cancer Inst.* **49:**1495.

Glade, P. R., and Chessin, L. N., 1968, Synthesis of $B1_c/B1_a$ globulin (C'3) by human lymphoid cells, *Internat. Arch. Allergy* **34:**181.

Glade, P. R., Hirshaut, Y., Douglas, S. D., and Hirschhorn, K., 1968, Lymphoid suspension cultures from patients with viral hepatitis, *Lancet* **2:**1273.

Glade, P. R., Hirschhorn, K., and Douglas, S. D., 1969*a*, Herpes-like virus (letter to editor), *Lancet* **1:**1049.

Glade, P. R., Paltrowitz, I. W., and Hirschhorn, K., 1969*b*, Lymphoproliferative potential in infectious diseases, *Bull. N.Y. Acad. Med.* **45:**647.

Gordon, J., and Maclean, L. D., 1965, A lymphocyte-stimulating factor produced *in vitro*, *Nature (Lond.)* **208:**795.

Gough, J., Elves, M. W., and Israels, M. C., 1965, The formation of macrophages from lymphocytes *in vitro*, *Exp. Cell Res.* **38:**476.

Granger, G. A., and Kolb, W. P., 1968, Lymphocytes *in vitro* cytotoxicity: Mechanisms of immune and non-immune small lymphocyte mediated target L cell destruction, *J. Immunol.* **101:**111.

Green, J. A., Cooperband, S. R., and Kibrick, S., 1969, Immune specific induction of interferon production in cultures of human blood lymphocytes, *Science* **164:**1415.

Gruenwald, M., Kiossoglou, K. A., Mitus, W. J., and Dameshek, W., 1965, Philadelphia chromosome in eosinophilic leukemia, *Am. J. Med.* **39:**1003.

Gyorkey, and Sinkovics, J. G., 1971, Microtubules of systemic lupus erythematosus, *Lancet* **1:**131.

Ham, R. G., 1963, An improved nutrient solution for diploid Chinese hamster and human cell lines, *Exp. Cell Res.* **29:**515.

Hampar, B., Derge, J. G., Martos, L. M., and Walker, J. L., 1971, Persistence of a repressed Epstein–Barr virus genome in Burkitt lymphoma cells made resistant to 5-bromodeoxyuridine, *Proc. Natl. Acad. Sci.* **68:**3185.

Haran-Ghera, N., and Peled, A., 1973, Thymus and bone marrow derived lymphatic leukaemia in mice, *Nature (Lond.)* **241:**396.

Harris, J., and Freireich, E. J., 1970, *In vitro* growth of myeloid colonies from bone marrow of patients with acute leukemia in remission, *Blood* **35:**61.

Hellström, I., and Hellström, K. E., 1971, Cellular immunity and blocking antibodies to tumors, *Res. J. Reticuloendothel. Soc.* **10:**31,

Henle, W., Diehl, V., Kohn, G., Zur-Hausen, H., and Henle, G., 1967, Herpes-type virus and chromosome marker in normal leukocytes after growth with irradiated Burkitt cells, *Science* **157:**1064.

Hersh, E. M., L-Glutaminase: Suppression of lymphocyte blastogenic response *in vitro*, *Science* **172:**736.

Horoszewicz, J. S., Dunkel, V. C., Avila, L., and Grace, J. T., Jr., 1970, EB virus infection and propagation in human hematopoietic cells, *Bibl. Haematol.* **36:**722–738.

Huang, C. C., Imamura, T., and Moore, G. E., 1969, Chromosomes and cloning efficiencies of hematopoietic cell lines derived from patients with leukemia, melanoma, myeloma, and Burkitt lymphoma, *J. Natl. Cancer Inst.* **43:**1129.

Imamura, T., Huang, C. C., Minowada, J., Takahashi, M., and Moor, G. E., 1970, Cloning of human hematopoietic cell lines, *J. Natl. Cancer Inst.* **44:**845.

Imrie, R. C., and Mueller, G. C., 1968, Release of a lymphocyte growth promoter in leukocyte cultures, *Nature (Lond.)* **219:**1277.

Ioachim, H. L., 1965, Emperiopolesis of lymphoid cells in mixed cultures, *Lab. Invest.* **14:**1784.

Iscove, N. N., Senn, J. S., Till, J. E., and McCulloch, E. A., 1971, Colony formation by normal and leukemic marrow cells in culture: The effect of conditioned medium from leukocytes, *Blood* **37:**1.

Iwakata, S., and Grace, J. T., Jr., 1964, Cultivation *in vitro* of myeloblasts from human leukemia, *N.Y. State. J. Med.* **64:**2279.

Kasakura, S., and Lowenstein, L., 1965, Hematology—A factor stimulating DNA synthesis derived from the medium of leukocyte cultures, *Nature (Lond.)* **208:**794.

Kiossoglou, K. A., Mitus, W. J., and Dameshek, W., 1966, Cytogenetic studies in the chronic myeloproliferative syndrome, *Blood* **28:**241.

Klein, G., Pearson, G., Henle, G., Henle, W., Diehl, V., and Niederman, J. C., 1968, Relation between Epstein–Barr viral and cell membrane immunofluorescence in Burkitt tumor cells. II. Comparison of cells and sera from patients with Burkitt's lymphoma and infectious mononucleosis, *J. Exp. Med.* **128:**1021.

Kohn, G., Mellman, W. J., Moorehead, P. S., Loftus, J., and Henle, G., 1967, Involvement of C group chromosomes in five Burkitt lymphoma cell lines, *J. Natl. Cancer Inst.* **38:**209–222.

Lamelin, J. P., and Vassalli, P., 1971, Inhibition of macrophage migration by a soluble factor from lymphocvtes stimulated with PHA or ALS, *Nature (Lond.)* **229:**426.

Lawrence, H. S., 1970, Transfer factor, *Advan. Immunol.* **11:**196.

Ling, N. R., and Holt, P. J. L., 1967, The activation and reactivation of peripheral lymphocytes in culture, *J. Cell Sci.* **2:**57.

Lucas, L. W., Whang, J. J., Tjio, J. H., Manaker, R. A., and Zeve, V. H., 1966, Continuous cell culture from a patient with myelogenous leukemia. I. Propagation and presence of Philadelphia chromosome, *J. Natl. Cancer Inst.* **37:**753.

Mann, D. L., Rogentine, G. N., Halterman, R., and Leventhal, B., 1971, Detection of an antigen associated with acute leukemia, *Science* **174:**1136.

Matsuoka, Y., Yagi, Y., Moore, G. E., and Pressman, D., 1969, Isolation and characterization of free chain of immunoglobulin produced by an established cell line of human myeloma cell origin. I. Chain in culture medium, *J. Immunol.* **102:**1136.

Maximow, A. A., 1963, in: *Special Cytology* (E. V. Cowdry, ed.), p.601, Hafner, New York.

Metcalf, D., Moore, M. A. S., and Warner, N. L., 1969, Colony formation *in vitro* by myelomonocytic leukemic cells, *J. Natl. Cancer Inst.* **43:**982.

Miles, C. P., and O'Neill, J. F., 1967, Chromosome studies of *in vitro* lines of Burkitt's lymphoma, *Cancer Res.* **27:**392.

Miller, G., Enders, J. F., Lisco, H., and Kohn, H. I., 1969, Establishment of lines from normal human blood leukocytes by co-cultivation with a leukocyte line derived from a leukemic child, *Proc. Soc. Exp. Biol. Med.* **132:**247.

Minowada, J., Klein, G., Clifford, P., Klein, E., and Moore, G. E., 1967, Studies of Burkitt lymphoma cells. I. Establishment of a cell line (B35M) and its characteristics, *Cancer* **20:**1430.

Minowada, J., Moore, G. E., Gerner, R. E., Toshima, S., Takagi, N., and Sandberg, A. A., 1968, in: *Cancer in Africa*, p. 177, East Africa Publishing House, Nairobi, Kenya.

Minowada, J., Ohnuma, T., and Moore, G. E., 1972, Rosette-forming human lymphoid cell lines. I. Establishment and evidence for origin of thymus-derived lymphocytes, *J. Natl. Cancer Inst.* **49:**891 (brief communication).

Mitchen, J. R., Moore, G. E., Gerner, R. E., and Woods, L. K., 1973, Interaction of human melanoma cell lines with autochthonous lymphoid cells, *Yale J. Biol. Med.*, **46:**669–680.

Miyakawa, Y., Tanigaki, N., Yagi, Y., and Pressman, D., 1971, An efficient method for isolation of HL-A antigens from hematopoietic cell lines, *J. Immunol.* **107:**394.

Moore, G. E., 1972, Cultured human lymphocytes, *J. Surg. Oncol.* **4:**320.

Moore, G. E., and Gerner, R. E., 1970, Cancer immunity-hypothesis and clinical trial of lymphocytotherapy for malignant diseases, *Ann. Surg.* **172:**733.

Moore, G. E., and Gerner, R. E., 1971, Malignant melanoma, *Surg. Gynecol. Obstet.* **132:**427.

Moore, G. E., and Glick, J. L., 1967, Perspective of human cell culture, *Surg. Clin. North Am.* **47:**1315.

Moore, G. E., and Kitamura, H., 1968, Cell line derived from patient with myeloma, *N.Y. State J. Med.* **68:**2054.

Moore, G. E., and Minowada, J., 1973, Letter to the editor, *New Engl. J. Med.* **288:**106.

Moore, G. E., and Pickren, J. W., 1967, Study of a virus-containing hematopoietic and a melanoma cell line derived from a patient with a leukemoid reaction, *Lab. Invest.* **16:**882.

Moore, G. E., Gerner, R. E., and Franklin, H. A., 1967, Culture of normal human leukocytes, *JAMA* **199:**519.

Moore, G. E., Gerner, R. E., and Minowada, J., 1968*a*, Studies of normal and neoplastic human hematopoietic cells *in vitro*, in: *The Proliferation and Spread of Neoplastic Cells*, pp. 41–63, Williams and Wilkins, Baltimore.

Moore, G. E., Kitamura, H., and Toshima, S., 1968*b* Morphology of cultured hematopoietic cells, *Cancer* **22:**245.

Moore, G. E., Kitamura, H., and Minowada, J., 1970, The incidence of "leukovirus" in cultured human hematopoietic cells, *J. Surg. Oncol.* **2:**385.

Moorhead, P. S., Nowell, P. C., Mellman, W. J., Battips, D. M., and Hungerford, D. A., 1960, Chromosome preparations of leukocytes cultured from human peripheral blood, *Exp. Cell Res.* **20:**613.

Nillsson, K., 1971*a*, Characteristics of establishment of myeloma and lymphoblast cell lines derived from an E myeloma patient: A comparative study, *Internat. J. Cancer* **7:**380.

Nilsson, K., 1971*b*, Histological changes in long term explants of human lymph nodes during lymphoblastoid transformation, *Acta Pathol. Microbiol. Scand.* **79:**243.

Nilsson, K., 1971*c*, Human hematopoietic cells in continuous culture, Abstract of Uppsala Dissertations from the Faculty of Medicine, Vol. 107, *Acta Univ. Uppsal.*

Nilsson, K., Pontén, J., and Philipson, L., 1968, Development of immunocytes and immunoglobulin production in long-term cultures from normal and malignant human lymph nodes, *Internat. J. Cancer* **3:**183.

Nilsson, K., Bennich, H., Johansson, S. G. O., and Pontén, J., 1970, Established immunoglobulin producing myeloma (IgE) and lymphoblastoid (IgC) cell lines from an IgE myeloma patient, *Clin. Exp. Immunol.* **7:**477.

Paran, M., Sachs, L., Barak, Y., and Resnitsky, P., 1970, *In vitro* induction of granulocyte differentiation in hematopoietic cells from leukemic and non-leukemic patients, *Proc. Natl. Acad. Sci.* **67:**1542.

Paucker, K., Cantell, K., and Henle, W., 1962, Quantitative studies on viral interference in suspended L-cells, III. Effect of interfering viruses and interferon on the growth rate of cells, *Virology* **17:**324.

Pike, B. L., and Robinson, W. A., 1970, Human bone marrow colony growth in agar gel, *J. Cell. Physiol.* **76:**77.

Pontén, J., 1967, Spontaneous lymphoblastoid transformation of long-term cell cultures from human malignant lymphoma, *Internat. J. Cancer* **2:**311.

Pope, J. H., 1967, Establishment of cell lines from peripheral leukocytes in infectious mononucleosis, *Nature (Lond.)* **216:** 810.

Pope, J. H., Horne, M. K., and Scott, W., 1968, Transformation of foetal human leukocytes *in vitro* by filtrates of a human leukaemic cell line containing herpes-like virus, *Internat. J. Cancer* **3:**857.

Possnerova, V., Smetana, K., Krecek, M., Hermansky, F., and Fortynova, J., 1970, Long-term culture of human leukaemic leukocytes, *Neoplasma* **17:**513.

Pulvertaft, R. J. V., 1964, Cytology of Burkitt's tumor (African lymphoma), *Lancet* **1:**238.

Rabin, E. R., Benyesh-Melnick, M., and Brunschwig, J., 1967, Studies on acute leukemia and infectious mononucleosis of childhood. II. Ultrastructure of cultured lymphoblastoid cells, *Exp. Molec. Pathol.* **7:**196.

Reisfeld, R. A., Pellegrino, M., Papermaster, B. W., and Kahan, B. D., 1970, HL-A antigens from continuous lymphoid cell line derived from normal donor. I. Solubilization and serologic characterization, *J. Immunol.* **104:**560.

Reisfeld, R. A., Pellegrino, M. A., and Kahan, B. D., 1971, Salt extraction of soluble HL-A antigens, *Science* **172:**1134.

Rosenfeld, C., Macieria-Coelho, A., Venuat, A. M., Jasmin, C., and Tuan, T. Q., 1969, Kinetics of the establishment of human peripheral blood cultures, *J. Natl. Cancer Inst.* **43:**581.

Sandberg, A. A., Moore, G. E., and Schubarg, J. R., 1959, "Atypical" cells in the blood of cancer patients—Differentiation from tumor cells, *J. Natl. Cancer Inst.* **22:**555.

Smith, J. W., Steiner, A. L., Newberry, W. M., Jr., and Parker, C. W., 1971, Cyclic adenosine 3',5'-monophosphate in human lymphocytes: Alterations after phytohemagglutinin stimulation, *J. Clin. Invest.* **50:**432.

Southam, C. M., Burchenal, J. H., Clarkson, B., Tanzi, A., Mackey, R., and McComb, V., 1969, Heterotransplantation of human cell lines from Burkitt's tumors and acute leukemia into newborn rats, *Cancer* **23:**281.

Steel, C. M., and Hardy, D. A., 1970, Evidence of altered antigenicity in cultured lymphoid cells from a patient with infectious mononucleosis, *Lancet* **1:**1322.

Stevens, D. P., Barker, L. F., Fike, R., Hopps, H. E., and Meyer, H. M., Jr., 1969, Lymphoblastoid cell cultures from patients with infectious hepatitis, *Proc. Soc. Exp. Biol. Med.* **132:**1042.

Suárez, H. G., de Sahum, S. B., Pavlovsky, S. Ruibal, B., and Pavlovsky, A., 1969, Culture *in vitro* d'une lignee cellulaire provenant d'un lymphosarcome humain. I. Cytogenetique et ultrastructure cellulaire, *Internat. J. Cancer* **4:**880.

Svet-Moldavsky. G. J., and Kadaghidze, Z. G., 1968, Anti-tumor effect of activated lymphocytes, *Lancet* **2:**641.

Swart, B. D., and Young, B. G., 1969, Inverse relationship of interferon production and virus content in cell lines from Burkitt's lymphoma and acute leukemias, *J. Natl. Cancer Inst.* **42:**941.

Takahashi, M., Takagi, N., Yagi, Y., Moore, G. E., and Pressman, D., 1969, Immunoglobulin production in cloned sublines of a human lymphocytoid cell line, *J. Immunol.* **102:**1388.

Tanagaki, N., Kreiter, V. P., Moore, G. E., and Pressman, D., 1972, HL-A zygosity, *Transplantation* **14:**793.

Toshima, S., Takagi, N., Minowada, J., Moore, G. E., and Sandberg, A. A., 1967, Electron microscopic and cytogenetic studies of cells derived from Burkitt's lymphoma, *Cancer Res.* **27:**753.

Trujillo, J. M., Drewinko, B., and Ahearn, M. J., 1972, The ability of tumor cells of the lymphoreticular system to grow *in vitro, Cancer Res.* **32:**1057.

Wilson, D. B., 1966, Analysis of some of the variables associated with the proliferative response of human lymphoid cells in culture, *J. Exp. Zool.* **162:**161–170.

Yoffey, J. M., Thomas, D. B., Moffatt, D. J., Sutherland, I. H., and Rose, C., 1961, in: *Biological Activity of the Leucocyte*, p. 45, Ciba Foundation Study Groups No. 10, Little, Brown, Boston.

Zur Hausen, H., 1967, Chromosomal changes of similar nature in seven established cell lines derived from the peripheral blood of patients with leukemia, *J. Natl. Cancer Inst.* **38:**683.

Zur Hausen, H., and Schulte-Holthausen, H., 1970, Presence of EB virus nucleic acid homology in a "virus-free" line of Burkitt tumor cells, *Nature (Lond.)* **227:**245.

Zur Hausen, H., Schulte-Holthausen, H., Klein, G., Henle, W., Henle, G., Clifford, P., and Santesson, L., 1970, EBV DNA in biopsies of Burkitt tumors and anaplastic carcinomas of the nasopharynx, *Nature (Lond.)* **228:**1056.

Cytological Characterization of Human Tumor Cells from Monolayer Cultures 12

MICHAEL A. BEAN AND STEVEN I. HAJDU

1. Introduction

Classically, when using the technique of monolayer tissue culture, an investigator describes the cytology of the tumor cells he is studying by referring either to a fixed and stained slide, to a coverslip preparation of the adherent cells or to the phase contrast appearance of these cells while living and attached to either a glass or plastic surface (see the listing of published human tumor cell lines, Chapter 5). The observer is then able to assign certain cytological characteristics to the cells such as epithelioid, spindle cell, fibroblastic, or pleomorphic. Because these cells are attached to glass and have been actively growing, a considerable amount of information can be gathered in terms of growth pattern, such as the degree of contact inhibition, piling up, colony formation, cohesiveness, and focus formation, all of which may be useful in distinguishing neoplastic from benign cells.

The development of specific cytological criteria of malignancy *in vivo* by pathologists and cytotechnologists (Papanicolaou, 1942; Koss, 1968) has largely been based on exfoliated human tumor cells studied in cases where there was adequate histopathology to guide interpretation. The state of the art is now sufficiently precise to allow a decision as to whether certain

MICHAEL A. BEAN AND STEVEN I. HAJDU Memorial Sloan-Kettering Cancer Center, New York exfoliated cells are malignant. In many cases, a comment as to the most likely derivation of the neoplasm can be made. These cytological criteria derive from the relationship of the nucleus to the cytoplasm (i.e., altered nuclear–cytoplasmic ratio and altered position of the nucleus within the cytoplasm) and changes within the nucleus itself (i.e., variation in size between cells, increase in nuclear volume and changes in shape, changes in the nuclear membrane such as furrowing and clumping, alterations in chromatin such as clumping and hyperchromasia, and abnormalities of size, shape, or number of nucleoli).

The application of these cytological criteria to the study of human tumor cells *in vitro* attached to a surface has many inherent limitations. Cells growing in monolayer culture will show changes in shape and size and nuclear appearance as a direct consequence of that attachment. For example, estimation of shape and of nuclear cytoplasmic ratio will vary widely from cell to cell because of flattening, attachment, and locomotion (Hlinka and Sanders, 1972). In a time-lapse cinematographic study of prostatic epithelial cells, Lerch *et al.* (1970) found that single epithelial cells varied from triangular, to round, to elongate, to polygonal depending on attachment and the stress placed on this attachment during movement of the cell.

TABLE 1

Staining Procedure for Smears with Papanicolaou Stain[a]

1.	80% ethyl alcohol	5 dips
2.	70% ethyl alcohol	5 dips
3.	50% ethyl alcohol	5 dips
4.	Distilled water	a few dips
5.	Harris's hematoxylin[b] (without acetic acid)	5 min
6.	Distilled water	a few dips
7.	0.5% aqueous solution of hydrochloric acid	5 dips
8.	Running tapwater	5 min
9.	50% ethyl alcohol	5 dips
10.	70% ethyl alcohol	5 dips
11.	80% ethyl alcohol	5 dips
12.	95% ethyl alcohol	5 dips
13.	Orange G[b]	2 min
14.	95% ethyl alcohol	5 dips
15.	95% ethyl alcohol	5 dips
16.	EA 65[b]	2 min
17–19	Ethyl alcohol (three changes)	5 dips in each
20–21.	Absolute ethyl alcohol (two changes)	5 dips in each
22.	Equal parts of absolute ethyl alcohol and xylol	5 dips
23–29.	Xylol (seven changes)	5 dips in each

[a] Adapted from Koss (1968) by permission of Lippincott Co., Philadelphia, Pa.

[b] Formula for preparation of stains listed separately (Tables 2, 3, 4).

TABLE 2
Preparation of Harris's Hematoxylin without Acetic Acid[a]

Hematoxylin crystals	8 g
95% ethyl alcohol	80 ml
Aluminum ammonium sulfate	160 g
Distilled water	1600 ml
Mercuric oxide	6 g

Procedure

1. Dissolve aluminum ammonium sulfate in distilled water by heating.
2. Dissolve hematoxylin crystals in 95% alcohol.
3. Add hematoxylin solution to sulfate solution and bring mixture to 95°C.
4. Remove from flame and add mercuric oxide while stirring.
5. Put into cold water bath and filter when cool.
6. Store in dark-brown bottles.
7. For use, dilute the required amount with an equal part of distilled water and filter again.

[a] Adapted from Koss (1968) by permission of Lippincott Co., Philadelphia, Pa. The necessary dyes may be purchased from National Aniline Division, Allied Chemical and Dye Company, New York, N.Y.

And, as cells moved both the nuclei and the nucleoli changed shape, size, and position.

Given these limitations, we decided that a cytological examination of the monolayer tumor cells released from their attachment was of interest. As trypsinization of monolayer cultures is widely used in order to transfer cultures and to prepare cell suspensions for electron microscopic and cytogenetic studies, we decided to fix, smear, and stain these trypsinized cell suspensions exactly as one would process a pleural or peritoneal effusion or sputum sample from a patient. After one washing, the trypsinized suspension of tumor cells was fixed in an equal volume of 70% alcohol, and the cells were sedimented by centrifugation and smeared on glass slides in preparation for Papanicolaou stain. This technique is not meant to replace the stained coverslip technique but rather to provide some additional information pertinent to the cytological characterization of human monolayer tumor cell lines.

2. Materials and Methods

Monolayer cultures of human tumor cells and normal cells were provided for this study by Dr. Jørgen Fogh (see Chapter 5). Monolayer cultures of the human cells in glass or plastic T-30 flasks were trypsinized [0.25% trypsin,

TABLE 3
Preparation of Orange G[a]

Orange G crystals	10 g
Distilled water	100 ml
95% ethyl alcohol	950 ml
Phosphotungstic acid	0.15 g

Procedure

1. Stock solution No. 1: 10 g Orange crystals in 100 ml distilled water. Allow to stand for a few days.
2. Stock solution No. 2: 50 ml stock solution No. 1 in 950 ml 95% ethyl alcohol.
3. To 1000 ml stock solution No. 2 add 0.15 g phosphotungstic acid. Mix well and store in dark-brown bottles.
4. Filter before using.

[a] Adapted from Koss (1968) by permission of Lippincott Co., Philadelphia, Pa. The necessary dyes may be purchased from National Aniline Division, Allied Chemical and Dye Company, New York, N.Y.

Bacto 1:250 or 0.05% Tryptar (Armour) in balanced salt solution] at near confluency up to 15 min. in order to release the cells from the monolayer. The trypsin solution containing the free cells was then neutralized by the addition of medium containing 15% fetal calf serum (FCS) and was centrifuged at 1000 rpm for 10 min in a 50 ml conical glass or plastic centrifuge tube in order to pellet the cells. The cell pellet was resuspended in 15 ml of balanced salt solution, and a few drops of the cell suspension was added to tissue culture chamber slides (Lab–Tek Products, Naperville, Ill.) in order for the cells to attach and grow for 1–2 days prior to fixation with 70% alcohol and appropriate staining. The tissue culture chamber slides were always prefilled with medium containing 15% FCS prior to the addition of the cell suspension so that the final concentration of FCS after the addition of the cell suspension was greater than 10%. The remaining cell suspension was then fixed by the addition of an equal volume of 70% ethyl alcohol. The alcohol-fixed cell suspension was then sent to the Cytology Department for processing after a minimum of at least overnight fixation. The choice of a protein-free medium for resuspension of the trypsinized cell pellet was dictated by the fact that alcohol fixation of cells resuspended in medium containing FCS produced large protein precipitates.

The chamber slides were harvested 1–2 days after seeding by gently washing twice with 37°C phosphate-buffered saline and then fixing with 70% EtOH or by air drying. Those fixed with alcohol were then stored in 70%

EtOH until they were stained either with Papanicolaou stain (Papanicolaou, 1942), as described in Tables 1–4, or with hematoxylin and eosin (Table 5). Tables 1–4 list the recipes and procedures used for staining routine human cytology preparations at Memorial Hospital (Durfee, 1968). Table 5 lists the recipe for hematoxylin and eosin stain as used by Memorial Hospital Pathology Department.

The alcohol-fixed tissue culture cell suspensions were processed according to the usual procedure for making a smear from a patient's specimen (Durfee, 1968). That is, the cells were pelleted by centrifugation at 2000 rpm for 15 min. and four to six smears were made from the pellet on albuminized microscopic slides. These slides were then postfixed in 80% EtOH before Papanicolaou stain or air dried prior to staining with hematoxylin and eosin. Extra smears for use with special stains were retained in alcohol prior to use.

3. *Results and Discussion*

It is readily apparent from the figures that this technique of Papanicolaou staining a smear of an alcohol-fixed suspension of a trypsinized monolayer.

TABLE 4
Preparation of EA 65[a]

Eosin Y	10 g
Bismark brown Y	10 g
Light green SF	10 g
Distilled water	300 ml
95% ethyl alcohol	2000 ml
Phosphotungstic acid	4 g
Saturated lithium carbonate solution in distilled water	20 drops

Procedure

1. Stock solution No. 1: 10 Eosin Y in 100 ml distilled water.
2. Stock solution No. 2: 10 g Bismark brown Y in 100 ml distilled water.
3. Stock solution No. 3: 10 g Light-green SF in 100 ml distilled water.
4. Mix 50 ml stock solution No. 1 with 10 ml stock solution No. 2 and add 5.5 ml stock solution No. 3.
5. Take mixture up to 2000 ml with 95% ethyl alcohol.
6. Add 4 g phosphotungstic acid.
7. Add 20 drops saturated lithium carbonate solution. Mix well and store in dark-brown bottles.
8. Filter before using.

[a] Adapted from Koss (1968) by permission of Lippincott Co., Philadelphia, Pa. The necessary dyes may be purchased from National Aniline Division, Allied Chemical and Dye Company, New York, N.Y.

FIG. 1 (a) WI-38 embryonic lung fibroblasts (Hayflick and Moorhead, 1961) fixed while growing as a monolayer. These uniform spindly fibroblasts with regular oval nuclei exhibit the well-known morphology of benign fibroblasts. Papanicolaou stain. ×460. (b) WI-38 fibroblasts in a smear prepared from a trypsinized suspension of a monolayer culture. The fibroblasts have round, well-outlined cytoplasm. The nuclei are displaced in the cytoplasm and they are oval or semilunar in shape. Note the tendency to form small loose clusters and the uniform small size of the cells. Papanicolaou stain. ×460.

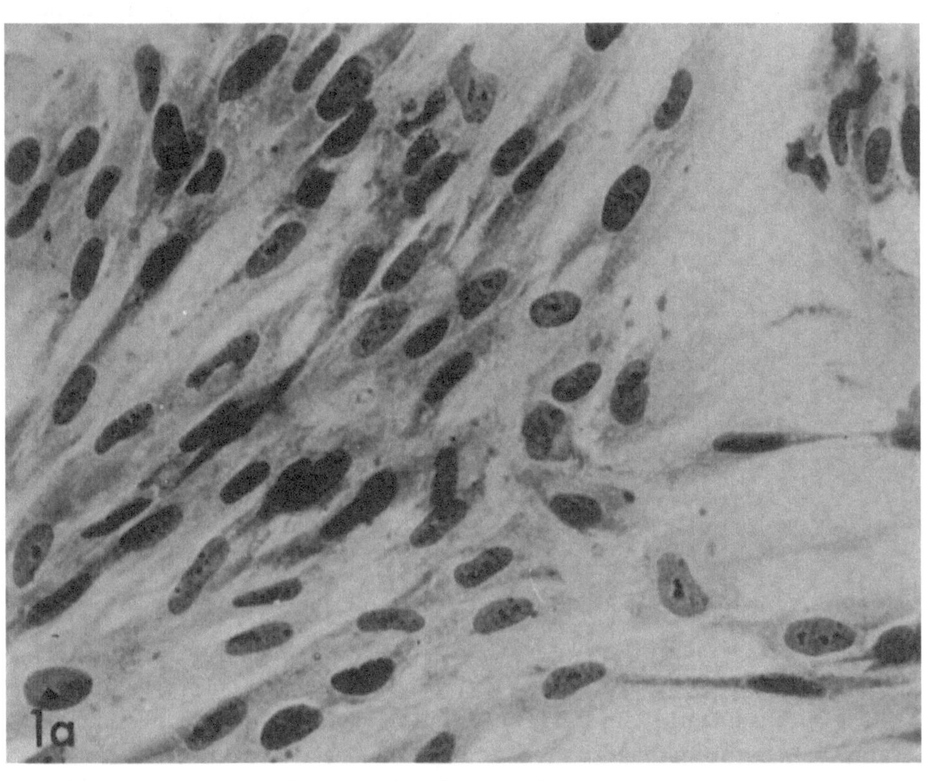
1a

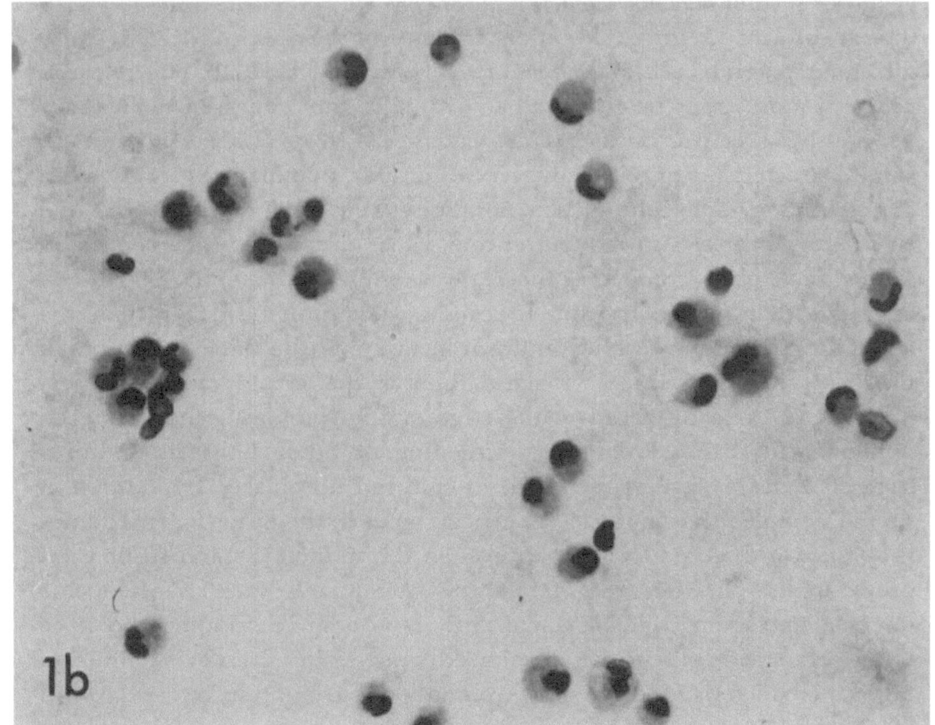
1b

TABLE 5

Staining Process for Air-Dried Smears with Hematoxylin and Eosin

Step	Time
1. Absolute alcohol	1 min
2. 95% alcohol	1 min
3. Tapwater	few dips
4. Harris's hematoxylin	2 min
5. Tapwater	few dips
6. 0.2% ammonium hydroxide	1–2 dips
7. Distilled water	few dips
8. Eosin	30 sec
9. Tapwater	few dips
10. 95% alcohol	few dips
11. 95% alcohol	few dips
12. Absolute alcohol	few dips
13. Acetone	few dips
14. Xylol	1 min
15. Mount in Permount	

culture results in a preparation for cytological examination which is considerably different from that usually examined. We feel that it is of considerable value for several reasons. Detachment of cells from the substrate on which they are attached reduces alterations in shape of the cell produced by those attachments (Hlinka and Sanders, 1972; Lerch *et al.*, 1970). The released cells can more easily be evaluated according to the criteria of malignancy previously developed on *in vivo* exfoliated cells (Koss, 1968). In addition, some characteristics of cells in this type of preparation may be very useful in distinguishing tissue culture cell types. For example, Fig. 1 shows the same culture of fibroblasts in monolayer and smear preparation, Papanicolaou stained, and photographed at the same magnification (×460). The difference is striking. The trypsinized cells appear much smaller than the adherent cells and are rather uniform in size, and the nucleus occupies a unique position within the cytoplasm. That is, the darkly stained uniform nuclei tend to be displaced to the edge of the cytoplasm and many are semilunar in shape. Preliminary screening of other fibroblast cultures suggests that this is a characteristic of cultured fibroblasts. In addition, it should be noted that most neoplastic cell types in the other figures do not show such a discrepancy in size between the monolayer and suspension preparations. On the other hand, the tumor cells such as osteogenic sarcoma, melanoma, glioblastoma, and some adenocarcinomas do have some very small cells in the trypsinized smears; in addition to differing nuclear characteristics, they show tremendous variation in cell size within the same smear.

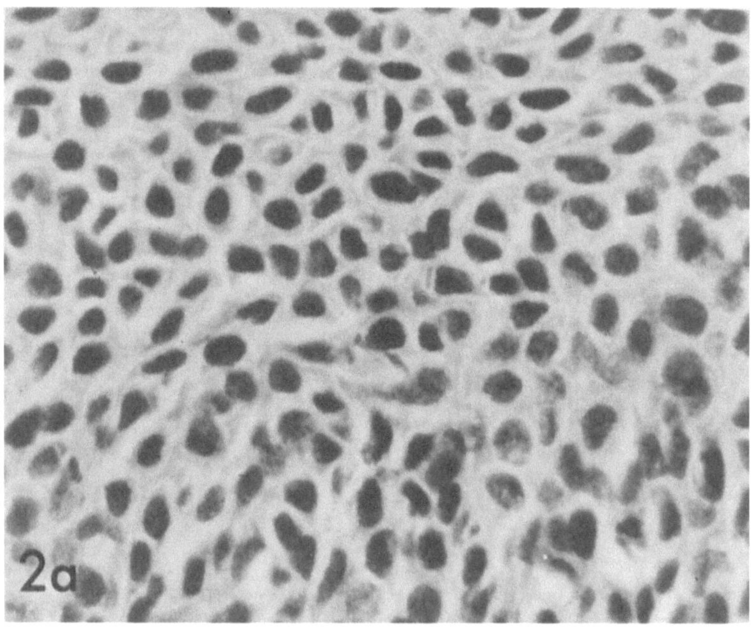

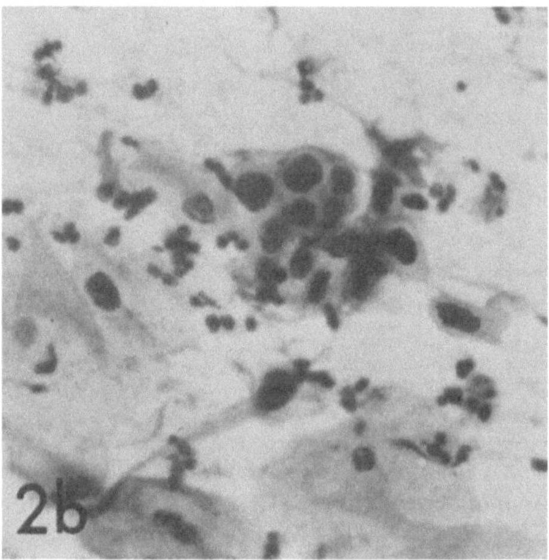

FIG. 2. *Malignant Epithelial Tumors (Carcinoma), Epidermoid Derivation* (a) Epidermoid carcinoma *in situ.* Tissue section prepared from cervical biopsy specimen of a 29-yr-old patient. After formalin fixation and paraffin embedding, a 6-μm section was cut with a microtome and stained with hematoxylin and eosin. The entire thickness of the epithelium is shown and is replaced by hyperchromatic and pleomorphic, mostly ovoid cancer cells. However, there are many elongated spindle cells. The cytoplasm is scanty and not well preserved. There is an alteration in the nuclear-cytoplasmic ratio in favor of the nucleus. Hematoxylin and eosin. ×380 (b) Epidermoid carcinoma *in situ.* A vaginal smear from the same patient as in Fig. 1a obtained prior to biopsy of the cervix. There are hyperchromatic and pleomorphic epidermoid tumor cells as they usually appear in a Papanicolaou-stained smear. Note five benign epithelial cells adjacent to the cluster of cancer cells. In the background are numerous inflammatory cells, mainly polymorphonuclear leukocytes. Papanicolaou stain. ×380.

FIG. 3. *Malignant Epithelial Tumors, Epidermoid Derivation* (a) 9812 bronchogenic carcinoma cells (Aaronson *et al.*, 1970) in monolayer culture. There are oval and spindle cells growing in a tight mosaic pattern. There is evidence of cell-to-cell contact and areas of overgrowth indicating some loss of contact inhibition. Mono- or multinucleated giant cells were rarely seen in smears of tumor cells of epidermoid derivation. Similarly, tumor cells in mitosis were observed only occasionally. Papanicolaou stain. ×380. (b,c,d,e) Papanicolaou smear of trypsinized monolayer cultures of epidermoid carcinoma cells [b; 9812; c, HT-3, cervical cancer (J. Fogh, Chapter 5); d,e, Chelo-1 alveolar cell cancer of the lung (R. E. Coalson and R. E. Nordquist, Chapter 5)]. There are sharply outlined nuclear and cytoplasmic membranes. The tumor cells are hyperchromatic and round or oval with little variation in size and shape. The nuclear–cytoplasmic ratio is increased in favor of the nucleus. These cells show a striking similarity to the tumor cells illustrated in Fig. 2a,b. There is a marked morphological difference, on the other hand, between these smears and the monolayer preparations in (a) and (f). Papanicolaou stain. ×460. (f) Monolayer culture of Chelo-1 alveolar cell carcinoma cells of the lung. These are fairly uniform elongated spindle cells. Note the few double and multinucleated tumor cells. (The morphology of the same tumor cells is shown in (d) and (e) in a Papanicolaou smear of the trypsinized suspension.) Papanicolaou stain. ×380.

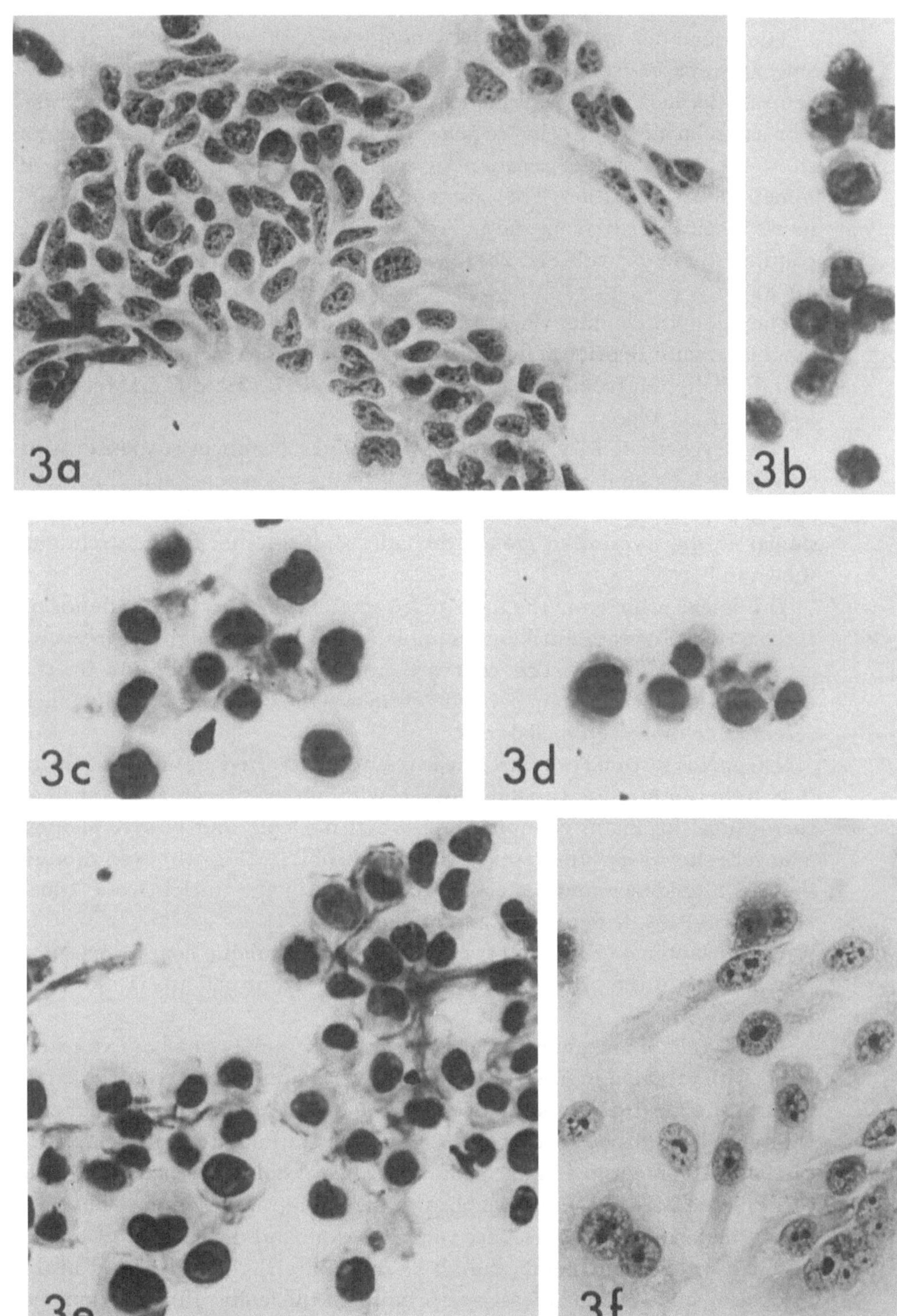
3a
3b
3c
3d
3e
3f

The squamous epithelial derived neoplastic cultures (Figs. 2 and 3) in smears prepared from suspensions of trypsinized monolayer cultures show centrally located nuclei with increased nuclear–cytoplasmic ratio and nuclear irregularities. The cells are generally larger than fibroblasts and do not show the considerable variation in cell size seen in the tumor cells of nonepithelial derivation. They also appear very similar to the cells in fixed tissue taken directly from the patient (compare Fig. 3b–e with Fig. 2b in contrast to Fig. 3a with Fig. 2b) (Spjut *et al.*, 1955; Wied *et al.*, 1962; Koss, 1968).

The adenocarcinomas (Figs. 4 and 5) prepared by trypsinization of the monolayer culture prior to fixation also bear a striking resemblance to tissue examined directly from the patient (Rosen *et al.*, 1972; Hajdu and Melamed, 1973, Zajicek, 1965).

That trypsinization of the monolayer culture produces suspensions of cells which look similar to cells normally growing in suspension is illustrated by Fig. 4c, which is a smear of a suspension culture of breast cancer. It is similar to the trypsinized monolayer culture of another adenocarcinoma shown in Fig. 5d.

The smear made from the trypsinized monolayer of a colonic adenocarcinoma (Fig. 5b) bears a striking resemblance to what one might see in *in vivo* cytology (Koss, 1968). The cells are not completely separated by the trypsinization and maintain papillary clusters. One can easily see cells which resemble columnar epithelial cells.

Osteogenic sarcoma cells in a smear from a trypsinized monolayer culture (Fig. 6) have a striking variability in size with nuclear irregularities such as furrowing, chromatin clumping, abnormal nucleoli, and bizarre shapes. The cells show very little resemblance to fibroblasts (Fig. 1b) even though there is a tendency towards eccentric position of the nuclei (Koss, 1968; Hajdu and Koss, 1969; Hajdu and Melamed, 1971).

The melanomas (Figs. 7–9) prepared by this technique bear a very close resemblance to the cytology of exfoliated cells from patients (Hajdu and Savino, 1973).

Tumor cells of malignant melanoma can be extremely small or extremely large, with variation in size from a few to several hundred micrometers. It is not unusual for the cytoplasm of the cell to be abundant and pleomorphic with a tendency to be round or oval. Occasional granular deposits of melanin can be clearly identified in the cytoplasm. Special stains, for example, ferric ferricyanide stain, make the pale brown melanin granules intense blue.

The majority of the nuclei are round or oval, and the cells have sharply outlined cytoplasmic membranes. The nuclei are slightly displaced in the cytoplasm, and contain at least one prominent nucleolus. Binucleation and multinucleation are common features. Cells in mitosis are not uncommon nor are intranuclear vacuoles of cytoplasmic contents (Figs. 7a, 8a, and 9b).

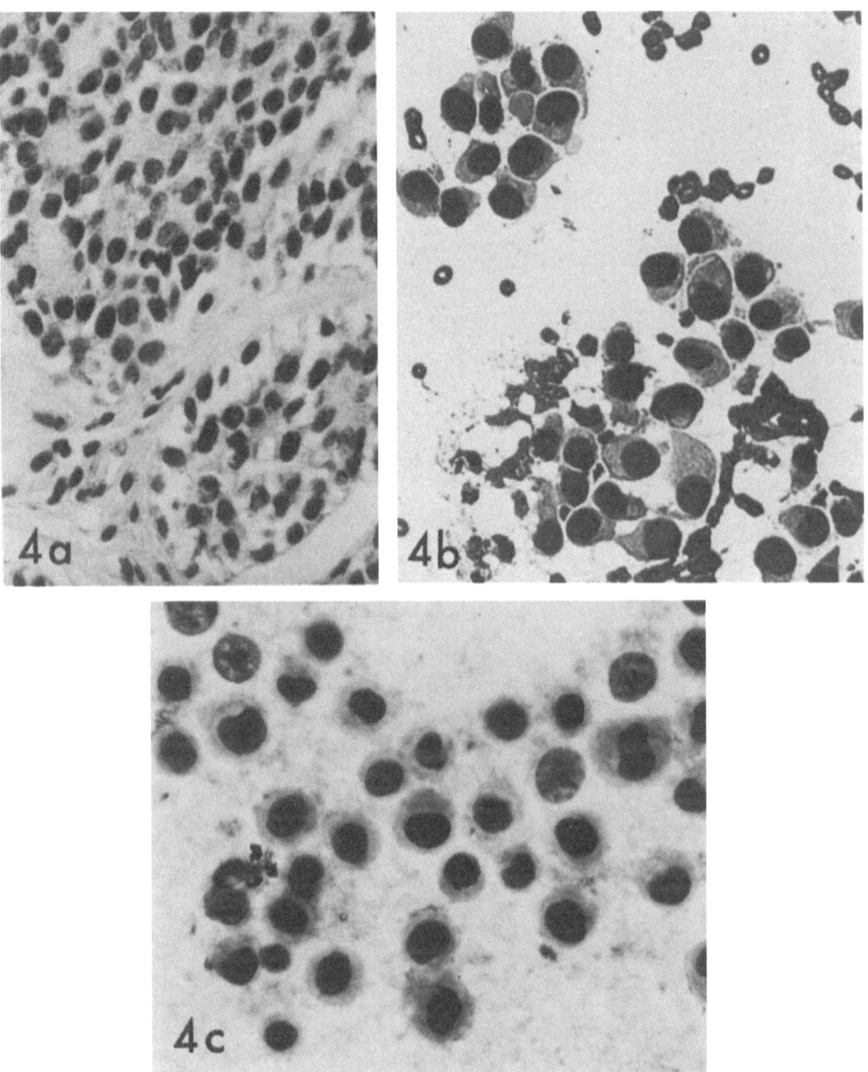

FIG. 4. *Malignant Epithelial Tumors, Adenocarcinoma* (a) Tissue section of a biopsy specimen of a mammary carcinoma. Hematoxyline and eosin. ×250. (b). Air-dried smear prepared from an aspiration biopsy of a mammary carcinoma. There are hyperchromatic round or oval cells, single and in clusters. There is significant variation in the size of nuclei and amount of cytoplasm. The nuclei are uniformly dark, and the cytoplasm is sharply demarcated because there was no fixative used. Hematoxylin and eosin. ×460. (c) Hematoxylin and eosin stained smear prepared from nontrypsinized suspension culture of SK-BR-1 mammary carcinoma cells (Giraldo *et al.*, 1971). The tumor cells smear out singly with ill-defined cytoplasm. There is marked nuclear pleomorphism, but there is no tendency to form spindle or elongated cells. The tumor cells are mostly ovoid or round in shape. Note the marked similarity to the tumor cells in the aspiration smear (b). Papanicolaou stain. ×460.

FIG. 5. *Malignant Epithelial Tumors, Adenocarcinoma.* (a) Monolayer culture of SW-48C, colonic adenocarcinoma cells (Leibovitz *et al.*, 1973). The tumor cells exhibit a strong tendency to grow in clusters or in nests. The nuclei are round or oval with one or two prominent nucleoli. Numerous cells could be observed in mitosis. Papanicolaou stain. ×460. (b) Smear prepared from a suspension of trypsinized cells from a monolayer culture of SW-48C. The cells tend to cluster even after trypsinization. There are well-preserved glandular and papillary clusters of round or oval, hyperchromatic tumor cells. A few large mononuclear cells had cytoplasmic vacuoles. These were positive with mucicarmine stain. Papanicolaou stain. ×460. (c) SK-OV-1 adenocarcinoma cells in monolayer culture (G. Trempe and L. J. Old, Chapter 5). The tumor cells are in pairs or single. There are numerous double nucleated cells. Two or more prominent nucleoli are easily visible, and there is marked nuclear pleomorphism. The cytoplasm is abundant and pleomorphic without a tendency to be elongated. Papanicolaou stain. ×460. (d) Papanicolaou smear of SK-OV-1 adenocarcinoma cells prepared from a suspension of a trypsinized monolayer culture. Note the marked variation of the size of darkly stained, hyperchromatic nuclei. The shape of the nuclei and cytoplasm is uniformly oval, which is in contrast to the polymorphic cytoplasm seen in monolayer (c). Papanicolaou stain. ×460.

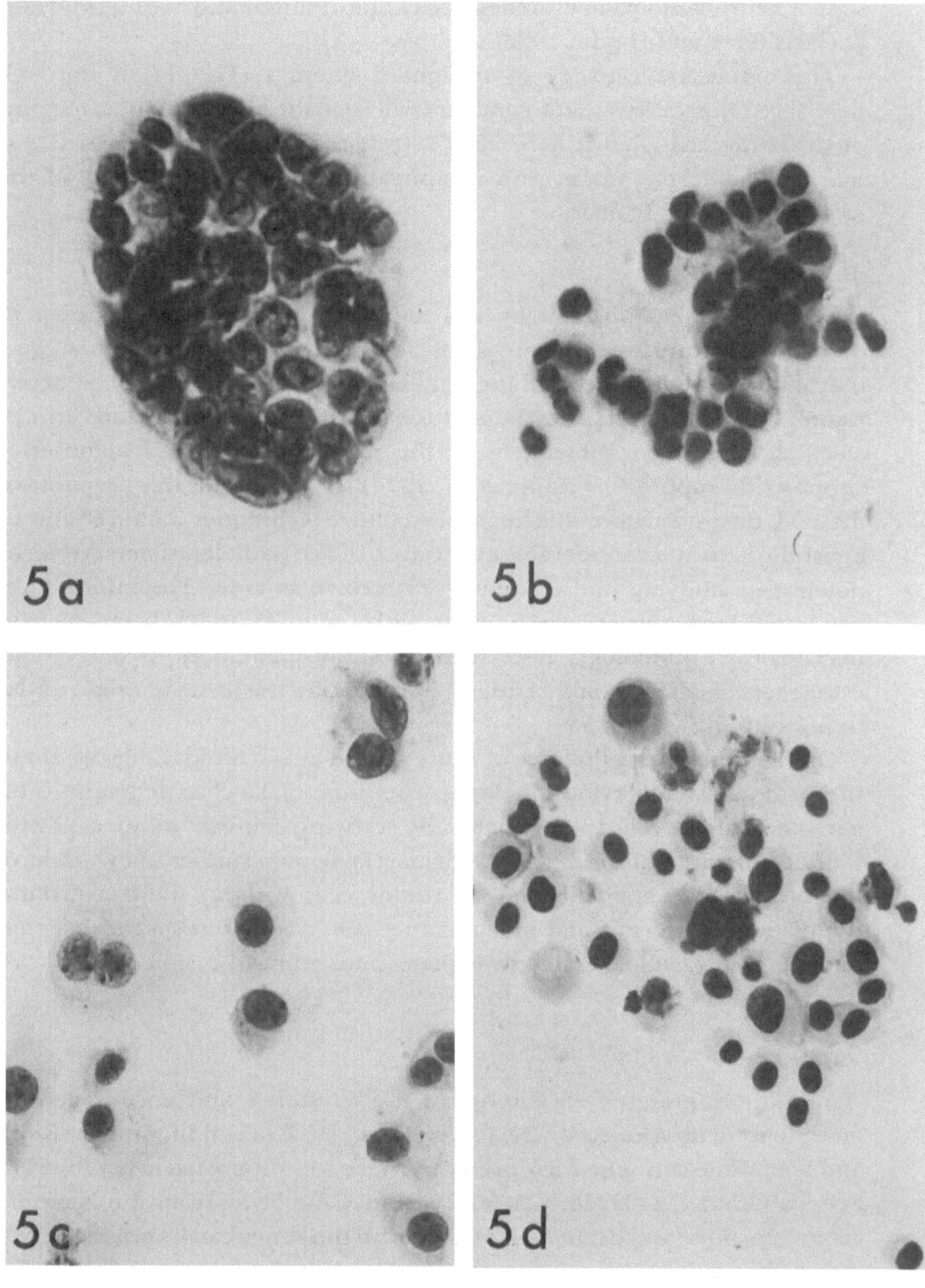
5a
5b
5c
5d

The exfoliative cytology of neuroblastoma (Fig. 10) is well illustrated by the somewhat pleomorphic spindle and round cells in monolayer culture which round up in the trypsinized suspension smear and even tend to form so-called rosettes, which are well known to the pathologist as a diagnostic sign of neuroblastoma in histological sections of tumor and body fluids from patients (Farr and Hajdu, 1972).

The exfoliative cytology of malignant gliomas (Fig. 11) is not well described (Koss, 1968). Little comment will be made here other than to point out that the cells shown here have a tremendous variability in size and markedly abnormal nuclei with an appearance somewhat like that of the melanomas and sarcomas.

4. Conclusion

Based on our examination by this technique of tumor cells grown in monolayer culture, we feel there is sufficient preliminary evidence to suggest that this technique will contribute significantly to the cytological characterization and identification of human tumor cells. Additional study of cell cultures performed subsequent to the preparation of this manuscript supports this approach (Hajdu *et al.*, 1974). By the use of this preparative method, the investigator utilizing tissue culture techniques should be able to enlist the help and considerable experience of the pathologist and cytotechnologist in studying human tumor cells grown *in vitro*. The information generated from this approach, along with the information from electron microscopy, enzymology, histochemistry, transplantation, serology, and cytogenetic studies, should be useful in validating the tissue of origin of the tumor cells grown *in vitro*.

On the other hand, this type of study should be of considerable benefit to the pathologist and cytotechnologist who must make clinical diagnosis on exfoliated tumor cells from patients. By studying cultured tumor cells with well-documented histories and confirmatory *in vitro* studies, they will have the benefit of examination of the tumor cells without the background populations of normal and inflammatory cells present in specimens from patients and should be able to expand and refine the subtle criteria of diagnostic cytology.

ACKNOWLEDGMENTS

The authors gratefully acknowledge the assistance and encouragement given to us in this project by Dr. Jørgen Fogh, Dr. Eva Hajdu, Andrew Ricci, and Maia Newman. The work presented here was supported in part by PHS Service Grant CA–08748, CA–05110, and CA–05826 from the National Cancer Institute and Grant No. IM 26A from the American Cancer Society.

(References follow on p. 358.)

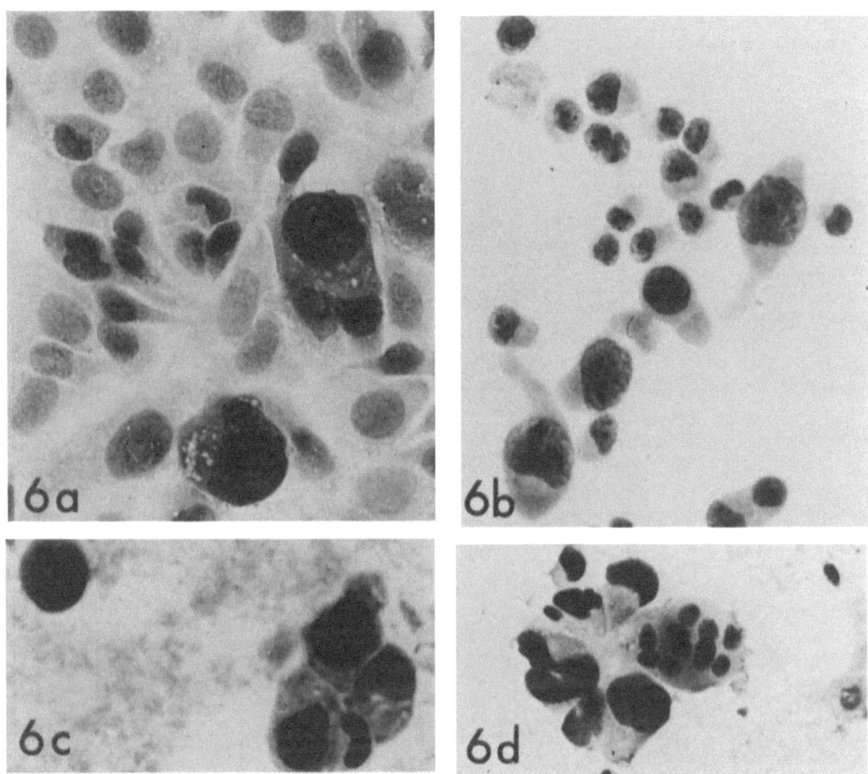

FIG. 6. *Nonepithelial Malignant Tumors, Osteogenic Sarcoma* (a) Air-dried slide of 2 T osteogenic sarcoma cells in monolayer culture (Pontén and Saksela, 1967). Numerous spindly and bizarre ovoid giant cells are present in tight clusters. The prominent nucleoli and the granular cytoplasm of the tumor cells are visible. Papanicolaou stain. ×460. (b) Smear prepared from a suspension of the trypsinized monolayer culture of 2 T cells. Here the tumor cells appear as elongated spindle cells and small round cells. Note the extreme variation in size of the tumor cells and the numerous folds or indentations of the nuclear membranes. Papanicolaou stain. ×460. (c) Alcohol-fixed smear prepared from a suspension of a trypsinized monolayer culture of 2 T osteogenic sarcoma cells and stained with hematoxylin and eosin. There is a tight cluster of peculiarly shaped cancer cells. Here again the coarsely granular cytoplasm is well demonstrated. Hematoxylin and eosin. ×460. (d) Air-dried smear prepared from an aspiration biopsy of the tibia of a 12-year-old boy with osteogenic sarcoma. There is a striking similarity between this and (c). It is of interest that the so-called epulis type of multinucleated giant cells, commonly seen in tissue sections and in aspiration biopsies of osteogenic sarcomes, were not observed in any of the cultures we examined. One of these multinucleated cells is clearly visible in this figure. Hematoxylin and eosin. ×460.

FIG. 7. ***Nonepithelial Malignant Tumors, Malignant Melanoma*** (a) Histological section of malignant melanoma excised from the skin of a patient. Note the extreme variation in the size and shape of these cancer cells. Binucleated and multinucleated tumor cells are very common. Note the intranuclear vacuoles consisting of cytoplasmic contents. Hematoxylin and eosin. ×380. (b,c) Malignant melanoma in a smear prepared from a pleural effusion of a patient with disseminated malignant melanoma. The exfoliated tumor cells appear similar to the tumor cells seen in the tissue section (a). Papanicolaou stain. b, ×380; c, ×460. (d) Malignant melanoma in a smear prepared from an effusion of a patient and stained with ferric ferricyanide, melanin stain. The intracytoplasmic granules are melanin pigment. ×580.

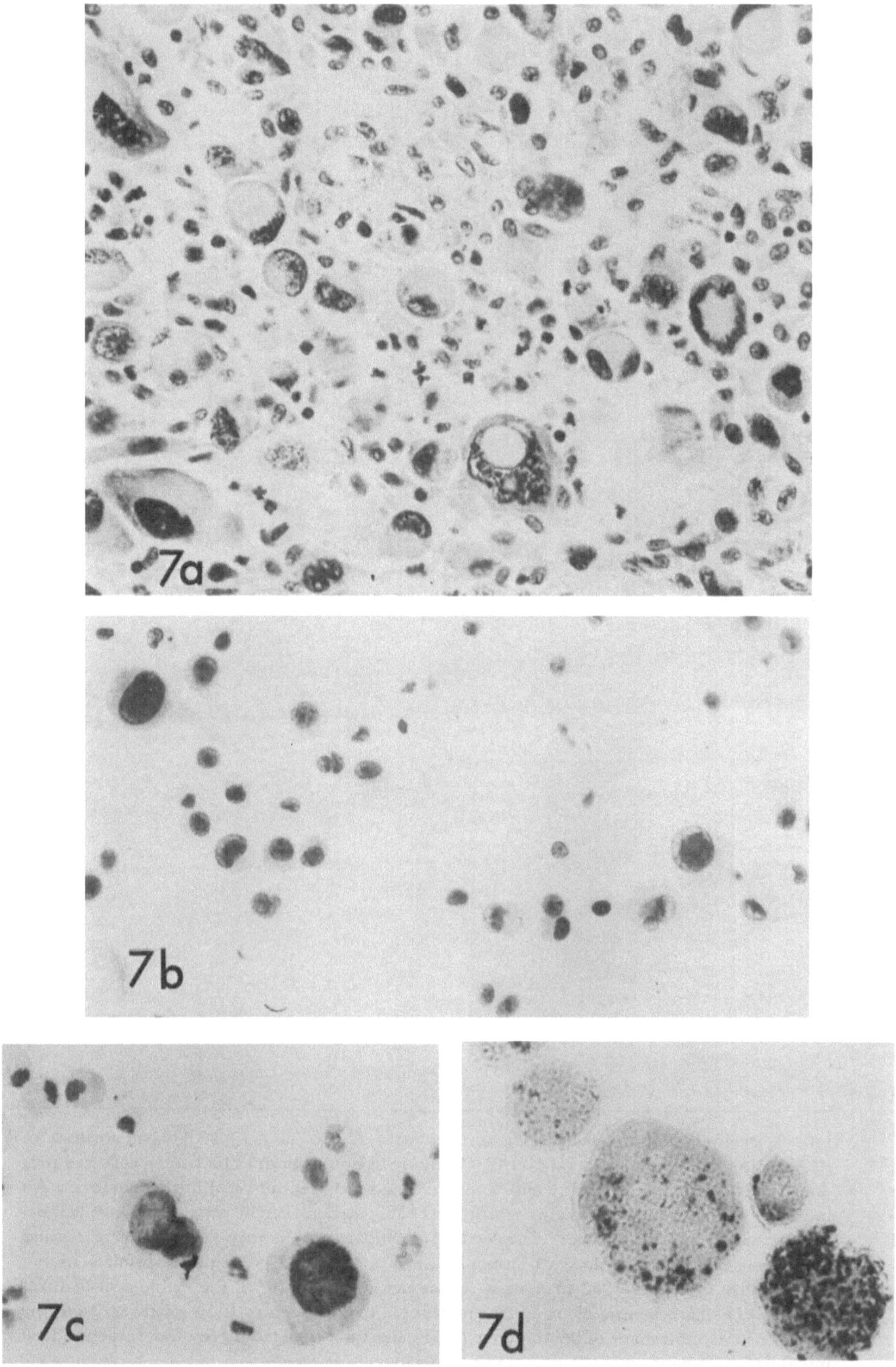

7a

7b

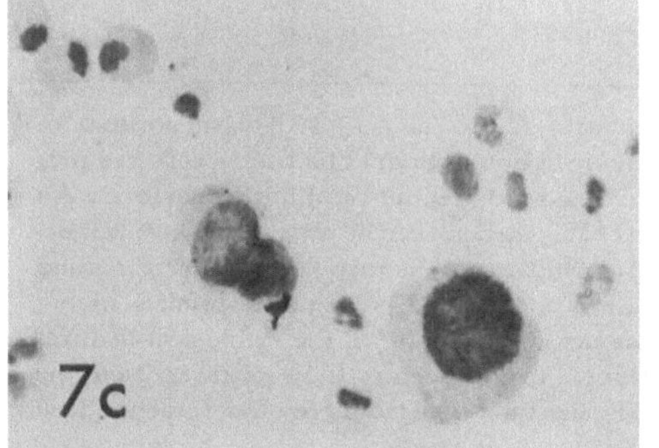

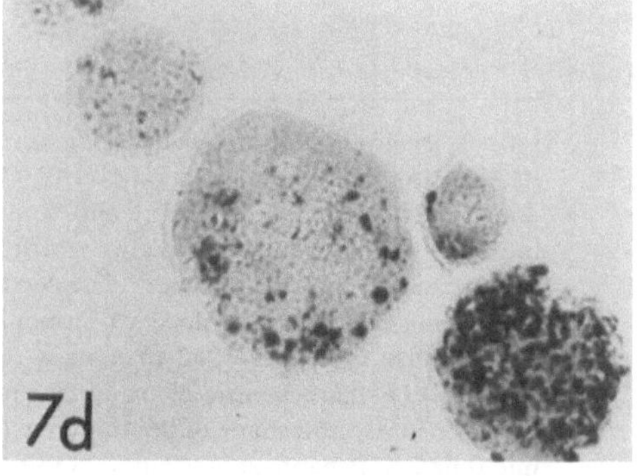

FIG. 8. *Nonepithelial Malignant Tumors, Malignant Melanoma* (a,b) Monolayer culture of RPMI–8252 malignant melanoma cells (G. Moore, unpublished). The tumor cells are predominantly spindly or polyhedral and mononucleated with frequent multinucleated forms. An intracytoplasmic granular substance which is probably melanin can be seen. Note the intranuclear vacuole in one of the cancer cells in (a) and its similarity to the vacuoles seen in Figs. 7a and 9b. Papanicolaou stain. ×460. (c,d) Tumor cells in a smear prepared from a trypsinized monolayer culture of RPMI–8252 malignant melanoma cells. Almost all the cytological features known to be characteristic of malignant melanoma can be seen in these pictures. Note the variation in size and shape of the tumor cells. The size can range from a few to several hundred micrometers. Papanicolaou stain. c; ×380; d, ×460.

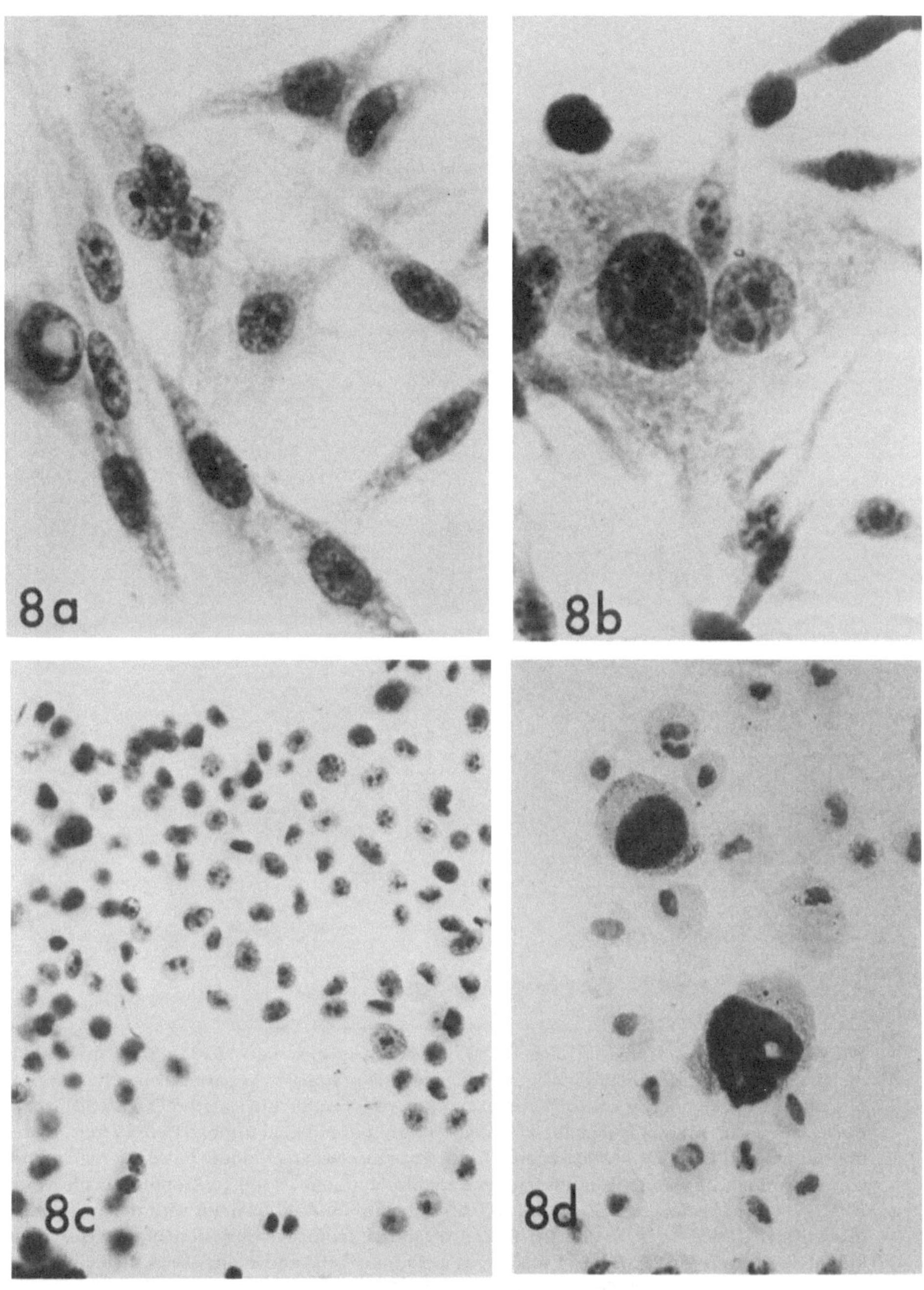
8a
8b
8c
8d

FIG. 9. *Nonepithelial Malignant Tumors, Malignant Melanoma* (a,b) RPMI–8072 malignant melanoma cells (G. Moore, unpublished) in Papanicolaou smears prepared from a suspension of a trypsinized monolayer culture. There are numerous double nucleated cells with displaced nuclei, a feature commonly seen in exfoliated cells of nonepithelial tumors. Cells in mitosis are not common findings in smears prepared by the Papanicolaou technique; however, melanoma is an exception with frequent mitotic figures. Papanicolaou stain. ×460. (c) Monolayer culture of RPMI–7931 malignant melanoma cells (G. Moore, unpublished) stained with melanin stain. Ferric ferricyanide stain. ×460. (d) Smear prepared from a suspension of a trypsinized monolayer culture of RPMI–7931 malignant melanoma cells and stained with melanin stain. Compare this with Fig. 7d. Ferric ferricyanide. ×460.

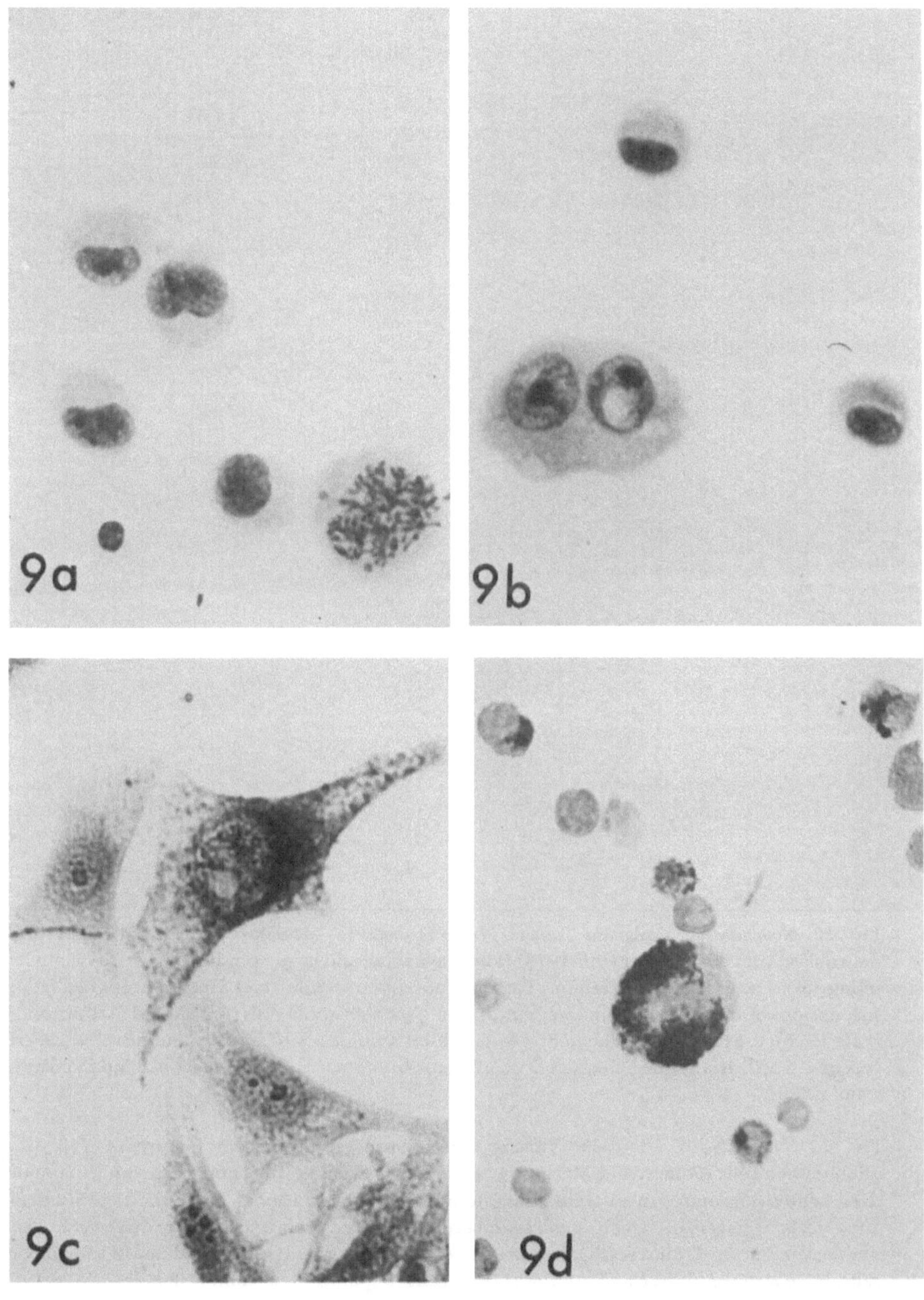
9a
9b
9c
9d

FIG. 10. *Nonepithelial Malignant Tumors, Neuroblastoma.* (a) Monolayer culture of SK–N–MC neuroblastoma cells (Biedler *et al.*, 1973). There are small and large spindle cells with oval nuclei piling up in a disorganized fashion. Papanicolaou stain. ×380. (b,c) Smears prepared from suspensions of trypsinized monolayer cultures of neuroblastoma cells [b, IMR–32 (Tumilowicz *et al.*, 1970); c, SK–N–MC]. The neuroblasts exhibit a tendency to form round nests, so-called rosettes, which is a known characteristic of neuroblastomas in tissue sections. Papanicolaou stain. ×380.

FIG. 11. *Nonepithelial Malignant Tumors, Glioblastoma* (a) Monolayer culture of 118 MG glioblastoma cells (Pontén and Macintyre, 1968). The extreme variation in size and shape of these tumor cells makes them quite similar to melanoma cells. Papanicolaou stain. ×380. (b,c) Papanicolaou smears of 118 MG glioblastoma cells prepared from a suspension of a trypsinized monolayer culture. Of interest again is the extreme variation in the size and shape of the cancer cells. Note also the bizarre and multinucleated cells. Papanicolaou stain. ×380.

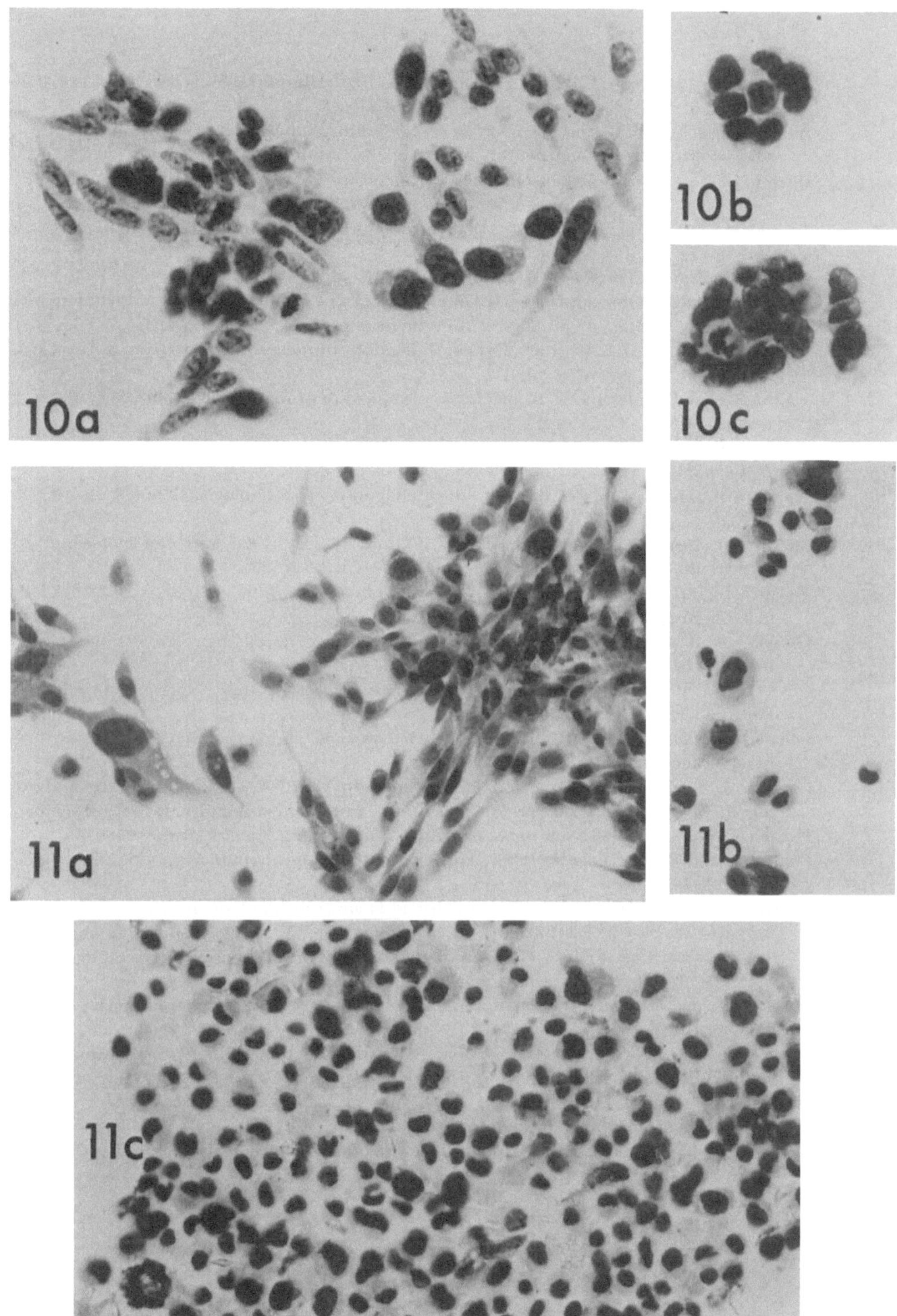
10a
10b
10c
11a
11b
11c

5. References

Aaronson, S. A., Todaro, G. J., and Freeman, A. E., 1970, Human sarcoma cells in culture, *Exp. Cell Res.* **61**:1.

Biedler, J. L., Helson, L., and Spengler, B. A., 1973, Morphology and growth, tumorigenicity, and cytogenetics of human neuroblastoma cells in continuous culture, *Cancer Res.* **33**:2643.

Durfee, G. R., 1968, Cytologic techniques, in: *Diagnostic Cytology and Its Histopathologic Bases*, 2nd ed. (L. G. Koss, ed.), pp. 597–628, Lippincott, Philadelphia.

Farr, G. H., and Hadju, S. I., 1972, Exfoliative cytology of metastatic neuroblastoma, *Acta Cytol.* **16**:203.

Giraldo, G., Beth, E., Hirshaut, Y., Aoki, T., Old, L. J., Boyse, E. A., and Chopra, H. C., 1971, Human sarcomas in culture: Foci of altered cells and a common antigen; induction of foci and antigen in human fibroblast cultures by filtrates, *J. Exp. Med.* **133**:454.

Hajdu, S. I., and Koss, L. G., 1969, Cytologic diagnosis of metastatic myosarcoma, *Acta Cytol.* **13**:545.

Hajdu, S. I., and Merlamed, M. R., 1971, Needle biopsy of primary bone tumors, *Surg. Gynecol. Obstet.* **133**:829.

Hajdu, S. I., and Melamed, M. R., 1973, The diagnostic value of aspiration smears, *Am. J. Clin. Pathol.* **59**:350.

Hajdu, S. I., and Savino, A., 1973, Cytologic diagnosis of malignant melanoma, *Acta Cytol.* **17**:320.

Hajdu, S. I., Bean, M. A., Fogh, J., Hajdu, E. O., and Ricci, A., 1974, Morphology of cultured human tumor cells in Papanicolaou smear, *Acta Cytol.* **18**:327.

Hayflick, L., and Moorhead, P. S., 1961, The serial cultivation of human diploid cell strains, *Exp. Cell Res.* **25**:585.

Hlinka, J., and Sanders, F. K., 1972, Real and reflected images of cells in profile. I. A method for the study of cell movement and adhesion, *J. Cell Sci.* **11**:221.

Koss, L. G., 1968, *Diagnostic Cytology and Its Histopathologic Bases*, 2nd ed., Lippincott, Philadelphia.

Leibovitz, A., McCombs, W. B., Johnston, D., McCoy, C. E., and Stinson, J. C., 1973, Two new human cancer cell lines, *in vitro* **8**:433.

Lerch, V. L., Todd, J., Lattimer, J. K., and Tannenbaum, M., 1970, A technique for the study of human prostatic epithelial cells *in vitro* by time-lapse cinematography, *J. Urol.* **104**:564.

Papanicolaou, G. N., 1942, New procedure for staining vaginal smears, *Science* **95**:438.

Pontén, J., and Macintyre, E. H., 1968, Long term culture of normal and neoplastic human glia, *Acta Pathol. Microbiol. Scand.* **74**:465.

Pontén, J., and Saksela, E., 1967, Two established *in vitro* cell lines from human mesenchymal tumours, *Internat. J. Cancer.* **2**:434.

Rosen, P., Hajdu, S. I., Robbins, G. F., and Foote, F. W., 1972, Diagnosis of carcinoma of the breast by aspiration biopsy, *Surg. gynecol. Obstet.* **134**:837.

Spjut, H. J., Fier, D. J., and Ackerman, L. V., 1955, Exfoliative cytology and pulmonary cancer, *J. Thorac. Surg.* **30**:90.

Tumilowicz, J. J., Nichols, W. W., Cholon, J. J., and Greene, A. E., 1970, Definition of a continuous human cell line derived from neuroblastoma. *Cancer Res.* **30**:2110.

Wied, G. L., Legoretta, G., Mohr, D., and Rauzy, A., 1962, Cytology of invasive cervical carcinoma and carcinoma *in situ*, *Ann. N.Y. Acad. Sci.* **97**:759.

Zajicek, J., 1965, Sampling of cells from human tumors by aspiration biopsy for diagnosis and research, *Eur. J. Cancer* **1**:253.

Chromosome Abnormalities in Human Tumor Cells in Culture

13

JUNE L. BIEDLER

1. *Introduction*

1.1. *Some Questions*

The ever-increasing availability of human tumor lines in continuous culture poses questions of pertinence to those interested in chromosomes of cancer cells as well as to those interested in the biology of cancer in a more general way. A cursory glance at reports detailing the establishment *in vitro* of a tumor line reveals that many include karyotype analysis. A simple but central question is, therefore, Is knowledge of the chromosome constitution of the cultured cells useful? That question can be answered intuitively with a yes, or otherwise, it could be said, chromosomal analysis would not be so frequently utilized as an ancillary descriptive method. However, it is possible that cytogeneticists are rather like squirrels who instinctively collect and store away acorns, sometimes for others eventually to retrieve and to make use of ineffectually if at all. Alternatively, the objectives of chromosome analysis of tumor cell cultures may be quite clear in the mind of the initiator. Whichever is the prevailing approach, it appears worthwhile to elaborate and to consider some possible objectives of chromosome studies of human tumor cells *in vitro*.

JUNE L. BIEDLER Memorial Sloan-Kettering Cancer Center, New York

The hope that many continuous cell lines established in culture from a wide variety of solid tumors of man would become available for investigative purposes is turning inexorably into reality. One of the first questions asked by anyone with some experience in the culturing of cells and in analyzing the chromosomes of cancer cells is, Is the karyotype abnormal? Lurking even deeper than sheer interest may be a suspicion that the cells are not the putative tumor cells at all, but rather normal stromal cells or even a ubiquitous cell contaminant. Despite an assumption on the part of some investigators that a unique, abnormal chromosome constitution is a rather reliable indicator of the tumor origin of the cells growing *in vitro*, there are others who are cautious about arriving at such a conclusion. An essential question thus is, Does an abnormal karyotype, when observed in human cells in culture, denote a malignant tumor cell? Although it may not be possible to arrive at a definitive and final answer, there are now an adequate number of published reports to permit assessment.

There are several additional considerations of relevance to chromosome characterization of tumor cells *in vitro*. It can be asked, Of what significance is the type or extent of chromosomal abnormality to the expression of the malignant phenotype of cells in culture? This is a difficult question to answer. There may be no (discernible) relationship between karyotype and malignant behavior of cultivated cells, but the possibility is to be dealt with. A less esoteric question and one of practical import is, With what degree of confidence may we assume that the chromosome constitution manifested *in vitro* represents that of the tumor in its host environment?

The aim in this chapter is to evaluate the use of karyotype analysis in determining the origin of putative human tumor cells in culture, i.e., whether derived from normal or malignant tissue, as well as in gaining fundamental knowledge in cancer biology.

1.2. Scope

It is well known that solid tumors are generally refractory to standard methods of metaphase chromosome preparation both because of the technical difficulties attendant on the mechanical separation of cells for adequate fixation and spreading and because of the paucity of mitotic cells relative to the numbers to be found in more freely associating cell populations such as malignant effusions and leukemias. Thus culture techniques are sometimes employed in order to enhance the number of dividing cells. Short-term culture, usually carried out over a period of about 4 h to 7 days, may be distinguished from long-term culture, which refers to cells maintained for several months or more, although sometimes with few intervening culture transfers. The latter group is comprised of diploid strains which appear to have a finite life span *in vitro* and tumor cell populations which cease to proliferate after a number of months without obvious reason. In a third, unique category, then, are continuous cell lines which have the capacity to proliferate indefinitely in the *in vitro* environment.

This discussion will be concerned primarily with karyological observations of apparently permanent *in vitro* cell populations derived from primary or metastatic solid tumors (carcinomas, sarcomas, melanomas, and neuroblastomas) and, more rarely, from cancerous effusions. Cell lines deriving from other types of malignancies such as leukemia, lymphoma, and Hodgkin's disease are not included here. Published reports dating from about 1960 are generally more useful than earlier ones, in large part because of advances in cytological techniques and standardization of chromosome analysis. Thus tumor cell lines may be characterized by kind and extent of numerical and structural chromosome abnormality and, where possible, by degree of stability of karyotype with time in culture. As with *in vivo* tumor cell populations, most lines appear to be composed of cells with predominating chromosome numbers that sometimes form sharp modes and sometimes fall within a range loosely termed "modal."

The chromosome constitution of all of the tumor lines included in the present survey has been analyzed by the now "conventional" methods of fixation and staining, whereby metaphase chromosomes are arranged according to a classification codified at several conferences on human cytogenetics (e.g., Chicago Conference, 1966). The "newer" banding methods for chromosome individualization (Paris Conference, 1972) await application to a vast number of malignant populations including human tumor lines *in vitro*.

2. *Early Studies of Human Tumor Lines*

Probably the earliest established human tumor line on record is the now famous and infamous HeLa, derived from a cervical adenocarcinoma (Gey *et al.*, 1952). It is believed to have been a ubiquitous contaminant or unwitting substitute for variously designated cultured cells in many laboratories throughout the world. Early chromosomal studies of this line (Hsu, 1945*a*; Hsu and Moorhead, 1957; Chu and Giles, 1958) revealed a wide range of chromosome numbers from about 71 to 90, with hypotetraploid modes (Table 1). In addition, several derived clonal lines, each generally showing a narrower range, taken together had an even greater span of chromosome numbers (Puck and Fisher, 1956; Chu and Giles,

TABLE 1

Modal Chromosome Numbers of Some Human Tumor Lines Established in Continuous Culture in 1951–1955

Cell line designation	Date established *in vitro*	Modal chromosome numbers	Reference for chromosome study
HeLa	1951	80–90	Hsu (1954*a*)
		80–84	Chu and Giles (1958)
HEp-2	1952	77	Norryd and Fjelde (1963)
HEp-1	1953	72	Norryd (1959)
Maben	1953	82[a]	Hsu and Moorhead (1957)
KB	1954	83[a]	Hsu and Moorhead (1957)
HEp-3	1954	68–71	Levan (1956)
HS-1	1955?	49–51	Levan (1956), Miles (1965)

[a]Number represents mean chromosome number rather than modal number.

1958). Thus the idea that tumor lines in continuous culture show extensive aneuploidy and wide karyotypic variation was introduced early. This idea appears to have grown into an erroneous generality that should, in specific instances, be discarded. At that time, the concept of marker chromosomes as distinctive, structurally abnormal chromosomes which may be a stable feature of a tumor cell population and may therefore have a fingerprint function had not yet evolved. It is remarkable that careful enumeration of chromosomes and some degree of karyotype analysis could be reported in those years, 1954–1958, when it is considered that the diploid number for man was not corrected from 48 to 46 until 1956 (Tjio and Levan, 1956; Ford and Hamerton, 1956). In further confirmation of the wide variation of chromosome numbers of HeLa are the results of a much later study of seven lines from different sources (Bottomley *et al.*, 1969). Modal numbers ranged from 65 to 81, approximately, and there were some differences as well in distribution of chromosome types and of markers. However, as Bottomley *et al.*, discuss, certain clones had sharp modal numbers which remained stable for at least 6 months of subculturing. Similarly, Chu and Giles (1958) and Vogt (1959) reported that several clones had sharp modes, while Spurna and Hill (1966) described a line of HeLa numerically stable for 7 months. Although Hsu (1961), in an extensive and illuminating review, emphasized the alterability of chromosome constitution of tumor cells in culture, he also noted the striking homogeneity of certain clonal lines of HeLa. An important conclusion, and one that emerges also from a survey of published reports of human tumor lines, was that "Some genomes are more stable than others."

The value of cell culturing methods for study of karyotypes of human tumors was early recognized by Dr. Hsu. Short-term cultures giving good yields of metaphase cells were established from a liposarcoma with a reported mode of 70 and from a metastatic melanoma with a "dipoid" mode (Hsu, 1954*b*). However, at that time the diploid chromosome number was still believed to be 48. In the following year came a report of new, permanent human tumor lines established in culture in the laboratory of Dr. Alice E. Moore at the Sloan-Kettering Institute (Moore *et al.*, 1955; Fjelde, 1955) from tumors first grown in conditioned rats (Toolan, 1954). Several of these lines, HEp-1, HEp-2, HEp-3, and HS-1, are listed in Table 1, as are also the line Maben, established by Frisch *et al.* (1955) from a lung adenocarcinoma, and the KB line, established by Eagle (1955) from an epidermoid carcinoma. With the clear exception of the HS-1 tumor line, modal chromosome numbers were generally in the hypertriploid–hypotetraploid range. Based on these findings as well as on studies of the extensively heteroploid lines obtained as the result of culturing normal tissues, it was considered that the heteroploidy (which in the 1950s generally meant hypotriploidy to hypotetraploidy) exhibited by fast-growing cell lines was due to its selective advantage under conditions of culture.

3. Normal Human Cells in Culture

During the earlier period of cultivation of human tumor lines, starting with HeLa and including those listed in Table 1, establishment of continuous lines from normal human tissues was reported by a number of workers in the field. Again, the lines were found to be heteroploid, in the sense of having hypotriploid to hypotetraploid modes or multiples thereof. Since the now prevailing doubt about the origin of many of these cell lines may becloud results of karyotypic and other studies of more recently established tumor lines, it seems of value to review attempts to establish permanent lines of diploid cells.

3.1. Stability of the Diploid Karyotype

In studies carried out by T. T. Puck and his associates (Tjio and Puck, 1958; Puck *et al.*, 1958), cells with fibroblast-like morphology were cultivated from various tissues of normal human subjects and could be maintained for at least 5 to about 9 months. It was stated that for seven different strains chromosome counting and analysis of more than 2000 cells revealed a chromosome number of 46, except for a small proportion of polyploid cells. Exact counts and karyotype analyses of 13 of 25 strains cultured from fetal tissues were reported by Hayflick and Moorhead (1961). The level of aneuploidy was low and could be ascribed to technical artifact. The level of tetraploidy was also low, ranging from 1.2 to 6.4%. Similarly, retention of a diploid chromosome complement in normal fibroblast-like cells *in vitro* has been demonstrated by others (Chu and Giles, 1959; Makino *et al.*, 1962). As discussed by Hayflick (1965), the diploid karyotype of human fibroblasts in cell culture appears to be stable during the period of active growth. A notable example is the widely utilized WI-38 strain. Aneuploidy and other aberrations occur chiefly in phase III, the degenerative phase of normal cell cultures. For example, in a chromosome study of two human cell strains carried out through the entire period of cultivation *in vitro*, aneuploid changes and chromosome breaks and rearrangements occurred only during decline of proliferative capacity (Saksela and Moorhead, 1963). Heteroploid transformation was not observed even though nonproliferative cultures were carefully maintained for 1–3 months following cessation of growth. Thus from these studies it is clear that the chromosome constitution of fibroblastic cells, at least, is remarkably stable even in long-term cultures. Furthermore, spontaneous transformation, in the sense of either heteroploid (i.e., chromosomal), morphological, or malignant, resulting in an established line did not occur in the studies described.

Of pertinence to the question of spontaneous conversion of normal to continuously growing cells are the results of *in vitro* studies with oncogenic viruses. It has been known since the early 1960s that SV40 virus could induce morphological transformation of human fibroblast-like cells (Shein and Enders, 1962; Koprowski *et al.*, 1962). Rapid transformation of WI-26 and WI-38 cultures approaching the end of their expected *in vitro* lifetime was noted by Jensen *et al.* (1963), and apparently pure cultures of transformed cells were obtained. One substrain was observed to have a high frequency of dicentrics, minutes, and other obvious chromosome changes, which did not appear until 4 wk after morphological transformation.

It was later demonstrated that permanent cell lines could be readily obtained by SV40 infection of diploid fibroblasts, which resulted in increase of proliferative capacity of a small number of cells (Girardi *et al.*, 1965). About 2 wk to 5 months was required for recovery after crisis. At this stage, there was increase in chromosome breakage and tetraploidy and alteration of cell morphology, with eventual establishment of a highly mixoploid cell line (Weinstein and Moorhead, 1967). Most studies have been directed toward relating chromosomal alteration to the transforming event. Thus chromosome analysis is generally carried out soon after viral infection, during the period when transformed cells appear, and rather soon after permanent cell lines are obtained (see reviews by Moorhead and Weinstein, 1966: Harnden, 1973). Unfortunately, there are few karyological studies of well-established SV40-transformed lines. One such permanent line exhibited a hypodiploid chromosome mode, with variable numbers and types of chromosomes (Weinstein and Moorhead, 1965). Each of four clones of the W-18VA2 line continued to exhibit instability of number and form even though infectious virus was no longer detectable. In a more recent series of investigations, established cell lines recovered from SV40-transformed human amnion cells were examined (Fogh *et al.*, 1969; Gaffney *et al.*, 1970). Two lines were hyperdiploid, while the others had hypotriploid, hypotetraploid, and near-tetraploid modal chromosome numbers in rather broad ranges. All of the lines had new chromosome varieties as well as a high frequency of cells with either acentric fragments or multicentric chromosomes, or both. A possible generalization is that transformation by SV40 results in cell lines characterized by karyotype instability. It appears, however, that there are new insights to be gained concerning the significance of chromosomal alteration to alteration of growth control as manifested both *in vitro* and *in vivo*. Considerably more persistent investigation will be required to determine whether a new chromosome constitution is specifically related to the transforming virus. For example, it was reported that adenovirus type 12 could induce focus formation in cultures of human fibroblasts (Todaro and Aaronson, 1968). Whether permanent cell lines can be established thereby and whether their karyotypes would differ in specific ways from those of SV40-transformed cells are topics for the future.

In contrast to findings with SV40-transformed populations and in keeping with observations of stability of euploid cells is the degree of karyotype stability of strains with constitutionally abnormal karyotypes (Fraccaro *et al.*, 1968). Long-term cultures with finite life spans were established from two chromosomal mosaic subjects, one with Turner's syndrome (45,X0/46,X,i(Xq)) and one with Down's syndrome (46,XX/47,XX,+G). During the period of analysis, 44–462 days, most cells of the first subject had 46 chromosomes, all of which possessed the isochromosome. In the second subject, cells with both karotypes, normal and trisomic, were in approximately equal proportion at day 124. Thus, as reviewed and discussed by these investigators, abnormal karyotypes do not necessarily predispose to instability and, more importantly, cells in long-term culture may be a true representation of the tissue of origin.

3.2. Continuous Cell Lines of Normal Tissue Origin

Among the first cell lines originating from normal human tissues were the Chang epithelial lines (Chang, 1954) and the numerous Detroit epithelial-

TABLE 2

Modal Chromosome Numbers of Some Continuous Cell Lines Established in Vitro from Nonmalignant Tissues

Cell line designation	Date established *in vitro*	Modal chromosome numbers	Reference for chromosome study
Chang liver	1954	77[a]	Hsu and Moorhead (1957)
Chang conjuctiva	1954	82[a]	Hsu and Moorhead (1957)
Detroit-98	1955	61–64	ATCC[b] (1972)
FL	1956	72–76	Petursson and Fogh (1963)
Mayes	1956	133	Hsu *et al.* (1957)
Girardi heart	1956	81	ATCC (1972)
WISH	1958	74	ATCC (1972)
MA 160	1966?	64	Fraley *et al.* (1970)

[a]Number represents mean chromosome number rather than modal number.
[b]American Type Culture Collection.

like lines described by Berman (Berman and Stulberg, 1956; Berman *et al.*, 1957). Several representative lines are listed in Table 2, with reference to sources of modal chromosome number determination. The Chang and Detroit lines as well as the cell lines described by Syverton and McLaren (1956) were also analyzed by others (Levan, 1956; Syverton, 1957; Ruddle *et al.*, 1958). The remarkable findings at that time were the degree of departure from diploidy and the epithelioid morphology of cells arising even from initially fibroblastic cultures. Several other early lines are listed in Table 2. The FL line was established from human amnion cells (Fogh and Lund, 1957). Strain Mayes showed both morphological transformation from spindle-shaped to epithelioid cells and "heteroploid transformation" (Hsu *et al.*, 1957). Girardi heart (Girardi *et al.*, 1958) and WISH cells derived from human amnion tissue (Hayflick, 1961) are described by the American Type Culture Collection (1972). A more recently reported line is MA 160 derived from a benign prostatic adenoma (Fraley *et al.*, 1970).

So far, most or all of the continuous lines described as deriving from noncancerous tissue, including MA 160, show the kind of extensive heteroploidy typified by modes of approximately 60–80 or double. An obvious conclusion is that the culture environment favors selection of cells with this range of chromosome number. However, the authenticity of some of these earlier findings is under question for several reasons. As discussed by Hsu (1961), many instances of cell contamination are known, and even the "heteroploid transformation" of Mayes (Hsu *et al.*, 1957) might be an example of replacement of normal cells by invader HeLa. Fraley *et al.* (1970) have given thoughtful consideration to this possibility, with respect to MA 160 cells, although it is believed unlikely. It is noteworthy that all of the continuous lines mentioned here were described as epithelial in appearance. Several years ago Dr. S. M. Gartler shocked the tissue culture establishment by presenting biochemical evidence to suggest that some of the lines listed in Table 2 and others as well are HeLa contaminants (Gartler, 1967, 1968). He rightly pointed out that there have been very few reports of so-called spontaneously transformed human cell cultures since about 1960. However, cell contamination is unfortunately not a rare phenomenon, and awareness of it, especially in consideration of more recently established human tumor lines, should better serve to caution than to accuse. New examples of spontaneous and induced malignant transformation of normal human cells of different types are awaited with interest. Investigative effort in this direction would have fundamental and practical consequences.

4. *Human Tumor Lines, 1960 Onward*

Owing to experience that establishment of continuous lines of tumor cells in culture is not an easy task and perhaps also to an entrenched assumption that human tumor cells are apt to exhibit the extensive heteroploidy and chromosomal variability of HeLa, karyotype analysis has seldom been a primary aim of such endeavors. Many descriptions of tumor lines nevertheless include determination of chromosome constitution. There are by now a sufficient number of descriptions in the literature for evaluation of trends with respect to the chromosome complements of human tumor lines and their stability during prolonged cultivation *in vitro*. However, there are still too few data to be able to discern patterns relating to tumor type or site. A still small group of neuroblastoma lines with near-diploid karyotypes may serve to exemplify some potentialities of the cytogenetics of human tumor cells in culture.

4.1. *Survey of Chromosome Characteristics*

An extensive but not exhaustive survey of tumor cell lines whose karyotypes are adequately described in published reports is presented chronologically in Table 3. Not included in this list of 34 lines are nine of various types established at Roswell Park Memorial Institute (Ishihara *et al.*, 1962; Moore and Koike, 1964), seven melanoma lines established at M. D. Anderson Hospital and Tumor Institute (Romsdahl and Hsu, 1967, 1972), and several neuroblastoma lines to be discussed separately.

Perhaps the first report in the decade of the 1960s, marking renewed interest and success in obtaining continuously growing human tumor cells, is

TABLE 3

Survey of Modal Chromosome Numbers and Presence of Consistent Abnormal Chromosomes in Some Human Tumor Cell Lines Established in Continuous Culture, 1960–1973

Cell line designation	Diagnosis and/or source	Modal chromosome numbers	Consistent chromosome markers	Reference
MAC-21	Mucoid lung adenocarcinoma	79[a]	?	Cailleau (1960)
L-16	Carcinoma of liver	63[a]	?	Chen *et al.*(1962)
Bl-II	Papilloma of bladder	78	?	Norrby *et al* (1962)
C3-II	Carcinoma of cervix	78	?	Norrby *et al* (1962)
CaMa	Mammary	62	?	Dobrynin (1963)
CaVe	Gastric carcinoma	58,60	Yes	Ugryumov and Tsoneva—Maneva (1963)
C-4 I and II	Invasive cervical carcinoma	44,45	Yes	Auersperg (1964)
C-33 I and II	Invasive cervical carcinoma	44–47	Yes	Auersperg (1964)
C-27	Invasive cervical carcinoma	43,44 73,74	Yes	Auersperg (1964)
RPMI-2650	Anaplastic squamous cell carcinoma	46	Yes	Moore and Sandberg (1964) Moorhead (1965)
C-12 I and II	Invasive cervical carcinoma	120–130 85–90	Yes	Auersperg (1966)
CM	Metastatic clear-cell carcinoma	69	Yes	Ishii and Nishimura (1966)
—[b]	Anaplastic thyroid carcinoma	77–92	Yes	Jones *et al.* (1967)
2 T	Osteogenic sarcoma	34–37 64–67	Yes	Pontén and Sassela (1967)
4 T	Synovioma	72–85	Yes	Pontén and Sassela (1967)
—	Rhabdomyosarcoma	56–57	Yes	White and Cox (1967)
PS	Thyroid cancer; pleural fluid	95–103	?	Hirose (1968)
TR	Thyroid cancer; pleural fluid	93,98	?	Hirose (1968)
TS	Thyroid cancer; pleural fluid	65,66	?	Hirose (1968)
BeWo	Choriocarcinoma	86	?	Pattillo and Gey (1968)

TABLE 3—(*cont'd*)

Cell line designation	Diagnosis and/or source	Modal chromosome numbers	Consistent chromosome markers	Reference
RD-1	Pelvic rhabdo-myosarcoma	51	Yes	McAllister *et al.* (1969)
RD-2	Pelvic rhabdo-myosarcoma	47–49	Yes	Nelson-Rees *et al.* (1972)
Det. 562	Adenocarcinoma of throat; pleural fluid	64–65	Yes	Peterson *et al.* (1970)
—	Transitional cell tumor of bladder	48	No	Rigby and Franks (1970)
ME-180	Metastatic cervical carcinoma	Subtriploid	No	Sykes *et al.* (1970)
Nagoya-78	Mixed tumor of salivary gland	62–65	Yes	Kondo *et al.* (1971)
MT	Osteosarcoma	58–65	?	McAllister *et al.* (1971)
OAT	Oat-cell lung carcinoma	47	Yes	Oboshi *et al.* (1971)
HBT-3	Breast adeno-carcinoma	65–70	Yes	Bassin *et al.* (1972)
—	Mixed parotid tumor	66	Yes	Duran-Troise and DeLustig (1972)
HEC-1	Endometrial adeno-carcinoma	47	Yes	Kuramoto *et al.* (1972)
T 187	Osteogenic sarcoma	56,110	?	Maunoury *et al.* (1972)
T_2	Neurofibro-sarcoma	100–103	Yes	Trujillo *et al.* (1972)
HBT-39	Ductal cell breast carcinoma	62–64	Yes	Plata *et al.* (1973)

[a]Number represents mean chromosome number rather than modal number.
[b]No designation given in cited report.

that by Cailleau (1960). A feature of the MAC-21 line as well as of those described in years immediately following is a hypotriploid–hypotetraploid modal or mean chromosome number. Norrby *et al.* (1962) point out that 78 (see Table 3) is a stemline number which recurs in clonal lines of HeLa as well. The intention here is not to dwell on the ubiquity of HeLa but rather to pause by the formerly entrenched idea that all human cells in culture are destined for extensive heteroploidy. Although the HS-1 line (Levan, 1956) was already a clear if little noted exception, a turning point was the description of epithelial cell cultures, obtained from invasive cervical carcinomas, which maintained hypodiploidy up to at least 33 months of cultivation (Auersperg and Hawryluk, 1962; Auersperg, 1964). Thus extensive heteroploidy was clearly demonstrated to be neither a prerequisite nor a necessary consequence of *in vitro* cultivation of human cells. The near-diploid or hyperdiploid chromosome numbers of the approximately six other lines also listed in Table 3 support this observation. Until many more lines are available for study, this is perhaps the single most important conclusion to be drawn from karyotype analyses of human tumor cells *in vitro*.

4.2. *In Vitro Stability of Tumor Cell Karyotype*

There are a sufficient number of published studies to enable some assessment of the stability of the chromosome constitution of tumor cells with time in culture. Whereas most of the tumor lines have been characterized in a single examination, there are several that have been carefully followed during prolonged cultivation *in vitro*.

The epithelioid cell line RPMI-2650, examined on several occasions during the period of a year, showed little deviation from a mode of 46 (Moore and Sandberg, 1964). Initially thought to have a normal karyotype, it was reexamined after more than 2 yr in culture (Moorhead, 1965). At least one distinctly abnormal chromosome and a sharp mode at 46 indicated that it was a remarkably stable line with a pseudodiploid karyotype. Ishii and Nishimura (1966) found that approximately 40% of their CM cells had a chromosome number of 69 within a fairly narrow range, in six determinations from 239 to 433 days of cultivation. In almost all cells, three distinctive marker chromosomes were present. The epithelial-like tumor line described by Rigby and Franks (1970) showed a sharp mode at 48, with extra chromosomes in groups C and D persisting over a period of $2\frac{1}{2}$ yr. Similarly, there was little variation in chromosome findings at different passage levels of the Det. 562 line (Peterson *et al.*, 1970). For 2 yr, the modal numbers were 64 and 65, and close to 100% of cells contained a large subtelocentric marker chromosome. Little variation in chromosome number was noted by Duran–Troise and DeLustig (1972) for their hypotriploid line, while the HBT-39 cells described by Plata *et al.* (1973) had mostly 62–64 chromosomes during 10 months of culture. The hypodiploid tumor lines of Auersperg (1964) likewise fall into the category of stable lines with respect to numbers of chromosomes per cell. Variation was limited to a narrow range of numbers and centered around distinctive karyotypes. Thus contrary to expectations deriving from the sometimes widely divergent modal chromosome numbers of HeLa cells, in different laboratories and in different years human tumor cells may show stability with respect to number of chromosomes and persistence of marker chromosomes.

In contrast to the somewhat larger group of tumor lines with generally stable karyotypes, a few instances of numerical drift have been reported. A melanoma line, MeGo, was observed to lose its hypodiploid stemline within 3 months of propagation *in vitro*, the chromosome number becoming hypotetraploid with a range of 78–81 (Romsdahl and Hsu, 1972). Auersperg (1966) described the gradual downward drift of chromosome numbers of a pair of lines, C-12 I and C-12 II, established from a cervical carcinoma. Both cultures initially had chromosome modes of 120–130, declining gradually to 85–90 over a period of 26 months. Likewise, the rhabdomyosarcoma line of White and Cox (1967) showed a downward shift of modal chromosome number from 66–67 at 2 wk to 64 at 4 months, 57–59 at 12 months, and 56–57 at 18 months. This is one of the few studies where comparisons were made with the original tumor specimen, which had an accumulation of counts of 67 and 68. A slight increase in number of chromosomes per cell with time in culture was reported for the HBT-3 line (Bassin *et al.*, 1972), with modes at 65–66 at 21 wk, 68–69 at 25 wk, and 69–70 at 45 wk. Although marker chromosomes were consistent, there was a decrease in the proportion of marker-containing cells with passage *in vitro*. As can be seen from Table 3, most of the listed tumor lines described in sufficient detail were comprised of cells with consistent, distinctly abnormal chromosomes. However, one line appeared to have only numerical deviations (Rigby and Franks, 1970) while another, the ME-180 line, showed occasional but differing markers (Sykes *et al.*, 1970). In addition to being consistent within a population at a given time, marker chromosomes generally persisted during the period of study. As might be expected, however, published reports vary in their descriptive detail, and the stability of marker chromosomes sometimes cannot be easily assessed. In the carefully followed rhabdomyosarcoma line of White and Cox (1967), a similar set of markers was observed in cultured cells as in direct preparations of the tumor. However, these markers shifted in their distribution with time, and apparently new ones were seen after 4 months of cultivation.

Another feature of several, but not most, of the tumor lines listed in Table 3 was a moderately high frequency of cells exhibiting a variety of abnormalities such as chromosome breaks and fragmentation, dicentric and ring chromosomes, and high degree of polyploidy. In these instances, there was apt to be a wide distribution of chromosome numbers, without a sharp mode. For example, the 2 T line (Pontén and Saksela, 1967) exhibited extensive chromosome destruction, particularly at early passage levels when there was also considerable variation in number. No modal chromosome number was established for the thyroid carcinoma line of Jones *et al.* (1967), which exhibited a high frequency of cells with chromosome breaks and gaps as well as dicentric and ring chromosomes and consistent markers. Approximately 50% of metaphase cells were in the range of octaploidy or greater. The carcinoma line ME-180 is described as having chromosome numbers ranging from 48 to 130, fragmentation, dicentrics, and other inconsistent chromosome rearrangements (Sykes *et al.*, 1970). The MT cell line derived from an osteogenic sarcoma by McAllister *et al.* (1971) showed a wide variability of karyotype, also with inconsistent marker chromosomes, occasional dicentrics, and a breakage frequency of 30%.

4.3. *Neuroblastoma Cells in Continuous Culture*

An interesting group of tumor cell lines, which may facilitate correlations between karyotype and functional and behavioral aspects of the cell and which may provide useful information regarding specificity of chromosome alteration *per se* in tumor cells, is comprised of those derived from patients with neuroblastoma. Listed in Table 4 is a group of four well-established

TABLE 4

Modal Chromosome Numbers and Saturation Densities of Continuous Human Neuroblastoma Cell Lines and Diploid Fibroblast-Like Cell Strains

Cell line designation	Source	Modal chromosome numbers	Number of cells per $cm^2 \times 10^4$	Reference
IMR-32	Abdominal tumor	48,49		Tumilowicz *et al.* (1970)
SK-N-SH	Bone marrow metastasis	47	110	Spengler *et al.* (1973), Biedler *et al.* (1973*b*)
SK-N-MC	Metastatic tumor of orbit	46,47	114	Spengler *et al.* (1973), Biedler *et al.* (1973*b*)
SK-N-BE(2)	Bone marrow metastasis	44	241	Biedler *et al.* (1973*a*)
F-ECH	Mediastinal cyst	46	9	Biedler *et al.* (1973*b*)
F-LSO	Intestine	46	6	Biedler *et al.* (1973*b*)
F-TGL	Ovary	46	13	Biedler *et al.* (1973*b*)

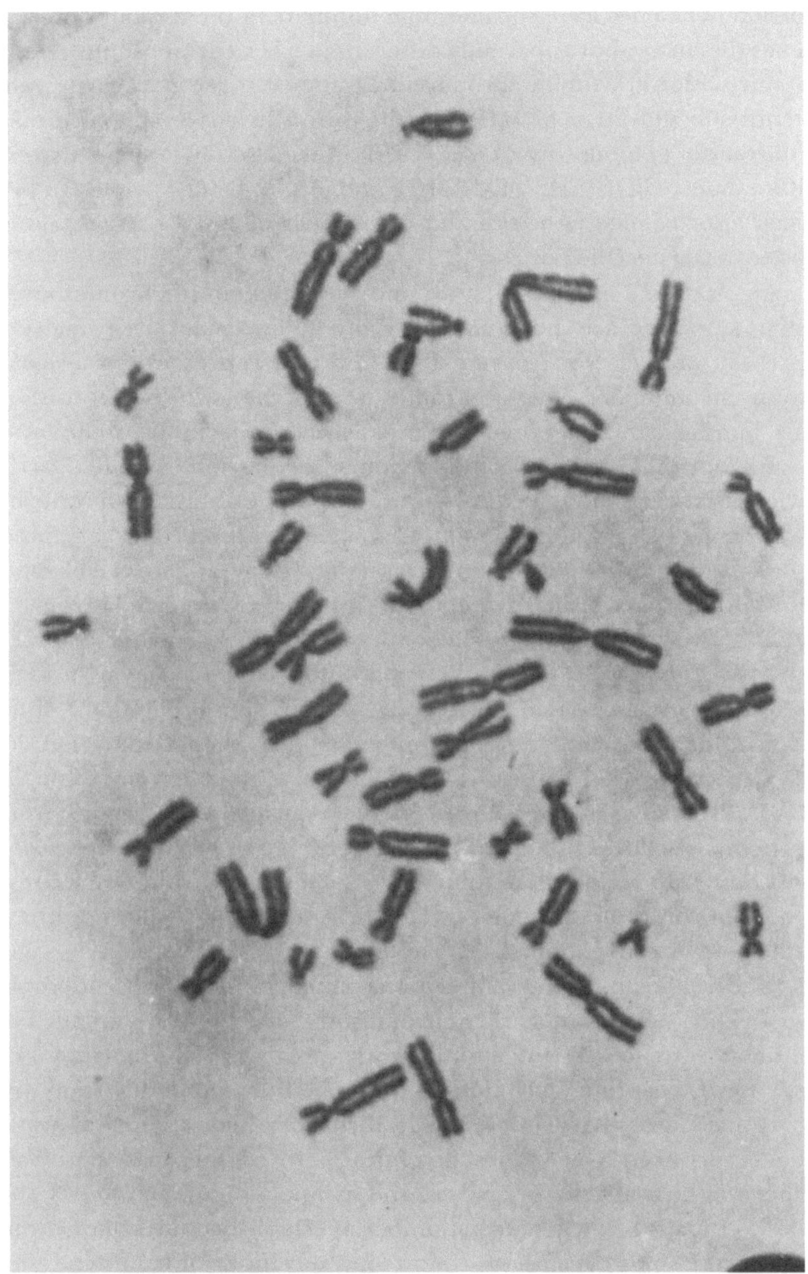

FIG. 1. A metaphase cell of the SK-N-SH neuroblastoma line.

lines whose chromosome constitution is described elsewhere and/or in this discussion. The lines have chromosome numbers in the diploid range, and each has distinctive but apparently different marker chromosomes. Despite slight fluctuation in stemline chromosome number, three markers present at the tenth subcultivation of IMR-32 cells were still observable at the 56th subcultivation (Tumilowicz *et al.*, 1970). Likewise, the Sloan-Kettering Institute lines, SK-N-SH, SK-N-MC, and SK-N-BE(2), when analyzed between approximately the 6th and 35th weeks of serial passage, showed consistent markers (Biedler *et al.*, 1973*a,b*).

A metaphase cell of SK-N-SH and the arrangement of chromosomes to reveal its karyotype are shown in Figs. 1 and 2. Two marker chromosomes are present. Marker No. 1 has satellites and may represent a translocated G-group chromosome since a chromosome of that group is consistently absent. Marker No. 2 has a secondary constriction proximal to the centromere and may thus consist of some portion of chromosome No. 1, 9, or 16. It is obvious that even though conventional karyotype analysis can contribute some information regarding identification of chromosome markers, precise assignments require newer staining techniques. A metaphase cell of subline SK-N-MC-IX, cloned from parental SK-N-MC cells, is depicted in Fig. 3. By inspection, two consistently present, abnormal chromosomes can be recognized with some ease. The karyotype of this line has been described elsewhere in greater detail (Biedler *et al.*, 1973*b*). Preliminary studies utilizing quinacrine fluorescence techniques suggest that the unusually long submetacentric marker consists in some part of a No. 3 chromosome. The SK-N-BE(2) subline likewise is characterized by an abnormally long chromosome, in this instance a subtelocentric marker (Fig. 4). A No. 1 chromosome is consistently absent in cells of this line. If the marker chromosome consists of some portion of a chromosome No. 1, as might be suspected, it is not ascertainable by conventional methodologies.

Thus nearly homogeneous populations of near-diploid or pseudodiploid cells with consistent large marker chromosomes available in virtually limitless number seem ideally suited for karyotype analysis of human tumor cells by the newer banding techniques. Minimal numerical deviation from diploidy facilitates the search for specificity of chromosomal alteration. Since it is very likely a mere question of time before additional neuroblastoma lines will be available for analysis and comparison of karyotypes, there should eventually be an adequate number of established lines of one tumor type to permit some conclusions concerning specificity of karyotype alteration. Moreover, since neuroblastoma cells have biochemical markers such as neurotransmitter-synthesizing enzymes, their origin can be ascertained. It may be questioned at this point whether the "diploid" karyotypes truly represent the tumor cells *in vivo*. It is unfortunate that for these four lines

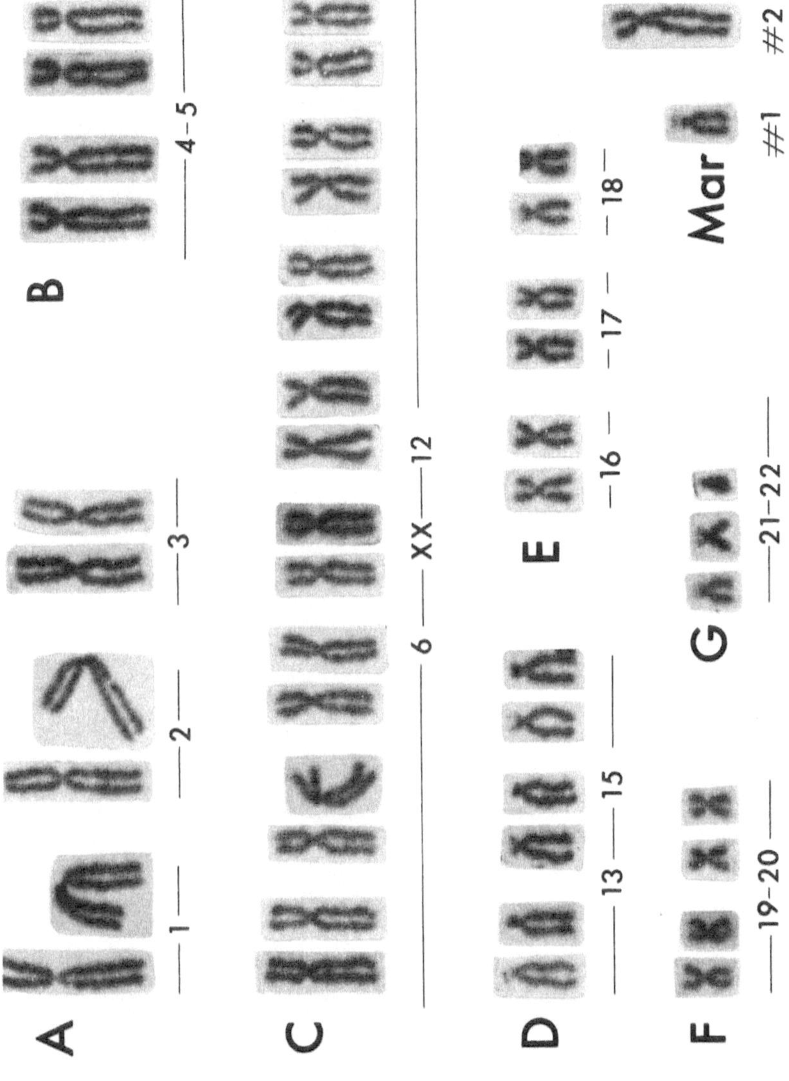

FIG. 2. Karyotype of metaphase cell depicted in Fig. 1. Marker No. 1 is probably a translocated G-group chromosome. marker No. 2 has a secondary constriction on its long arm proximal to the centromere.

direct preparations were not successful. However, from other reports it is known that neuroblastoma cells obtained from patients both before and after treatment with chemotherapeutic agents and radiation may have abnormal karyotypes with pseudodiploid or near-diploid modal chromosome numbers (Sandberg *et al.*, 1972; Wakonig–Vaartaja *et al.*, 1971; Mark, 1970; Levan *et al.*, 1968; Cox *et al.*, 1965; Makino *et al.*, 1965). Consistent marker chromosomes were detectable in tumor cells in at least five of the eight well-documented cases. It thus seems probable that the chromosome constitutions of the four established cell lines do indeed represent those of the tumor cells *in vivo.* Whether the selection pressures exerted by the explantation process and the culture environment induced further alterations is not known. Again, it would be of considerable value to have direct metaphase preparations for future comparisons with established cell lines. However, from comparisons of karyotypes of the four neuroblastoma lines with those found in the cited instances utilizing direct preparations it seems likely that the striking aberrations manifested as marker chromosomes represent those present in the tumor cells *in vivo.*

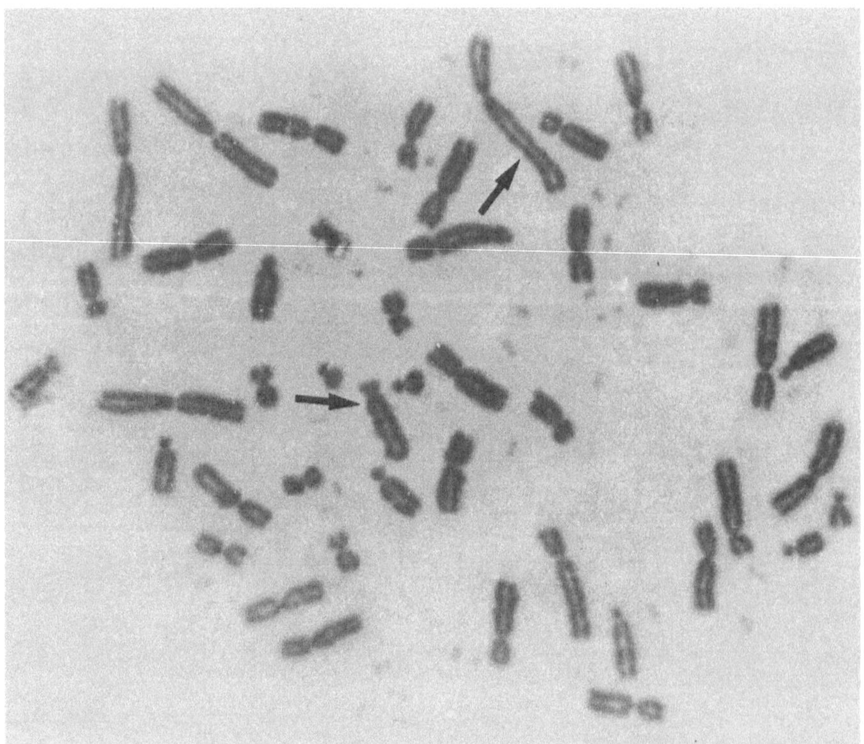

FIG. 3. Metaphase cell of subline SK-N-MC-IX, cloned from neuroblastoma line SK-N-MC. Two readily discernible marker chromosomes are indicated by arrows.

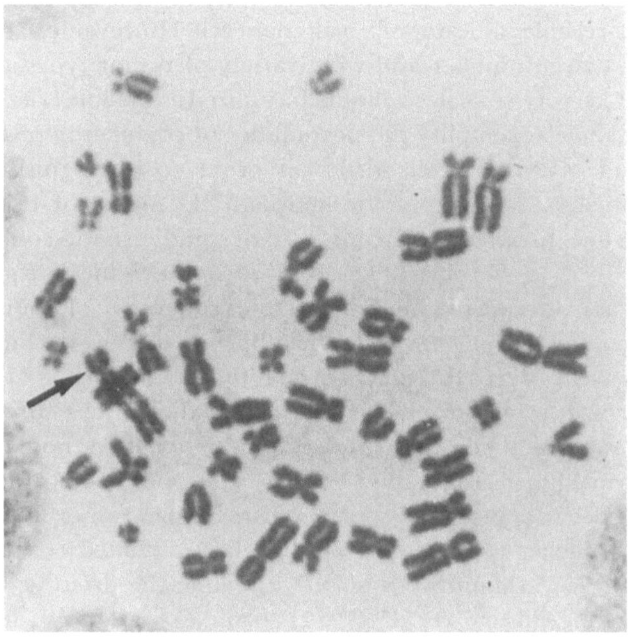

FIG. 4. Metaphase cell of neuroblastoma line SK-N-BE(2). An abnormally long subtelocentric marker is indicated by an arrow.

The usefulness of karyotype analysis for distinguishing between normal and malignant cells in culture is illustrated by the following example. In the continuing effort to derive tumor lines from patients with disseminated neuroblastoma, a line designated SK-N-WE was established. It was initially thought to be composed of neuroblastoma cells (Biedler *et al.*, 1973*a*). From several different bone marrow samples from one patient, cells which grew readily in clusters unattached to substrate were obtained. However, when the chromosome constitution of SK-N-WE cells was examined after approximately 1 year in culture, 46 apparently normal chromosomes were observed. This finding in conjunction with suspicions raised by the behavior of the cells in culture prompted investigation of immunoglobulin production. Growth medium purified 67-fold and analyzed by immunodiffusion testing was strongly positive for κ-immunoglobulin antigens and μ-immunoglobulin antigens and weakly positive for γ-immunoglobulin antigens; a low percentage of cells had κ-antigens on their surface (T. H. Hütteroth and H. Cleve, personal communication). Thus karyotypic analysis led to rectification of an erroneous identification of a lymphocyte line as a tumor cell line.

It is obviously important to differentiate between malignant and normal cells in culture by criteria other than morphological. From the evidence presented so far, it would appear that the karyotype, i.e., a grossly abnormal karyotype, is a reliable indicator of a malignant cell. However, establishment and study of a large number and wide variety of tumor types are not so advanced that karyotype analysis should be utilized as the sole criterion. The neuroblastoma lines exemplify the possibilities of correlating several morphological and growth characteristics in order to distinguish between normal and malignant cells and to pinpoint the tissue of origin. The SK-N-MC cell line, for example, is composed of spindle-shaped cells and can best be described as fibroblast-like. It does not exhibit morphological features such as extension of long cell processes suggestive of neural origin. However, when this cell line as well as the other two lines were compared to fibroblast-like cells derived from normal tissues in terms of density-dependent growth inhibition, it was found that the three neuroblastoma lines grew to saturation densities 8- to 40-fold higher than those of several putatively normal fibroblast strains (Table 4). Determinations of saturation densities have been reported for several of the human tumor lines listed in Table 3. The fibroblast-like osteosarcoma line T 187 attained a cell density of at least $10 \times 10^4/cm^2$ (Maunory *et al.*, 1972), while the osteosarcoma cells described by McAllister *et al.* (1971) had a saturation density of 14×10^4 cells/cm^2 in the 16th passage. Values of $16 \times 10^4/cm^2$ and $48 \times 10^4/cm^2$ were reported for RD-1 and RD-2, respectively (McAllister *et al.*, 1969). In none of these studies were comparisons made with normal cells under similar experimental conditions. However, an illustrative example of the value of such comparison is provided by Plata *et al.* (1973) from their experience in obtaining a cultured cell line, HBT-39, derived from human breast carcinoma. The primary culture gave rise to three proliferative populations, two epithelial-like and one fibroblast-like. Epithelial-like cells of both lines, karyotypically abnormal, grew to densities of 41×10^4 cells/cm^2, while for the fibroblast-like cells the saturation density was 8×10^4. The latter cells had a normal karyotype and were limited to 15–20 passages without occurrence of spontaneous transformation. From these few instances, it would appear that estimation of saturation density, in controlled conditions, may be a useful and technically simple method for assessing malignancy, in conjunction with karyotype analysis.

Since human neuroblastoma cells display differentiated functions concomitant with their capacity for continued proliferation, these cells may provide a means of correlation of karyotype with other phenotypic expressions. It has been found that SK-N-SH cells have elevated levels of dopamine-β-hydroxylase while SK-N-MC cells do not (Freedman *et al.*, 1973; Biedler *et al.*, 1973*b*). Similarly, the SK-N-BE(2) line shows high activity (L. S. Freedman, personal communication). However, SK-N-MC cells have high choline acetyltransferase activity, thereby distinguishing this cell line from both SK-N-SH and SK-N-BE(2) (M. Schachner, personal communication). IMR-32 cells also possess neurotransmitter-synthesizing enzyme activity (Prasad *et al.*, 1973). Similarly, the human malignant melanoma lines described by Romsdahl and Hsu (1967, 1972) appear to offer possibilities for correlations between karyotype and pigment production. However, as these investigators point out, many biochemical processes, i.e., many genes, may be involved. The genetic basis for expression of differentiated functions by malignant cells of neurogenic origin may also be highly complex. Nevertheless, karyotypically abnormal near-diploid or pseudodiploid cells which synthesize differentiated products such as pigments, hormones, or neurotransmitters may have potential for correlating karyotype and phenotype.

Finally, another type of chromosomal abnormality has been reported for tumor cells but not, to date, for normal cells. Small, paired chromatin bodies, often referred to as double-minute chromosomes, are most often found in tumors of neurogenic origin but have been described also in other types of human cancer cells. As first reported by Spriggs *et al.* (1962), and subsequently studied in greater detail by Cox *et al.* (1965), double-minute chromosomes were present in cells in the pleural fluid of a 58-yr-old patient with carcinoma of the lung. Occurrence and possible derivation of these small chromatin bodies have been discussed recently (Mark, 1970; Sandberg *et al.*, 1972). Double-minute chromosomes were also found in SK-N-MC cells (Biedler *et al.*, 1973*b*). Examples are given in Figs. 5 and 6. The metaphase cell of the clonal subline SK-N-MC-IX (Fig. 5) has more than 60 pairs of very small chromatin bodies of similar size, while another cell shows the size variation which may occur (Fig. 6). At least two additional accounts of cultured human tumor cell lines comprised of some proportion of cells with double-minute chromosomes are known (White and Cox, 1967; Jones *et al.*, 1967). Although an infrequent phenomenon, it is one which has value for distinguishing malignant from normal cells.

4.4. *Comparisons with* in Vivo *Data*

There continues to be substantial effort toward assessment of the chromosome status of the many varieties and phases of human tumors. Possible trends, patterns, specificities, and significance are the subjects of a number of helpful reviews (see, e.g., Atkin, 1973; Hamerton, 1971; Koller, 1972; Nowell, 1965; Levan, 1967, 1969; Sandberg and Hossfeld, 1970). By comparing the results of chromosome studies of human tumor lines *in vitro* with data obtained from direct chromosome preparations or short-term cultures, it may be possible to make certain inferences concerning whether the *in vitro* chromosome complement reflects that which obtained *in vivo*. A clear-cut finding for the 54 tumor lines described since 1960 and included in this discussion is that none is predominantly euploid, i.e., diploid, triploid, or tetraploid numbers and apparently normal karyotypes. A question that always intrigues cytogeneticists is whether malignant tumor cells of man can be diploid. In this consideration, as elsewhere in this discussion, leukemias and lymphoma cells are deliberately excluded. Disparity of results, owing undoubtedly to the prevailing difficulties of obtaining large numbers of photogenic metaphases, contributes to confusion in answering this question. While Sandberg and Hossfeld (1970) state that they have not observed diploid primary or metastatic tumors in their extensive studies, studies by Miles (1967*a,b*; Miles and Wolinska, 1973) of a large series of solid tumors and effusions from cancer patients give emphasis to the possible existence of diploid tumor cells.

It is informative to look at the distribution of modal chromosome numbers observed for tumor lines in continuous culture and to compare this distribution with that found for solid tumors. In Table 5, the 54 human tumor lines have been categorized according to their chromosome modes. There appear to be two major categories of tumor lines in terms of chromosome ploidy, one that is near-diploid and the other covering a wider range of modal numbers which may be designated as hypo-hypertriploid.

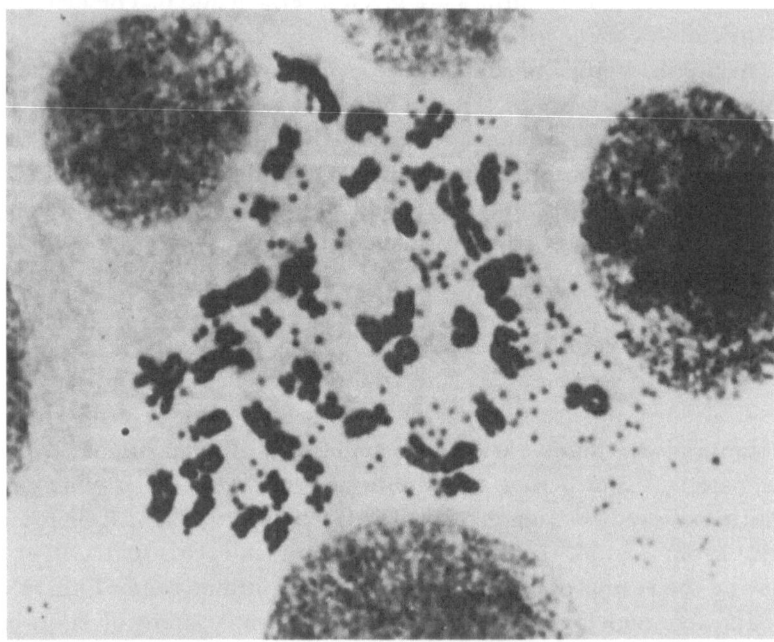

FIG. 5. An SK-N-MC-IX cell with more than 60 double-minute chromosomes. The subline had been maintained in culture for 5 months.

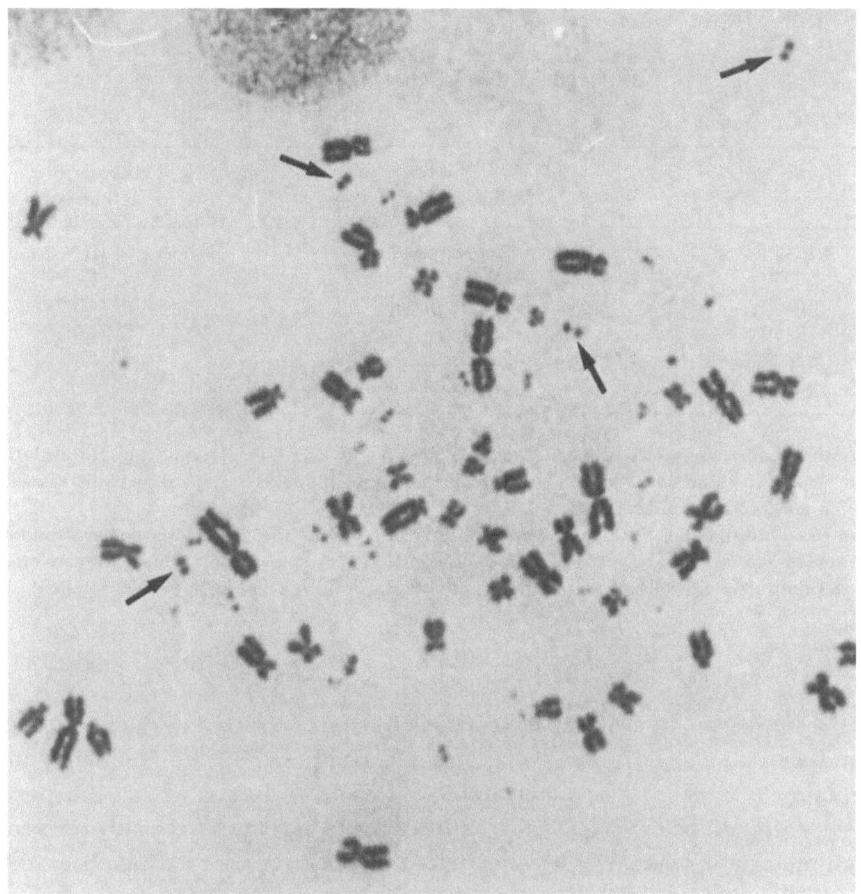

FIG. 6. An SK-N-MC-IX cell showing the size variation of double-minute chromosomes which may occur. Several of the largest pairs of chromatin bodies are indicated by arrows.

Of the 15 lines classed as near-diploid, six are hypodiploid. These findings may be compared with the distributions of modal numbers of chromosomes in 91 cases of human primary cancers reported in the literature and summarized by Yamada *et al.* (1966). Interestingly, there are points of similarity. In the latter survey, 61% of tumors were "diploid" (modal chromosome numbers of 40–57), 28% "triploid" (modal numbers of 58–80), and 11% "tetraploid" (modal numbers of 81–103). With the only slightly different modal number ranges utilized here (Table 5), the breakdown is 41% "diploid," 50% "triploid," and 9% "tetraploid." Among the solid tumors, 17% were reported to be hypodiploid, while 9% of tumor lines surveyed here have modal number below 46. In both surveys, the number of tumor populations in the tetraploid range is relatively small.

TABLE 5

Distribution of Modal Chromosome Numbers of 54 Human Tumor Cell Lines[a] Cited in the Literature

Number of chromosomes	Ploidy designation[b]	Number of cell lines
<46–49	Near-diploid	15
50–59	Hyperdiploid	6
60–69	Hypotriploid	14
70–80	Hypertriploid	13
81–91	Hypotetraploid	3
92–110	Hypertetraploid	3

[a]Tumor lines are comprised of the 38 cited in Tables 3 and 4, seven melanoma lines (Romsdahl and Hsu, 1972), and nine established from various tumor types as described by Ishihara *et al.* (1962) and Moore and Koike (1964).

[b]The ploidy designations are somewhat arbitrary since some lines do not have sharp modal chromosome numbers and many lines have obviously rearranged chromosomes. For convenience, pseudotriploid cells are classed as hypotriploid, pseudotetraploid as hypertetraploid.

In a similar analysis of 129 cancerous effusions reported in the literature (Sandberg *et al.*, 1967; Sandberg and Hossfeld, 1970), the frequency of "diploidy," "triploidy," and "tetraploidy" was 48%, 40%, and 12%, respectively. As might be expected, since many of the tumor lines were also derived from metastatic tissue, this latter distribution is even closer to that observed for the *in vitro* cell lines. In a more recent review of modal chromosome numbers of malignant tumors of man, Atkin (1973) has shown that most tumors tend to fit into two groups, a near-diploid group, often the major one, and another in the hypertriploid–hypotetraploid region. However, tumors in the higher range are commonly near-triploid rather than near-tetraploid, which follows closely the pattern discerned for the *in vitro* tumor lines.

Another point made by Atkin (1973) in his extensive appraisal of chromosome findings in human cancers is that the pattern for each tumor is indicative of a clonal relationship. Of the *in vitro* tumor lines included in the present survey, each appears to be comprised of cells with karyotype characteristics such as consistent numerical and/or structural deviations or persistent variability around a stemline likewise indicative of clonal origin. Thus although selection resulting in relative homogeneity of karyotype cannot be rigidly excluded by analogy or even by chromosome analysis of the cells themselves, it seems reasonable that the *in vitro* cell populations may in large part represent the tumor tissue of origin.

5. Perspectives

Several questions concerning karyotype analysis and chromosome abnormalities of human tumor lines in cell culture were posed in the introductory section of this discussion. Since all of the studies included in the present survey relied on conventional staining techniques, it seems appropriate to note or illustrate opportunities afforded by newer techniques before summarizing findings and prospects. The far greater resolution to be gained in analysis of chromosome complements should enhance understanding and usefulness of human tumor lines, particularly as related to the phenomenon of cancer.

5.1. New Techniques for Chromosome Identification

In recent years, technical advances have made possible the unequivocal identification of each pair of normal autosomes and the sex chromosomes. A standardized system of nomenclature has been developed whereby metaphase chromosomes may be described by banding patterns along their length, as exposed by several methods of treatment and staining (Paris Conference, 1972). Applications of techniques such as quinacrine fluorescence and Giesma banding for delineation of the human karyotype have been reviewed by Hirschhorn (1973) and Miller *et al.* (1973). Despite the passing of this methodological milestone, there are to date few published reports dealing with tumor cells in culture. Utilizing quinacrine fluorescence banding techniques, Miller *et al.* (1971) observed that the chromosome complement of WI-38 cells, in terms of banding pattern, was indistinguishable from that of cultured human leukocytes. They also studied three HeLa lines obtained from different sources as well as D98/AG cells received from the American Type Culture Collection. Apparently identical markers were found in the various HeLa populations, thus indicating their relatedness. Three of these markers were present in D98/AG cells, supporting thereby an earlier contention that several well-known lines are in fact HeLa contaminants (Gartler, 1968). In a recent study (Walker, 1973) of HeLa cells of unknown history, comparisons were made between conventional, unbanded karyotypes and banded karyotypes prepared by the trypsin–Leishmann staining method described by Seabright (1971). It was found that 16 structurally abnormal chromosomes, as determined from banding patterns, were incorrectly included in normal groups when karyotype analysis was carried out by conventional methods. Several of the marker chromosomes corresponded to those described by Miller *et al.*

(1971), illustrating and emphasizing that the study of marker chromosomes can serve to identify tumor cell lines.

In another report (Chen and Shaw, 1973), metastatic melanoma cells were analyzed by several of the newer staining methods during 11 wk following explantation. Although possibly not yet established as a continuous cell line, these cells are ideally suited for comparative karyotype analyses of human tumor cells. The modal chromosome number of the melanoma cells, which could be distinguished from fibroblasts on the basis of morphology, was 45. Only one identifiable member of pairs No. 1, 2, 8, 9, 10, 11, and 13 was present. Six or seven marker chromosomes could be distinguished and the origin of their component parts identified with some degree of certainty. Two unusual and stable markers, observable during the time period of study, were a ring chromosome and an unusually long chromosome with an interstitial C-band. Both chromosomes were seen in metaphase preparations made 4 h after explantation, strongly suggesting that they had been present also in the tumor cells *in vivo.*

It is revealing that the earliest group of published reports dealing with analysis of human chromosome complements of malignant cells by banding methods was restricted primarily to tumor cells in continuous or long-term culture, as discussed, or to lymphoblastoid cell lines and lymphomas with modal numbers in near-diploid range (Fleischmann *et al.*, 1971, 1972; Manolov *et al.*, 1971*a,b*; Manolov and Manolova, 1972; Steel, 1971; Petit *et al.*, 1972). In a single study, hypodiploid and hypotriploid cells of malignant effusions from two patients with ovarian adenocarcinomas were analyzed (Tiepolo and Zuffardi, 1973). Thus the newer methodologies have been successfully applied initially to cells in continuous culture or in effusions where the mitotic index is apt to be high and/or to cells with minimal deviations of chromosome number. Some of the findings illustrate possibilities, needs, and advantages of utilizing banding techniques for analysis of human tumor cells *in vitro.*

Fluorescence staining of short-term cultures of lymph node cells from patients with malignant lymphomas was used to look for and analyze marker chromosomes (Fleischmann *et al.*, 1971). Stable markers were observed, and one particular type of marker was present in each of four cases. In a detailed study of a lymphosarcoma with a modal number of only 48, cells with five to six marker chromosomes were found (Fleischmann *et al.*, 1972). While some markers could be identified as rearrangements of normal chromosomes, others were unidentifiable isochromosomes. Studies of Burkitt tumors showed that the normal fluorescence pattern was maintained for most chromosomes (Manolov *et al.*, 1971*a,b*). Three different markers characterizing one tumor population could be shown to be composed of portions of chromosomes No. 1 and 3. However, one segment of the largest marker could not be identified. Of 12 different Burkitt tumors or tumor cell lines, ten were positive for one chromosome No. 14 with an extra band at the distal end of the long arm. The significance of this observation resulting from the use of newer staining techniques is not yet known. In contradistinction to the few findings of identical markers was the lack of identity of like-appearing markers, as determined by conventional staining methods, among 14 near-diploid lymphoblastoid lines of normal and malignant origin (Steel, 1971). For example, the abnormally long D-group chromosomes characterizing four different cell lines were by fluorescence analysis found to be either different chromosomes or the same chromosome with segments having differing banding patterns. Thus in these populations aneuploidy appeared to have arisen by a variety of nondisjunctional and breakage and reunion events. Similarly, two additional chromosomes present in a Burkitt cell line could not be termed markers because their fluorescence pattern appeared to vary from cell to cell (Petit *et al.*, 1972). Finally, illustrative of both the magnitude of difficulties and the possibilities of banding analysis is the study of cancerous effusions (Tiepolo and Zuffardi, 1973). In one population with a chromosome mode of 72–75, 24 different, new chromosomes could be recognized, of which four had no banding pattern similar to that of any segment of a normal chromosome. The other adenocarcinoma population had 39–41 chromosomes, 14 of which were abnormal but could be identified completely or in part. The normal chromosomes could be sorted out with certainty. Abnormal chromosomes could be distinguished as products of deletions, translocations, and inversions.

Thus for utilizing to advantage the newer techniques the requirement for numerous metaphase cells of good morphology is as great or greater than when conventional techniques were the only resort. This requirement can best be met by the use of *in vitro* cell lines whereby the number of suitable metaphases may be amplified. It would appear that in some instances the extent of abnormality and/or variability of tumor cell chromosome complements may be so great that the search for specificity of abnormality may be temporarily encumbered rather than implemented. Banding analysis of near-diploid tumor lines could be an initially practical and informative approach.

5.2. *Usefulness of Karyotyped Human Tumor Cell Lines*

For many sorts of studies of mammalian cells including cytogenetic investigation *per se*, well-growing chromosomally characterized human tumor lines appear advantageous. There are areas of endeavor where karyotype analysis of cells under study is also of practical importance. Some points will be briefly examined here, some have been detailed elsewhere in this discussion.

Most useful, perhaps, is the fingerprint function that analysis of karyotype may have. Since, as a generality, chromosome constitutions of cultured cells are fairly stable and since human tumor lines have unique, abnormal karyotypes, it is often possible to distinguish one cell line from another as well as from normal, stromal cells. The occasional need to verify species should not have to be mentioned, but cross-species cell contamination is a distressful and not uncommon event. In this regard, the simplicity and reliability of chromosomal analysis are not to be overlooked.

The use of karyotype analysis of a continuous line as the sole means of chromosomal characterization of a tumor is certainly not advocated. However, the difficulties of obtaining adequate numbers of morphologically acceptable metaphases directly from solid tumors are well known. In most instances, the tumor lines included in the present survey were not successfully studied prior to establishment in culture. Whether karyotypes of continuous lines may often represent *in vivo* patterns has been considered in detail. In general, the answer is in the affirmative, with the qualifications noted. Although most cytogeneticists prefer direct preparation of metaphases from tumor tissue, the need for short-term culture as a supplement or substitute is recognized. A comparative study of these two techniques was carried out by Kotler and Lubs (1967). Selection for or against cells having normal karyotypes or abnormal karyotypes with particular chromosome numbers and markers was not demonstrated. However, for proper estimates of similarities or differences between *in vivo* tumor cells and their progeny in continuous culture, comparative analysis of chromosome complements of cells before and after establishment *in vitro* is needed.

The facility with which adequate numbers of morphologically suitable metaphases can be obtained from cell cultures is a major advantage in utilization of chromosome banding methods. In view of the sometimes extensive chromosome rearrangements that have been revealed by the newer techniques, and in consideration of their potential for cytogenetic analysis of cancer cells, the quality of metaphase preparations is an important factor. Similarly, availability of nearly homogeneous tumor cell populations free of contaminating stromal cells is helpful.

Populations of tumor cells with marker chromosomes but with otherwise minimal numerical and structural deviations and restricted karyotype variability would seem of value for somatic cell genetic studies. As noted in the preceding discussion of neuroblastoma lines, such near-diploid tumor lines have been described. More are expected to become available as more tumor lines are successfully established *in vitro*, since approximately 40% of the already surveyed lines have near-diploid modal chromosome numbers.

Furthermore, cells such as neuroblastoma and melanoma which express differentiated functions have added usefulness. Investigations with these types of cells utilizing cell hybridization techniques or even perhaps banding analysis alone could enhance the possibility of correlation of karyotype with a variety of phenotypic characters and have implications for gene mapping.

Finally, chromosome analysis is a simple means of assessing homogeneity of cells in order to obtain large numbers of reasonably pure cell types for biochemical and biological studies.

5.3. *Some Answers, More Questions*

From appraisement of chromosome abnormalities of human tumor cells *in vitro*, of karyotype stability of normal cells in culture, and of chromosome abnormalities of human tumors in the host environment, at least tentative answers to certain questions may be made. (1) Knowledge of the chromosome constitution of tumor lines is useful in a variety of ways (Section 5.2). (2) The *in vitro* karyotype usually represents the karyotype of the original tumor tissue (Section 4.4). (3) Karyotype abnormality of human cells in culture may be a reliable indicator of their malignant origin.

In support of the third "answer," various observations can be summarized. Continuous lines of human diploid fibroblasts have not been reported as yet. Spontaneous transformation of diploid fibroblasts to permanently growing (aneuploid) cells has not been authenticated. It is possible to transform human fibroblasts and epithelial cells by exposure to SV40 virus and perhaps other oncogenic viruses in the sense of obtaining morphologically altered cells with increased proliferative capacity and new, or newly expressed, antigens. However, karyotype studies of long-established, virally transformed cell lines with demonstrable oncogenic potential are rare or nonexistent. Neither continuous lines nor long-term cell cultures, i.e., strains, of human diploid epithelial cells are available. Similarly, chromosomally normal parenchymal cells cannot be maintained in continuous culture. Many, but not all, tumor lines are described as epithelial-like, in accord with the fact that carcinoma is the most common form of human cancer. Thus it is unlikely that these lines are derived from normal cell precursors. Contrary to misleading reports that accumulated in the decade of the 1950s, nondiploid established cell lines deriving from normal tissue are exceptional. Whether normal human epithelial cells, as compared to fibroblasts, would have a higher frequency of spontaneous transformation to permanent *in vitro* lines or whether they are more susceptible to viral transformation in the sense of either conversion to malignancy or establishment of continuous lines with or without karyotypic alteration is a pertinent, pending question. Another line of evidence is that all of the surveyed tumor lines are noneuploid. The finding of a karyotypically normal tumor line would be of extreme interest and importance, although unfortunately difficult to authenticate. Both possibility and difficulty are exemplified by the cell line H. Emb. Rh. No. 1, derived from a rhabdomyosarcoma. It was maintained in conditioned rats and also established *in vitro* (Moore *et al.*, 1955). The line, after being carried exclusively in animal passage for about 260 transplant generations, was found to have a diploid chromosome number and no visible abnormalities (Miles, 1965). Even though banding techniques would have to be utilized to establish normality, this observation promotes speculation: tumor cells can have normal karyotypes; heterologous animal passage is more suitable than cell culture for maintaining diploidy; and, less likely, normal human cells can be maintained in animal passage. Even so, a large body of circumstantial evidence makes it seem unlikely that the aneuploid cell lines obtained in attempts to culture human tumor cells originated from normal cells which became karyotypically altered as a consequence of explantation. Also, despite the sometimes long period of time that elapses before chromosomal characterization, it appears unlikely that at least most described karyotypic abnormalities were induced by conditions of cell culture. This viewpoint is contrary to one which would result from experiences only with the culturing of mouse cells, where "spontaneous" transformation to heteroploidy as well as to malignancy is not uncommon. A pertinent observational generality is that most adequately studied solid tumors, primary or metastatic, and tumor cell effusions have structural and/or numerical chromosome abnormalities. An important attestation to the malignant origin of human cell lines is the observed parallel between the distribution of chromosome numbers of tumor populations and that of established tumor cell cultures. It appears that culture procedures have relatively little influence on karyotypes of tumor cells other than to present altered conditions for cell selection. Thus an accumulation of observations indicates that karyotypic abnormality, structural and numerical, is a criterion of malignancy or, more pertinent to this discussion, an indicator of malignant origin of cell lines. Concomitant examination of other cellular attributes and growth characteristics such as density-dependent inhibition of proliferation *in vitro* and transplantability in xenogeneic hosts is potentially just as informative or more so. Nevertheless, it would appear that karyotype analysis, in combination with experienced observation of cells *in vitro*, can adequately distinguish between normal and tumor cells in culture.

Assessment of the significance of numerical and/or structural alterations of chromosomes of human tumor cells, either *in vivo* or *in vitro*, is still in its early stages. The full import of the extraordinary advances in methods for chromosome identification has only begun to be realized. From some of the earliest reported banding studies, it is apparent that the degree of visible chromosome rearrangement even in near-diploid cells far exceeds that indicated by conventional methods, implying lack of functional relationship between segments of chromosomes. However, perhaps there are critical chromosomes or even combinations of chromosome segments involved in the regulation of malignant growth. Heretofore it has not been generally possible to distinguish between specific alteration, should it exist, and random, inconsequential alteration, should this, too, exist as a form of background noise characterizing malignant cells in their origination and evolution. Perhaps the meaning of markers can be elucidated at last. If instances of specificity associated with a certain type of cancer cell are found, more sophisticated approaches to the understanding of the significance of cytogenetic alteration in malignant transformation will undoubtedly evolve. Should answers emerge, the process may well be accelerated by the availability of human tumor lines *in vitro*.

Acknowledgments

Thanks are due Miss Barbara A. Spengler for her many contributions to the preparation of this manuscript. This work was supported in part by National Cancer Institute Grant CA 08748.

6. *References*

American Type Culture Collection, 1972, *Registry of Animal Cell Lines* (J. E. Shannon and M. L. Macy, eds.), Rockville, Md.

Atkin, N. B., 1974, Chromosomes in human malignant tumors: A review and assessment, in: *Chromosomes and Cancer* (J. German, ed.), pp. 375–422, Wiley, New York.

Auersperg, N., 1964, Long-term cultivation of hypodiploid human tumor cells, *J. Natl. Cancer Inst.* **32**:135.

Auersperg, N., 1966, Karyotype changes of near hexaploid carcinoma cells during adaptation in culture, *Nature (Lond.)* **212**:635.

Auersperg, N., and Hawryluk, A. P., 1962, Chromosome observations on three epithelial-cell cultures derived from carcinomas of the human cervix, *J. Natl. Cancer Inst.* **28**:605.

Bassin, R. H., Plata, E. J., Gerwin, B. I., Mattern, C. F., Haapala, D. K., and Chu, E. W., 1972, Isolation of a continuous epithelioid cell line, HBT-3, from a human breast carcinoma, *Proc. Soc. Exp. Biol. Med.* **141**:673.

Berman, L., and Stulberg, C. S., 1956, Eight culture strains (Detroit) of human epithelial-like cells, *Proc. Soc. Exp. Biol. Med.* **92**:730.

Berman, L., Stulberg, C. S., and Ruddle, F. H., 1957, Human cell culture: Morphology of the Detroit strains, *Cancer Res.* **17**:668.

Biedler, J. L., Helson, L., and Suciu-Foca, N., 1973*a*, Expression of HL-A antigens on human neuroblastoma cells in continuous culture, *In Vitro* **8**:410.

Biedler, J. L., Helson, L., and Spengler, B. A., 1973*b*, Morphology and growth, tumorigenicity, and cyto genetics of human neuroblastoma cells in continuous culture, *Cancer Res.* **33**:2643.

Bottomley, R. H., Trainer, A. L., and Griffin, M. J., 1969, Enzymatic and chromosomal characterization of HeLa variants, *J. Cell Biol.* **41**:806.

Cailleau, R., 1960, The establishment of a cell strain (MAC-21) from a mucoid adenocarcinoma of the human lung, *Cancer Res.* **20**:837.

Chang, R. S. M., 1954, Continuous subcultivation of epithelial-like cells from normal human tissue, *Proc. Soc. Exp. Biol. Med.* **87**:440.

Chen, J., Tang, S., Chu, T., and Shen, T., 1962, Preliminary report on the establishment of a strain of human liver cancer cells *in vitro*, in: *VIII International Cancer Congress*, p. 136, Moscow.

Chen, T. R., and Shaw, M. W., 1973, Stable chromosome changes in a human malignant melanoma, *Cancer Res.* **33**:2042.

Chicago Conference: Standardization in Human Cytogenetics, 1966, *Birth Defects: Original Article Series*, Vol. II, No. 2, The National Foundation, New York.

Chu, E. H. Y., and Giles, N. H., 1958, Comparative chromosomal studies on mammalian cells in culture. I. The HeLa strain and its mutant clonal derivatives, *J. Natl. Cancer Inst.* **20**:383.

Chu, E. H. Y., and Giles, N. H., 1959, Human chromosome complements in normal somatic cells in culture, *Am. J. Hum. Genet.* **11**:63.

Cox, D., Yuncken, C., and Spriggs, A. I., 1965, Minute chromatin bodies in malignant tumours of childhood, *Lancet* **2**:55.

Dobrynin, Y. V., 1963, Establishment and characteristics of cell strains from some epithelial tumors of human origin, *J. Natl. Cancer Inst.* **31**:1173.

Duran-Troise, G., and DeLustig, E. S., 1972, Cytogenetic studies on a cell line from a mixed parotid tumour, *Rev. Eur. Etudes Clin. Biol.* **17**:605.

Eagle, H., 1955, Propagation in a fluid medium of a human epidermoid carcinoma strain KB, *Proc. Soc. Exp. Biol. Med.* **89**:362.

Fjelde, A., 1955, Human tumor cells in tissue culture, *Cancer* **8**:845.

Fleischmann, T., Hakansson, C. H., and Levan, A., 1971, Fluorescent marker chromosomes in malignant lymphomas, *Hereditas* **69**:311.

Fleischmann, T., Hakansson, C. H., Levan, A., and Möller, T., 1972, Multiple chromosome aberrations in a lymphosarcomatous tumor, *Hereditas* **70**:243.

Fogh, J., and Lund, R. O., 1957, Continuous cultivation of epithelial cell strains (FL) from human amniotic membrane, *Proc. Soc. Exp. Biol. Med.* **94**:533.

Fogh, J., Ramos, L., and Fogh, H., 1969, Transformation of primary human amnion cells with simian virus 40, in: *Axenic Mammalian Cell Reactions* (G. L. Tritsch, ed.), pp. 59–116, Dekker, New York.

Ford, C. E., and Hamerton, J. L., 1956, The chromosomes of man, *Nature (Lond.)* **178**:1020.

Fraccaro, M., Lindsten, J., Mannini, A., Scappaticci, S., and Tiepolo, L., 1968, Stability of abnormal karyotypes in cell culture, *Hereditas* **62**:105.

Fraley, E. E., Ecker, S., and Vincent, M. M., 1970, Spontaneous *in vitro* neoplastic transformation of adult human prostatic epithelium, *Science* **170**:540.

Freedman, L. S., Roffman, M., Lele, K. P., Goldstein, M., Biedler, J. L., Spengler, B. A., and Helson, L., 1973, Further studies on dopamine-β-hydroxylase in neuroblastoma, *Fed. Proc.* **32**:708.

Frisch, A. W., Jentoft, V., Barger, R., and Losli, E. J., 1955, A human epithelium-like cell (Maben) derived from an adenocarcinoma of lung, *Am. J. Clin. Pathol.* **25**:1107.

Gaffney, E. W., Fogh, J., Ramos, L., Loveless, J. D., Fogh, H., and Dowling, A. M., 1970, Established lines of SV40-transformed human amnion cells, *Cancer Res.* **30**:1668.

Gartler, S. M., 1967, Genetic markers as tracers in cell culture, *Natl. Cancer Inst. Monogr.* **26**:167.

Gartler, S. M., 1968, Apparent HeLa cell contamination of human heteroploid cell lines, *Nature (Lond.)* **217**:750.

Gey, G. O., Coffman, W. D., and Kubicek, M. T., 1952, Tissue culture studies of the proliferative capacity of cervical carcinoma and normal epithelium, *Cancer Res* **12:**264.

Girardi, A. J., Warren, L., Goldman, C., and Jeffries, B., 1958, Growth and CF antigenicity of measles virus in cells deriving from human heart, *Proc. Soc. Exp. Biol. Med.* **98:**18.

Girardi, A. J., Jensen, F. C., and Koprowski, H., 1965, SV40-induced transformation of human diploid cells: Crisis and recovery, *J. Cell. Comp. Physiol.* **65:**69.

Hamerton, J. L., 1971, Chromosomes and neoplastic disease, in: *Human Cytogenetics*, Vol. 2, pp. 407–441, Academic Press, New York and London.

Harnden, D. G., 1974, Viruses, chromosomes and tumours: The interaction between viruses and chromosomes, in: *Chromosomes and Cancer* (J. German, ed.), pp. 151–190, Wiley, New York.

Hayflick, L., 1961, The establishment of a line (WISH) of human amnion cells in continuous cultivation, *Exp. Cell Res.* **23:**14.

Hayflick, L., 1965, The limited *in vitro* lifetime of human diploid cell strains, *Exp. Cell Res.* **37:**614.

Hayflick, L., and Moorhead, P. S., 1961, The serial cultivation of human diploid cell strains, *Exp. Cell Res.* **25:**585.

Hirose, M., 1968, Tissue culture of human thyroid cancer, *Acta Med. Okayama* **22:**185.

Hirschhorn, K., 1973, Chromosome identification, *Ann. Rev. Med.* **24:**67.

Hsu, T. C., 1954*a*, Cytological studies on HeLa, a strain of human cervical carcinoma. I. Observations on mitosis and chromosomes, *Texas Rep. Biol. Med.* **12:**833.

Hsu, T. C., 1954*b*, Mammalian chromosomes *in vitro*. IV. Some human neoplasms, *J. Natl. Cancer Inst.* **14:**905.

Hsu, T. C., 1961, Chromosomal evolution in cell populations, *Int. Rev. Cytol.* **12:**69.

Hsu, T. C., and Moorhead, P. S., 1957, Mammalian chromosomes *in vitro*. VII. Heteroploidy in human cell strains, *J. Natl. Cancer Inst.* **18:**463.

Hsu, T. C., Pomerat, C. M., and Moorhead, P. S., 1957, Mammalian chromosomes *in vitro*. VIII. Heteroploid transformation in the human cell strain Mayes, *J. Natl. Cancer Inst.* **19:**867.

Ishihara, T., Moore, G. E., and Sandberg, A., 1962, The *in vitro* chromosome constitution of cells from human tumors, *Cancer Res.* **22:**375.

Ishii, S., and Nishimura, N., 1966, Establishment and characteristics of a tissue culture strain from metastatic clear-cell carcinoma in human bone, *J. Jap. Orthop. Ass.* **40:**285.

Jensen, F., Koprowski, H., and Pontén, J., 1963, Rapid transformation of human fibroblast cultures by simian virus 40, *Proc. Natl. Acad. Sci* **50:**343.

Jones, G. W., Simkovic, D., Biedler, J. L., and Southam, C. M., 1967, Human anaplastic thyroid carcinoma in tissue culture, *Proc. Soc. Exp. Biol. Med.* **126:**426.

Koller, P. C., 1972, The role of chromosomes in cancer biology, *Rec. Results Cancer Res.* **38:**1.

Kondo, T., Muragishi, H., and Imaizumi, M., 1971, A cell line from a human salivary gland mixed tumor, *Cancer* **27:**403.

Koprowski, H., Pontén, J. A., Jensen, F., Ravdin, R. G., Moorhead, P. S., and Saksela, E., 1962, Transformation of cultures of human tissue injected with simian virus SV40, *J. Cell. Comp. Physiol.* **59:**281.

Kotler, S., and Lubs, H. A., 1967, Comparison of direct and short-term tissue culture technics in determining solid tumor karyotypes, *Cancer Res.* **27:**1861.

Kuramoto, H., Tamura, S., and Notake, Y., 1972, Establishment of a cell line of human endometrial adenocarcinoma *in vitro*, *Am. J. Obstet. Gynecol.* **114:**1012.

Levan, A., 1956, Chromosome studies on some human tumors and tissues of normal origin, grown *in vivo* and *in vitro* at the Sloan–Kettering Institute, *Cancer* **9:**648.

Levan, A., 1967, Some current problems of cancer cytogenetics, *Hereditas* **57:**343.

Levan, A., 1969, Chromosome abnormalities and carcinogenesis, in: *Handbook of Molecular Cytology* (A. Lima-de-Faria, ed.), pp. 717–731, North-Holland, Amsterdam and London.

Levan, A., 1969, Chromosome abnormalities and carcinogenesis, in: *Handbook of Molecular Cytology* (A. Lima-de-Faria, ed.), pp. 717–731, North-Holland, Amsterdam and London.

Makino, S., Kikuchi, Y., Sasaki, M. S., Sasaki, M., and Yoshida, M., 1962, A further survey of the chromosomes in the Japanese, *Chromosoma* **13:**148.

Makino, S., Sofuni, T., and Mitani, M., 1965, Cytological studies on tumors. XLIII. A chromosome condition in effusion cells from a patient with neuroblastoma, *Gann* **56:**127.

Manolov, G., and Manolova, Y., 1972, Marker band in one chromosome 14 from Burkitt lymphomas, *Nature (Lond.)* **237:**33.

Manolov, G., Manolova, Y., Levan, A., and Klein, G., 1971*a*, Fluorescent pattern of apparently normal chromosomes in Burkitt lymphomas, *Hereditas* **68:**160.

Manolov, G., Manolova, Y., Levan, A., and Klein, G., 1971*b*, Experiments with fluorescent chromosome staining in Burkitt tumors, *Hereditas* **68:**235.

Mark, J., 1970, Chromosomal characteristics of neurogenic tumors in children, *Acta Cytol.* **14:**510.

Maunoury, R., Arnoult, J., and Vedrenne, C., 1972, Etablissement et caractérisation d'une lignée cellulaire provenant d'un ostéosarcome humain, *Pathol. Biol.* **20:**369.

McAllister, R. M., Melnyk, J., Finklestein, J. Z., Adams, E. C., and Gardner, M. B., 1969, Cultivation *in vitro* of cells derived from a human rhabdomyosarcoma, *Cancer* **24:**520.

McAllister, R. M., Gardner, M. B., Greene, A. E., Bradt, C., Nichols, W. W., and Landing, B. H., 1971, Cultivation *in vitro* of cells derived from a human osteosarcoma, *Cancer* **27:**397.

Miles, C. P., 1965, Chromosomes of some heterotransplanted human tumors. I. H.Emb. Rh. No. 1, H.S. No. 1, and ME 1, *J. Natl. Cancer Inst.* **34:**103.

Miles, C. P., 1967*a*, Chromosome analysis of solid tumors. I. Twenty-eight nonepithelial tumors, *Cancer* **20:**1253.

Miles, C. P., 1967*b*, Chromosome analysis of solid tumors. II. Twenty-six epithelial tumors, *Cancer* **20:**1274.

Miles, C. P., and Wolinska, W., 1973, A comparative analysis of chromosomes and diagnostic cytology in effusions from 58 cancer patients, *Cancer* **32:**1458.

Miller, O. J., Miller, D. A., Allderdice, P. W., Dev, V. G., and Grewal, M. S., 1971, Quinacrine fluorescent karyotypes of human diploid and heteroploid cell lines, *Cytogenetics* **10:**338.

Miller, O. J., Miller, D., and Warburton, D., 1973, Application of new staining techniques to the study of human chromosomes, *Progr. Med. Genet.* **9:**1.

Moore, A. E., Sabachewsky, L., and Toolan, H. W., 1955, Culture characteristics of four permanent lines of human cancer cells, *Cancer* **15:**598.

Moore, G. E., and Koike, A., 1964, Growth of human tumor cells *in vitro* and *in vivo*, *Cancer* **17:**11.

Moore, G. E., and Sandberg, A. A., 1964, Studies of a human tumor cell line with a diploid karyotype, *Cancer* **17:**170.

Moorhead, P. S., Human tumor cell line with a quasi-diploid karyotype (RPMI 2650), *Exp. Cell. Res.* **39:**190.

Moorhead, P. S., and Weinstein, D., 1966, Cytogenetic alterations during malignant transformation, *Rec. Results Cancer Res.* **6:**104.

Nelson-Rees, W. A., McAllister, R. M., and Gardner, M. B., 1972, Clonal aspects of the C-type virus-releasing cells of a cultured human rhabdomyosarcoma line (RD 114) *in vitro*, *Nature New Biol.* **236:**147.

Norrby, K., Eriksson, O., and Mellgren, J., 1962, Growth, morphology, and karyotype in 2 pairs of human cell strains of malignant and benign origin from the same individuals, *Cancer Res.* **22:**147.

Norryd, C., 1959, The chromosomes of three human cell strains, *Hereditas* **45:**449.

Norryd, C., and Fjelde, A., 1963, The chromosomes in the human cancer cell tissue culture line H.Ep No. 2, *Cancer Res.* **23:**197.

Nowell, P. C., 1965, Chromosome changes in primary tumors, *Progr. Exp. Tumor Res.* **7:**83.

Oboshi, S., Tsugawa, S., Seido, T., Shimosato, Y., Koide, T., and Ishikawa, S., 1971, A new floating cell line derived from human pulmonary carcinoma of oat cell type, *Gann* **62:**505.

Paris Conference (1971): Standardization in Human Cytogenetics, 1972, *Birth Defects: Original Articles Series*, Vol. VIII, No. 7, The National Foundation, New York.

Pattillo, R. A., and Gey, G. O., 1968, The establishment of a cell line of human hormone-synthesizing trophoblastic cells *in vitro*, *Cancer Res.* **28:**1231.

Peterson, W. D., Stulberg, C. S., and Simpson, W. F., 1970, A permanent heteroploid human cell line with type B glucose-6-phosphate dehydrogenase, *Proc. Soc. Exp. Biol. Med.* **136:**1187.

Petit, P., Verhest, A., Lecluse v. d. Bilt, F., and Jongsma, A., 1972, The chromosomes of EB virus–positive Burkitt cell line P3J.HR1K studied by the fluorescent staining technique, *Pathol. Eur.* **7:**17.

Petursson, G., and Fogh, J., 1963, The chromosomes of primary human amnion cells and FL cells, *Cancer Res.* **23:**1021.

Plata, E. J., Aoki, T., Robertson, D. D., Chu, E. W., and Gerwin, B. I., 1973, An established cultured cell line (HBT-39) from human breast carcinoma, *J. Natl. Cancer Inst.* **50:**849.

Pontén, J., and Saksela, E., 1967, Two established *in vitro* cell lines from human mesenchymal tumours, *Int. J. Cancer* **2:**434.

Prasad, K. N., Mandal, B., and Kumar, S., 1973, Demonstration of cholinergic cells in human neuroblastoma and ganglioneuroma, *J. Pediat.* **82:**677.

Puck, T. T., and Fisher, H. W., 1956, Genetics of somatic mammalian cells. I. Demonstration of the existence of mutants with different growth requirements in a human cancer cell strain (HeLa), *J. Exp. Med.* **104:**427.

Puck, T. T., Cieciura, S. J., and Robinson, A., 1958, Genetics of somatic mammalian cells. III. Long-term cultivation of euploid cells from human and animal subjects, *J. Exp. Med.* **108:**945.

Rigby, C. C., and Franks, L. M., 1970, A human tissue culture cell line from a transitional cell tumour of the urinary bladder: Growth, chromosome pattern and ultrastructure, *Brit. J. Cancer* **24:**746.

Romsdahl, M. M., and Hsu, T. C., 1967, Establishment and biologic properties of human malignant melanoma cell lines grown *in vitro, Surg. Forum* **18:**78.

Romsdahl, M. M., and Hsu, T. C., 1972, Establishment and characterization of human malignant melanoma cell lines grown *in vitro*, in: *Pigmentation: Its Genesis and Biologic Control* (V. Riley, ed.), pp. 461–477, Appleton–Century–Crofts, New York.

Ruddle, F. H., Berman, L., and Stulberg, C. S., 1958, Chromosome analysis of five long-term cell culture populations derived from nonleukemic human peripheral blood (Detroit strains), *Cancer Res.* **18:**1048.

Saksela, E., and Moorhead, P. S., 1963, Aneuploidy in the degenerative phase of serial cultivation of human cell strains, *Proc. Natl. Acad. Sci.* **50:**390.

Sandberg, A. A., and Hossfeld, D. K., 1970, Chromosomal abnormalities in human neoplasia, *Ann. Rev. Med.* **21:**379.

Sandberg, A. A., Yamada, K., Kikuchi, Y., and Takagi, N., 1967, Chromosomes and causation of human cancer and leukemia. III. Karyotypes of cancerous effusions, *Cancer* **20:**1099.

Sandberg, A. A., Sakurai, M., and Holdsworth, R. N., 1972, Chromosomes and causation of human cancer and leukemia. VIII. DMS chromosomes in a neuroblastoma, *Cancer* **29:**1671.

Seabright, M., 1971, A rapid banding technique for human chromosomes, *Lancet* **2:**971.

Shein, H. M., and Enders, J. F., 1962, Multiplication and cytopathogenicity of simian vacuolating virus 40 in cultures of human tissue, *Proc. Soc. Exp. Biol. Med.* **109:**495.

Spengler, B. A., Biedler, J. L., Helson, L., and Freedman, L. S., 1973, Morphology and growth, tumorigenicity, and cytogenetics of human neuroblastoma cells established *in vitro, In Vitro* **8:**410.

Spriggs, A. I., Boddington, M. M., and Clarke, C. M., 1962, Chromosomes of human cancer cells, *Brit. Med. J.* **2:**1431.

Spurna, V., and Hill, M., 1966, Chromosomal composition of HeLa and L cells in tissue cultures, *Neoplasma* **14:**11.

Steel, C. M., 1971, Non-identity of apparently similar chromosome aberrations in human lymphoblastoid cell lines, *Nature (Lond.)* **233:**555.

Sykes, J. A., Whitescarver, J., Jernstrom, P., Nolan, J. F., and Byatt, P., 1970, Some properties of a new epithelial line of human origin, *J. Natl. Cancer Inst.* **45:**107.

Syverton, J. T., 1957, Comparative studies of normal and malignant human cells in continuous culture, *N.Y. Acad. Sci. Spec. Publ.* **5**:331.

Syverton, J. T., and McLaren, L. C., 1956, Stable and pure line human cells in continuous culture for studies of polioviruses, *Am. J. Pathol.* **32**:640.

Tiepolo, L., and Zuffardi, O., 1973, Identification of normal and abnormal chromosomes in tumor cells, *Cytogenet. Cell Genet.* **12**:8.

Tjio, J. H., and Levan, A., 1956, The chromosome number of man, *Hereditas* **42**:1.

Tjio, J. H., and Puck, T. T., 1958, Genetics of somatic mammalian cells. II. Chromosomal constitution of cells in tissue culture, *J. Exp. Med.* **108**:259.

Todaro, G. J., and Aaronson, S. A., 1968, Human cell strains susceptible to focus formation by human adenovirus type 12, *Proc. Natl. Acad. Sci.* **61**:1272.

Toolan, H., 1954, Transplantable human neoplasms maintained in cortisone-treated laboratory animals: H.S. No. 1, H.Ep. No. 1, H.Ep. No. 2, H.Ep. No. 3, and H.Emb. Rh. No. 1, *Cancer Res.* **14**:660.

Trujillo, J. M., Drewinko, B., Lichtiger, B., Ahearn, M. J., and Cork, A., 1972, Establishment *in vitro* of a human neurogenic sarcoma, *Cancer Res.* **32**:1066.

Tumilowicz, J. J., Nichols, W. W., Cholon, J. J., and Greene, A. E., 1970, Definition of a continuous human cell line derived from neuroblastoma, *Cancer Res.* **30**:2110.

Ugryumov, E. P., and Tsoneva-Maneva, M. T., 1963, Karyotype study of monolayer culture of human stomach cancer cells, *Byul. Eksperim. Biol. Med.* **55**:93.

Vogt, M., 1959, A study of the relationship between karyotype and phenotype in cloned lines of strain HeLa, *Genetics* **44**:1257.

Wakonig-Vaartaja, T., Helson, L., Baren, A., Koss, L. C., and Murphy, M. L., 1971, Cytogenetic observations in children with neuroblastoma, *Pediatrics* **47**:839.

Walker, J. R., 1973, Identification and misidentification of the chromosomes of heteroploid cell lines, *J. Natl. Cancer Inst.* **51**:1113.

Weinstein, D., and Moorhead, P. S., 1965, Karyology of permanent human cell line, W-18VA2, originated by SV40 transformation, *J. Cell. Comp. Physiol.* **65**:85.

Weinstein, D., and Moorhead, P. S., 1967, The relation of karyotypic change to loss of contact inhibition of division in human diploid cells after SV40 injection, *J. Cell Physiol.* **69**:367.

White, L., and Cox, D., 1967, Chromosome changes in rhabdomyosarcoma during recurrence and in cell culture, *Brit. J. Cancer* **21**:684.

Yamada, K., Takagi, N., and Sandberg, A. A., 1966, Chromosomes and causation of human cancer and leukemia. II. Karyotypes of human solid tumors, *Cancer* **19**:1879.

Ultrastructural Characteristics of Human Tumor Cells *in Vitro** 14

GABRIEL SEMAN AND LEON DMOCHOWSKI

1. *Introduction*

In this chapter, only tumor cells of human origin will be considered. Animal tumor cells will not be considered, except when a direct comparison between the results of ultrastructural studies of human cells and those of animal cells will help in furthering the discussion. The history of ultrastructural studies of human tumor cells grown *in vitro* has been determined by a number of important factors. The first was the development, in the late 1940s, of commercially available electron microscopes, followed by the development, in the early 1950s, of thin-sectioning procedures and fixation and embedding procedures (Palade, 1952; Porter and Kallman, 1953) for biological material that were suitable for electron microscopy. For several years, electron microscopists have been experiencing serious difficulties with fixative solutions and even more with media for embedding. Methacrylate, the plastic commonly used for embedding until 1963–1964, was a poor

* Some of the work described in this chapter was conducted under Contract NO1-CP-33304 with the Virus Cancer Program of the National Cancer Institute and was supported in part by Grants CA-05831 and RR-05511 from the National Cancer Institute, N.I.H., U.S.P.H.S., and by a grant from the Leukemia Society of America, Inc.

GABRIEL SEMAN AND LEON DMOCHOWSKI Department of Virology, The University of Texas, M. D. Anderson Hospital and Tumor Institute at Houston, Texas Medical Center, Houston, Texas medium. The understanding of cellular ultrastructure improved considerably when fixation in glutaraldehyde (Sabatini *et al.*, 1963), followed by fixation in osmic acid, and use of high-quality embedding resins such as Epon (Luft, 1961) and Araldite (Glauert *et al.*, 1956) were introduced for preparation of specimens. At the same time, the development of media for tissue culture (Eagle, 1955*b*; McCoy and Neuman, 1956) protected against contamination by a variety of antibiotics made possible the prolonged cultivation of human tumor cells with reasonable chances of success.

Since the beginning of the century, innumerable attempts have been made to grow human tumor cells and tissues *in vitro*. A variety of tissue culture systems were devised which usually resulted in growth of tumor-derived cells for only a short period of time. Long-term cultivation of tumor cells or tissues proved a difficult enterprise; the number of successes since the establishment of the first human tumor cell line, the HeLa strain (Gey *et al.*, 1952), is still limited. However, it is necessary to keep in mind that the purpose of growing human tumor cells may vary, and they determine the type and length of cultivation. For instance, the applications of organ cultures (see Easty, 1967; Lasfargues, 1957; Hagmuller and Leslie, 1962) are very different from those of monolayer cultures, in which the cells rapidly lose most of their original properties. This situation is reflected at the ultrastructural level. While cellular differentiation may occur in organ culture systems (see, e.g., Flaxman, 1972), human tumor cells in long-term monolayer or suspension cultures tend to resemble animal cells grown under the same conditions, to the point that their malignant or nonmalignant characters, or their organs of origin, become impossible to determine by ultramorphology alone (Dmochowski, 1960). A typical example is that of cells derived in continuous cultures of tumors of human hematopoietic tissues, which are indistinguishable from cells derived from cultures of normal human blood or bone marrow (Moore *et al.*, 1968; Chandra *et al.*, 1968). Therefore, it is not surprising that ultrastructural studies of human tumor cells turned very early to investigation of the relationship between function and ultrastructure and to examination of the morphological alterations induced by chemical and physical agents, by viruses, and by other factors, regardless of the origin of the cells. In many investigations, HeLa cells are simply (and somewhat confusingly) called "mammalian cells." But, as will be seen, human tumor cells retain *in vitro* a number of specific characters related to their tissues of origin, if not to malignancy.

The purpose of this chapter is to describe the most significant ultrastructural features of human tumor cells in culture, whether grown under optimal conditions or influenced by a variety of factors, as they appear from descriptions published in the literature and from observations made in this laboratory. First, the ultrastructure of cells derived from a number of human tumors (epithelial tumors, sarcomas, and neoplasms of the hematopoietic system) will be described. Next the effects of cultivation conditions, of chemical and physical agents, and of viruses and mycoplasmas on the fine structure of some of these cells will be considered. In view of the diversity of the subject, the references listed should not be considered exhaustive. They have been limited to morphological observations as much as possible, with a minimum of digressions into other fields whenever necessary.

It appears necessary to begin with a brief description of some of the procedures employed in preparation of tissue culture cells for electron microscopy.

2. *Preparation of Tissue Culture Cells for Electron Microscopy*

2.1. *Routine Techniques*

2.1.1. *Harvesting of Tissue Culture Cells*

Cells grown as monolayers are usually scraped off the substrate with a rubber policeman in a small amount of fresh medium. The cells may also be detached from the substrate by covering them with medium containing trypsin (0.25% trypsin in saline, in a proportion of 1:20 w/v, for 20–30 min at 37°C) or by versene (0.0037% in Hank's solution). The cells detached from the substrate are centrifuged at 700g for 15 min to form a pellet. When cells are grown in suspension, they are simply spun down from the medium with or without prior addition of fixative (of choice). Explants grown in organ cultures are prefixed before removal from the culture dish.

2.1.2. *Fixation and Embedding*

Cell pellets and specimens from organ cultures are processed the same way as tissue biopsy specimens. First they are fixed overnight in 2–3% buffered glutaraldehyde, and after a wash in buffer are postfixed for 2–3 h in 2% buffered osmic acid. The buffer most commonly employed is Millonig's phosphate buffer (Millonig, 1961). Next dehydration is carried out at half-hour intervals through a series of graded alcohols (50%, 70%, 95%, and absolute) followed by two changes of 15 min each in propylene oxide. The dehydrated specimens are stored overnight in a 1:1 mixture of propylene oxide and resin, and then embedded in fresh resin. A very satisfactory embedding resin formula, derived from formulas given by Luft (1961) and

Mollenhauer (1964), is the following mixture of Epon 812 and Araldite: Epon (25 ml), Araldite (20 ml), DDSA (60 ml), dibutylphthalate (4 ml), BDMA (3%). Specimens are embedded in special plastic capsules and allowed to harden for 2–3 days at 60°C in a vacuum oven.

2.1.3. Sectioning and Staining

Thin sections cut from the blocks with an ultramicrotome and collected on copper grids are stained for 10 min by floating the grids on a solution of saturated uranyl acetate in 50% ethanol (Watson, 1958) and, after a wash in distilled water, on a solution of lead citrate (Reynolds, 1963; Venable and Cogeshall, 1965), again for 10 min. The sections are then carbon-coated in an evaporator to give them stability in the electron beam.

2.2. Special Techniques

2.2.1. Cell Synchronization

Sometimes, for certain ultrastructural studies, the cultured cells exposed to chemical or physical agents have to be arrested at a determined stage of the cell cycle (see Whitmore, 1971). Simple methods to obtain mitotic or near-mitotic cells take advantage of the fact that such cells are easily detached from the substrate with simple mechanical devices. The "selected detachment" or "controlled agitation" techniques (Robbins and Marcus, 1964; Kim and Perez, 1965; Erlandson and De Harven, 1971) belong to this category. A more precise control over the cell cycle can be obtained by treating the cultured cells with colcemid (Robbins and Scharff, 1966), vinblastine sulfate (Kim and Stambuk, 1966; Pfeiffer and Tolmach, 1967*a*; Djordjevic and Tolmach, 1967), FUdR (Djordjevic and Tolmach, 1967), or hydroxyurea (Pfeiffer and Tolmach, 1967*b*) or by adding to the medium an excess of thymidine (Xeros, 1962; Bootsma *et al.*, 1964; Whitmore and Gulyas, 1966).

2.2.2. Oriented Embedding and Sectioning

Special procedures have been developed in attempts to study the fine structure of cells in culture in their actual shape and connections in monolayers. These procedures involve fixation of the cells on the substrate itself, covering them with embedding resin, peeling off the pre-embedded cells, and re-embedding them in the desired orientation for sectioning (Howatson and Almeida, 1958). Various modifications of this basic procedure have been used to study human tumor cells *in vitro* (Hendee *et al.*,

1963*a*; Robbins and Gonatas, 1964*a*; Willoch, 1967; Brinkley *et al.*, 1967; Moreno and Vinzens, 1969; Arstila *et al.*, 1971).

2.2.3. *Special Electron Microscopic Techniques*

Some particular techniques that are frequently used in other types of ultrastructural studies have been applied to examination of human tumor cells grown *in vitro*. Scanning electron microscopy of cell monolayers (see Hodges, 1970; Carr, 1971; Boyde *et al.*, 1972) was used by Strauli *et al.* (1971) to study the surface of HEp–2 cells. HeLa cells have been examined by freeze-etching (Bekerhi and Markani, 1970; Reith and Oftebro, 1971). Interesting observations about the surface of HeLa and HEp–2 cells have been made by the classical carbon replica method (Easty and Mercer, 1960; Willoch, 1967; Cooper and Fisher, 1968*a,b*). Negative staining of thin sections of herpesvirus–infected HeLa cells has shown in great detail the mode of formation of viral capsids in the nucleus (Miyamoto, 1971).

3. *General Aspects of Ultrastructure of Human Tumor Cells in Vitro*

3.1. *General Considerations*

Electron microscopic examination of the structure of human tumor cells grown *in vitro* reveals, as expected, all the fundamental components of animal cells grown in culture. A generally large nucleus, with one or more nucleoli, occupies part of the cytoplasm. In the cytoplasm are seen ribosomes, mitochondria, Golgi system, centrioles, vacuoles of different types, and osmiophilic inclusions representing lipidic material and lysosomes. Because of the thinness of the sections, and depending on the plane of sectioning, the nucleoli, the centrosome, and part or all of the Golgi system may be missed in a single section of a cell. It is therefore important to examine sections of many cells of a preparation to have an accurate representation of their structure.

The outlines of the cells examined in thin sections are influenced by the way they have been grown and then prepared for electron microscopy. Scraped or trypsinized cells from monolayers lose most of their intercellular connections; their cytoplasm is retracted and often broken into fragments. Cell retraction results in a redistribution of the cytoplasmic organelles. This is why no ultrastructural study of cells grown as monolayers is complete without their examination following fixation *in situ*. The anatomy of cells grown in suspension is certainly less disturbed, while that of cells in organ cultures, fixed the same way as biopsy tissues, is in theory perfectly preserved.

A detailed description of the fine structure of each of the cellular components mentioned above is irrelevant to this chapter, and will be found in specialized publications (e.g., Fawcett, 1966; Dalton and Haguenau, 1968; Dingle and Fell, 1969; Sandborn, 1970; Busch and Smetana, 1970; Toner and Carr, 1971). The principal components have the same structure in all cultured human tumor cells, with only minor variations. The nuclei are generally indented. Nuclear indentations and invaginations may be very pronounced (see Figs. 28 and 29) and appear as holes or slits in the nucleus when cross-sectioned, or give a false impression of multinucleation. However, true nuclear inclusions are frequently observed in nuclei of the cells in culture. They are usually limited by a membrane and contain vacuolar structures (Fig. 1). Large inclusions of this type may simulate viral or various cytopathic inclusions in the light microscope. The chromatin of interphase nuclei is lightly distributed, with little margination. As in cancer cells and in rapidly growing cells (Bernhard, 1966), one or several hypertrophied nucleoli are present; their structure is similar to that of the nucleoli of all other mammalian cells (Busch and Smetana, 1970). On the basis of their gross appearance in the cells in culture, nucleoli may be described as belonging to three different categories: (1) large nucleoli, frequently attached to the nuclear membrane, and consisting of a loose nucleolonemal network (see Fig. 28); (2) more compact nucleoli, where the nucleolonema is less distinct and interspersed with light areas (see Fig. 14); (3) dense, rounded nucleoli composed entirely of an aggregate of highly osmiophilic granules (Figs. 2 and 6). Dense nucleoli are frequently "capped" or partitioned by zones of light, fibrillar material (Fig. 2). The three broad categories of nucleoli can be observed in any tumor or nontumor human cell *in vivo* or *in vitro*; however, compact nucleoli seem to be more prevalent in tumor cells (Yasuzumi and Sugihara, 1965; Bernhard and Granboulan, 1968; Busch and Smetana, 1970).

Fibrillar or granular nuclear bodies appear to be a common observation in cultured human tumor cells (see Fig. 34). These structures are known to be more frequent in pathological conditions and are probably related to cellular hyperactivity (Bouteille *et al.*, 1967).

Perichromatin granules, about 200–500 Å in size (see Fig. 13), are often seen at the periphery of the nucleus. Their number increases from late S phase to early prophase (Erlandson and De Harven, 1971). The granules are definitely more frequent in tumor cells and are likely to contain nucleoprotein (Monneron and Bernhard, 1969).

"Giant cells" with multiple nuclei, or with a single but very large nucleus, are frequently observed in cultures of human tumor cells, in particular in the strains HeLa, KB, and Hep–2 (see Rose, 1970). They are apparently not formed by fusion of several cells. No signs of fusion through cytoplasmic

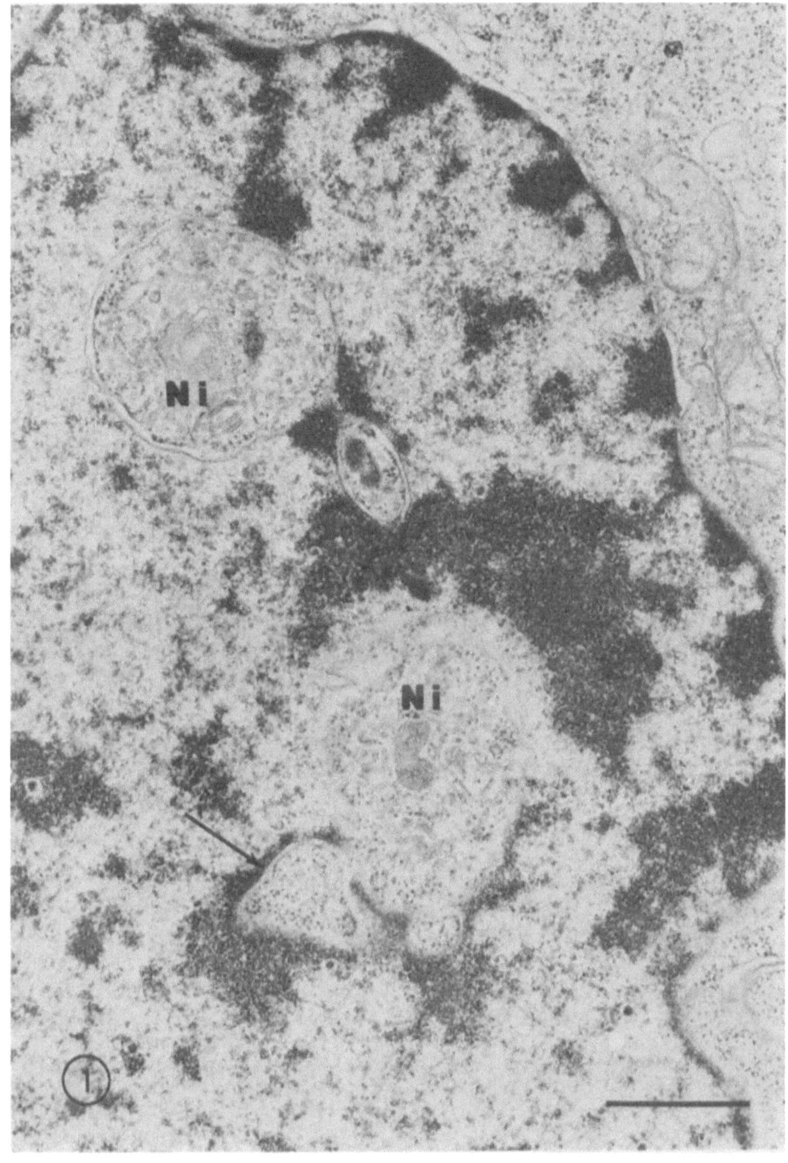

FIG. 1. Part of the nucleus of a HeLa cell showing nuclear inclusions (Ni) and cross-section of a nuclear invagination (arrow).

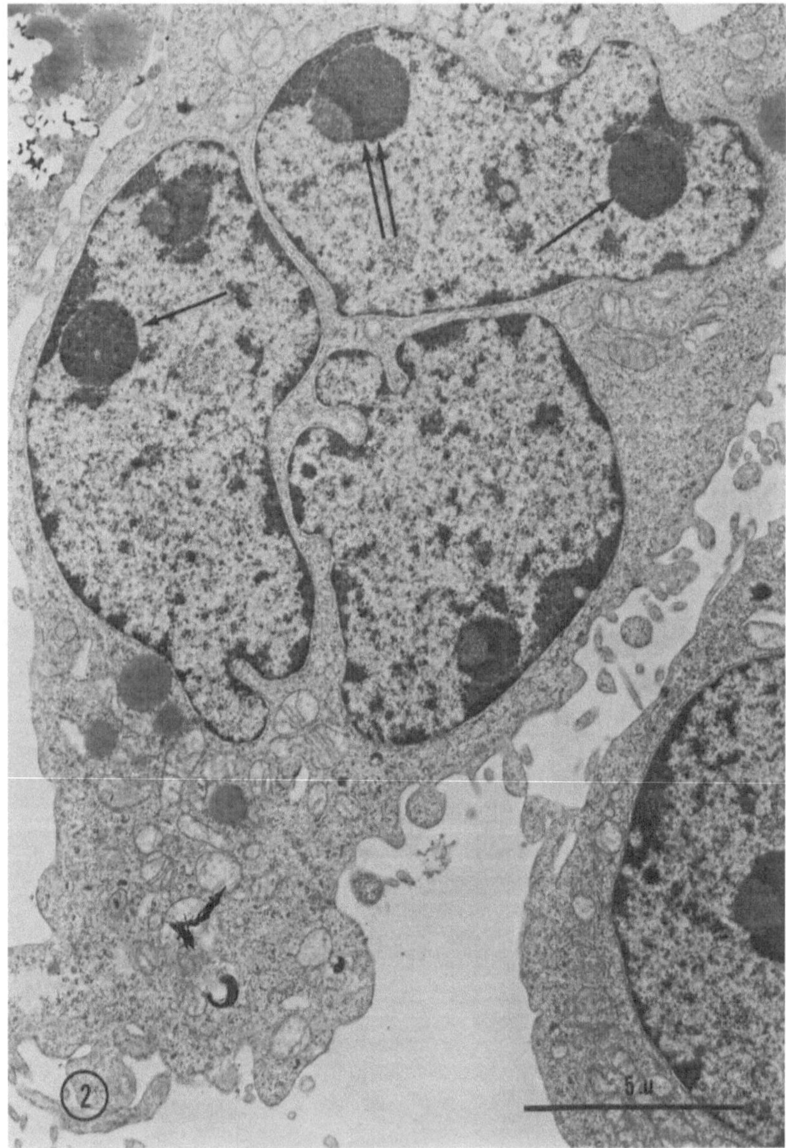

FIG. 2. Example of a "giant" HeLa. Nuclei show margination of chromatin and contain dense nucleoli (arrows). A nucleolus (double arrow) is "capped" by fibrillar material.

bridges have been observed, in this laboratory, by examination of "giant cells" in HeLa cell cultures (Fig. 2). Multinucleated "giant cells" could result, according to light microscopic observations of Rose *et al.* (1964) and Rose (1966), from the fragmentation of a large nucleus into several nuclei, following mitosis. Some of the nuclei thus formed may recombine into a single nucleus, while the others either degenerate or are eliminated from the cell.

Cultured tumor cells contain numerous mitochondria varying in shapes and sizes according to the origin of the cell line. Some mitochondria contain ribosome-like granules, and sometimes clusters of fine fibrils, probably representing DNA, are visible (Nass and Nass, 1963; Erlandson and De Harven, 1971) (see Fig. 12).

Ribosomes and polyribosomes are found in all phases of the life cycle of the cultured cells. The most common polysomes are tetrads. Circular polysomes consisting of five or six ribosomes, or linear polysomes disposed in a helical fashion, are also frequently observed (Erlandson and De Harven, 1971). Helical polysomes, mostly seen in S and in G_2 phase, are characteristic of cells actively synthesizing protein. Single ribosomes are prevalent in late prophase (Fig. 3), when protein synthesis decreases, and also during metaphase and telophase. Polysomes reappear in telophase and in G_1 phase (Scharff and Robbins, 1966; Hodge *et al.*, 1969; Erlandson and De Harven, 1971).

The Golgi system is represented by dictyosomes, usually several of them. Each dictyosome consists of a series of lamellae surrounded by vesicles and vacuoles. At both ends of the lamellae are found numerous coated vesicles, about 500 Å in diameter (Fig. 4).

The cytoplasm of the cultured cells always contains a variety of inclusions, generally more abundant in cells growing in monolayers. Inclusions are also more abundant in slow-growing or older cultures. The nature of these inclusions is not easy to establish. They are osmiophilic, dark-staining in thin sections, and bound by a single limiting membrane. Many are homogeneous, although varying in shapes and sizes, and correspond undoubtedly to the classical lysosomes (see Dingle and Fell, 1969). Other inclusions have a more complex appearance, with vacuoles and multilayered or multilaminated structures (Figs. 5, 28, and 29) sometimes including crystalloidic components. There seems to be no doubt, from studies by Arstila *et al.* (1971) on HeLa cells, that many of these complex inclusions are derived from autophagic or heterophagic cell activity. Cells in culture phagocytize and probably destroy parts of their own structures and a variety of materials present in the medium (Dourmashkin and Dougherty, 1961), derived from calf serum or from other cells, as for instance in the case of melanoma cells (Maul and Romsdahl, 1970) or of mycoplasma (see Fig. 41).

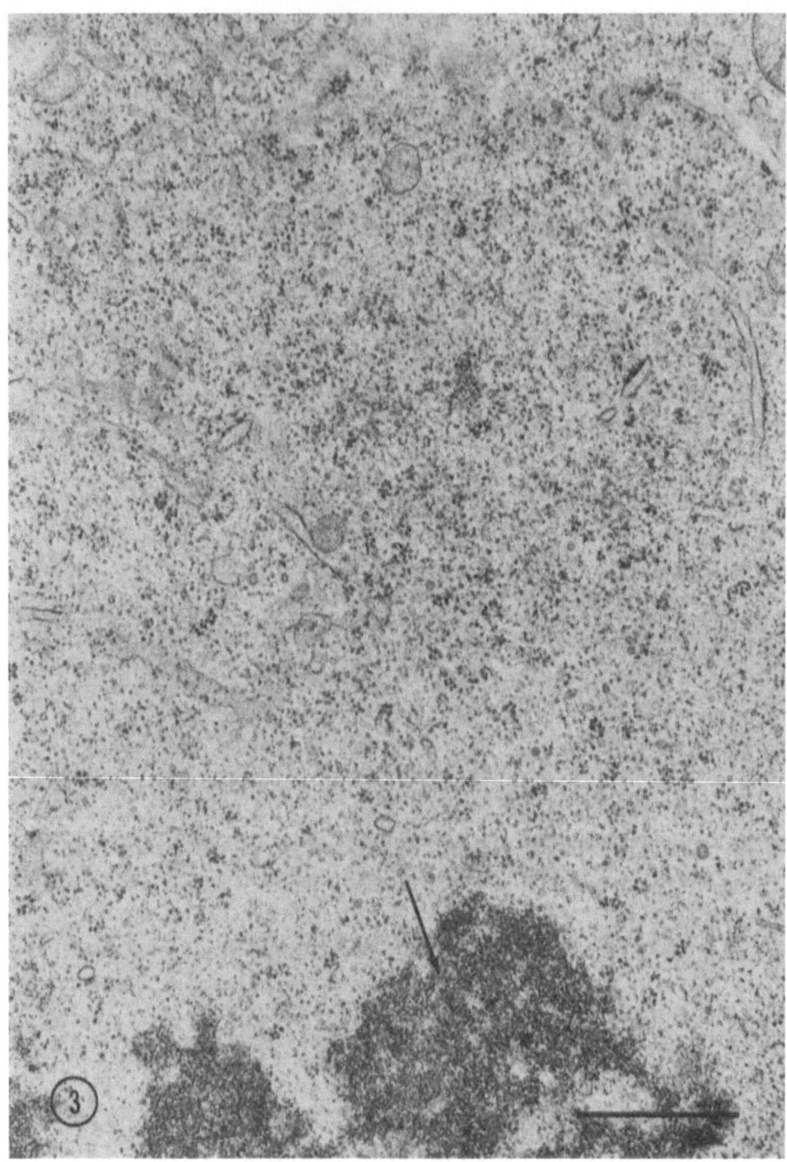

FIG. 3. Part of a KB cell in mitosis. There is a prevalence of single ribosomes. The dense patches represent chromosomal material (arrow).

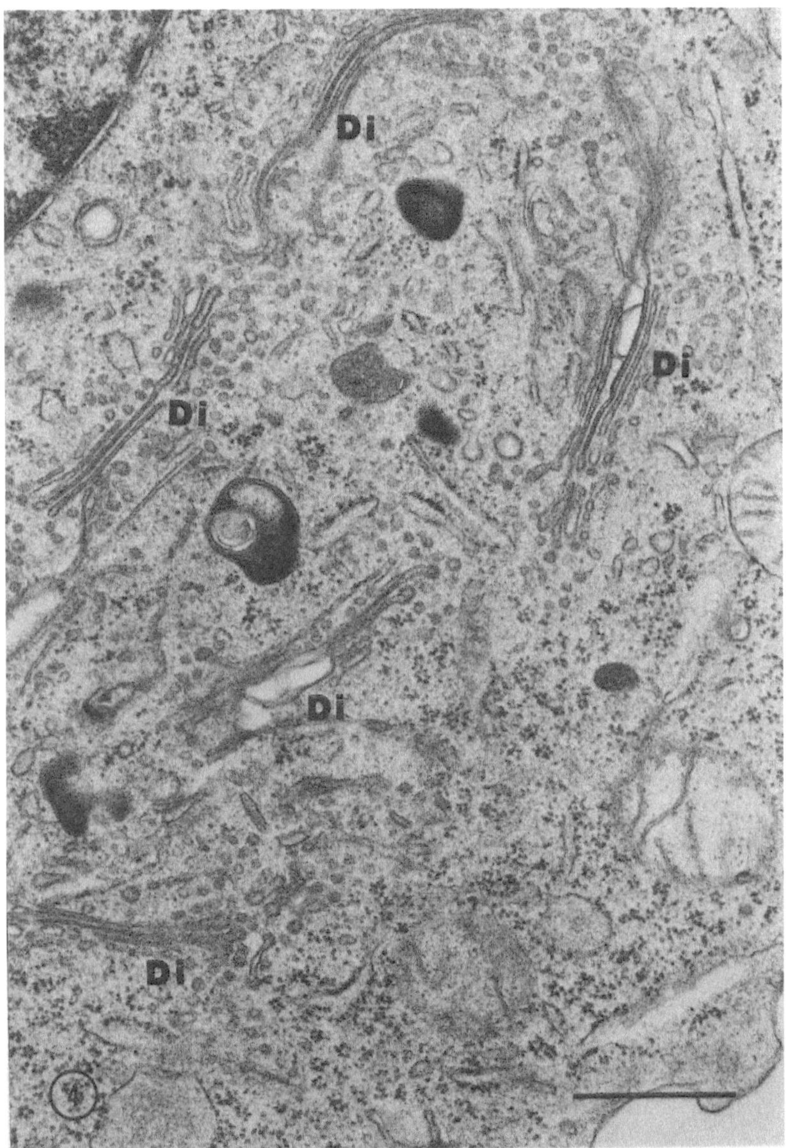

FIG. 4. Appearance of Golgi system of a KB cell. There are five dictyosomes (Di) composed of several lamellae surrounded at both ends by small coated vesicles.

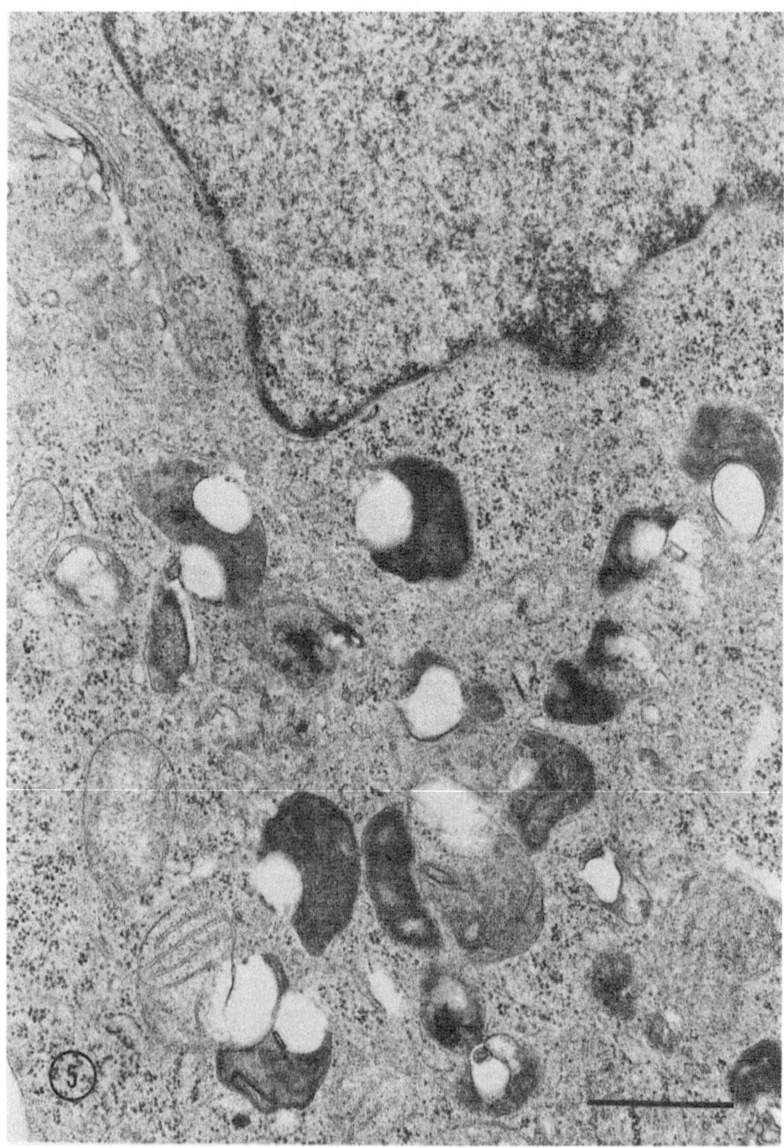

FIG. 5. Cytoplasm of a KB cell filled with osmiophilic inclusions of complex structure. This is the most common appearance of lysosomes in cells of established cultures.

3.2. Ultrastructure of Cells Derived from Epithelial Tumors

Cells of epithelial tumor origins best known for their ultrastructure in monolayer cultures are the HeLa, KB, and HEp–2 cells derived from carcinoma of the cervix, oral carcinoma, and laryngeal carcinoma, respectively. Cells of other established cell lines derived from melanomas, breast cancer, and lung cancer have also been examined by electron microscopy.

3.2.1. The HeLa Cells

HeLa cells, derived from a carcinoma of the cervix, were the first human tumor cells to be established as a line (Gey *et al.*, 1952). Although aneuploid and, at least in theory, malignant, these cells have been used in a considerable number of investigations in cell biology, cell biochemistry, and cellular ultrastructure.

The fine structure of interphase HeLa cells (Fig. 6) has been described in some detail in a number of publications. The cells have been examined in thin sections (Harford *et al.*, 1956*b*, 1957; Bruni *et al.*, 1961; Epstein, 1961; Journey and Goldstein, 1961; Fuse *et al.*, 1963; Robbins and Gonatas, 1964*a*; George *et al.*, 1965; Lettre *et al.*, 1966; Loni *et al.*, 1967; Lewin and Moscarello, 1968; Robbins *et al.*, 1970; Erlandson and De Harven, 1971; Arstila *et al.*, 1971) and by other ultramicroscopic techniques, such as carbon replicas (Easty and Mercer, 1960; Willoch, 1967; Fisher and Cooper, 1967) and freeze-etching (Bekerhi and Markani, 1970; Reith and Oftebro, 1971).

The ultrastructure of HeLa cells during the mitotic cycle has received particular attention, as a model for the study of mammalian cell replication (Blondel and Tolmach, 1965; Robbins and Gonatas, 1964*b*; Byers and Abramson, 1968; Robbins *et al.*, 1968; Robbins and Jentzsch, 1969; Erlandson and De Harven, 1971; McIntosh and Landis, 1971).

Ultrastructural differences among the substrains of HeLa cells, such as the HeLa S3 substrains (Puck *et al.*, 1956), HeLa JJ, and others, have not been reported.

a. The Nucleus. Nuclei of HeLa cells (Fig. 6) measure about 4–5 μm in diameter (Epstein, 1961); Fuse *et al.*, 1963). The structure of the nuclear envelope and of the nuclear pores does not differ from that of the same components in any other animal cell (Journey and Goldstein, 1961). The fine structure of HeLa cell nucleoli has been examined by Lettre *et al.* (1966) under various conditions of fixation in an attempt to identify the components of the nucleolonema and of the pars amorpha. The authors have confirmed the presence of DNA strands in the nucleolonema.

b. The Cell Surface. The periphery of HeLa cells presents two types of microextensions. The first is comprised of microvilli, relatively uniform in

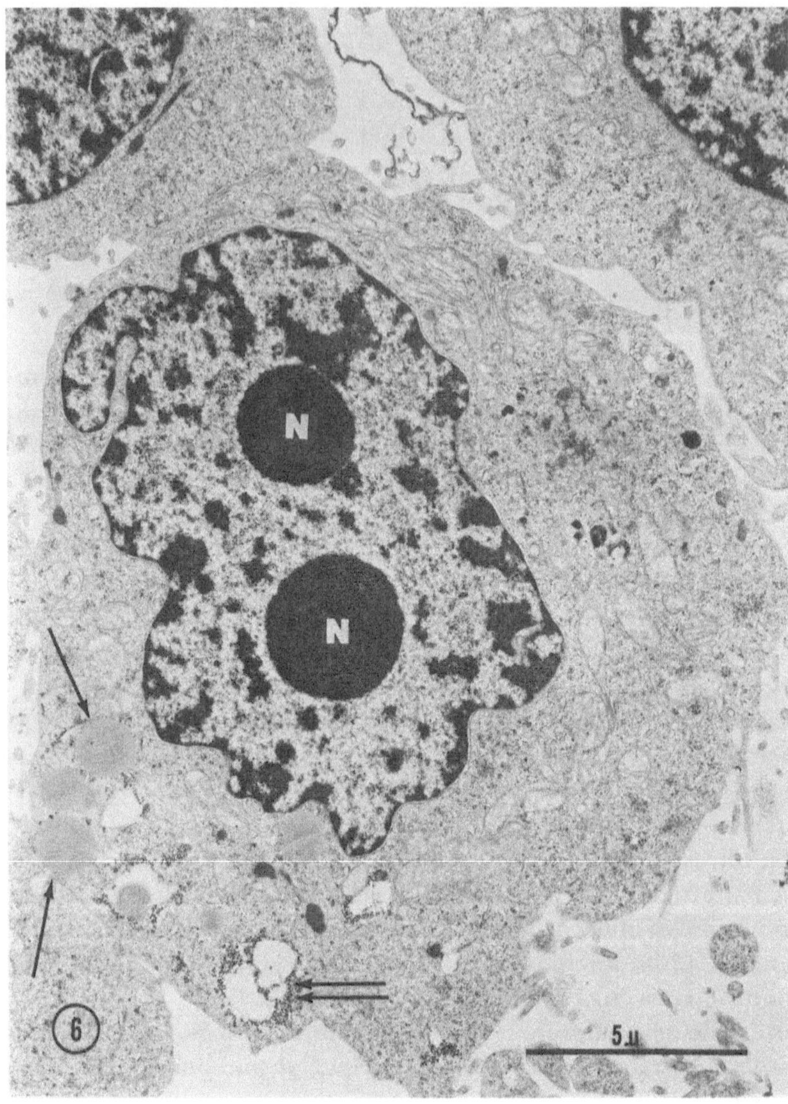

FIG. 6. Appearance of a HeLa cell at low magnification. Nucleoli (N) are very dense and rounded. The cytoplasm contains some lipid droplets (arrow) and islands of glycogen (double arrow) associated with empty cavities.

diameter (about 0.1 μm), extending as far out as 2 μm. Microvilli often have a narrow pedicle and contain fine axial fibers originating in deeper parts of the cytoplasm (Figs. 7a and 7b). They are usually implanted perpendicular to the cell surface, but an oblique insertion is fairly common. From Fisher and Cooper's calculations (1967), there are about 13 microvilli per square micrometer of the HeLa cell surface in monolayers. They are absent on the

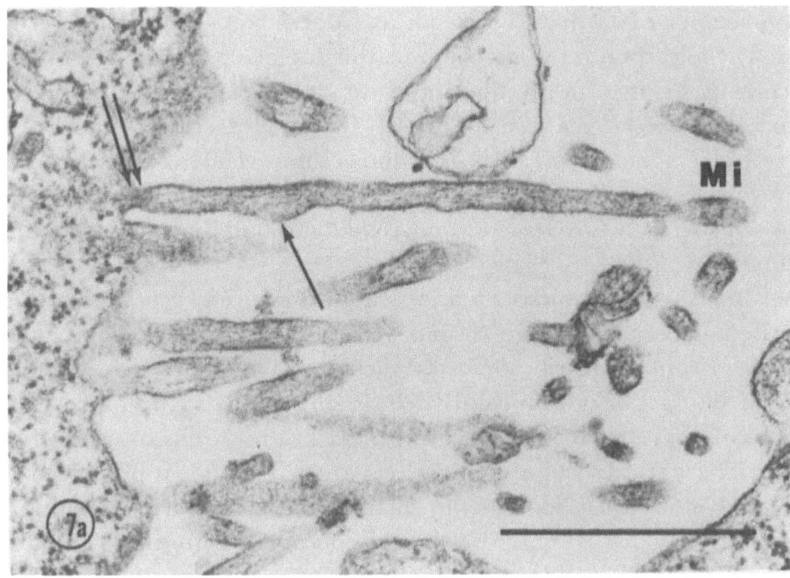

FIG. 7a. Microvilli at the surface of a HeLa cell. One of them (Mi) is sectioned through its full length and presents fine axial fibers (arrow) and a narrow pedicle (double arrow). Microvilli, in this micrograph, are implanted perpendicular to the cell surface.

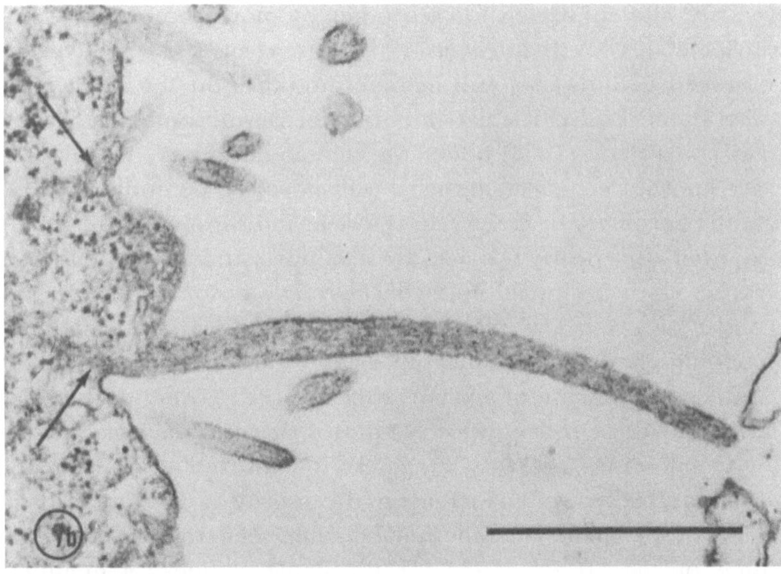

FIG. 7b. Microvilli at the surface of another HeLa cell. Their implantation is oblique as indicated by the orientation of the fine axial fibrils (arrows) originating far below the plasma membrane.

bottom surface of the cells. Instead, as Cooper and Fisher (1968*b*) have shown by the carbon replica technique, this surface presents short (800 Å) "attachment bridges" with the substrate, about 10–25 μm. The same technique, applied to the study of rapidly frozen HeLa cells (Willoch, 1967; Fisher and Cooper, 1967; Cooper and Fisher, 1968*a,b*), revealed that microvilli were frequently terminated by a dilatation and that certain zones of the cell surface were devoid of microvilli and had a peculiar reticulated structure.

The other type of microextensions at the periphery of HeLa cells is comprised of cytoplasmic protrusions of various shapes, sizes, and orientations, often containing ribosomes or vacuoles. These protrusions are observed in all types of cells in culture (see, e.g., Figs. 2, 28, and 29).

HeLa cells have few contact areas with each other. Cells fixed *in situ* and examined by vertical sectioning show long and tortuous cytoplasmic protrusions, and contact areas between the cells are limited to short segments of the protrusions (Willoch, 1967). The abutting plasma membranes run parallel to each other, and the contact zones are underlined, below the inner leaflet of the plasma membranes, by a diffuse band of dense cytoplasmic material (Fig. 8). A gap of 100–150 Å, filled with a fuzzy substance of variable electron density, may separate the outer leaflets. This type of attachment device, known to connect animal cells *in vivo* and *in vitro*, corresponds to the "zonula occludens" or "tight junctions" described in detail by Farquhar and Palade (1963), Kelly and Luft (1966), Flaxman *et al.* (1969), and others. HeLa cells, however, are also connected to each other by more complex attachment devices. Some authors (Bruni *et al.*, 1961; Fuse *et al.*, 1963; Willoch, 1967) have observed desmosomes and hemidesmosomes on the surface of the cells. This point is of particular importance. Desmosomes, described by Farquhar and Palade (1963) under the denomination of "maculae adherens," are known to connect epithelial cells *in vivo*. The finding of desmosomes at the periphery of HeLa cells is a clear indication that the cells have retained, even after nearly two decades in culture, an important ultrastructural marker characteristic of epithelial cells. Desmosomes connecting two cells consist of two short plaques parallel to the inner leaflet of the corresponding plasma membrane, separated by an interval of about 200 Å filled with a component of fibrous appearance. Frequently bundles of tonofibrils, 50 Å thick, converge toward the inner face of each plaque (Figs. 8 and 9). Desmosomes are easy to detect in cultured cells even at low magnifications, because of an increase in the density of the cytoplasm at the approaches of the plaques. Desmosomal plaques seem to persist, at least for some time, on the surface of HeLa cells. Single plaques (or hemidesmosomes) are frequently encountered on the plasma membrane of scraped or trypsinized HeLa cells (see Fig. 12). These structures are sometimes found in

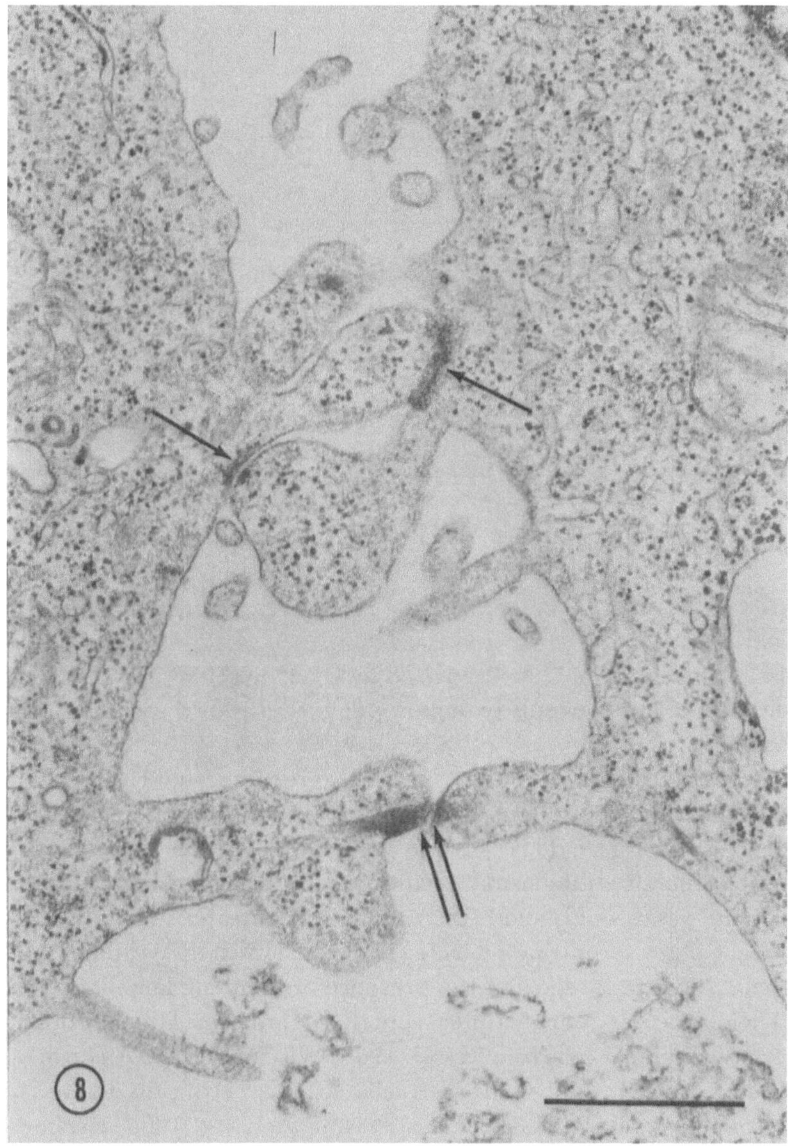

FIG. 8. Attachment devices between HeLa cells. Two "tight junctions" (arrows) and a desmosome (double arrow) may be seen.

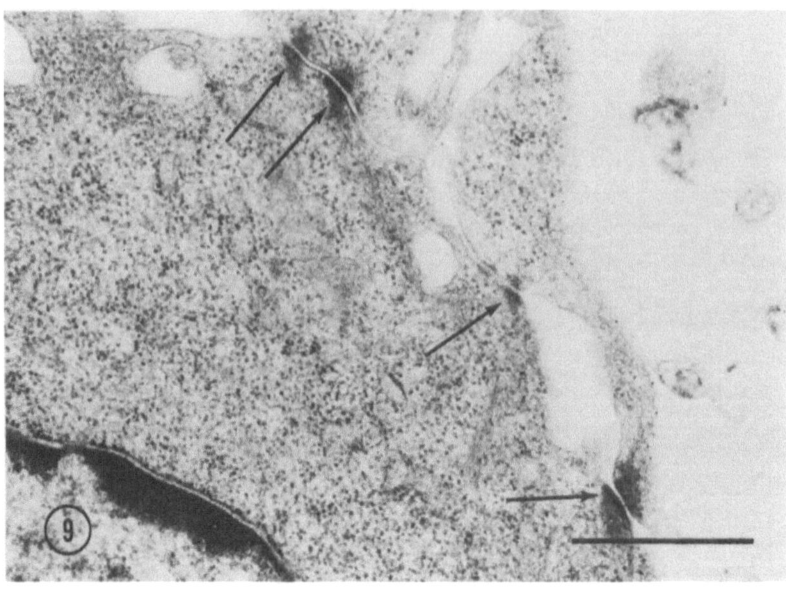

FIG. 9. A group of four desmosomes (arrows) joining a HeLa cell to cytoplasmic extensions of a neighboring cell.

cytoplasmic invaginations. As suggested by Overton (1968), invagination of hemidesmosomes may result from autophagocytosis of trypsin-dissociated desmosomes.

c. The Cytocavitary System. There is general agreement that HeLa cells have only a small amount of rough endoplasmic reticulum. The cisternae are short and narrow (see Figs. 11 and 12) and scattered throughout the cytoplasm. Smooth endoplasmic cavities are represented by a number of vacuoles and vesicles of limited size, usually concentrated around the Golgi zone. The Golgi system is well developed, with several dictyosomes.

Epstein (1961) first reported the presence of annulate lamellae in HeLa cells. Their structure does not differ from that of annulate lamellae observed in a variety of animal cells (see Kessel, 1968; Wischnitzer, 1970) or in other human cells grown *in vitro*, such as KB cells (see Fig. 21) or cells derived from normal or malignant leukocytes (Epstein and Achong, 1965; Gerber and Monroe, 1968).

Detailed studies have been carried out on the mode of formation of multivesicular bodies (MVBs) often encountered in the cytoplasm of HeLa cells (Hartford *et al.*, 1957; Bruni *et al.*, 1961; Robbins and Gonatas, 1964*a*; Arstila *et al.*, 1971). The bodies have a single limiting membrane (see Fig. 36b) coated on some parts of its cytoplasmic side, and contain a number of small vesicles, fairly uniform in size. The matrix of some of the bodies is

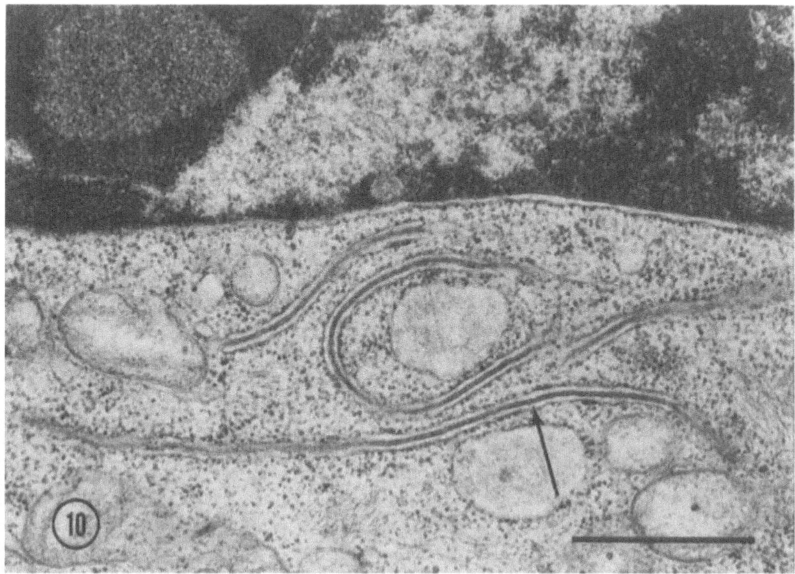

FIG. 10. "Confronting cisternae" in the cytoplasm of a HeLa cell, composed of rough endoplasmic cavities apposed by one of their membranes. The apposed membranes form an intermediate membrane (arrow) about 200 A thick.

darkened by an electron-dense material (see Fig. 36b). Arstila *et al.* (1971), studying the uptake of Thorotrast particles by HeLa cells, have concluded that MVBs actually represent part of a process of cytoplasmic autophagocytosis very commonly observed in a variety of cells in culture.

The cytoplasm of HeLa cells also shows the presence of two frequently encountered structures: "confronting cisternae" and "cytoplasmic fractures." "Confronting cisternae" have been observed in HeLa and KB cells by Kumegawa *et al.* (1968). They consist of two endoplasmic cisternae apposed by one of their membranes. Apposition of the two membranes results in the formation of an intermediate double membrane about 400 Å thick (Fig. 10). According to Kumegawa *et al.* (1968) and to Rose (1970), "confronting cisternae" form open arrangements in HeLa cells, while in KB cells these systems may form closed, ring-shaped structures. "Cytoplasmic fractures" appear as empty gaps in the cytoplasm, bordered by a membrane on one of their sides. There is no membrane or only an incomplete one on the other side. For some reason as yet undetermined, these empty spaces are frequently associated with lipid droplets (Fig. 11). Such structures are very often observed in other types of cultured cells (see Figs. 14 and 29) and, although present in apparently well-preserved cells, may represent an artifact.

d. Mitochondria. HeLa cells contain numerous mitochondria, variable in size and shape. They are usually elongated and frequently show branching

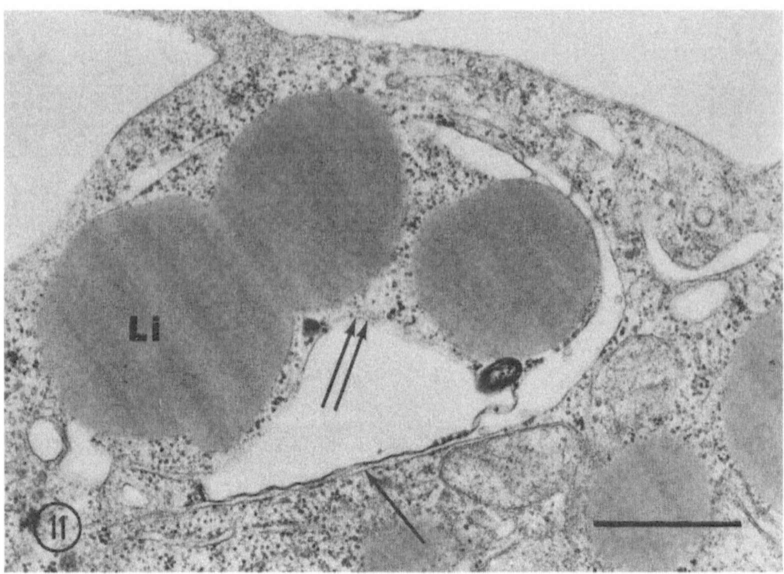

FIG. 11. "Cytoplasmic fracture" in a HeLa cell, associated with lipid droplets (Li). One side of the fracture is limited by a continuous membrane system (arrow). On the other side, interruptions in the membrane system bring the cytoplasm in direct contact with the cavity (double arrow).

(Fig. 12). According to Fuse *et al.* (1963), the mitochondria are distributed in layers, the larger being located near the nucleus and the smaller in the peripheral area of the cytoplasm.

e. Ribosomes. The structure and distribution of ribosomes correspond to the description given in Section 3.1.

f. Cytoplasmic Fibrils. As described by Bruni *et al.* (1961) and Fuse *et al.* (1963), the cytoplasm of HeLa cells contains bundles of filaments (Fig. 13). They are identical to the tonofibrils seen in cells of normal or malignant epithelium of the cervix (Hinglais–Guillaud, 1960; Luibel *et al.*, 1960) and to the tonofibrils characteristically present in a variety of epithelial cells *in vivo*. The fibrils are frequently seen ending on desmosomal plaques (see Figs. 8 and 9).

g. Glycogen. Accumulation of glycogen particles is commonly found in various areas of the cytoplasm of HeLa cells (Bruni *et al.*, 1961) (see Fig. 12). The particles average 230 Å in size. They either lie free in the cytoplasm or cluster in membrane-bound areas often associated with empty cavities (see Fig. 6).

h. Cytoplasmic Inclusions. Besides multivesicular bodies, the cytoplasm of HeLa cells contains lipid inclusions and electron-dense bodies. Lipid inclusions are generally rounded, with no limiting membrane, and have a light homogeneous content (see Figs. 6 and 11). Electron-dense bodies, sur-

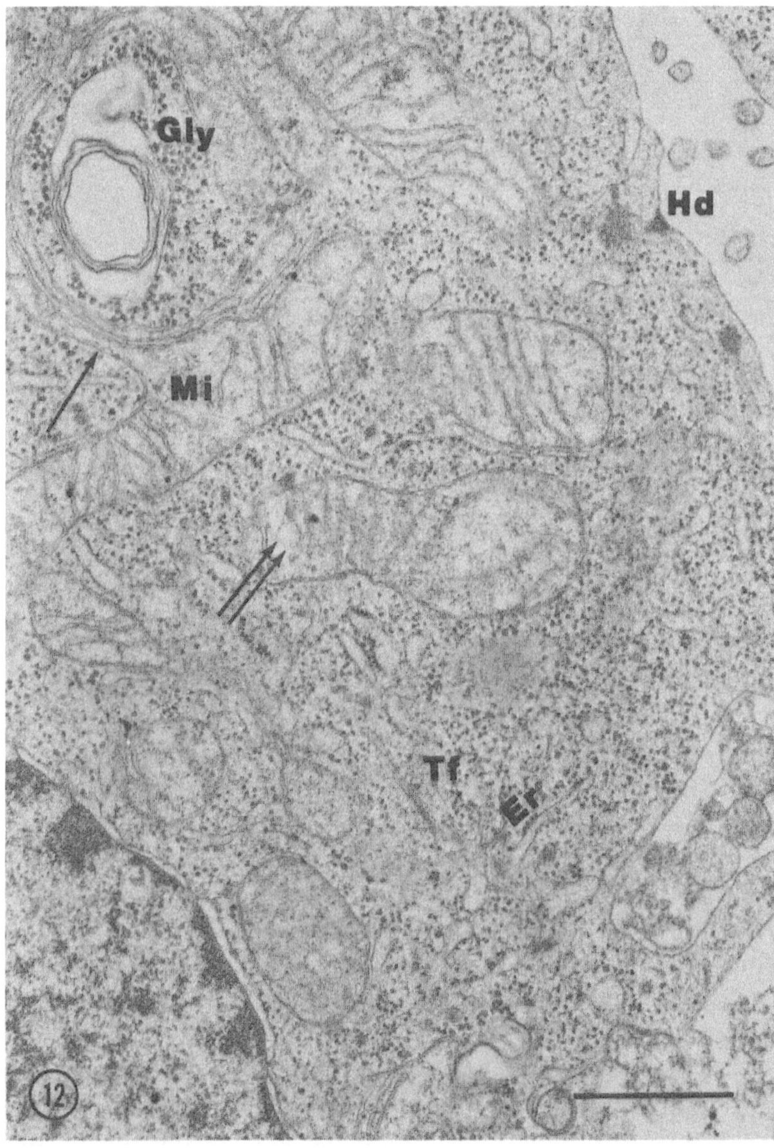

FIG. 12. Part of the cytoplasm of a HeLa cells, showing several mitochondria (Mi), one of them with branching (arrow) around a cavity surrounded by glycogen granules (Gly). Mitochondria contain small RNP granules, and sometimes fine DNA fibers (double arrow). Rough endoplasmic cavities are short (Er). A small bundle of tonofibrils (Tf) and a hemidesmosome (Hd) may be seen.

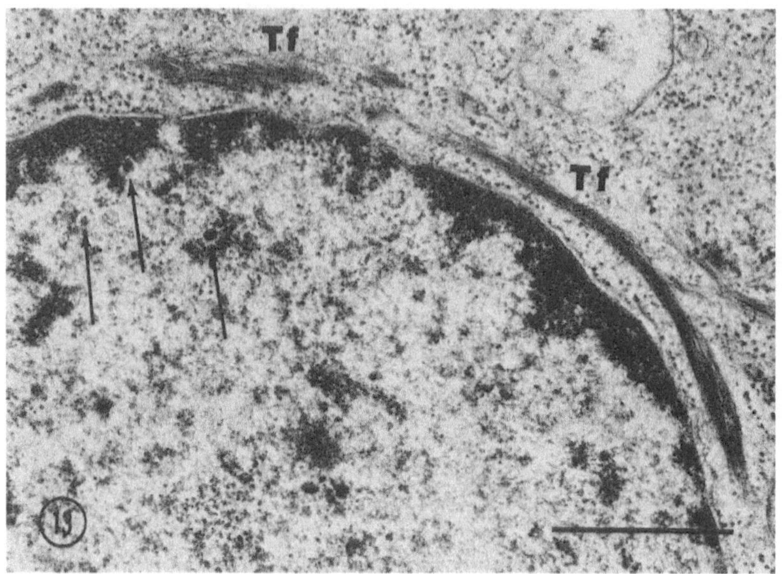

FIG. 13. Bundles of tonofibrils (Tf) around the nucleus of a HeLa cell. The nucleus contains some perichromatin granules (arrows).

rounded by a single membrane, may vary in shape and internal structure (see Fig. 6). These bodies have a dense matrix and frequently contain lamellar structures, sometimes arranged in paracrystalline fashion. These formations have been described as "globoid bodies" (Harford *et al.*, 1956*b*), "dense bodies," or "microbodies" (Journey and Goldstein, 1961). They correspond to primary lysosomes derived from the Golgi system, or to secondary lysosomes resulting from auto- or heterophagocytosis, as shown by Arstila *et al.* (1971).

i. Ultrastructure of HeLa Cells During the Mitotic Cycle. The ultrastructure of HeLa cells during the successive stages of mitosis has been thoroughly investigated and has served as a model for the "ultrastructure of mammalian cell during the mitotic cycle" (Robbins and Gonatas, 1964*b*).

The classical study of Robbins and Gonatas (1964b) has shown the principal sequence of events in the morphology of HeLa cells during mitosis. In prophase, the nucleoli dissolve and chromatin initiates its condensation. At the same time, an osmiophilic zone appears around the centrioles, which start replicating. Spindle tubules radiate from the centrosome in every direction. The nuclear membrane disappears in metaphase and the spindle tubules enter into contact with the chromosomes. During anaphase, the spindle tubules attach to the kinetochores, which are crescent-shaped osmiophilic bands found at the tip of the chromosomes. Then, at the stage of karyokinesis by elongation, the chromosomes fuse in a continuous mass, while reconstruction of the nuclear membrane proceeds from endoplasmic vesicles surrounding the chromosomes. About 6 min after the onset of anaphase, an equatorial constriction of the cytoplasm appears, forming the mid-body. The mid-body is filled with spindle tubules in close contact. Simultaneously with equatorial constriction, the plasma membrane shows an increase in density extending about one-quarter of the way around the cell periphery. Cytoplasmic blebs are frequency during anaphase. The nuclear membranes are completely reconstructed during telophase and chromosomes start uncoiling. The mid-body is finally eliminated by a symmetrical invagination of the plasma membrane.

Abramson and Byers (1966) have found that complete separation of the daughter cells, during late cytokinesis of HeLa cells, may take several hours. During that time, the cells remain connected by a long bridge containing the mid-body. As may be seen by light microscopy, the bridge is animated by a pulsating, wavelike movement. At the arrival of each wave to one of the cells, it starts blebbing for a while, then stops. The bridge slowly elongates, and finally, when the distance between cells and mid-body reaches 7–8 μm, the bridge pinches off. The authors have also followed these events by electron microscopy.

In further ultrastructural studies of HeLa cells, Robbins *et al.* (1968) have paid special attention to centriolar replication. The centrioles replicate by orthogonal budding from parent centrioles, during the periods of thesis (G_1) and syntheses (S). Replication of the centrioles is completed by G_2 and prophase, when the first symptoms of chromosome condensation are observed. At this stage, the migration of the centriole pairs has also been accomplished.

Robbins and Jentzsch (1969) have completed these studies of HeLa cells by examining in detail the behavior of spindle tubules during the metaphase-to-anaphase transition. The authors have shown that the numerous small vesicles that appear during late metaphase around the centriolar complex represent fragments of spindle tubules, encapsulated in endoplasmic cavities. Fragmentation and depolymerization of the tubules at their centriolar end probably allow migration of the chromosomes toward the cellular poles.

McIntosh and Landis (1971) have studied the distribution of spindle tubules along the spindle axis of HeLa and WI-38 cells during anaphase and telophase. As the anaphase chromosomes separate, spindle tubules remain in the interzone. Short segments of the interzone tubules are surrounded by a dense, amorphous material of unknown origin and significance. These segments embedded in the dense material correspond to the "stem bodies" seen by light microscopy. The authors have also demonstrated that, as already suspected by Robbins and Gonatas (1964*b*), spindle tubules pass not only between the chromosomes but also right through them. During the formation of the cleavage furrow, in late anaphase–telophase, the "stem bodies" shorten and assemble into a compact mid-body separating the daughter cells. The intrachromosomal spindle tubules slide past along the continuous spindle tubules as the chromatids move to the poles. There is apparently no initiation of new tubules in the interzone of WI-38 cells during telophase, while tubules grow in number and length in the interzone of HeLa cells. This observation indicates that it is possible to detect by electron microscopy differences between human cells in certain stages of their mitotic cycle.

Combining radioautography of synchronized HeLa cells labeled with ^{3}H-TdR and electron microscopy, Erlandson and De Harven (1971) have attempted to correlate structural variations in the cells in G_1, S, and G_2 with coexisting biochemical events. Colcemid was used to stop cells in G_2 from going into the next cycle. Cells in G_1 showed extensive cytoplasmic blebbing. Small patches of condensed chromatin, still visible in the nucleus of G_1 cells, decreased until S phase, and then progressively increased up to the end of G_2. At the same time, increased numbers of perichromatin granules, 50 mμm in diameter, were visible in the nucleolus-associated chromatin and in hetrochromatin. Nucleoli, still small and attached to the nuclear envelope in early G_1, increased in size, and by late G_1 most of the nucleoli lost contact with the nuclear envelope and remained unchanged for the rest of interphase. Fibrillar nuclear bodies were seen in many HeLa cells from mid-G_1 throughout interphase, while granular nuclear bodies were most prominent in S and G_2 cells. Nuclear bodies did not incorporate tritiated thymidine. The Golgi system and mitochondria did not show any major changes during phases G_1, S, and G_2. Annulate lamellae were also seen during these three phases.

3.2.2. The KB Cells

The ultrastructure of KB cells, derived from an epidermoid carcinoma (Eagle, 1955*a*), has not been investigated to the extent of that of HeLa cells. Some specific structures observed in KB cells grown under normal conditions have been reported by Rose *et al.* (1963), Kumegawa *et al.* (1967, 1968), and Rose (1970). Additional data on the fine structure of control KB cells may be found in experiments on the effect on KB cells of exposure to mitomycin C (Lapis and Bernhard, 1965), arginine deprivation and X-irradiation (Lane and Novikoff, 1965), ultraviolet irradiation (Lane and Novikoff, 1965; Moreno, 1971), ruby laser irradiation (Amy and Storb, 1965; Storb *et al.*, 1966), exposure to toyocamycin (Phillips and Phillips, 1971), and infection with herpes virus (Sirtori and Bosisio-Bestetti, 1967) and Newcastle disease virus (Loni, 1971).

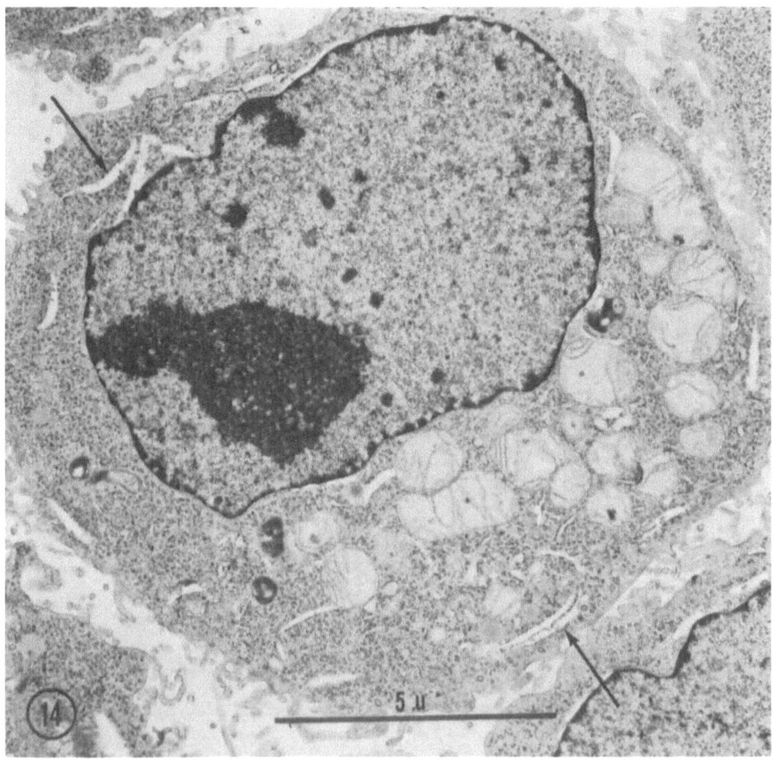

FIG. 14. Appearance of a KB cell in monolayer culture, after trypsinization. The nucleus contains a nucleolus with a tightly woven nucleolonema. A number of cytoplasmic "fractures" (arrows) are visible.

The general appearance of KB cells in thin sections (Fig. 14) does not differ much from that of HeLa cells. The nuclear structure is the same, and as pointed out by Phillips and Phillips (1971) so is the nucleolar structure, although in KB cells recently examined in this laboratory dense nucleoli were less frequent than in HeLa cells. As in HeLa cells, the cell periphery is marked by microvilli and cytoplasmic extensions, but in KB cells cytoplasmic extensions often take the form of cytoplasmic "blebs", sometimes of considerable size. Cytoplasmic blebbing or bubbling, also called "zeiosis" by Costero and Pomerat (1951), has been studied in KB cells by Rose *et al.* (1963). It consists of the formation of pseudopod-like projections containing ribosomes, segments of ergastoplasm, vacuoles, and sometimes mitochondria (Fig. 15). Blebbing, or so-called zeiotic activity, is not limited to KB cells. The phenomenon has been described in detail in HEp-2 cells (Price, 1967) and seen in a variety of normal or malignant cells grown *in vitro* (Bessis, 1964). Blebbing is commonly associated with cell activity during anaphase

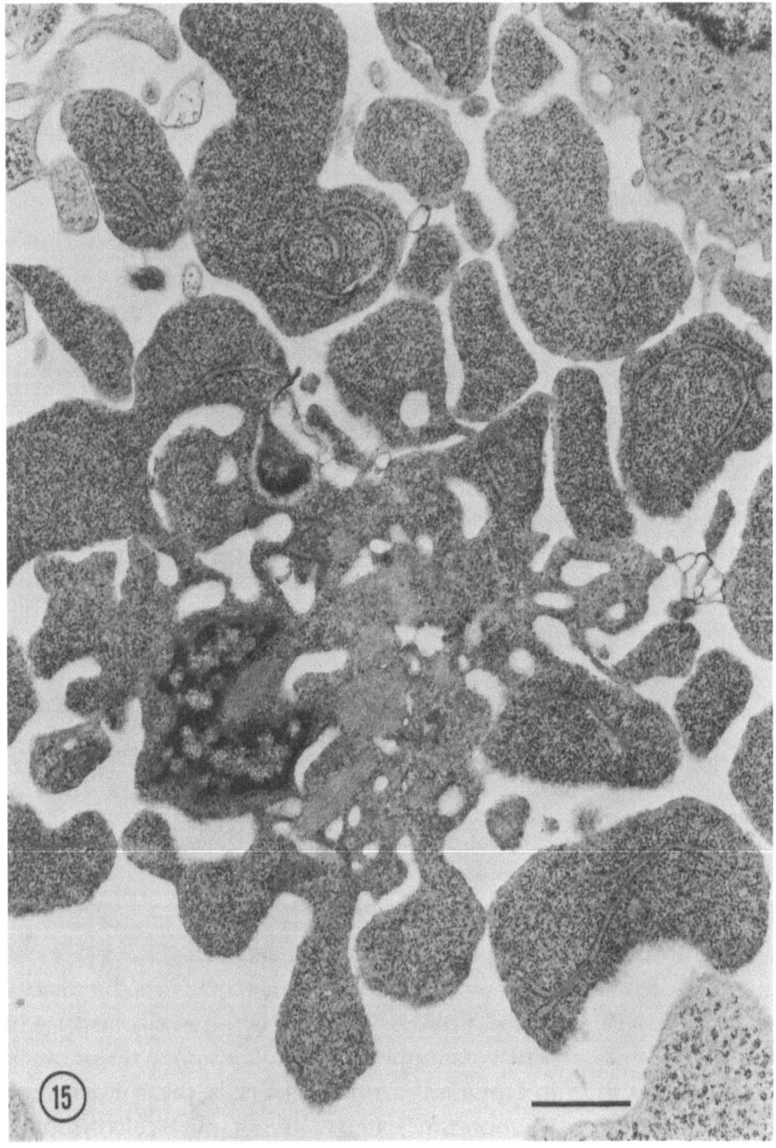

FIG. 15. Cytoplasmic blebbing of a KB cell from a trypsinized culture. The blebs are packed with ribosomes and contain segments of rough endoplasmic reticulum.

and separation of the daughter cells. It can also be artificially induced by a variety of agents or tissue culture conditions (see Price, 1967; Rose, 1970).

As in HeLa cells, the presence of desmosomes (Fig. 16) and hemidesmosomes (Fig. 17) (Lane and Novikoff, 1965), sometimes invaginated in cytoplasmic cavities (Fig. 18), indicates the epithelial origin of KB cells.

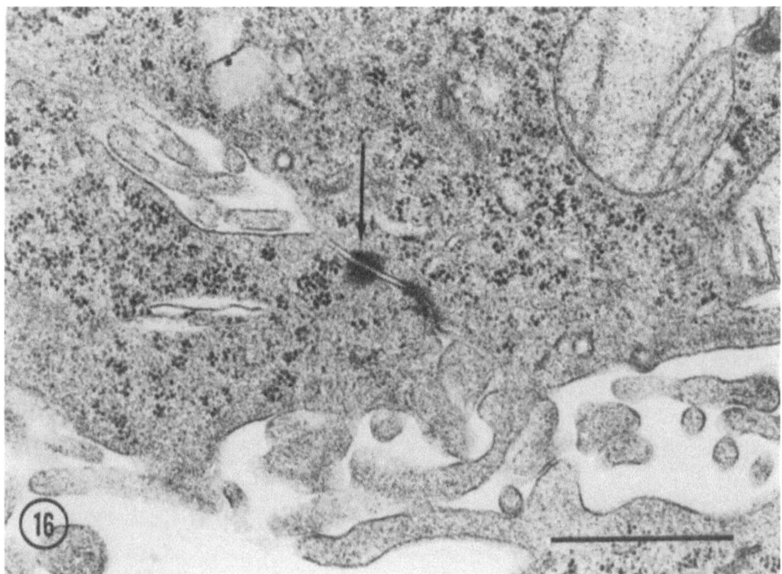

FIG. 16. Examples of desmosome (arrow) joining two KB cells in monolayer culture.

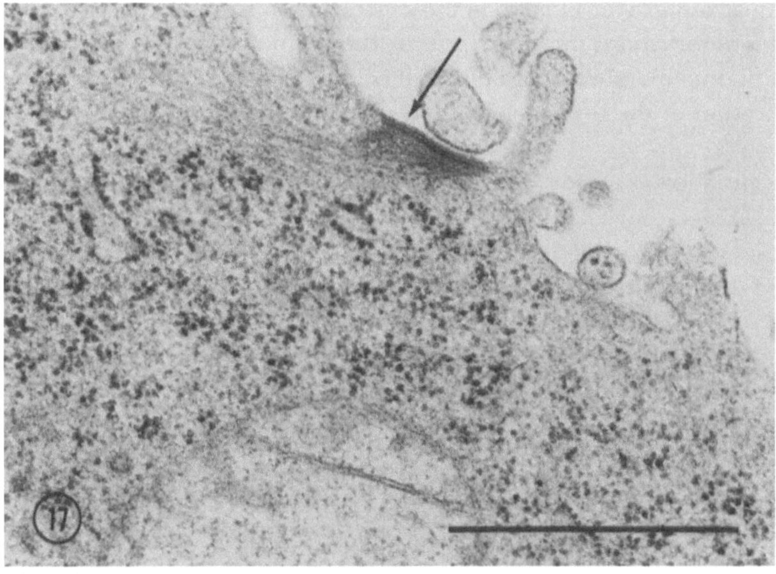

FIG. 17. Hemidesmosome (arrow) at the surface of a KB cell trypsinized culture. The structure of the desmosomal plaque and the system of fibrils converging to it are clearly visible.

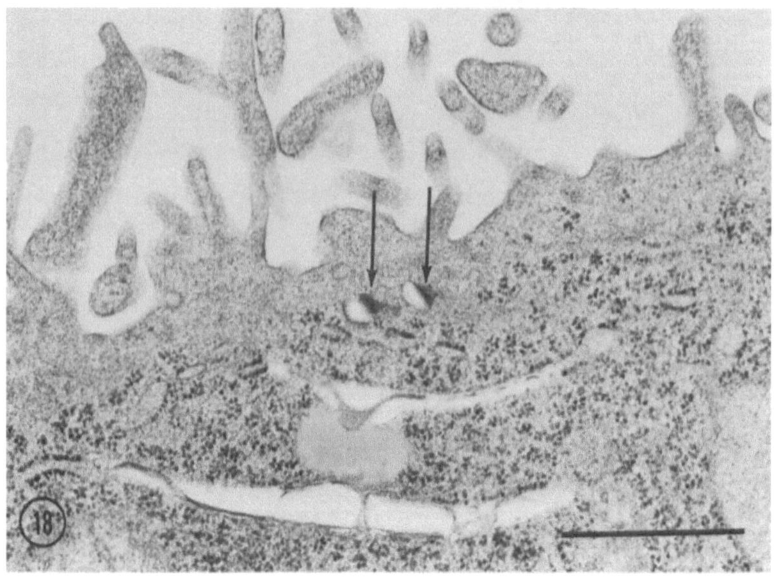

FIG. 18. Invaginated hemidesmosomes (arrows) at the periphery of a KB cell from a trypsinized culture.

Interestingly enough, hemidesmosomes are found not only in KB cells growing as monolayer but also in those growing in suspension (Figs. 19 and 20). This observation appears to indicate the permanence of these structures on the plasma membrane of epithelial cells grown in culture and provides an indication of the origin of cells maintained in culture for any period of time.

KB cells show, in addition to desmosomes, the presence of cytoplasmic tonofibrils suggestive of epithelial cells.

Ribosomes, mitochondria, and the Golgi system of KB cells have no features different from those of HeLa cells. Annulate lamellae (Fig. 21) are found in KB cells grown in monolayers (Lane and Novikoff, 1965; Kumegawa *et al.*, 1968) or in suspension. Lipid droplets, multivesicular bodies, and lysosomes are common constituents of the KB cell cytoplasm (Lane and Novikoff, 1965).

3.2.3. The HEp-2 Cells

Of the three human epithelial tumor cell lines established by Toolan (1954), only line HEp-2, derived from a carcinoma of the larynx, has been extensively used for biological and virus studies. Two publications, one by Price (1967) and a more important one by Strauli *et al.*. (1971), form the main body of our knowledge of the ultrastructure of HEp-2 cells.

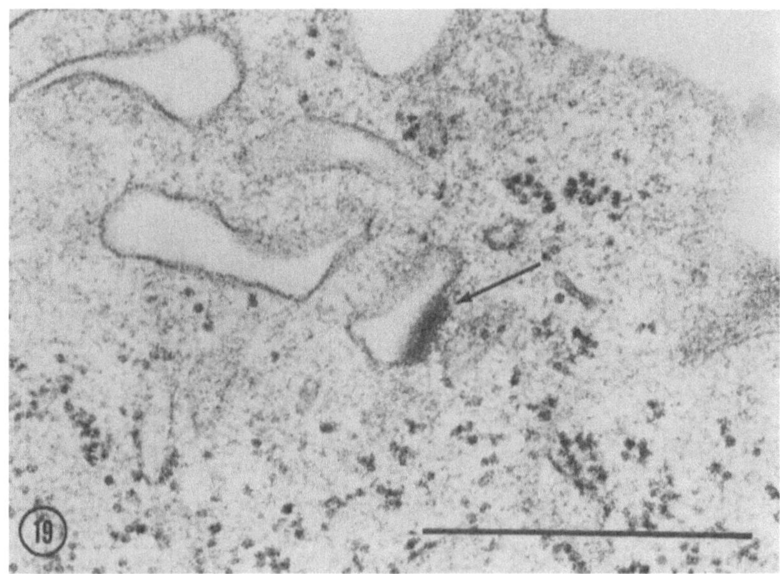

FIG. 19. Invaginated hemidesmosome (arrow) in the cytoplasm of a KB cell growing in suspension.

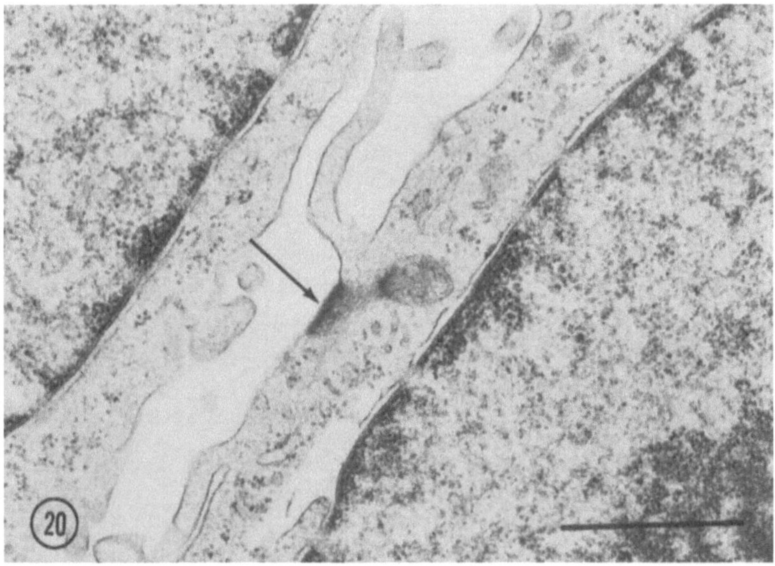

FIG. 20. A typical hemidesmosome (arrow) at the surface of a KB cell growing in suspension.

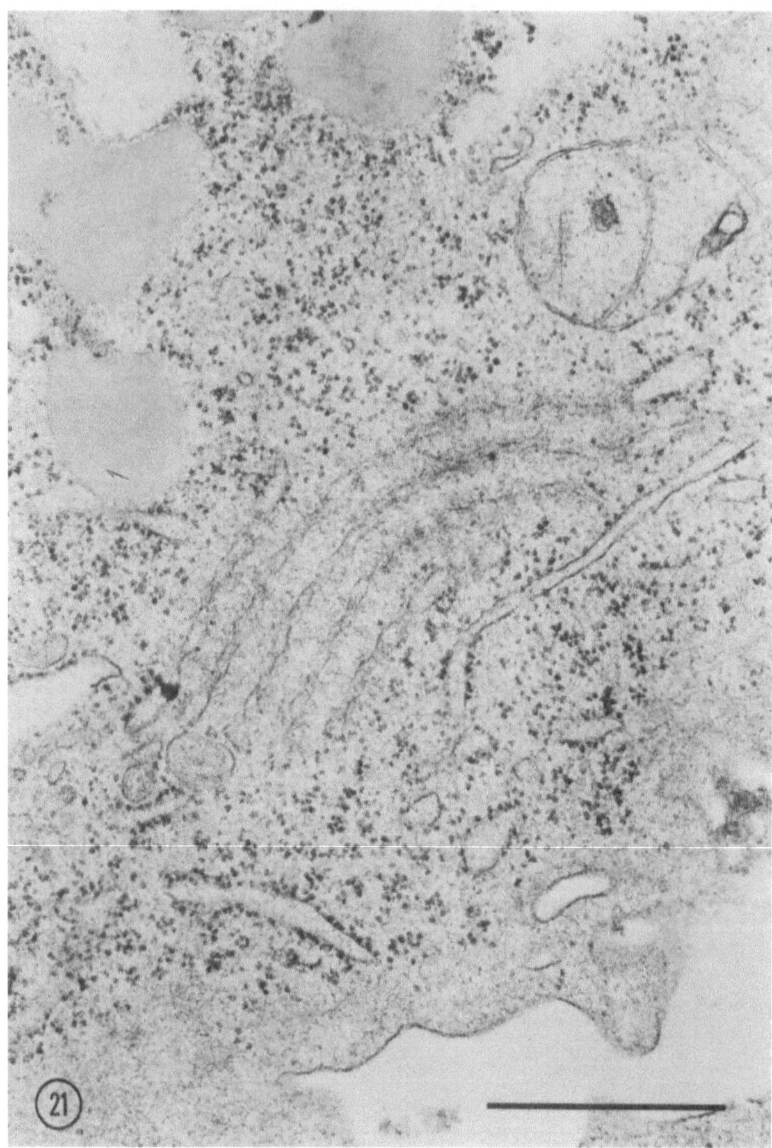

FIG. 21. A system of annulate lamellae in the cytoplasm of a KB cell growing in suspension.

Price (1967) was specifically interested in study of the fine structure of the "zeiotic blebs" displayed by HEp-2 cells growing as monolayers. Strauli *et al.* (1971), using light microscopy, microcinematography, and transmission and scanning electron microscopy, have elucidated many aspects of the surface structure and cell-to-cell contacts of HEp-2 cells during their settling on the substrate after trypsinization and seeding. Freshly seeded cells show an intense zeiotic activity along their entire surface. During elongation and flattening, microextensions of the cytoplasm start forming an intricate network linking the cells to the substrate and to neighboring cells. In spite of the complexity of the network, there is no cytoplasmic continuity between cells through the microextensions. Cell contacts occur through tight junctions and desmosomes. Hemidesmosomes and invaginated hemidesmosomes are, as in HeLa cells, observed at the cell periphery. Strauli *et al.* (1971) have also observed that the plasma membrane of cells entering the mitotic phase retracts but stays for a while connected to the substrate and to other cells by long extensions resembling a radiatings sun ("Strahlensonne"). Later in mitosis the cells lose most of their connections, and the mitotic cells may be easily detached by mechanical means in cultures.

3.2.4. Melanomas

Cells from a number of continuous cultures derived from human melanomas have been examined by electron microscopy. The cell lines examined include melanotic line RPMI-3236 and amelanotic line RPMI-5966, grown in monolayers (Toshima *et al.*, 1968), melanotic line SK-MEL-1, grown in suspension (Oettgen *et al.*, 1968), and melanotic line LeCa and amelanotic line MeGo, grown as monolayers (Romsdahl and Hsu, 1967; Maul and Romsdahl, 1970). Lines RPMI-3236, RPMI-5966, LeCa, and MeGo are derived from tumors or from metastatic tumors, while line SK-MEL-1 has been established as a suspension line of thoracic duct cells of a patient with melanoma.

The principal ultrastructural features of cells from line SK-MEL-1 can be summarized as follows: rounded nuclei with single or multiple nucleoli; abundance of free ribosomes; elongated mitochondria; prominent Golgi complexes; large numbers of microvilli at the cell periphery; and large quantities of dense, osmiophilic granules (Oettgen *et al.*, 1968). The granules are surrounded by a single membrane and most of them resemble lysosomes or phagosomes; others are pigmented but do not show the characteristic crystallike lattice of melanosomes.

The fine structure of melanin-producing apparatus and of melanosome formation has been extensively studied by Toshima *et al.* (1968) in cells of the RPMI lines. In these cells, premelanosomes and melanosomes are scattered in the entire cytoplasm, and appear to be associated with the endoplasmic reticulum. The earliest components of the melanin-producing system consist of lamellae and vesicles derived from the Golgi apparatus and from the endoplasmic reticulum. These structures develop into 0.3–0.5 μm "intermediate vesicles" filled with coarse granules about 200–300 Å in diameter. The granules conglomerate into larger granules, and the vesicle–granule system develops into premelanosomes, as seen by the appearance of a fibrillar structure in the dense matrix filling the vesicles (Fig. 22). At the point where pigment deposition obscures the fibrillar pattern,

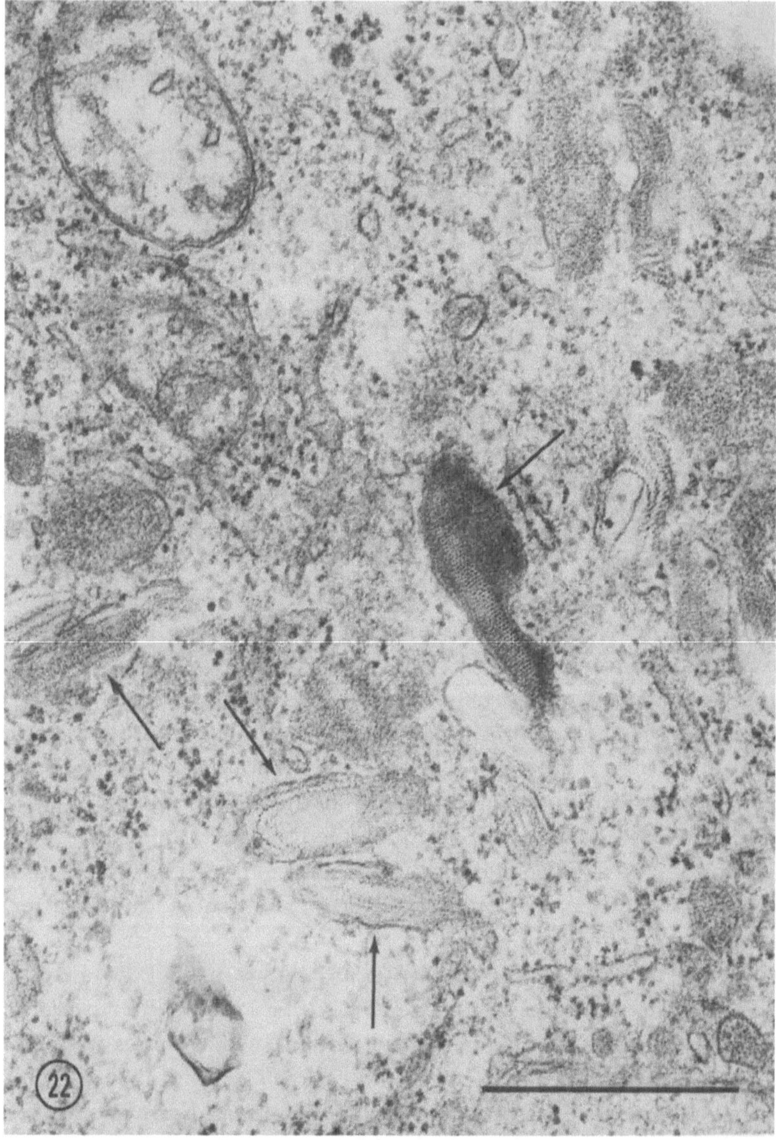

FIG. 22. Passage 35 of a culture derived from buffy coat cells of a patient with melanoma. The micrograph shows part of the cytoplasm of a pigment-producing cell, containing a number of premelanosomes (arrows).

premelanosomes become mature melanosomes. Melanosomes are generally oblong structures and are surrounded by an outer membrane, except when they are phagocytized. In the "amelanotic" line RPMI-5966, electron microscopy has revealed that the cells are actually synthesizing melanosomes but the fibrillar component is missing and the pigment deposition is very light.

Ultrastructural studies by Maul and Romsdahl (1970) of melanogenesis in cells from lines LeCa and MeGo confirmed the previous findings of Toshima *et al.* (1968). While in cells from line LeCa melanosomes show a characteristic helical fiber structure, the pigmented bodies of cells from the "amelanotic" subline AMEL-P4 and AMEL-4 and of the low-pigment-producing line MeGo lack this characteristic structure. In the absence of substructure, premelanosomes of the MeGo cells are difficult to differentiate from lysosomes. However, like lysosomes, pigment-producing bodies of the MeGo cells show acid phosphatase activity, and, like premelanosomes, they show tyrosinase activity, thus apparently confirming the hypothesis of Novikoff *et al.* (1968) that melanosomes are modified lysosomes.

Cells from line LeCa, like SK-MEL-1 cells, contain autophagic vacuoles filled with melanosomes. This observation may indicate either an uptake by some cells of melanosomes released by other cells or a phenomenon of autodigestion of melanosomes accumulating in the cytoplasm.

Maul and Brinkley (1970) have carried out a special ultrastructural study of the Golgi apparatus during mitosis in cells from line LeCa. They have observed that elements of the Golgi system may persist throughout mitosis, contrary to the findings of Robbins and Gonatas (1964) in dividing HeLa cells.

Melanocytes of the skin apparently have no desmosomes (Lentz, 1971). In our laboratory, desmosomes have not been seen in pigment-synthesizing melanoma cells grown *in vitro* and derived from buffy coat cells of a melanoma patient (M. F. Miller, unpublished observation).

3.2.5. Breast Cancer

Successful attempts to grow epithelial cells from breast tumors have until now been very limited, irrespective of the technique employed in preparing primary monolayer cultures of breast tumor tissues. In spite of the initial outgrowth of some kind of cells, generally fibroblastic, from biopsy tissues in about 60% of the cases (Feller *et al.*, 1972; Seman *et al.*, 1971; Bassin *et al.*, 1972), survival and multiplication of the cells did not generally extend to more than a few weeks or months. Nevertheless, prolonged or continuous cultivation of breast tumor cells has been reported in the literature. Line Detroit 30A has been obtained by Berman and Stulberg (1956) from the ascitic fluid of a patient with breast cancer. Brest tumor lines EG, EJ, EV, AR, and LR (Mustakallio and Gronroos, 1957) and CaMa (Dobrynin, 1963) are no longer available. The most interesting cell line, because of its epithelial morphology, is line BT-20, established in 1958 by Lasfargues and Ozzello, and still actively growing. More recent breast cancer lines are one established by Martorelli *et al.* (1969), line HBT-3 established by Bassin *et al.* (1972), from a mucus-producing adenocarcinoma, and line HBT-39 (Plata *et al.*, 1973) derived from a ductal carcinoma. Line HBT-39 has been cloned into three sublines: HBT-39A and HBT-39B of epithelial-like morphology, and HBT-39F of fibroblastic morphology. Cells from line HBT-39B have the ability to grow in suspension culture in the presence of aged human serum (Plata *et al.*, 1973).

Ozzello (1972) has published a comparative electron microscopic study of cells from the BT-20 line and of cells from short-term cultures of breast tumor biopsies. The BT-20 cells have retained, even after many years, their epithelial character, as shown by the presence of desmosomes and tonofibrils. The cells also possess ductlike vacuoles in their cytoplasm, structures that have been claimed to be very symptomatic of epithelial breast cancer cells *in vivo* (Sykes *et al.*, 1968; Seman *et al.*, 1971). Plata *et al.* (1973) have examined cells from the HBT-39 lines by electron microscopy. The authors do not mention having observed desmosomes, tonofibrils, or ductlike vacuoles in the epithelioid HBT-39A and HBT-39B cells. Flaxman and Van Scott (1972), examining vertical sections of normal human mammary epithelium grown on plasma clots, have observed desmosomes and tonofilaments in the epithelial cells, but no ductlike vacuoles.

A problem of particular difficulty is to determine the origin of cells derived from pleural effusions of breast cancer patients (Seman *et al.*, 1971). About 60% of the effusions contain islands of metastatic cells generally identifiable by routine cytological techniques, and therefore should be particularly suitable for the initiation of breast cancer cell cultures. However, pleural effusions also contain mesothelial cells, histiocytes, and fibroblasts, cells capable of temporary, if not continuous, growth in monolayers. Morphological diagnosis of a fibroblastic outgrowth is in general not difficult, by either light or electron microscopy. The growth potential of histiocytes of human pleural effusion is as yet unknown. The major diagnostic problem is caused by the presence of mesothelial cells, because of their ultrastructural similarities with other cells of epithelial origin. These cells are known to possess many microvilli, tonofilaments, and typical desmosomes (Stoebner *et al.*, 1970; Salazar *et al.*, 1972; Ferenczy *et al.*, 1972), all structural components shared with breast cancer cells *in vivo* or *in vitro*. It has been shown, however, that in about 50% of the breast cancers examined, mitochondria of the epithelial cells contain tubulofilamentous structures

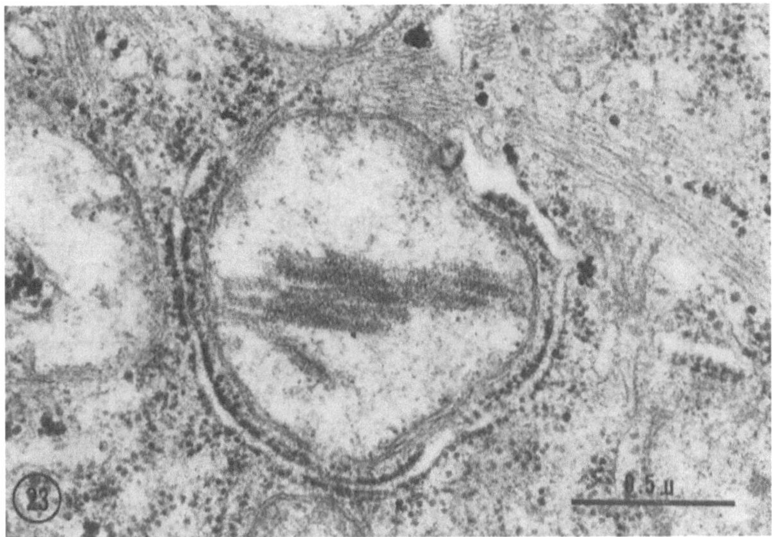

FIG. 23. Tubulofilamentous structures in mitochondrion of a tumor cell from a pleural effusion of a patient with breast cancer.

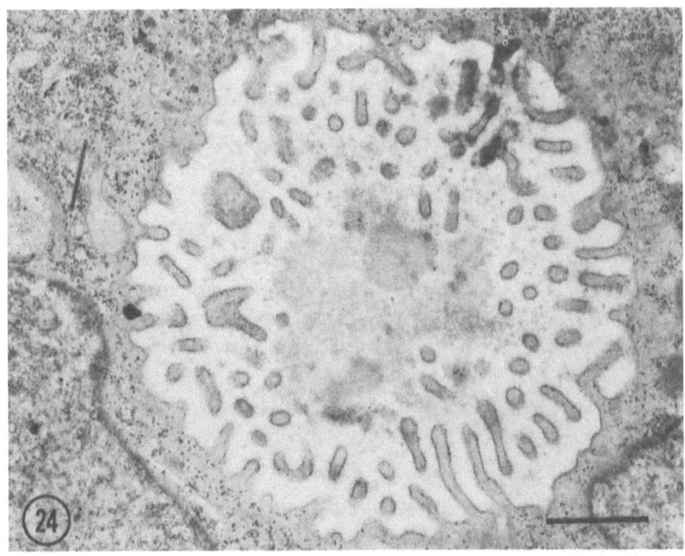

FIG. 24. A characteristic ductlike vacuole in a tumor cell from a pleural effusion of a patient with breast cancer.

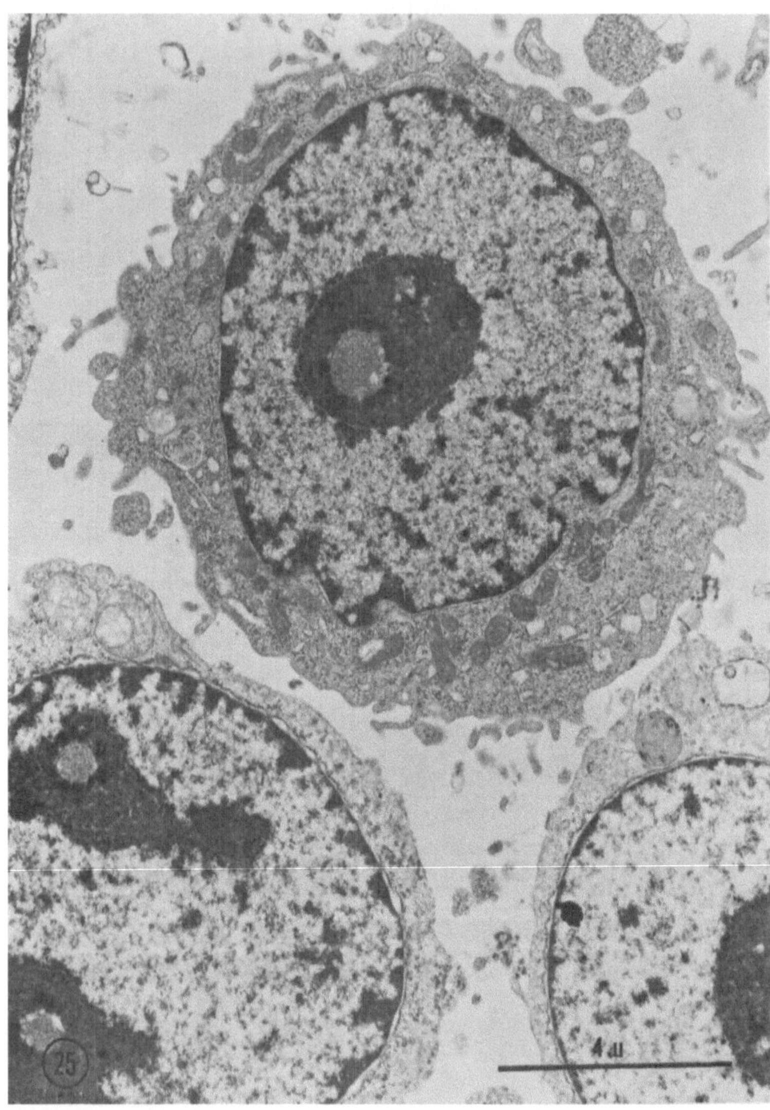

FIG. 25. View of a cell from passage 314 of the MAC-21 line derived from lung cancer.

(Seman *et al.*, 1971). The presence of such structures in cells of fresh pleural effusions (Fig. 23) and of ductlike vacuoles (Fig. 24) may help in identifying the cancer cells (personal observation). The destiny of these mitochondrial markers in long-term cultures is not yet known, however. Only a study of

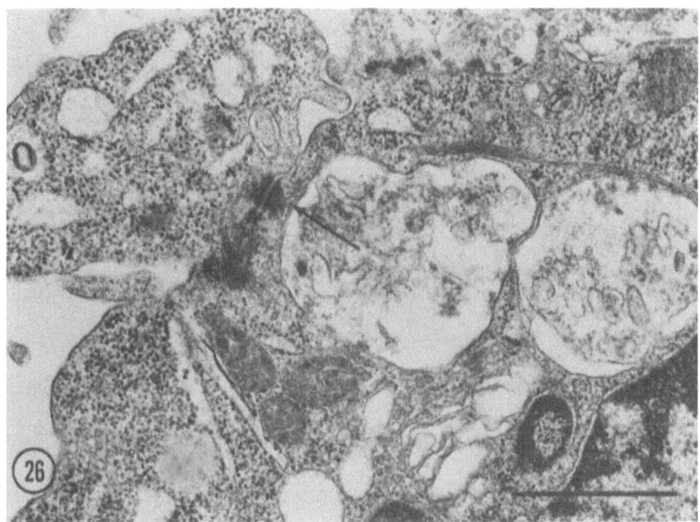

FIG. 26. Desmosome (arrow) joining MAC-21 cells.

more epithelial cell lines derived from breast cancer can help to solve these problems.

3.2.6. Lung Cancer

Several cell lines derived from lung adenocarcinoma have been reported: line LAC (Baron and Rabson, 1957), line MAC-21 (Cailleau, 1960), lines ThoCu, AlAb, and SaBa (Reed and Gey, 1962). The fine structure of cells from line MAC-21 has been reported by Fuse *et al.* (1963) in a comparative study of the ultrastructure of MAC-21 and HeLa cells. The authors have found that MAC-21 cells have larger nuclei, more microvilli, a better-developed Golgi system, and more endoplasmic reticulum and mitochondria than HeLa cells. They have seen very few tonofibrils and no desmosomes or hemidesmosomes. In view of the importance of the last point, a recent passage of the MAC-21 cell culture has been examined in this laboratory. The cells (Fig. 25) show the presence of small desmosomes (Fig. 26) and hemidesmosomes and of a well-developed endoplasmic reticulum filled with lightly staining material (Fig. 27). Many vesicles, probably multivesicular bodies, filled with rounded or elongated structures (Fig. 27) are present in the cytoplasm of the cells.

3.2.7. Acanthosis Nigricans

Dawe *et al.* (1964) have established a cell line, AN_3CA, from a uterine carcinoma of a patient with lesions of acanthosis nigricans. The cells show an

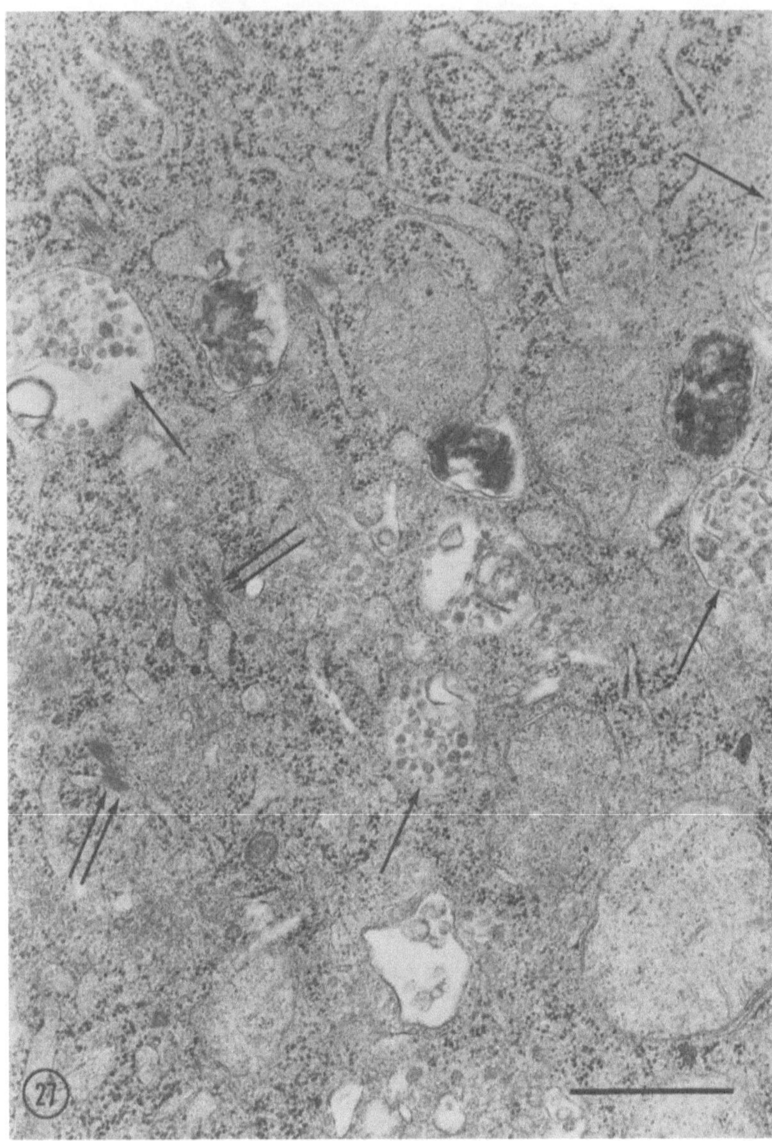

FIG. 27. Part of the cytoplasm of a cell from the MAC-21 line. Endoplasmic reticulum is well developed. The cisternae contain amorphous material. Multivesicular bodies (arrows) contain many rounded structures that could sometimes be mistaken for virus-like particles. Small bundles of tonofilaments (double arrows) are interspersed in the cytoplasm.

intense blebbing (zeiotic) activity. In the electron microscope, the blebs appear as pseudopods containing fibrils, ribosomes, mitochondria, and parts of the endoplasmic reticulum. The authors have not found clues to the true nature (epithelial or fibroblastic) of these cells.

3.3. *Cells Derived from Cultures of Sarcomas*

Published data on the ultrastructure of cells derived from human sarcomas and grown *in vitro* (osteosarcomas, fibrosarcomas, giant cell tumors, etc.) are very scarce, probably for lack of continuous cultures.

Many specimens of sarcoma tissues have been put in culture in this laboratory, and examined after growth in monolayers at various passage numbers. Whether the cells are derived from osteosarcomas (Fig. 28), fibrosarcomas (Fig. 29), giant cell tumors, or other tumors, they reveal considerable ultrastructural similarities. These similarities are shared, as expected, with other cells derived in culture from the stroma of epithelial tumors, lymph nodes, bone marrow, spleen, etc.

The cells are always fairly large, with deeply indented nuclei (Figs. 28 and 29). The cell periphery, probably because of retraction and tearing of the substrate of cytoplasmic extensions, shows many villosities and pseudopod-like protrusions, especially at the cellular end opposed to the nucleus. Nuclei appear light, with small clumps of chromatin packed along the nuclear borders. Nucleoli are generally large and multiple, usually consisting of a rather loose nucleolonemal network (Fig. 28). Compact, granular nucleoli are less frequent. Besides a Golgi system of moderate size, with one or two dictyosomes, the cytocavitary system of the cells is characterized by the appearance of the endoplasmic reticulum. The rough endoplasmic reticulum consists of an abundance of tortuous cavities spread throughout the cell without any definite orientation. The cavities, bordered by single rows of ribosomes (Fig. 30), are filled with an amorphous, slightly electron-dense material. There are also very numerous smooth vesicles of irregular shape (Fig. 31). Free ribosomes and a few polyribosomes, generally in rosettes, dot the cytoplasmic matrix.

The cytoplasm of the cells has two other important features. One is the abundance of fibrils running in every direction, resulting in a criss-cross, branching pattern (Fig. 31). Cross-sections of the fibres appear as small dots. Another feature, along the borders of the cytoplasm, especially where the protrusions are numerous, is the presence of zones devoid of organelles. In these zones, the cytoplasmic fibrils are seen embedded in patches of electron-dense material (Fig. 32). Many small, smooth vesicles are frequently

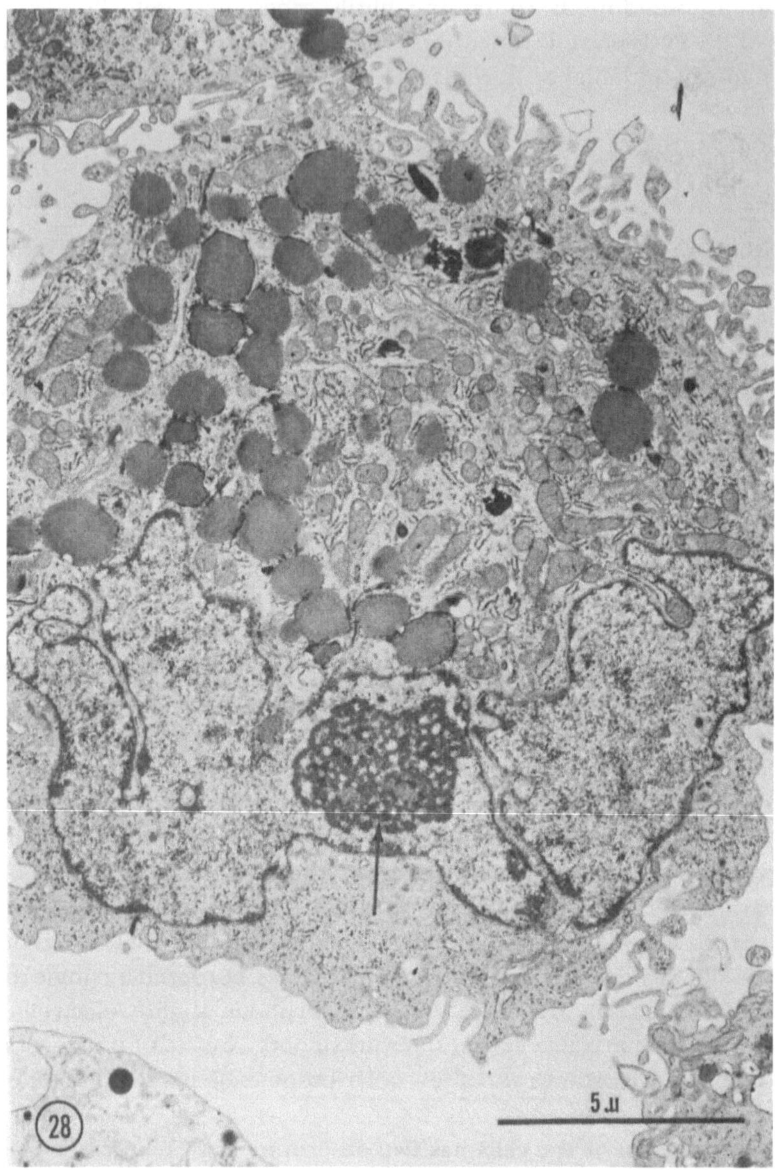

FIG. 28. Appearance of a cell from passage 33 of a culture derived from osteosarcoma. The nucleus is lobulated and indented. The nucleolus is composed of a loose nucleolonemal network (arrow). Many lipid droplets fill the cytoplasm.

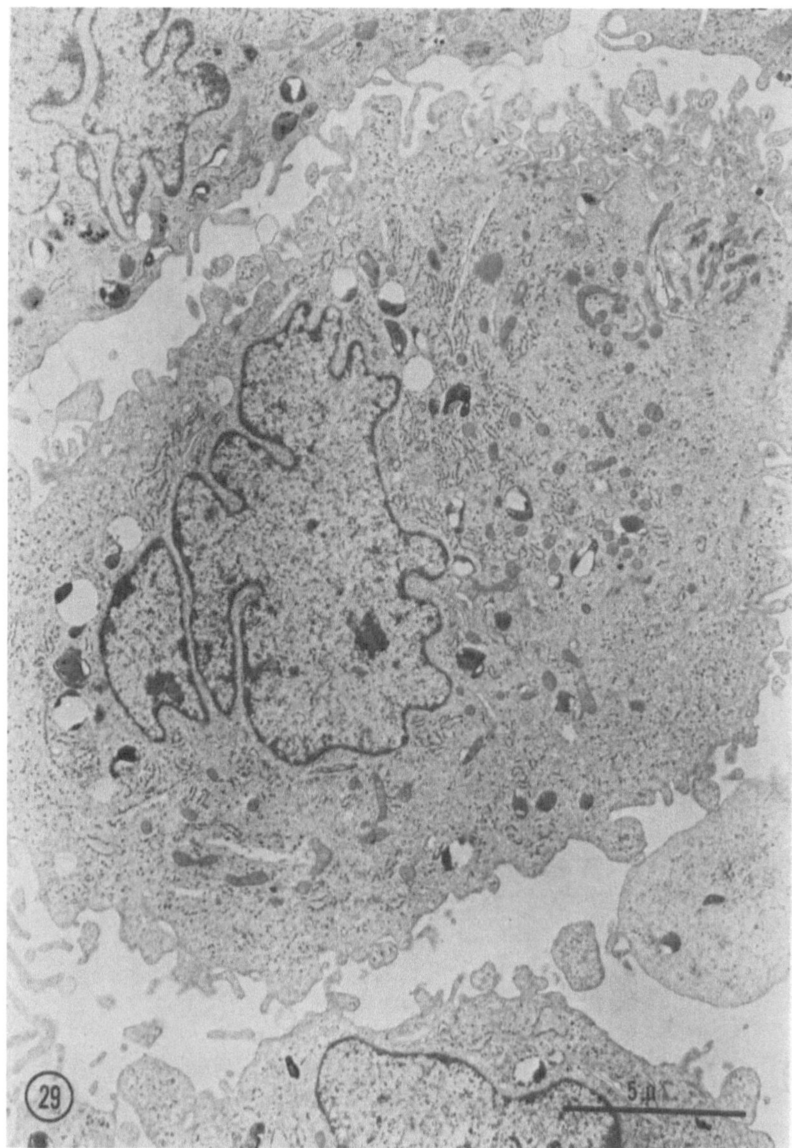

FIG. 29. Appearance of a cell derived from fibrosarcoma in monolayer culture.

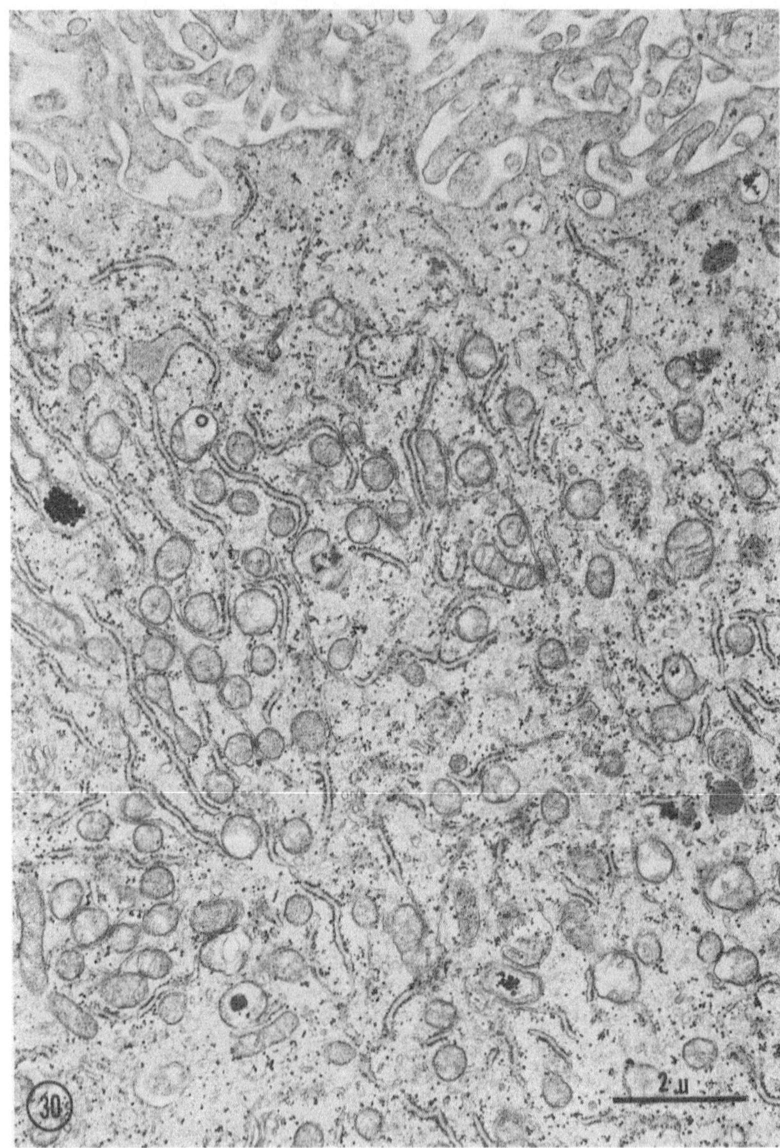

FIG. 30. Passage 19 of a culture derived from a stromal sarcoma of the breast. The micrograph shows part of the cytoplasm of a cell with elongated endoplasmic cisternae filled with lightly staining material. Single ribosomes are scattered in the cytoplasmic matrix.

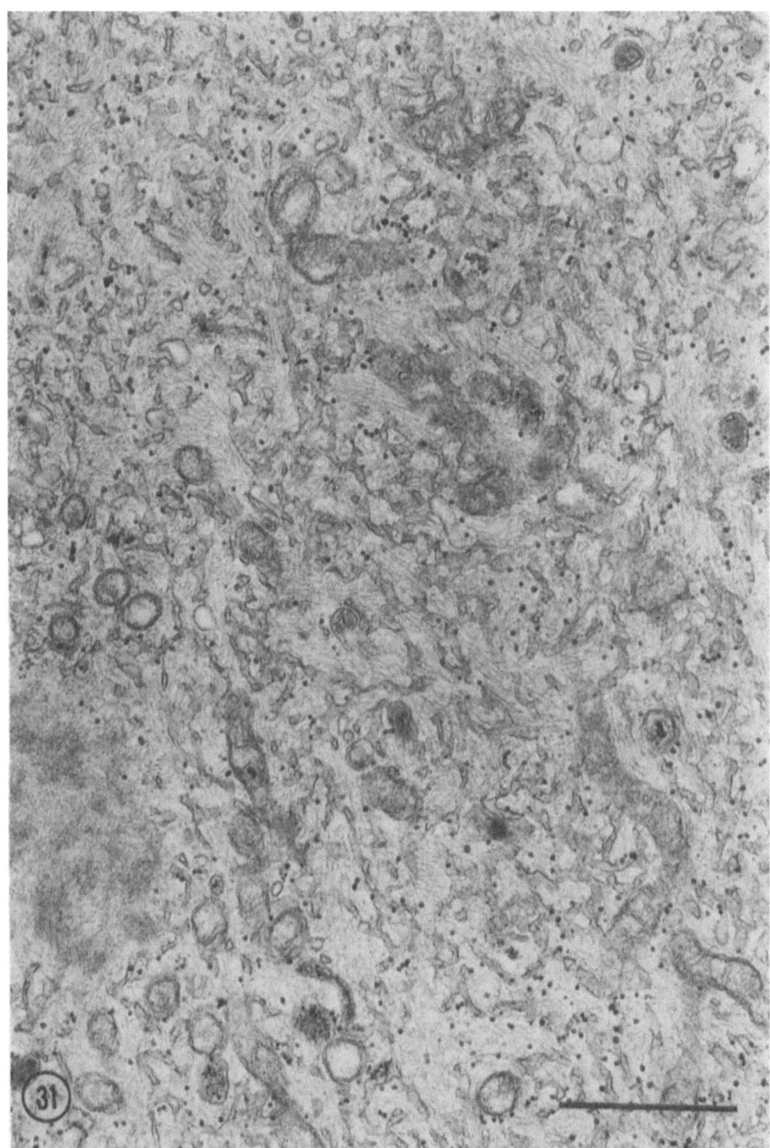

FIG. 31. Same culture as in Fig. 30. Part of the cytoplasm of a cell showing the fibrillar network and an abundance of small smooth cisternae of complex configuration.

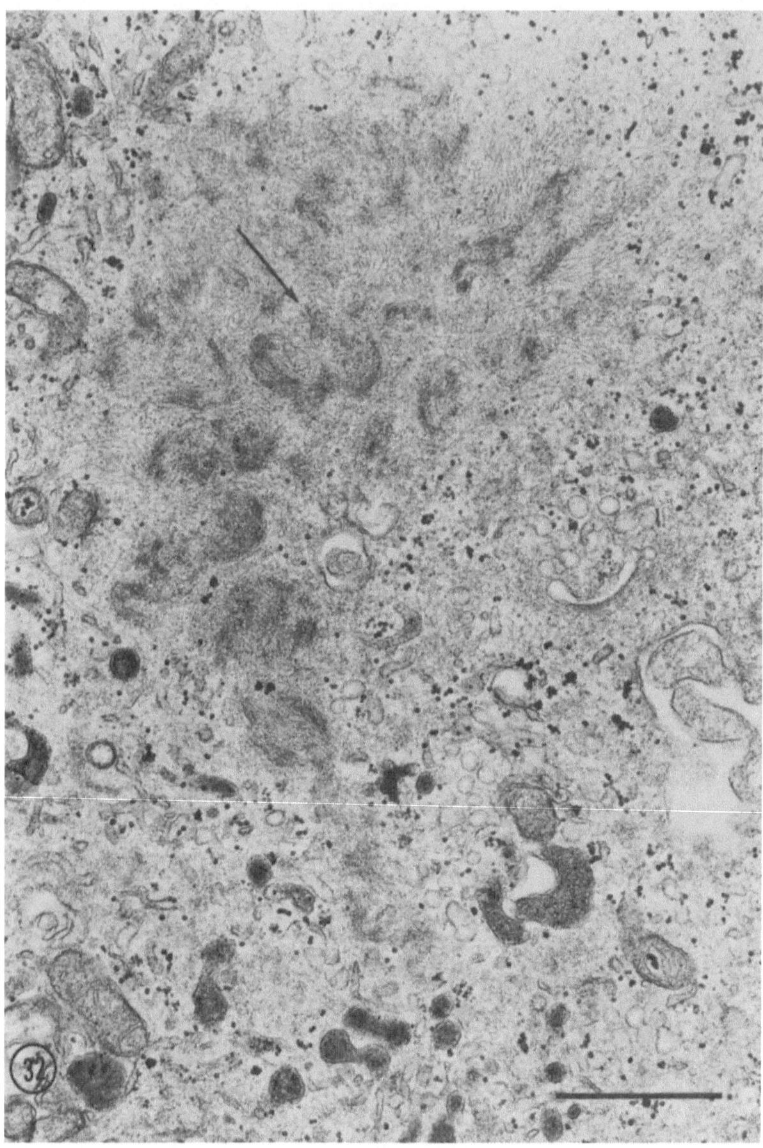

FIG. 32. Same culture as in Fig. 30. Fibrillar densifications (arrow) at the periphery of a cell. Many smooth vesicles are present between the densifications and the cellular borders.

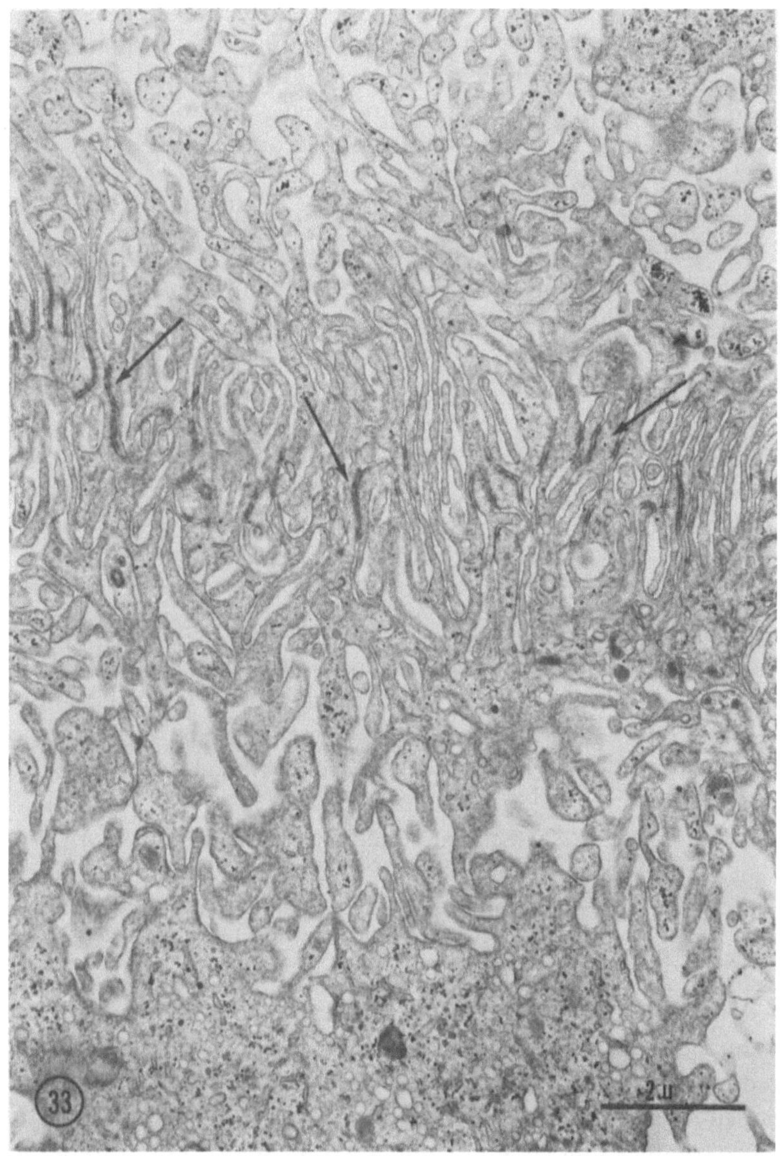

FIG. 33. Same culture as in Fig. 30. contacts between the cells occur through "tight junctions" (arrows) at the surface of intertwined cytoplasmic extensions.

interposed between these zones and the cell membrane (Fig. 32). Mitochondria may vary in shape. They are usually elongated, with irregular outlines, a relatively dense matrix, and oblique cristae (Fig. 31). Other cytoplasmic organelles are varying numbers of dense bodies, lipid droplets, and inclusions of heterogeneous structure (Figs. 30 and 32), sometimes extremely abundant and probably derived from phagocytic activity and autophagy.

The cells are in contact with each other through "tight junctions" only (Fig. 33). Desmosomes or hemidesmosomes are characteristically absent. Tonofibrils packed in bundles, as seen in epithelial cells, are never found.

Cells derived in culture from human sarcomas may differ in the amounts of some of their cytoplasmic structures (filaments, endoplasmic reticulum, vesicles, etc.), but even after many passages they retain the basic structure of actively growing fibroblasts (see Movat and Fernando, 1962) or of fibrosarcoma cells *in vivo*. Fibrosarcoma cells have large, indented nuclei, a well-developed endoplasmic reticulum filled with homogeneous material, elongated mitochondria, and many cytoplasmic fibrils.

Ultrastructural features of some sarcomas have been published by a number of authors, as mentioned below.

a. Neuroblastomas and Gliomas. Continuous cultures of cells derived from neuroblastomas have been reported by Goldstein *et al.* (1964) and by Tumilowicz *et al.* (1970), who established line IMR-2 from the tumor of a 13-month-old boy. Goldstein (1971) had grown cells derived from the tumors of four different children with neuroblastoma for periods of 10–160 days.

Cells from the line IMR-2, examined by electron microscopy between passages 54 and 63, were found to be composed of two morphologically different types. The predominant cell was small and refractile, and resembled a neuroblast. The second type of cell, less frequent, was relatively large, well spread, and fibroblast-like (Tumilowicz *et al.*, 1970). Cloning tests seemed to indicate that the second cell type, derived from the first by differentiation, had a limited life span. Cells of the predominant type showed little chromatin margination, elongated mitochondria, and poorly developed ergastoplasm. The other cells had a heavily marginated chromatin, more complex mitochondria, and a well-developed ergastoplasm filled with lightly electron-scattering material.

In two of the cultures of neuroblastoma cells grown by Goldstein (1971), annulate lamellae have been frequently found.

In a study on the effect of nerve growth factor (NGF) on HEp-2 cells and on cells derived from glioblastoma multiforme, Pinkerton *et al.* (1971) have published an electron micrograph of an untreated cell of the glioblastoma line C356. The cell showed features apparently no different from those of any mesenchymal cell in culture.

b. Retinoblastomas. Some ultrastructural features of cells derived from retinoblastomas in culture are shown in the atlas of Rose (1970). Retinoblasts lose their neurofibrils after several months in culture and resemble fibroblasts.

c. Synovial Sarcomas. Cells from monolayer cultures of human synovial sarcomas have been examined in the electron microscope by Buonassisi and Ozzello (1973). The cells are fibroblastic and resemble the original tumor cells. Collagen synthesis has not been observed.

d. Ewing Sarcoma of the Bone. Tumor specimens from seven different patients have been grown in this laboratory for 8 wk to 6 months. In the electron microscope (Hou-Jensen *et al.*, 1972), the cells appeared different from the original tumor cells in that they resembled fibroblastic cells of other sarcomas. Desmosomes have not been seen in these cells.

3.4. *Cells Derived from Tumors of the Hematopoietic Tissues*

The first long-term cultures of human cells derived from tumors of the hematopoietic tissues were established by Epstein and Barr (1964) and by Pulvertaft (1964, 1965) from tissues of Burkitt's lymphoma. At about the same time, Iwakata and Grace (1964) reported the successful establishment of the RPMI-6410 cell line, derived from the peripheral blood of a patient with acute myelogenous leukemia. Improvements in the generally simple cultivation methods required to grow cells from hematopoietic tissues have led since then to a proliferation of so-called lymphoblastoid cell lines. They all have in common the ability to grow preferably in suspension. Many lines have been originated from the peripheral blood of patients with leukemia, such as lines SB-2 (Foley *et al.*, 1965), M2 (Lucas *et al.*, 1966), LK1D, LK57, and LK60 (Armstrong, 1966), CCRF-CEM (Uzman *et al.*, 1966), SK-L1 to SK-L9 (Clarkson *et al.*, 1967), a series of RPMI lines (Moore *et al.*, 1968), and CoA-2 and HUM-1 (Steel and Edmond, 1971). A series of other lines have been derived from tissues of patients with Burkitt's lymphoma: EB-1 and EB-2 (Epstein *et al.*, 1965), P-1-Raji, P-2-Kudi, P-3-Jijoye, and P-4-Ogun (Pulvertaft, 1965), SL_1 (Stewart *et al.*, 1965), AL-1 (Rabson *et al.*, 1966), P-3J-HR1-K and P-3-HR5, derived from line P-3-Jijoye (Hinuma and Grace, 1967), and the 35 NK lines (Nadkarni *et al.*, 1969).

Many attempts have been made to serially propagate bone marrow cells from patients with leukemia or other malignancies (Berman and Stulberg, 1958; Benyesh–Melnick, 1967; Rabin *et al.*, 1967; Mouriquand and Mouriquand, 1968). These attempts have met with little success, however, and only a few lines have been established: Detroit 6, 32, and 34 (Berman and Stulberg, 1956), L 1-BM6, L 1-BM15, and L 1-BM18 (Rabin *et al.*, 1967), and C529 and C566 (Benyesh–Melnick, 1967). Some lines have been established from other tissues. Line SK-RCS-1 was derived from a pleural effusion of a patient with reticulum cell sarcoma (Clarkson *et al.*, 1969). Line IM-1 (Finegold *et al.*, 1968) and another line (Trujillo, 1966) have been established from lymph node tissues of patients with lymphoma, while lines LY are derived from tumor tissues of patients with nasopharyngeal carcinoma (De The *et al.*, 1969, 1970).

From the first ultrastructural studies of cells derived from Burkitt's lymphoma and from peripheral blood of leukemic patients (Epstein and Achong, 1965; Uzman *et al.*, 1966), and from those studies that followed, it soon became apparent that the fine structure of the cells established in culture was always the same, whether the cultures were derived from tumor tissues, peripheral blood, or bone marrow of patients with Burkitt's lymphoma, leukemia, infectious mononucleosis, or a variety of malignancies, or from the blood of apparently healthy subjects.

The general ultrastructure of lymphoblastoid cells in long-term cultures became known from the following studies: electron microscopic examination of cells from the M2 line by Zeve *et al.* (1966); cells from lines derived from leukemic bone marrows and bone marrow from children with infectious mononucleosis by Rabin *et al.* (1967); the SKL-1 cells and cells from a series of RPMI lines derived from leukemic bloods and Burkitt's tumor by De Harven (1967) and De Harven *et al.* (1967); cells from lines AL-1 and EB-2 and from PHA-stimulated normal lymphocytes by Douglas *et al.* (1967); cells from a series of cultures of hematopoietic cells by Moore *et al.* (1968) and Chandra *et al.* (1968); cells from the NHDL lines derived from the blood of normal human donors by Gerber and Monroe (1968); cells from lines AL–1 and AL-3 by Bedoya *et al.* (1969); cells from line SK-RCS-1 by Clarkson *et al.* (1969); cells established from the lymph node of a patient with chronic lymphocytic leukemia by Trujillo *et al.* (1966); cells derived from cultures of bone marrow, lymph node, and spleen of patients with leukemia by Recher *et al.* (1969).

The cells resemble lymphoblasts or large lymphocytes, as described by Anderson (1970) in his important ultrastructural survey of normal and leukemic blood cells. As stated by Moore *et al.* (1968): "There are no microscopic or ultramicroscopic characteristics that permit separation of cultured human lymphoblastoid cells derived from normal individuals and from patients with leukemia, Burkitt's lymphoma, and infectious mononucleosis" (see also Dalton and Zeve, 1967).

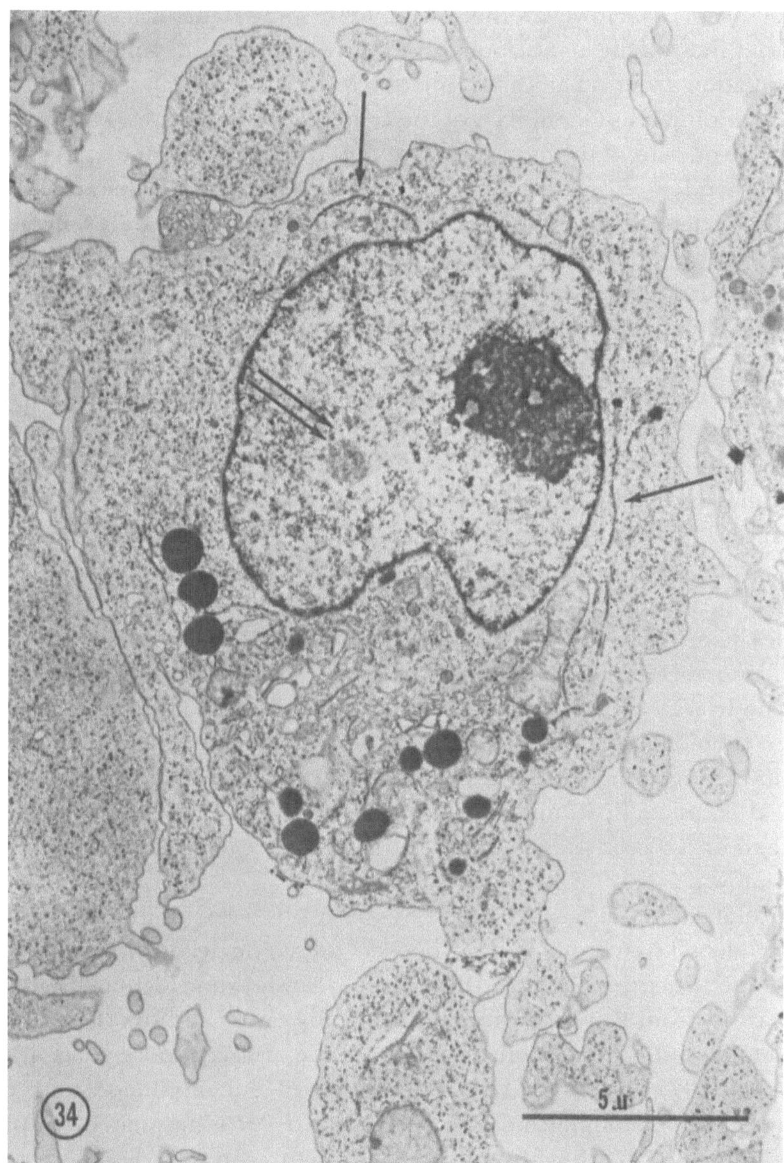

FIG. 34. A typical "lymphoblastoid cell" from a suspension culture of buffy coat cells from a patient with lymphoblastic leukemia. Endoplasmic cisternae are long and narrow (arrows). Several lipid droplets are present in the cytoplasm. A nuclear body (double arrow) may be seen in the nucleus.

The lymphoblastoid cells have the general appearance of undifferentiated blast cells (Fig. 34). However, there seem to be some structural variations of the nuclei that might be attributed, in a given culture, to some degree of differentiation from an undifferentiated reticulum cell (about 5% of the cells) to lymphoblasts (about 85% of the cells) and lymphocytes (Moore *et al.*, 1968). The nucleus of the most primitive cells is large and irregular in shape, with little condensed chromatin. More "mature" cells are smaller and have a rounded nucleus and a more condensed chromatin. These differences are reflected in the appearance of the cytoplasm. The most primitive cells have a clear and large cytoplasm with many ribosomes in rosettes, and a well-developed Golgi apparatus. The other cells, with more even distribution of ribosomes, a smaller surface, and a less conspicuous Golgi system, appear darker. In all the cells, the endoplasmic reticulum is limited to a few narrow channels, except in a small number of cells where the endoplasmic reticulum is more abundant and has a plasmacytoid disposition. The endoplasmic reticulum is exceptionally well developed, however, in lines EB-3 and SKL-3 (De Harven, 1967). Annulate lamellae are frequent in cells of all the cultures (De Harven, 1967). Mitochondria are generally rounded, less frequently fusiform; giant forms are not uncommon. They may contain dense granules, about 150 Å in size, resembling ribosomes as described by Andre and Marinozzi (1965), and tenuous fibers, 30 Å wide, probably representing mitochondrial DNA. Mitochondria of cultured hematopoietic cells may also contain tubulofilamentous structures 400 Å in diameter, consisting of subunits arranged in a helical pattern (De Harven, 1967), identical to those observed occasionally in mitochondria of breast cancer cells (Seman *et al.*, 1971) and of KB cells (Rose, 1970). The significance of the last structures is still unknown.

Particular attention has been paid by many observers to nuclear projections or "blebs," frequently seen as "pockets" of the nuclei of lymphoblastoid cells. These structures have been described by Epstein and Achong (1965) in cells derived from Burkitt's lymphoma, and by other authors (Foley *et al.*, 1965; Mollo and Stramignoni, 1967; McDuffie, 1967; Moore *et al.*, 1968; Burns *et al.*, 1971) in cells derived from cultures of leukemic blood, leukemic lymph nodes, or Hodgkin's disease and also in PHA-stimulated lymphocytes. Anderson (1970) has observed these structures in fresh leukemic cells. However, it appears from studies by Smith and O'Hara (1968) that the formation of nuclear "pockets" is not characteristic of leukemic cells and can readily be observed in normal leukocytes as well. The significance of the nuclear projections remains undetermined.

According to Moore *et al.* (1968), lymphoblastoid cells of continuous cultures possess phagocytic activity, as evidenced by their ability to ingest ink and plastic spheres. Although the cells frequently contain fragments of other cells in their cytoplasm, the fragments are not digested, denoting the absence of true macrophagy.

Lymphoblastoid cells do not contain specific granules similar to those of granulocytes. Instead, their cytoplasm generally contains spherical globules filled with light-staining material, probably lipidic in nature. The globules are not limited by a membrane. They probably correspond to the "vacuoles" so often seen by light microscopy in leukemic cells or in PHA-stimulated lymphocytes. These inclusions are particularly prominent in cultures derived from Burkitt's lymphoma (Toshima *et al.*, 1967; Douglas *et al.*, 1967).

The cytoplasm of the lymphoblastoid cells contains a few scattered lysosomes. Also, microtubules, 200 Å in diameter, may be seen associated with the centrosomes of interphase cells.

Chandra *et al.* (1968) have noticed in the cytoplasm of cultured leukocytes from patients with cancer or from normal individuals the presence of bundles of cylindrical fibers, 300 Å in diameter, sometimes aggregated to form paracrystalline structures. The structures show cross-striations with a periodicity of about 200 Å, similar to that of fibrin. However, their true nature has not yet been determined.

Emphasis has been put by several authors on peculiar tubular arrays frequently observed in the endoplasmic reticulum of the lymphoblastoid cells. They consist (Fig. 35) of branching tubular units about 200 Å in diameter. The membrane limiting the tubules is in continuity with the rough

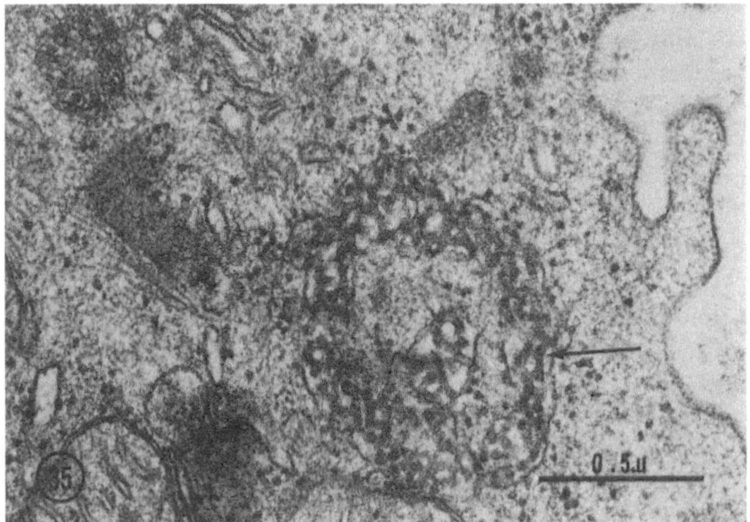

FIG. 35. Tubuloreticular arrays (arrow), similar to those observed in cultures of hematopoietic cells, present in a blast cell from the buffy coat of a patient with acute myelogenous leukemia.

endoplasmic reticulum. The tubular arrays are identical to those found in the kidney or skin cells of patients with lupus erythematosus; or collagen diseases (Gyorkey *et al.*, 1969). They have been seen in cultured cells from peripheral blood of cancerous and noncancerous patients (Chandra *et al.*, 1968, Uzman *et al.*, 1971), and also in a wide variety of animal and human cells *in vivo* (see Uzman *et al.*, 1971), for instance, epithelial and lymphoid cells of breast tumors (Seman *et al.*, 1971). Interpreted at first to represent nucleocapsids of paramyxoviruses, the tubular arrays are probably the result of cellular reaction to antigenic stimulation (Baringer and Swoveland, 1972).

The questions related to the origin and to the malignant or nonmalignant character of the lymphoblastoid cells have been much debated (see Clarkson, 1967; Benyesh–Melnick, 1967; Mouriquand and Mouriquand, 1968; Moore *et al.*, 1968; Chandra *et al.*, 1968) but so far have not met with satisfactory answers. A particularly puzzling problem is the origin of lymphoblastoid cells derived from cultures of bone marrow and of lymphoid tissues. Primary cultures of bone marrow aspirates and of trypsinized lymphoid tissues always yield spindle-shaped elements resembling fibroblasts (Ang *et al.*, 1962; Berg and Rosenthal, 1961) mixed with lymphocytic cells. Lymphocytic cells are often seen enclosed in the cytoplasm of spindle-shaped cells that resemble reticulum cells. This phenomenon has been called "emperipolesis" (Humble *et al.*, 1956; Pulvertaft and Humble, 1962). Electron microscopy has shown (Shelton and Dalton, 1959; Klug, 1962) that the lymphocytic cells sequestrated by emperipolesis have an intact cell membrane and some cytoplasmic bridges with the host cells. The cultures always degenerate after some weeks of cultivation, leaving only fibroblastic cells. However, in a limited number of cases, blast cells appear in the cultures after 50–60 days in the form of clusters of rounded cells, with prominent nucleoli and hyperbasophilic cytoplasm. The cells are loosely attached to the underlying fibroblasts and can be grown in suspension. The origin of the blast cells which appear during this phenomenon of "spontaneously lymphoblastoid transformation" (Benyesh-Melnick, 1967) remains obscure. Electron microscopic examination of stationary bone marrow or lymph node cultures has shown, in this laboratory, a predominance of fibroblast-like elements.

The problem of the origin of the cells also arose in the case of ten prolonged suspension cultures derived by Dalton *et al.* (1973) from biopsy tissues of melanomas, rhabdomyosarcomas, and lymphomas. By electron microscopy, the cells resembled the "lymphoblastoid cells" described above. The cells contained tubuloreticular structures in their ergastoplasm and synthesized Epstein–Barr virus. Dalton *et al.* assumed that, in the case of melanomas and rhabdomyosarcomas, the cells originated from the tumoral stroma. Whether lymphoblastoid cells derived from lymphomas were malignant or normal could not be determined.

Following the finding by Morgan (1968) and by Martinez-Palomo *et al.* (1969) of an increased thickness of the glycocalix (cell coat) of hamster and chicken embryo cells transformed by oncogenic viruses, Paintrand and Rosenfeld (1972) have applied the ruthenium red technique (Luft, 1966) to study the glycocalix of lymphoblastoid cells derived from buffy coat cultures of two normal donors and of two patients with acute myeloid and chronic myeloid leukemia, respectively. The glycocalices of lymphoblastoid cells derived from the normal donors and from the patient with chronic myeloid leukemia had the same average thickness (35 mμm), while that of the cells derived from the patient with acute myeloid leukemia measured 68 mμm. The significance of this observation remains to be ascertained by longer studies.

4. *Ultrastructure of Human Tumor Cells According to Conditions of Cultivation*

There is a considerable body of published data on factors influencing growth and morphology of cells grown *in vitro*. However, information on ultrastructural changes in human tumor cells depending on cultivation conditions is very fragmentary and limited to well-established cells such as HeLa or KB cells. The ultrastructural differences between cells grown as monolayer cultures and the same cells grown in suspension cultures have practically not been investigated. Very few ultrastructural studies of human tumor cells in organ cultures have so far been published, probably because of the difficulties encountered in attempts to grow human tumors in organ cultures and because no fundamental changes in the structure of tumor cells are expected to occur in short-lived tumor explants.

a. Fine Structure of HeLa Cells in Relation to Growth. Bruni *et al.* (1961) have examined by cytochemistry and electron microscopy the glycogen content of HeLa cells at intervals of 24–72 h after renewal of the medium. The cells were grown either on glass, on collagen, or on plasma clots. Cells with high content of glycogen were predominant at 24 h. A sharp drop in the amount of glycogen occurred between 24 and 48 h, and glycogen content decreased slowly between 48 and 72 h. It is obvious that studies along these lines are needed, and many types of human tumor cells will have to be examined in order to obtain some information on the relationship of growth and structure of cells.

b. Structure of HeLa Cells Grown in Serum-Free Medium. When serum was replaced by polyvinylpyrrolidone, many lamellar bodies, with central vacuolated areas, appeared in HeLa cells (Kojima and Kozuka, 1962), probably indicating cell degeneration.

c. Effect of Arginine Deprivation on KB Cells. Lane and Novikoff (1965), using cytochemistry and electron microscopy, have examined the effects of arginine deprivation on KB cells. Deprivation induced nucleolar segregation and the appearance of tubular structures in mitochondria, while the cytoplasm and the endoplasmic reticulum filled with lipid-rich vesicles. Lamellated dense bodies increased in number with time, and acquired rectangular or triangular shapes. Cells exposed to arginine deprivation usually recovered, but the structural alterations persisted for some days after restoration to complete medium.

d. Effect of Reduced Glucose Supply on HeLa Cells. Willoch (1967) has shown that under conditions of reduced glucose supply (less than 9 mg % or 0.5 mM present in the medium) HeLa and Chang liver cells still grow well in roller tubes but, as revealed by electron microscopy, have a smoother cellular border fewer microvilli, and less contact between adjacent cells, resulting in an increase of the total cell surface.

e. Effect of Changes in Tonicity on HeLa Cells. Robbins *et al.* (1970) attempted to show ultrastructural similarities between interphase HeLa cells treated with hypertonic solutions and untreated HeLa cells entering prophase. HeLa cells were submitted to conditions of 1.6–2.8 times isotonicity by addition to the medium, for 2–4 min, of KCl, $MgCl_2$, or NaCl.

At 1.6 times isotonicity, the normally fibrillar chromatin is condensed in masses arranged around the nucleolus as in prophase cells. Also as in prophase cells, the nuclear envelope becomes irregular, and polyribosomes are dispersed. At 2.8 times isotonicity, the nuclear membranes have disappeared and the scattered condensed chromatin resembles chromatin of cells arrested in metaphase by colchicine. Mitochondrial membranes become indistinct by a narrowing of the space between the membranes. Changes induced by hypertonic solutions are apparently rapidly reversible, and the nuclei go through a recovery phase morphologically resembling changes which occur in telophase. Hypertonic solutions markedly but temporarily depress macromolecular synthesis. Disaggregation of polysomes can be prevented by prior exposure of the cells to high magnesium ion concentrations.

f. Organ Culture of Human Tumors. Problems involved in successful growth of human tumor explants in organ culture systems have been investigated by a number of authors (see Rovin, 1962; Wolff, 1962, 1966; Easty, 1967; Archer, 1968). Except for two specimens of cancer of the colon, successfully maintained in continuous organ culture by Wolff and Wolff (1966), attempts to grow explants of human tumors have resulted until now only in temporary growth or simple survival of these explants for a short period of time. Recently, however, Flaxman (1972) has studied by electron microscopy explants of human basal cell cancer growth in plasma clots for up to 50 days. Basal cell carcinoma of the skin invades the surrounding tissues but metastasizes very little, and does not show keratinization *in vivo* only *in vitro* (Flaxman and Van Scott, 1968). There is an epithelial outgrowth from the explants after 3–4 days, progressing for 30 days, then slowing down, with corresponding opacification of the cells indicating keratinization. The outgrowing epithelial cells resemble normal keratinizing cells of skin, with massive accumulation of tonofilaments, nuclear degeneration, and disappearance of the ribosomes in cells of the upper layers. It would therefore appear that *in vivo* keratinization is inhibited for some reason not yet determined.

Gazzolo *et al.* (1972), in a study of explants of nasopharyngeal carcinoma (NPC) growing for 2–4 wk in tissue culture, have found a typical epithelial outgrowth in 15 out of 18 cultures. The short-term cultures also showed the presence of lymphoreticular cells mixed with the epithelial cells. This "early lymphocytic production" (De The *et al.*, 1970) is different from the "lymphoblastoid transformation" which occurs later in some cultures derived from hematopoietic cells or tissues. Gazzolo *et al.* (1972) have observed that in some cultures of NPC some cells which appeared to be epithelial by light microscopy were cells with an ultrastructure intermediate between epithelial and fibroblastic, showing no desmosomes but tonofibrils. In view of this observation, the authors have suggested that, in some instances, cultured tumorous epithelial cells are able to dedifferentiate and gain a fibroblastoid morphology, and perhaps evolve into "lymphoblastoid" cells (Gazzolo *et al.*, 1972).

g. Cell Fusion. Harris *et al.* (1966) first succeeded in fusing HeLa cells with mouse Ehrlich ascites cells in the presence of ultraviolet-inactivated Sendai virus. Schneeberger and Harris (1966) carried out an extensive electron microscopic study of the formation of heterokaryons between HeLa cells and Ehrlich ascites cells, HeLa cells and Mouse lymphocytes, HeLa cells and hen erythrocytes, and HeLa cells and HeLa cells, using ultraviolet-inactivated Sendai virus to promote fusion. Fusion with Ehrlich ascites cells started in a few minutes at 37°C, through cytoplasmic bridges. The cells rounded up after fusion. Fusion with mouse lymphocytes resulted in a passage of the nuclei of the mouse cells into HeLa cells. A reverse phenomenon was observed during fusion of HeLa cells with hen erythrocytes. Hen erythrocytes were hemolyzed at 37°C; the HeLa cells fused with them by filling their ghosts. The mechanism of fusion remains obscure because, as it appeared by electron microscopy, there was no interposition of Sendai virus between fusing cells. What seemed to be essential was the integrity of the viral membranes.

5. *Ultrastructural Effects of Chemical and Physical Agents*

HeLa, KB, and cells from a few other continuous lines derived from human tumors have frequently been used in studies of the effects of chemical and physical agents on cell function and structure. The correlation between biochemical events and ultrastructural changes in the cells exposed to the agents has been investigated in many experiments. The results of these studies have demonstrated the outstanding possibilities of the electron microscope in helping to understand the cellular effects of anticancer drugs. These experiments have also shown that the behavior of human tumor cells in continuous cultures does not significantly differ from that of other mammalian cells exposed to similar agents *in vitro*, thus justifying the use of human cells as model systems.

First the effects on human tumor cells *in vitro* of chemical substances, some of which are employed in cancer therapy, will be considered. Next the effects on human tumor cells of some important physical agents such as X-rays, ultraviolet light, and supraoptimal temperatures will be discussed.

5.1. *Chemical Agents*

5.1.1. *Poisons to the Mitotic Spindle*

Poisons to the mitotic apparatus (colchicine, colcemid, and alkaloids of *Vinca rosea*) are known to arrest dividing cells in metaphase. The effects of these chemical agents on the ultrastructure of HeLa cells have been studied by a number of workers: Robbins and Gonatas (1964*b*), using colchicine and vinblastine sulfate; George *et al.* (1965), using vincristine; Erlandson and De Harven (1971), using colcemid. In cells blocked in metaphase, spindle tubules were absent and the chromosomes were scattered throughout the cytoplasm. Although duplication of centrioles proceeded normally, migration of the daughter centrioles to the opposite poles of the cell was inhibited (George *et al.*, 1965). An increase in the amount of ergastoplasm and in the numbers of annulate lamellae was also noted. The cytoplasm of colchicine-treated cells contained increased numbers of 60–80 Å fibrils, presumably tonofibrils, packed in bundles running parallel to the surface of the cells (Robbins and Gonatas, 1964).

The appearance of intracytoplasmic paracrystals in cells treated with vinblastine and vincristine was reported only in 1968 by Bensch and Malawista. In this laboratory, paracrystals have been readily induced in HeLa or AKR mouse embryo cell cultures by exposing the cultures to vinblastine sulfate (Oncovin) at a concentration of 0.1 μg/ml for 24 h. The

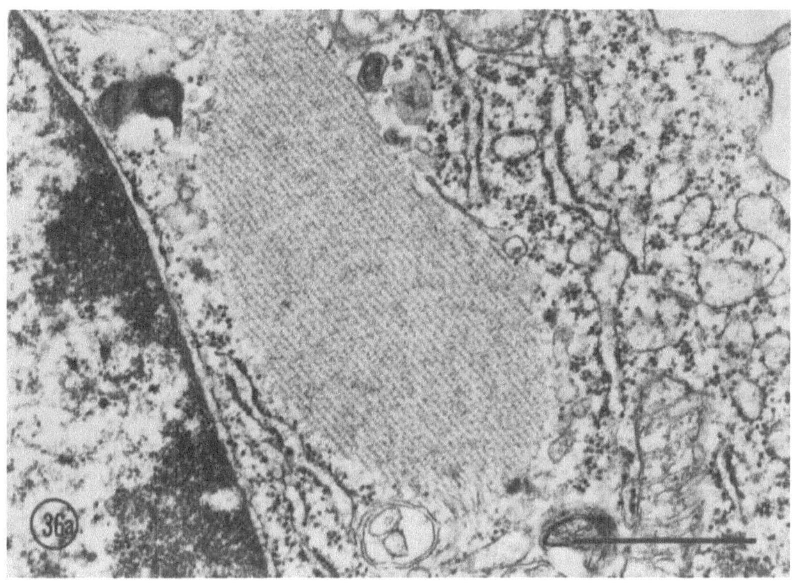

FIG. 36a. Longitudinal section of a crystalline structure appearing in the cytoplasm of a HeLa cell after a 24-h exposure to Oncovin.

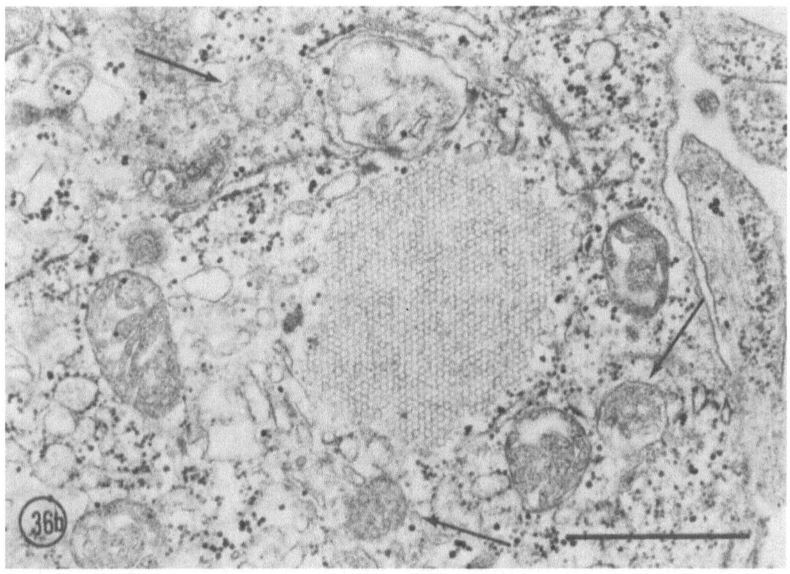

FIG. 36b. Same preparation. Cross-section of a crystalline structure showing polyhedral arrangement of the tubular subunits. Arrows indicate multivesicular bodies.

paracrystals are composed of an assembly of rodlike structures, about 300 Å in diameter, packed together, as seen in cross-sections, in a hexagonal pattern (Figs. 36a and 36b). The rodlike units present, along their longitudinal sections, a periodic substructure every 200–300 Å. Nagayama and Dales (1970) have extracted paracrystals induced by vinblastine in mouse L fibroblasts and immunized rabbits with the purified product. Rabbit antisera to the paracrystals have been found to react in the immunofluorescence test with the mitotic apparatus of HeLa cells, of chicken embryo cells, and of mouse L fibroblasts, thus demonstrating the existence of a common antigen in the spindle tubules of vertebrate cells. Furthermore, Krishan and Hsu (1971*a,b*) showed that ^{3}H-labeled colchicine fixed selectively on vinblastine–induced paracrystals of HeLa cells, which indicated the presence of a colchicine-binding protein in these structures.

McGill and Brinkley (1972) have examined the ultrastructure of normal and leukemic human cells in short-term cultures after treatment with colcemid. Cells from cultures of normal PHA-stimulated leukocytes, arrested in metaphase, progressed through anaphase and telophase after removal of colcemid from the medium. Cells from the blood of patients with chronic myeloid leukemia recovered only slowly, while cells from the blood of patients with acute myeloid leukemia did not recover from metaphase arrest after removal of the drug. Electron microscopy revealed severe alterations in many of the cells: multipolar spindles, anaphase bridges, abnormal centrioles, and lagging of chromosomes. Large numbers of multivesicular bodies indicated degeneration of the affected cells.

5.1.2. Drugs Interfering with DNA and RNA Synthesis

Journey and Goldstein (1961) were first to study the effects of actinomycin D on HeLa cell ultrastructure. HeLa cell sublines were exposed constantly or intermittently to the drug at a concentration of 0.1 μg/ml. In cells sensitive or only partially resistant to actinomycin D, the main lesions consisted of fragmentation of the nucleoli, which appeared as small, rounded bodies with no substructure. Resistant cells were smaller and had prominent, intensely osmiophilic nucleoli.

Ultrastructural changes produced by actinomycin D in nucleoli of a variety of cells have received considerable attention (see reviews by Bernhard and Granboulan, 1968; Simard, 1970). Using the human tumor cell line ME-180, derived from carcinoma of the cervix, Recher *et al.* (1971) have examined in detail the effects of various concentrations of actinomycin D on nucleolar ultrastructure, and compared them with the effects of proflavin, puromycin, and cycloheximide on nucleoli of the same cells. The most important alteration observed was "nucleolar segregation" (Simard and Bernhard, 1966), consisting of a dissociation of the nucleolonema into fibrillar centers and granular portions. The granular portions in turn gave rise to two fractions: P 1 granules attached to a fibrous component and P 2 granules, derived from P 1 granules, which lacked fibrous support. The authors assumed that P 1 granules contain 32S RNA and P 2 granules 28S RNA, and believe that the fibrillar component of the nucleolonema is derived from chromatin. Actinomycin D, like the other drugs, is known to block DNA-dependent RNA synthesis, and probably dissociates the nucleolonemal structure by producing a condensation of the dispersed chromatin.

The effects of proflavin on nucleoli of ME–180 cells were similar to those of actinomycin D (Recher *et al.* 1971*b*). However, the P 1 granules did not evolve into P 2 granules. Low concentrations of proflavin led to the formation of fibrillar nodules similar to the dense fibrillar substance of normal nucleoli. The nodules were in close association with interchromatin granules, and have been shown, by enzymatic digestion, to be composed of pepsin-digestible proteins and of fibrils of unknown nature. Similar nodules were induced by cycloheximide and by cordycepin (3-deoxyadenosine).

Nucleolar segregation has also been observed in ME-180 cells treated with the alkaloid camptothecin (Recher *et al.*, 1972), known to inhibit ribosomal RNA synthesis and to some extent DNA and protein synthesis.

The effects of mitomycin C on nucleoli of KB cells have been studied by Lapis and Bernhard (1965). Nucleolar redistribution and segregation could be observed at about 9 h after the beginning of the treatment with the drug. The morphological alterations in nucleoli were similar to those induced by actinomycin D and 4-nitroquinoline-*N*-oxide in animal tissues and cultured cells (Reynolds *et al.*, 1963, 1964).

The effects of the antibiotic toyocamycin, a selective inhibitor of ribosomal RNA synthesis on HeLa cells grown in suspension, have been examined by Heine (1969) and by Philips and Phillips (1971) on KB cells. In HeLa cells, low doses of the drug induced an enlargement of the nucleoli, with increase of the fibrillar component and decrease of the granular component, resulting in time in the appearance of round nucleoli of high electron density. At doses 20 times higher, nuclear segregation very similar to that induced by actinomycin D occurred, generally followed by cell degeneration, as indicated by an increase in the numbers of lysosomes, breakdown of polysomes, and cytoplasmic blebbing. The effects on KB cells observed with this drug were the same as on HeLa cells.

Nucleolar segregation was also observed in HeLa cells treated with the aminonucleoside of puromycin (Lewin and Moscarello, 1968), which preferentially inhibits ribosomal 45S RNA synthesis. At the concentrations used (100 μg/ml), growth of the cells was strongly inhibited, but the cells remained viable. These ultrastructural changes were observed as early as 12 h following exposure to the drug, and were maximum at 72 h.

5.1.3. *Inhibitors of Mitochondrial Synthesis*

Chloramphenicol, like ethidium bromide, inhibits autonomous mitochondrial synthesis (Smith *et al.*, 1970). The structure of HeLa cells (Lenk and Penman, 1970) and of HeLa and L cells (King *et al.*, 1972) treated with both drugs has been examined by electron microscopy. Both drugs induce similar mitochondrial alterations: swelling of the inner chamber and reduction of the number of cristae, which become disoriented and whorling. In HeLa cells, numerous lipid droplets and osmiophilic inclusions appear following treatment (Lenk and Penman, 1970). The cytochrome oxidase activity, like the cytochrome content of mitrochondria, is largely reduced (King *et al.*, 1972).

5.1.4. *Effects of 5-Bromodeoxyuridine*

Incorporation of 5-BUdR into cellular DNA suppresses *de novo* thymidine synthesis in cells. Hendee *et al.* (1963*a*) attempted to determine whether the drug induced infrastuctural alterations in HeLa cells exposed to concentrations of 10–7 M to 10–4 M for 1–7 days. The principal change observed was an important increase in the numbers of dense osmiophilic bodies in the cytoplasm of the cells, indicative of cellular degeneration.

5.1.5. *Effects of Acridine Orange (AO)*

In order to determine the nature of the brilliantly fluorescent juxtanuclear granules that appear in cultured cells exposed to acridine orange, Robbins *et al.* (1964) have followed by electron microscopy the uptake of AO in HeLa cells. The authors have shown that the "acridine orange particles" actually are acid phosphatase–positive multivesicular bodies (MVBs), presumably lysosomes. Exposure of the cells to low concentrations of the dye (1 part per million) led to hypertrophy of the MVBs and accumulation of myelin figures within them, the acid phosphatase activity being retained. Cells stained for a short time in high concentrations of the dye (1 part per 20,000) showed a diffuse cytoplasmic staining, and when they were incubated in dye-free medium the dye segregated rapidly into MBVs. This phenomenon of segregation did not occur if cells stained in high concentrations of the dye were incubated in glucose-free medium; instead, the cells rapidly degenerated.

5.1.6. *Effects of Chloroquine*

Bedoya (1970) has examined by electron microscopy the effects of chloroquine on cells of the AL-1 line, derived from Burkitt's lymphoma, and on cells of the Cloudman S–91 malignant mouse melanoma line. The effects of single or repeated doses, from 10 to 300 μg/ml, were similar on cells of both lines and very cytotoxic. By light microscopy, the cells appeared pyknotic. Electron microscopy revealed ruptures of the nuclear membrane, reduction in the size of nucleoli, dilatations of the Golgi and endoplasmic cavities, decrease in the number of ribosomes, and presence of many dense bodies with myelin figures or with lamellar structure. Ultrastructural lesions were in proportion to the dose employed.

5.1.7. *Effects of Glycerol*

The technical problems involved in freezing tissue culture cells for storage or freeze-etching have been investigated by Reith and Oftebro (1971) on HeLa cells grown as monolayers. The cells were examined by electron microscopy either after addition to the medium of various concentrations of glycerol varying from 5 to 30% or after a gradual increase in 2 h of the glycerol concentration to a final value of 30%. The quality of fixation was also compared by fixing the cells in glutaraldehyde after or during addition of glycerol. Best preservation was obtained by putting gradually increased concentrations of glycerol on the cells and by fixing in glutaraldehyde containing 30% glycerol.

5.2. *Physical Agents*

5.2.1. *X-Irradiation*

Very few studies have been published describing the effects of X-irradiation on the fine structure of cells derived from human tumors. HeLa and to a lesser extent KB cells have been used as model cells in a great number of investigations in the field of radiobiology. Yet from the available literature, it appears that the effects of X-rays on the ultrastructure of these cells have been described only by Hendee *et al.* (1963*b*) for HeLa cells and by Lane and Novikoff (1965) for KB cells. From electron microscopic observations of HeLa cells irradiated with doses ranging from 150 to 1700 r and examined between 12 h and 4 days, Hendee *et al.* (1963*b*) concluded that the cellular lesions induced were not characteristic of radiation damage. Similar lesions, indicating nonspecific cell degeneration, may be observed following the initial action of a variety of agents interfering with cell survival. The major cellular alterations observed consisted of vacuolization of the cytoplasm, peripheral blebbing, and increase in the number of osmiophilic inclusions. There were, in addition, zones of cytoplasmic dislocation, with loss of identifiable substructures. Mitochondria lost their dense matrix and most of their cristae.

With improved electron microscopic techniques, Lane and Novikoff (1965) studied the effect of a dose of 1300 r on the structure of KB cells. This dose has been shown to be lethal for most HeLa cells in about 15 days (Tolmach and Marcus, 1960). Dramatic changes occurred in the cells in about 5 days. They consisted of disorganization of the nucleoli, appearance of many osmiophilic inclusions in the cytoplasm, and whorling of the rough endoplasmic reticulum. Many of the dense osmiophilic bodies probably represented residual bodies as a consequence of cell degeneration and autophagocytosis.

5.2.2. Ultraviolet Irradiation

As for X-irradiation, study of the effects of ultraviolet light on fine structure of human tumor cells *in vitro* has until now been limited to HeLa and KB cells. Using whole-cell irradiation with ultraviolet light, Djordjevic and Tolmach (1967) compared in great detail the biological effects of ultraviolet and X-irradiation on HeLa cells. They found that many aspects of the effects of ultraviolet light on these cells differ qualitatively from those of X-rays. HeLa cells have two sensitivity peaks to X-rays, one in M phase, and one in late G_1, and only one sensitivity peak to ultraviolet at about 15 h after mitosis. X-irradiated HeLa cells are able to enter and complete mitosis following irradiation at a dose leaving only a few percent of viable cells, while ultraviolet irradiation, administered in G_1, destroys the majority of the cells within 30 h. In addition, DNA synthesis is much more depressed after ultraviolet irradiation.

Lane and Novikoff (1965) compared by electron microscopy the changes in KB cells following X-ray and ultraviolet irradiation. Ultraviolet irradiation of interphase cells induced, with only quantitative differences, nucleolar and cytoplasmic lesions very similar to those produced by X-irradiation or arginine deprivation.

The use of an ultraviolet microbeam has permitted a more precise ultrastructural study of lesions induced by ultraviolet light in nuclei, nucleoli, and cytoplasm of KB cells (Moreno *et al.*, 1969; Moreno and Vinzens, 1969; Moreno, 1971). Irradiation of parts of the cytoplasm at 2570 Å with a 12-μm spot (Moreno *et al.*, 1969) produced a swelling of mitochondria and vacuolization in the irradiated region. Irradiation of the nucleoli at 2570 and 2313 Å produced a disaggregation of the nucleolar components, observed by light microscopy as a phenomenon of nucleolar "paling" and a dispersion of chromatin clumps throughout the nucleoplasm. Dispersion of chromatin was also observed after partial irradiation of the nucleus excluding the nucleoli. In further experiments, Moreno (1971) used a 5-μm beam to study the morphological and metabolic effects of partial irradiation of KB cell nuclei. Nuclear spots irradiated for 2 min showed immediate damage as seen from their decreased electron density. At the same time, there was an aggregation of chromatin into small clumps in the remainder of the nuclei. Following incubation of the irradiated cells with ^{3}H-TdR, Moreno (1971) showed that cells irradiated in S phase contained radioactive label everywhere in the nucleus except in the irradiated spot, while in interphase cells the label was present only in the irradiated spot. The labeling of chromatin in interphase cells following ultraviolet irradiation is known to correspond to DNA repair by a phenomenon called "unscheduled DNA synthesis" (Rasmussen and Painter, 1966).

5.2.3. Ruby Laser Irradiation

The effect of laser beam has been studied on KB cells after vital staining with Janus green B, which increases sensitivity of mitochondria to this type of light (Bessis and Storb, 1965). Primary and secondary damage to the cells depended on the intensity of irradiation (Amy and Storb, 1965; Storb *et al.*, 1966). Light irradiation produced only mitochondrial lesions: appearance of electron-dense material in the mitochondrial matrix, degeneration of the matrix, swelling, and loss of cristae. However, lightly irradiated cells appeared normal after 24 h. Heavy irradiation was fatal to the cells. The irradiated spot was destroyed and the cellular structures showed serious damage: empty areas in the cytoplasm, partial disruption of the nuclear membrane, disaggregation of the polyribosomes, swelling and cavulation of mitochondria, and dispersion of nuclear chromatin into small, dense islands. Heat, production of gas bubbles, and rupture of the cell membrane appeared to be the main causes for the secondary lesions.

5.2.4. Effects of Supraoptimal Temperatures

Cancer cells are apparently more sensitive to supraoptimal temperatures than normal cells (Cavaliere *et al.*, 1967). The mechanism of cell injury by hyperthermia has been investigated by electron microscopy (Simard and Bernhard, 1967; Simard *et al.*, 1969) and biochemical analysis (Amalric *et al.*, 1969; Warocquier and Scherrer, 1969). Hyperthermia disrupts the nucleolar architecture and selectively inhibits 45S and 30S nucleolar RNA synthesis, leading to a failure of maturation of rRNA. In an extensive electron microscopic study, combined with cytochemistry, Love *et al.* (1970) investigated the effect of exposure of HeLa, WI–38, and human embryo cells to temperatures of 45–46°C. Cells growing in petri dishes were floated on heated water for periods of 15–60 min. Using acid phosphatase reaction, lead staining, and the toluidine blue–molybdate (TBM) method, the authors have observed, by light microscopy, disappearance of the nucleus of the heated cells. Electron microscopy showed that the fibrillar component and the nucleolini became diffusely distributed throughout the nucleolus and that the granular component of the nucleolus disappeared. Inclusions made of ribosome-like granules, similar to those observed in the nucleoli, were found in the cytoplasm of all the heated cells. These inclusions were evidently derived from the nucleoli by extrusion through the nuclear envelope. Hyperthermia also produced a disaggregation of the polysomes. The effects of a 15-min heating were entirely reversible. Responses to hyperthermia were similar in all three strains of cells.

6. Viruses, Mycoplasmas, and Cell Transformation

6.1. Virus Infection of Human Tumor Cells in Vitro

Tissue cultures have been extensively used for isolation, identification, and propagation of viruses and for analysis of the relationship of viruses to the host cells. The contribution of electron microscopy has been invaluable in this field, not only by revealing the fine structure of many viruses, but also by showing the correlations between ultrastructural changes in virus-infected cells and the biochemical events accompanying virus infection and replication.

The human tumor cells selected for virus studies are chiefly cells from well-established lines, such as HeLa, KB, and HEp-2. The probable malignant character of the cells has apparently not interfered with their ability to replicate many kinds of viruses. The contrary might be true. The scope of this chapter makes it impossible to report in detail the many ultrastructural observations published on virus infection and replication in human tumor cells *in vitro*, even though the number of tumor cell lines employed has been very limited. In Table 1 are summarized the references on electron microscopic studies of virus infection and replication. The table indicates the virus and the human cells studied and the names of the authors.

6.1.1. Infection with Adenoviruses

HeLa, HEp-2, or KB cells infected with various strains of adenoviruses have been examined frequently by electron microscopy: for example, strains 1, 2,

TABLE I

Ultrastructural Studies of Human Tumor Cells Infected with Viruses in Vitro

Virus	Human tumor cells	Authors	Year
Adenoviruses	HeLa	Harford *et al.*	1956
	HeLa	Bloch *et al.*	1957
	HeLa	Tousimis and Hilleman	1957
	HeLa	Gregg and Morgan	1959
	HeLa, HEp-2	Morgan *et al.*	1959
	HeLa	Mayor *et al.*	1964
	HeLa	Tawara *et al.*	1966
	KB	Martinez-Palomo *et al.*	1967
Herpes simplex	HeLa	Stoker *et al.*	1958
	HeLa	Morgan *et al.*	1959
	HeLa	Epstein *et al.*	1962 1964
	KB	Sirtori and Bosisio-Bestetti	1967
	HeLa	Morgan *et al.*	1968
	HeLa	Nii *et al.*	1968
	HEp-2	Schwartz and Roizman	1969
	HeLa	Miyamoto	1971
Vaccinia	HeLa	Morgan *et al.*	1961
	HeLa	Nielsen and Peters	1962
	HeLa, KB	Easterbrook and Davern	1963
	HeLa, HEp-2	Harford *et al.*	1966
	HeLa	Grimley *et al.*	1970
	HeLa	Grimley and Moss	1971
Poliovirus	HeLa	Fogh and Stuart	1960
	HeLa	Fogh	1961
	HeLa	Mattern and Daniel	1965
Influenza	HeLa	Birch-Anderson and Paucker	1959
	HeLa	Kendall *et al.*	1971
Parainfluenza	HeLa, HEp-2	Kuhn and Harford	1963
	KB	Bonissol *et al.*	1971
Measles	HeLa	Kallmann *et al.*	1959
	HeLa	Tawara *et al.*	1961
Newcastle disease virus	HeLa	Silverstein and Marcus	1964
	KB	Loni	1971
Vesicular stomatitis	RPMI-6410, SKL-1	Zajac and Hummeler	1970
Coxsackie	HeLa	Morgan *et al.*	1959
Yellow fever	HeLa	Bayer and Nielsen	1961
	HeLa, KB	Bergold and Weibel	1962
Venezuelan equine encephalitis	KB	Mussgay and Weibel	1962
Semliki forest	HEp-2	Erlandson *et al.*	1967
Mayaro	KB	Saturno	1963
Parvoviruses	KB	Siegl *et al.*	1971
	KB	Siegl *et al.*	1972

and 3 (Hartford *et al.*, 1956*a*); strains 3, 4, and 5 from the RI-PAC group (Bloch *et al.*, 1957); strain 4 from group RI-67 (Tousimis and Hilleman, 1957); strain 3 (Gregg and Morgan, 1959); strain 5 (Morgan *et al.*, 1960); strains 12 and 18 (Mayor *et al.*, 1964); strain 12 (Tawara *et al.*, 1966; Martinez-Palomo *et al.*, 1967). The cellular alterations observed are very similar with all the strains.

In KB cells (Martinez-Palomo *et al.*, 1967), the earliest change, 8 h after infection, consists of hypertrophy of nuclei and nucleoli of some of the cells. After 16 h, the nucleolonema begins to loosen, and long, thin fibers appear in the nucleoplasm. At 18 h, irregular, dense inclusions of two different types appear in the nucleus: type I inclusions made of dense granules about 100 Å in diameter and type II inclusions appearing as large patches of fine fibrils 40–60 Å thick. After 24 h, virus particles appear near type II inclusions, and at the same time clear, rounded zones of loosely stained fibrils appear (type III inclusions). Nuclear fibers become more and more abundant, and the clear zones of loose fibrils finally fill the nucleus by 36 h, virus particles start to agglomerate in crystal-like formations, while inclusions made of a dense reticulated substance (type IV inclusions) form at the same time. Lysis of the cells begins on the third day. Nuclear fibers and the various inclusions have been shown to contain viral proteins.

6.1.2. *Infection with Vaccinia Virus*

Vaccinia virus synthesis in HeLa or KB cells has been followed by electron microscopy by Morgan *et al.* (1961), Nielsen and Peters (1962), Easterbrook and Davern (1963), Harford *et al.* (1966), Grimley *et al.* (1970), and Grimley and Moss (1971). The virus is synthesized in cytoplasmic inclusions (viroplasms) more or less completely surrounded by a membrane. Virus particles form by the appearance of a coating around the membrane, then separation of the virus particle from the viroplasm, with a still immature nucleoid. The virus particle matures in the cytoplasm. Grimley *et al.* (1970) and Grimley and Moss (1971) have studied the effect of rifampin and its derivatives on vaccinia virus synthesis in HeLa cells and have shown that the drugs inhibit virus assembly during the stage of envelope formation. Rifampin derivatives also produce in vaccinia-infected HeLa cells mitochondrial swelling with considerable distortion of cristae.

6.1.3. *Infection with Herpes Virus*

The cellular events that follow herpes simplex virus entry and replication have received considerable attention. Electron microscopy has not revealed fundamental differences in the behavior of the various animal or human cells infected with the virus. The entry and replication of herpes simplex virus in HeLa cells have been followed in great details by Morgan *et al.* (1968), Nii *et al.* (1968), and Miyamoto (1971). Schwartz and Roizman (1969) used HEp-2 cells to study differences among laboratory or freshly isolated herpes virus strains. Nucleolar changes induced by the virus in KB cells have been examined by Sirtori and Bosisio-Bestetti (1967).

The most striking alterations that follow herpes virus infection are observed in the nuclei of the cells. A few hours after infection, the nuclear components are displaced to the periphery by a large electron-lucent inclusion that corresponds to the classical inclusion seen by light microscopy. At the same time, granular, irregular structures form in apposition to the nuclear membrane, and filaments resembling microtubules, arranged in parallel bundles, are also seen. After 8 h, viral nucleocapsids appear at the periphery of the clear inclusion associated aggregates of dense 150-Å granules arranged in rosettes and with 250-Å granules interspersed with the nucleocapsids. As soon as the first immature virus particles appear in the nucleus, the nucleolar components segregate into a dense, round mass of RNP granules capped by a fibrillar substance. Later the nucleolar structures disaggregate into fragments of unidentifiable composition. Segregation of the nucleolus is very similar to the nucleolar segregation induced by a number of chemical agents interfering with DNA synthesis, such as actinomycin D, mitomycin C (Lapis and Bernhard, 1965), or nitroquinoline-*N*-oxide. As shown by Miyamoto (1971) by negative staining of thin sections of virus-infected cells, the nucleocapsids form from the granular aggregates and accumulate in a crystalline pattern. Nucleocapsids are packed near the thickened areas of the inner lamellae of the nuclear membrane, which at the same time has started breaking down. Nucleocapsids are enveloped near the nuclear membrane.

Major alterations seen in the cytoplasm of the virus-infected cells are reduplication of the nuclear membrane and the appearance of long, membrane-bound tubules. Viral nucleocapsids are seen opposed to those tubules. Infected cells are lysed between 50 and 72 h and viruses are released in the medium.

6.1.4. *Infection with Influenza and Parainfluenza Viruses*

The structure of influenza virus, strain PR 8 from group A, grown in HeLa cells was examined by Birch-Anderson and Paucker (1957). Kuhn and Harford (1963) examined by electron microscopy the cytoplasmic inclusions produced in HeLa cells and HEp-2 cells by infection with parainfluenza 2 virus. Cytopathic effect, in the form of rounding of the cells, appeared in 2–9 days. In the cytoplasm were seen aggregates of closely intertwining filaments and granules, about 100 Å in diameter. There were no intranuclear aggregates. The filaments contained viral antigen, as demonstrated by immunofluorescence, but mature viruses were absent.

Bonissol *et al.* (1967) studied the morphology of KB cells after infection with parainfluenza virus 2 and observed three types of cytoplasmic inclusions: (1) homogeneous, perinuclear inclusions of light density; (2) networks of 120-Å filaments mixed to ribosomes and to mitochondria; (3) inclusions surrounded by a double limiting membrane and filled with 120-Å filaments with helicoidal substructure, representing viral capsids.

6.1.5. Infection with Measles Virus

It was recognized as early as 1939 that measles virus determines the appearance in the infected cells of nuclear and cytoplasmic inclusion bodies, staining pink by hematoxylin and eosin. In HeLa cells infected with the Edmonton strain, numerous giant cells appear after 5 days (Kallmann *et al.*, 1959). In the cytoplasm and in the nuclei of the cells, large, irregular, and refringent areas may be seen by light microscopy. In the electron microscope, these inclusions consist of filamentous structures sometimes arranged in parallel strands, about 200 Å in diameter. These observations have been confirmed by Tawara *et al.* (1961) in HeLa cells infected by measles (Edmonton strain) and distemper viruses.

6.1.6. Infection with Newcastle Disease Virus

The mechanism of entry of Newcastle disease virus (NDV) into HeLa cells by viropexis has been described in detail by Silverstein and Marcus (1964). Loni (1971) examined the fine structure of KB cells infected with high concentrations of NDV. Six hours after infection, clear areas filled with homogeneous material appeared in the cytoplasm of the cells. At 8 h, cytoplasmic inclusions, increasing in size up to several micrometers with time, were seen containing filamentous structures. Virus particles started budding from the plasma membrane at 21 h. In many cells, abundant perichromatin granules appeared in the nucleus, preceding the disintegration of the whole cell. Ultraviolet microirradiation of the nucleolus for 10 s at 2750 Å, 1–3 h after infection, did not influence virus synthesis. But irradiation for 2 min produced margination of chromatin and disorganization of the cytoplasm; however, synthesis of nucleocapsids was still visible after 8 h. The comparison with cytoplasmic lesions observed by Moreno (1967) by ultraviolet microirradiation under similar conditions has demonstrated that virus-infected KB cells are more sensitive to ultraviolet irradiation than noninfected cells.

6.1.7. Infection with Poliovirus

Poliovirus-infected HeLa cells contain, 17 h after infection, cytoplasmic crystals of the virus (Fogh and Stuart, 1960; Fogh, 1961). The crystals, sometimes 2.5 μm in size, are made of aggregated 270-Å virus particles. In a more detailed ultrastructural study of HeLa cells infected with poliovirus type I, Mattern and Daniel (1965) have observed that the first changes, 2–4 h after infection, are represented by nuclear protrusions produced by pulling apart of the two membranes of the nuclear envelope. The protrusions contain 200-Å ribosome-like granules, and as their number increases they separate from the nucleus and become enveloped by the cytoplasm. Also, around the fourth hour, aggregates of small vesicles appear close to the nucleus and around mitochondria. Regular arrays of virus particles form in the cytoplasmic vesicles. At 8 h there are large accumulations of virus particles, many of them arranged in paracrystalline lattices.

6.1.8. Infection with Other Viruses

HeLa cells infected with Coxsackie virus B-5 have been examined by Morgan *et al.* (1959*a*). The development of the following viruses, with few detailed studies of cellular alterations proper, has been examined by electron microscopy in HeLa, KB, or HEp-2 cells (see also Table 1): Semliki forest virus (Elandson *et al.*, 1970); Venezuelan equine encephalitis virus (Mussgay and Weibel, 1962); yellow fever virus (Bayer and Nielsen, 1961; Bergold and Weibel, 1962); mayaro virus (Saturno, 1963); vesicular stomatitis virus (Zajac and Hummeler, 1970); simian foamy virus (Clarke *et al.*, 1970).

6.1.9. Spontaneous Appearance of Viruses in Cultures of Human Tumors

A most intriguing problem has arisen from the discovery of a herpes-type virus in a small proportion of the cells of the first established culture derived from Burkitt's lymphoma (Epstein *et al.*, 1964*a*). The virus has been designated as Epstein–Barr virus (EBV). The same virus was later identified by electron microscopy in other continuous cultures of Burkitt's tumor: EB-2, EB-3, SL_1 and P-3-Jijoye (see De Harven, 1967; Toshima *et al.*, 1967). However, it was discovered at the same time that established suspension cultures of leukocytes from the blood or the bone marrow of patients suffering from malignant or nonmalignant diseases or from normal subjects frequently shed a morphologically identical virus. This virus has been seen by electron microscopy in cultures of leukemic leukocytes (Iwakata and Grace, 1964; Zeve *et al.*, 1966), leukocytes from patients with infectious mononucleosis and solid tumors (see Moore *et al.*, 1968; Chandra *et al.*, 1968;

Steel and Edmond, 1971), and leukocytes from normal subjects (Moore *et al.*, 1967). The same virus has been observed in lymphoblastoid cells of tissue culture lines derived from nasopharyngeal carcinoma (De The *et al.*, 1970) and, in this laboratory, in a culture of buffy coat cells from a patient with rhabdomyosarcoma. The virus is found only in suspension cultures, once they are established, and is readily detected by immunofluorescence with anti-EBV serum. According to Steel (1972), irradiated EBV-containing cells have the property of inducing long-term growth of fresh leukocytes from patients with infectious mononucleosis and leukemia. Whether EBV is an etiological agent in human leukemias and lymphomas has as yet not been determined.

One of the major purposes for growing leukemic or other types of human malignant cells *in vitro* is to retrieve a viral agent similar to the type C viruses implicated in the etiology of leukemias and solid tumors in a variety of vertebrates (see Dmochowski, 1973). The morphological identification of type C viruses is based on two criteria: budding of the viruses from the plasma membrane and structure of the "mature" extracellular virions (see Dalton and Stewart, 1972). While a budding virus is practically unmistakable when seen by electron microscopy, "mature" virions, when there are only few of them, may be confused with structures derived from cellular decay or "degeneration" having, like type C particles, a diameter between 1000 and 1300 Å, an outer unit membrane, and an electron-dense core. These structures have been called "virus mimickers" by Uzman *et al.* (1966) in a study on the ultrastructural effects of a variety of drugs in cells of the lymphoblastoid line CCRF-CEM. A group of similar particles, very closely resembling type C viruses, has been demonstrated by Trujillo *et al.* (1966) in their long-term culture derived from a lymph node of a patient with lymphoma. The nature of the particles has not been determined. Neither in the case of Uzman *et al.* nor in that of Trujillo *et al.* have budding virus particles been seen. In this laboratory, occasional structures resembling type C virus, but not budding, have been encountered in electron microscopic examination of cultures derived from human tumors, but the particles could not be isolated or propagated. The first culture producing a significant amount of type C virus particles, sufficient for isolation and propagation, was ESP-1 (Fig. 37), derived in monolayer culture of pleural effusion cells from a patient with Burkitt's lymphoma (Priori *et al.*, 1971). In 1969, Morton *et al.* reported the finding of budding C-type viruses in cultures of human liposarcoma, and more recently Stewart *et al.* (1972) observed similar particles in cultures of lung adenocarcinoma. These virus particles have so far not been fully characterized.

In 1971, Hallauer *et al.* reported the frequent isolation of viral agents from stable human cell lines, such as KB, HeLa, and HEp-2. The isolated viruses

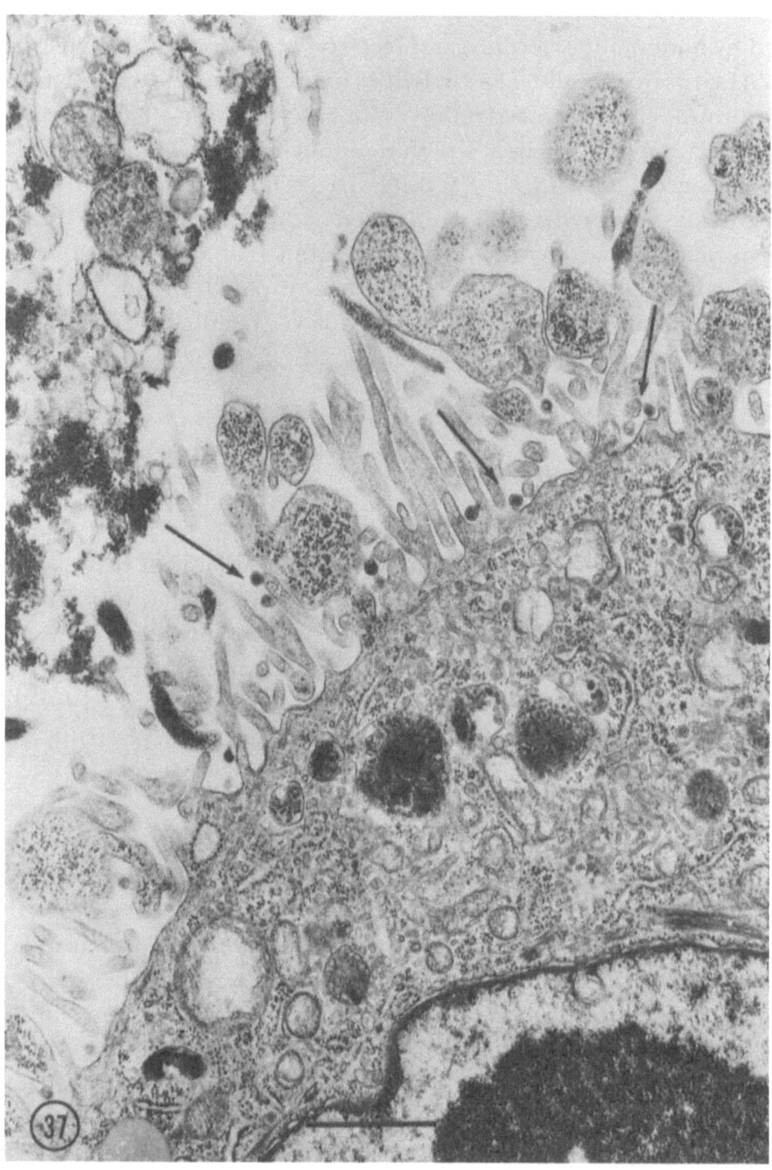

FIG. 37. Partial view of a cell from the ESP-1 line, in passage 19. Type C particles, some of them budding from the plasma membrane, are present among microvilli (arrows).

(strains KBSH, TVX, and Lu III) are said to be small DNA viruses with cubic symmetry, about 190–210 Å in diameter, belonging to the group of parvo (picodna) viruses (Mayor and Melnick, 1965). Siegl *et al.* (1971, 1972) have studied by immunofluorescence and electron microscopy the development of KBSH virus in KB cells. The virus does not produce a clear-cut cytopathic effect in routinely maintained cultures, but a cytopathic effect does appear after inoculation of KB cells at a high multiplicity of infection. There is also strong evidence that synthesis of KBSH-virus is favored by cells undergoing active growth. Virus synthesis is completed within the nucleus, producing a disorganization of chromatin and the appearance of aggregates of densely staining very small particles. The presence of small viruses in nuclei of established human tumor cell lines has not yet been confirmed by other observers.

6.2. *Infection by Mycoplasmas*

Mycoplasmas are very frequently found as contaminants of tissue cultures. While primary cultures are seldom contaminated (Rothblat, 1960; Gori and Lee, 1964), the risk of contamination increases considerably with the number of passages, a clear indication of the exogenous origin of mycoplasmas, although in some cases, such as in human leukemia, a preexisting contamination should not be disregarded (see Macpherson, 1966; Dmochowski *et al.*, 1965).

The effects of mycoplasmal infection on the cells in culture are most of the time minimal or inapparent, at least on morphological grounds, to the extent that frequently the organisms are detectable only by electron microscopy. Chronic infection of human tumor cells in serial passages is discovered, in the electron microscope, by the observation of characteristic, generally darkly staining mycoplasmal bodies in extracellular spaces and sometimes inside the cells. The bodies are rounded or more often elongated, filament-like structures clustering around the cell surfaces (Fig. 38). They are limited by a unit membrane and filled with granules and filaments representing mostly nucleoproteins. Mycoplasmal bodies are in frequent contact with the plasma membrane of the cells through a pedicle or by an apparent coalescence with the cytoplasm itself (Fig. 39). Electron microscopic studies (Edwards and Fogh, 1960; Fogh and Hacker, 1960; Dmochowski *et al.*, 1965) have shown that the presence of mycoplasmal bodies is associated with that of their elementary bodies, small reproductive units capable of passing through Millipore filters of 0.22-μm porosity (Morowitz *et al.*, 1963).

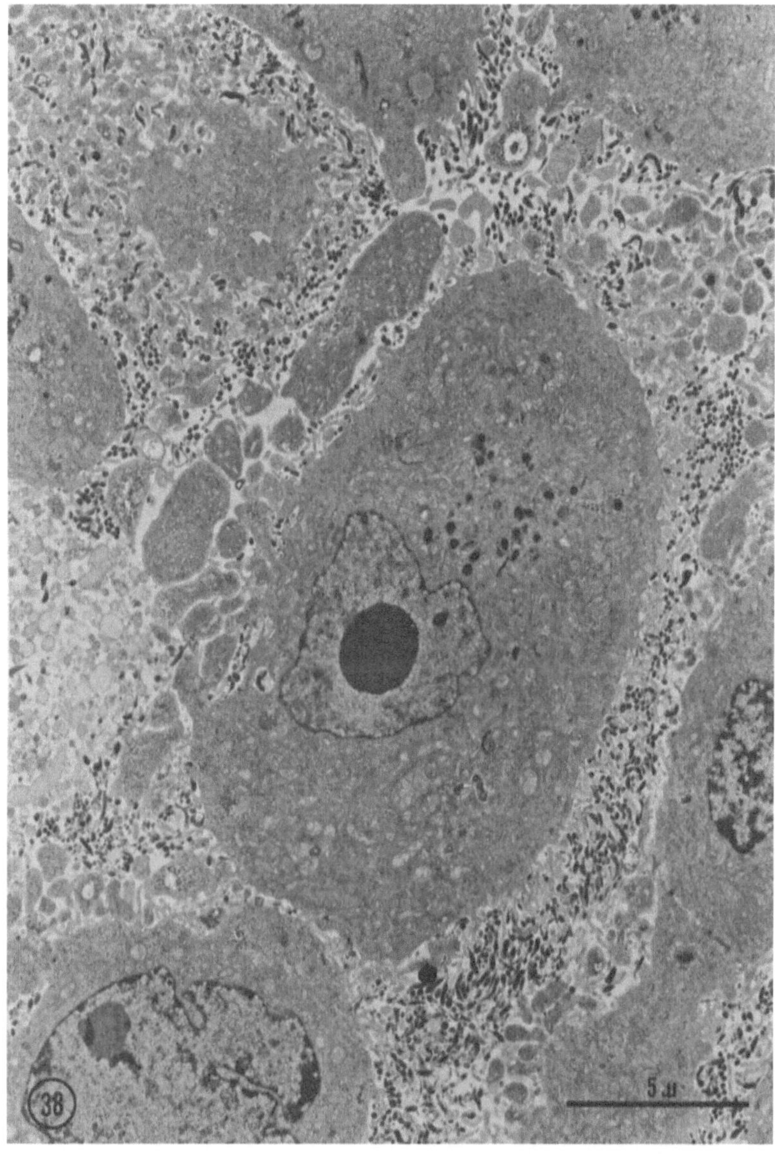

FIG. 38. Monolayer culture derived from a leukemic bone marrow. Round or filamentous dark-staining mycoplasmal bodies are easily spotted in the intercellular spaces in this low-magnification micrograph. The cells appear unaltered.

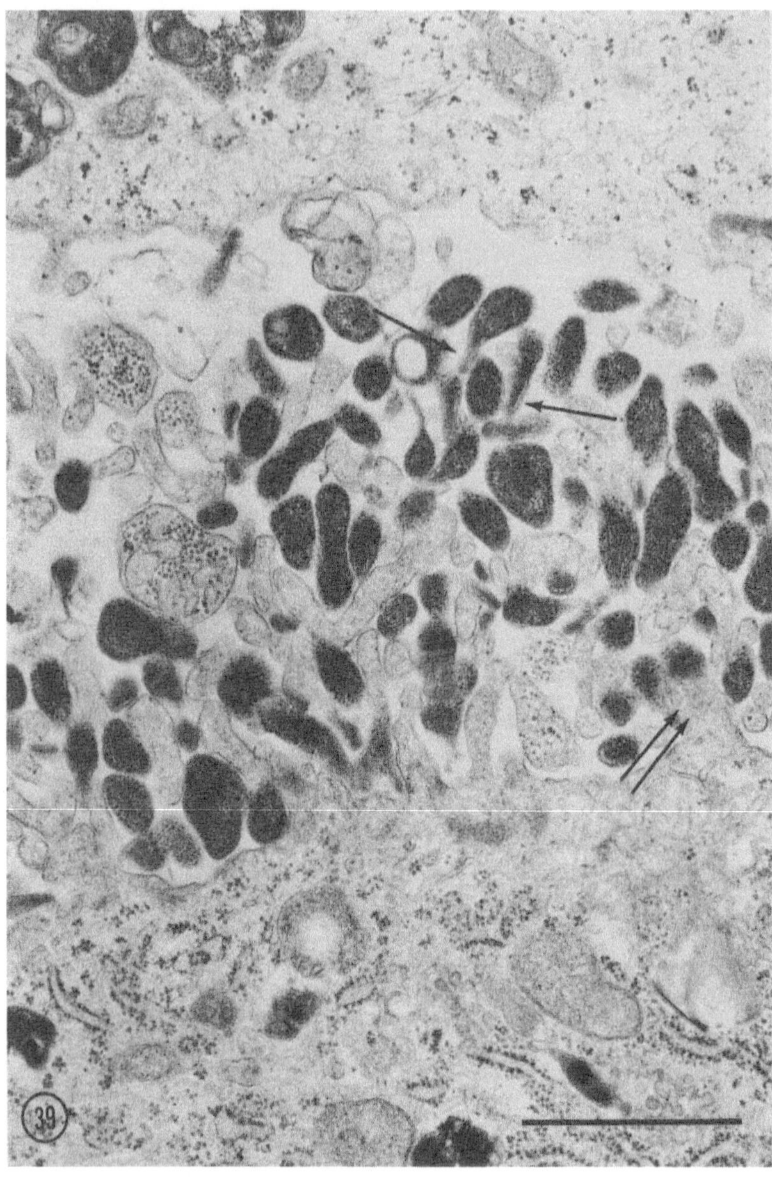

FIG. 39. Monolayer culture derived from fibrosarcoma. The dark-staining mycoplasmal bodies are in intimate contact with cellular microvilli and projections. Several of the bodies disclose a pedicle (arrows). At the place marked by a double arrow, the mycoplasma is apparently fused to a cellular projection.

It has been found that HeLa cells or other cells in established cultures derived from human tumors fail to grow in suspension in the presence of mycoplasmal infection, but still grow well in monolayers under the same conditions (Macpherson and Allner, 1960; Moore *et al.*, 1963). However, ultrastructural alterations caused by mycoplasmas in these cells are very little known. According to Jezequel *et al.* (1967), experimental infection of human embryonic lung cells and of Chang liver cells with mycoplasmas determines a segregation of granular and filamentous components of nucleoli very similar to segregation caused by a series of drugs and by arginine deprivation (see above). Nucleolar segregation precedes cytoplasmic changes (fragmentation of the endoplasmic reticulum, swelling of mitochondria, and increase in the number of electron-dense inclusions and of lysosomes) which in many cases lead to cell lysis in the absence of appropriate antibiotics. The cytopathic effect may be prevented or occasionally suppressed by kanamycin.

The mechanism(s) of the lytic effects of mycoplasmas on cells is not well understood. Jezequel *et al.* (1967) have not observed intracytoplasmic mycoplasmal bodies in their experiments. Mycoplasmas are known to interfere with DNA synthesis (Nardone *et al.*, 1965) and to deplete the medium of its amino acids (Hayflick, 1965). It has been found, in this laboratory, that human cells of infected cultures showing cytopathic effect accumulate large quantities of mycoplasmal bodies in cytoplasmic vacuoles (Fig. 40) and that dying cells are completely invaded by the organisms (Fig. 41). Whether the cells die first from the toxic effects of the mycoplasmas or die because of their intracellular proliferation has not been determined yet. Limited numbers of mycoplasmas were frequently observed in cytoplasmic inclusions of cells from nonlytically infected cultures, which evidently indicates that in the absence of toxic effects some kind of coexistence is established between the cells and the organisms (Fogh *et al.*, 1965).

6.3. *Cell Transformation in Vitro*

A considerable amount of literature exists on the subject of spontaneous or induced cell transformation *in vitro* (see reviews by Sanford, 1965; Abercrombie, 1970). However, the ultrastructural criteria indicative of transformation have not been to this point clearly demonstrated. A number of the attempts to determine these criteria have been carried out on cultures of animal cells (mouse, rat, and guinea pig) using scanning electron microscopy (Hodges, 1970; Privat *et al.*, 1971; Boyde *et al.*, 1972). No clear-cut morphological clue of transformation has so far been found. The reason for it, in our opinion, is a persistent uncertainty about the nature (epithelial,

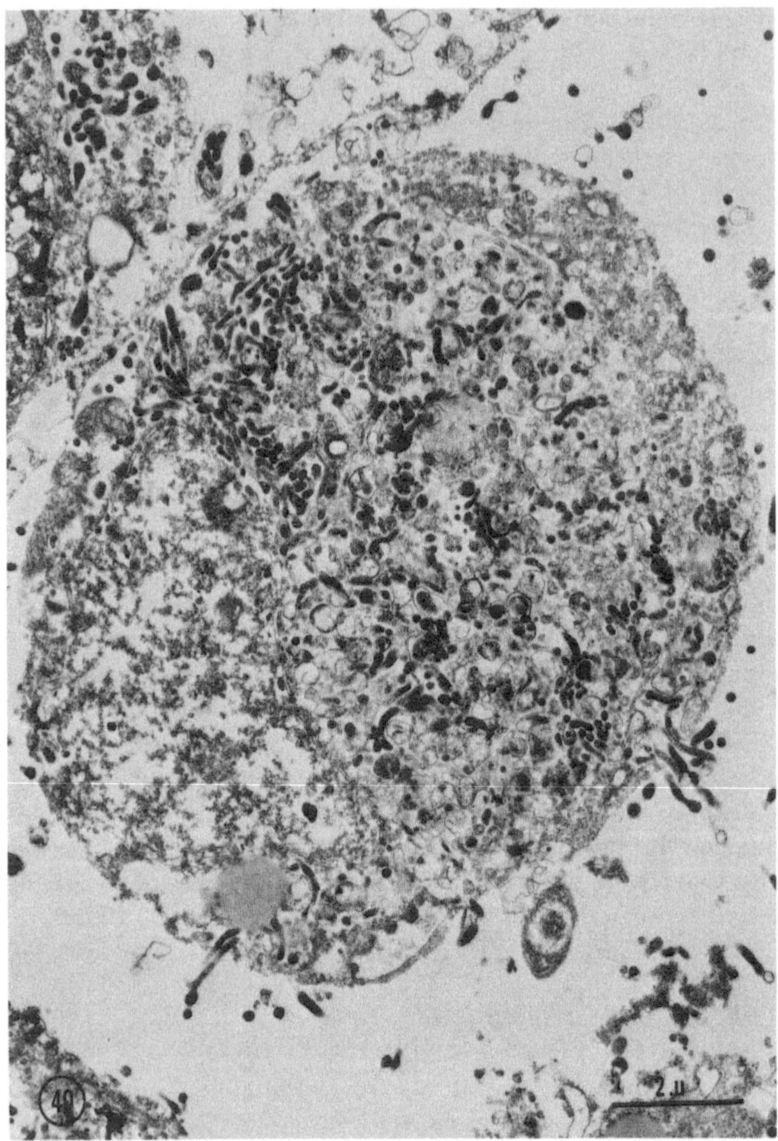

FIG. 40. Cell from a culture of fibrosarcoma cells, undergoing complete lysis caused by mycoplasmal infection. The microorganisms have entirely invaded the dead cell.

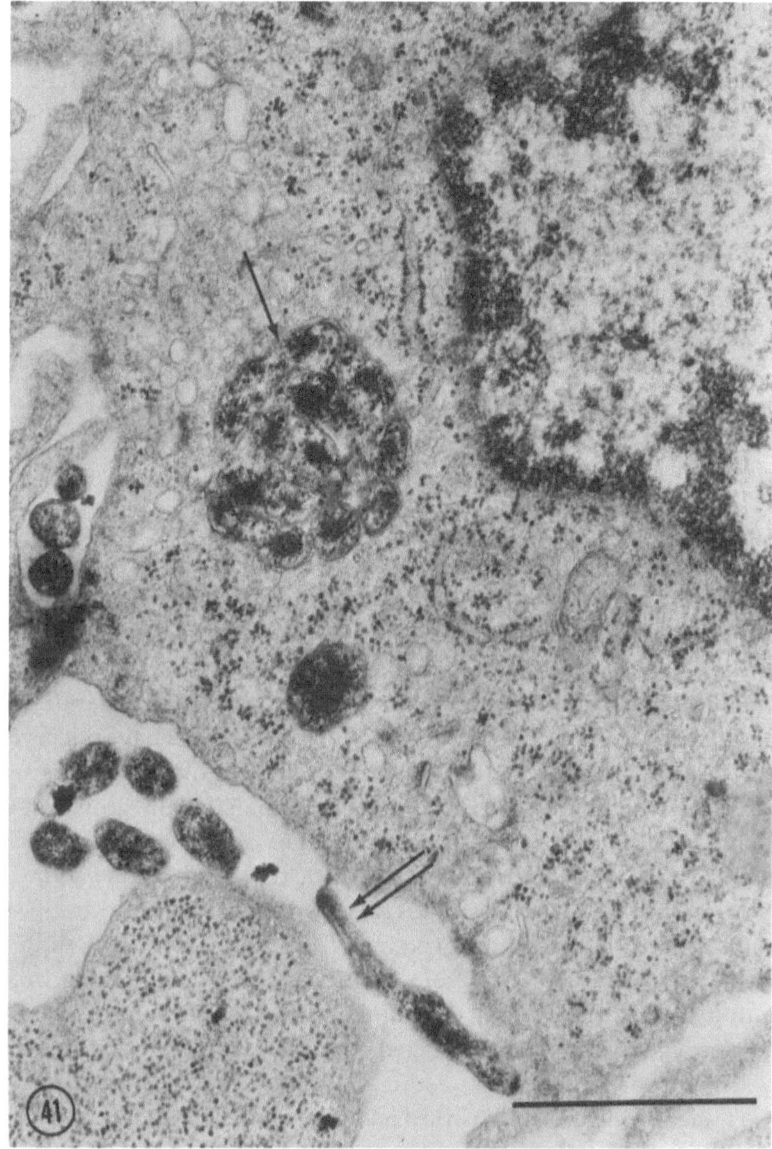

FIG. 41. Intracytoplasmic mycoplasma (arrow) in an apparently well-preserved cell from a culture derived from fibrosarcoma. There are several extracellular mycoplasmas, one of them showing a distinct pedicle (double arrow).

fibroblastic, or other) of the cells growing in culture. Yet the nature of the cells entirely conditions their behavior in cultures, especially the types of contacts between them (see also Abercrombie, 1970). As far as human tumor cells *in vitro* are concerned, most of the cells have been handled under many experimental conditions just as any ordinary cells. Studies of the surface and cell contacts of HeLa cells by Cooper and Fisher (1968*a,b*) and of HEp-2 cells by Strauli *et al.* (1971) have not shown the presence of structural conformations attributable to the transformed state. These rather negative results probably indicate that the symptoms of transformation have to be found by using more sophisticated electron microscopic approaches, such as study of the properties of the surface of the cells (see Martinez-Palomo *et al.*, 1969; Paintrand and Rosenfeld, 1972; Shigematsu and Dmochowski, 1973).

7. *Conclusions*

The results of ultrastructural studies of human tumor cells *in vitro* are, except for HeLa cells, still fragmentary. However, it is possible to draw some conclusions of general value from the accumulated data. These conclusions may be related to two different aspects of these studies: (1) cellular ultrastructure and (2) cytological diagnosis.

From the information already collected, it appears, as mentioned in Section 3.1, that human tumor cells in prolonged cultures have not revealed so far any specific morphological markers indicative of malignancy, when compared with other normal animal and mammalian cells grown *in vitro*. This failure of electron microscopy in the field of tissue culture is parallel to the impossibility of demonstrating, by ultrastructural studies alone, the cancerous nature of cells *in vivo*. This situation is probably only temporary. Although constantly being improved, electron microscopic techniques are still crude in comparison with biochemical or biomolecular techniques presently available. In addition, the number of successful cultures of human tumor cells examined so far by so-called conventional electron microscopy is notoriously insufficient.

Nevertheless, electron microscopy has shown that human tumor cells *in vitro* follow, with time, a pattern of morphological simplification which in most cases might be called dedifferentiation, provided that the origin of the cells in culture has been correctly identified. This is frequently not the case. The lineage of the lymphoblastoid cell cultures of hematopoietic tissues is still not known, and the study of cells derived from pleural or ascitic effusions is only beginning. Be that as it may, cells in prolonged cultures have essentially quite similar structures from one culture to another, whatever the tumor tissue of origin; for that matter, the ultrastructure of HeLa cells may serve as a model.

On the other hand, electron microscopy has also revealed that human tumor cells in culture retain certain structural characteristics which provide important clues to the origin of the cells. The practice of tissue culture quickly allows one to recognize, under the light microscope, cells of epithelial, fibroblastic, or other type, but in the electron microscope differential diagnosis is more accurate. Examination of cells from well-known lines such as HeLa, HEp-2, KB, MAC-21, or BT-20 has clearly demonstrated that epithelial cells in culture can be identified from ultrastructural markers such as desmosomes, hemidesmosomes, tonofibrils, and microvilli, while cells derived from soft tissues or bone tumors can be recognized from the features they share with actively growing fibroblasts. Still, identification does not go beyond the possibility of telling an epithelial cell from another type of cell—in other words, of recognizing the tissue of origin but not the organ or origin of the cells, especially when the culture has been initiated from a metastatic tumor. In addition, established cultures are too few, at the moment, for differential diagnostic criteria concerning the organs of origin to be established on solid grounds. The contribution of electron microscopy in solving the particular and very serious problem of the contamination of human cultures with unrelated cells (see Sanford, 1965) is for that reason rather limited.

The most rewarding approach in studying the ultrastructure of human tumor cells grown *in vitro* is undoubtedly the combination of ultramorphology with biochemistry, that is, a simultaneous analysis of structure and function. Several examples of this type of approach have been given in this chapter. However, here again the various experiments have so far not indicated any clear-cut difference in the behavior of human tumor cells grown *in vitro* from that of other normal animal or human cells grown under the same conditions, when exposed to chemical or physical agents. Further experiments utilizing more refined methods and a broader variety of cultured human tumor cells may conceivably enable investigators to recognize some characteristic properties of malignant cells.

8. *Addendum*

Some recent data dealing with ultrastructural observations of viruses in tissue cultures of human tumor cells should be included in this chapter. Virus particles morphologically similar to the Mason–Pfizer virus (MP-MV) isolated in 1970 from a spontaneous mammary tumor of a rhesus monkey

(Chopra and Mason, 1970) have been found by electron microscopy in some human tumor cell lines. The particles have been observed by Russian authors in HeLa and HEp-2 (Zhdanov *et al.*, 1973), by Hooks *et al.* (1972) in a tissue culture derived from human brain, and by Gelderblom *et al.* (1972, 1974) in one of four HeLa cell strains grown in Germany, the so-called Dusseldorf strain (HeLa D). These particles have biophysical and biochemical properties of oncornaviruses and may be specific for primates (Bauer *et al.*, 1974).

9. *References*

Abercrombie, M., 1970, Contact inhibition in tissue culture, *In Vitro* **6:**128–142.

Abramson, D. H., and Byers, B., 1966, Morphological changes in HeLa cells during late cytokinesis, in: 6th Annual Meeting of the American Society for Cell Biology, Nov. 17–19, Houston, Texas, *J. Cell Biol.* **31:**3A (abst.).

Amalric, F., Simard, R., and Zalta, J.-P., 1969, Effets de la temperature supra-optimale sur les ribonucleoproteines et le RNA nucleolaire. II. Etude biochimique, *Exp. Cell Res.* **55:**370–377.

Amy, R. L., and Storb, R., 1965, Selective mitochondrial damage by a ruby laser microbeam: An electron microscope study, *Science* **150:**756–757.

Anderson, D. R., 1970, Ultrastructure of normal and leukemic leukocytes in human peripheral blood, *J. Ultrastruct. Res.* **30:**1–42 (Suppl. 9).

Andre, J., and Marinozzi, V., 1965, Presence, dans les mitochondries, de particules ressemblant aux ribosomes, *J. Microsc.* **4:**615–626.

Ang. B., Jaross, L., and McAllister, R. M., 1962, Studies of fibroblast-like cells from the bone marrow of leukemic and non-leukemic children, *Proc. Soc. Exp. Biol. Med,* **109:**467–471.

Archer, F. L., 1968, Normal and neoplastic human tissue in organ culture, *Arch. Pathol.* **85:**62–71.

Armstrong, D., 1966, Serial cultivation of human leukemic cells, *Proc. Soc. Exp. Biol. Med.* **122:**475–481.

Arstila, A. U., Jauregui, H. O., Chang, J., and Trump, B. F., 1971, Studies on cellular autophagocytosis: Relationship between heterophagy and autophagy in HeLa cells, *Lab. Invest.* **24:**162–174.

Baringer, J. R., and Swoveland, P., 1972, Tubular aggregates in endoplasmic reticulum: Evidence against their viral nature, *J. Ultrastruct. Res.* **41:**270–276.

Baron, S., and Rabson, A., 1957, A culture strain (LAC) of human epithelial-like cells from an adenocarcinoma of the lung, *Proc. Soc. Exp. Biol. Med.* **96:**515–518.

Bassin, R. H., Plata, E. J., Gerwin, B. I., Mattern, C. F., Haapala, D. K., and Chu, E. W., 1972, Isolation of a continuous epitheloid cell line, HBT-3, from a human breast carcinoma (36850), *Proc. Soc. Exp. Biol. Med.* **141:**673–680.

Bauer, H., Daams, J. H., Watson, K. F., Molling, K. Gelderblom, H., and Schafer, W., 1974, Oncornavirus-like particles in HeLa cells. II. Immunological characterization of the virus, *Int. J. Cancer* **13:**254–261.

Bayer, M. E., and Nielsen, G., 1961, Zur Morphologie des Gelbfiebervirus, *Arch. Ges. Virusforsch.* **11:**303–306.

Bedoya, V., 1970, Effect of chloroquine on malignant lymphoreticular and pigmented cells *in vitro, Cancer Res.* **30:**1262–1275.

Bedoya, V., Grimley, P. M., and Rabson, A. S., 1969, Ultrastructural evidence of *in vitro* interaction among Burkitt lymphoma cells: Possible relevance to the "phagocytic" activity of starry sky histiocytes *in vivo, Cancer Res.* **29:**753–762.

Bekerhi, A., and Markani, K., 1970, Etude des cellules HeLa par le cryodecapage, *J. Ultrastruct. Res.* **32:**23–31.

Bensch, K. G., and Malawista, S. E., 1968, Microtubule crystals: A new biophysical phenomenon induced by *Vinca* alkaloids, *Nature (Lond.)* **218:**1176–1177.

Benyesh-Melnick, M., 1967, Formal discussion: Continuous lymphoid cell cultures from human bone marrow, *Cancer Res.* **27:**2504–2506.

Berg. R. B., and Rosenthal, M. S., 1961, Studies of fibroblastic cells from bone marrow of leukemic and non-leukemic patients, *Proc. Soc. Exp. Biol. Med.* **106:**614–617.

Bergold, J. H., and Weibel, J., 1962, Demonstration of yellow fever virus with the electron microscope, *Virology* **17:**554–562.

Berman, L., and Stulberg, C. S., 1956, Eight cultures (Detroit) of human epithelial-like cells, *Proc. Soc. Exp. Biol. Med.* **92:**730–735.

Bernhard, W., 1966, Ultrastructural aspects of the normal and pathological nucleolus in mammalian cells, *Natl. Cancer Inst. Monogr.* **23:**13–38.

Bernhard, W., and Granboulan, N., 1968, Electron microscopy of the nucleolus of vertebrate cells, in: *Ultrastructure in Biological Systems*, Vol. 3 (A. J. Dalton and F. Haguenau, eds.), pp. 81–149, Academic Press, New York.

Bessis, M., 1964, Studies on cell agony and death: An attempt at classification, in: *Cellular Injury* (A. V. S. De Reuck and J. Knight, eds.), pp. 287–328, Little, Brown, Boston.

Bessis, M., and Storb, R., 1965, Sensibilite des leucocytes au laser a rubis apres differentes colorations vitales, *Nouv. Rev. Fr. Hematol.* **5:**459–474.

Birch-Anderson, A., and Paucker, K., 1959, Studies on the structure of influenza virus. II. Ultrathin sections of infectious and noninfectious particles, *Virology* **8:**21–40.

Bloch, D. P., Morgan, C. Godman, G. C., Howe, C., and Rose, H. M., 1957, A correlated histochemical and electron microscopic study of the intranuclear crystalline aggregates of adenovirus (RI-APC virus) in HeLa cells, *J. Biophys. Biochem. Cytol.* **3:**1–8.

Blondel, B., and Tolmach, L. J., 1965, Studies on nuclear fine structure: Three phases of the HeLa cell cycle, *Exp. Cell Res.* **37:**497–501.

Bonissol, C., Sisman, J., and Lepine, P., 1968, Etude preliminaire au microscope electronique du myxovirus parainfluenza. II, *Ann. Inst. Pasteur* **114:**551–554.

Bootsma, D., Budke, L., and Vos. O., 1964, Studies on synchronous division of tissue culture cells initiated by excess thymidine, *Exp. Cell. Res.* **33:**301–309.

Bouteille, M., Kalifat, S. R., and Delarue, J., 1967, Ultrastructural variations of nuclear bodies in human diseases, *J. Ultrastruct. Res.* **19:**474–486.

Boyde, A., Weiss, R. A., and Vesely, P., 1972, Scanning electron microscopy of cells in culture, *Exp. Cell Res.* **71:**313–324.

Boyer, G. S., Leuchtenberger, C., and Ginsberg, H. S., 1957, Cytological and cytochemical studies of HeLa cells infected with adenoviruses, *J. Exp. Med.* **105:**195–216.

Brinkley, B. R., Murphy, P., and Richardson, L. C., 1967, Procedure for embedding *in situ* selected cells cultured *in vitro, J. Cell Biol.* **35:**279–283.

Bruni, C., Gey, M. K., and Svotelis, M., 1961, Changes in the fine structure of HeLa cells in relation to growth, *Bull. Johns Hopkins Hosp.* **109:**160–177.

Buonassissi, V., and Ozzello, L., 1973, Sulfated mucopolysaccharide production by synovial sarcoma cells *in vivo* and in tissue culture, *Cancer Res.* **33:**874–881.

Burns, E. R., Soloff, B. L., Hanna, C., and Buxton, D. F., 1971, Nuclear pockets associated with the nucleolus in normal and neoplastic cells, *Cancer Res.* **31:**159–165.

Busch, H., and Smetana, K., 1970, *The Nucleolus*, Academic Press, New York.

Byers, B., and Abramson, D. H., 1968, Cytokinesis in HeLa: Post-telophase delay and microtubule-associated motility, *Protoplasma* **66:**413–435.

Cailleau, R., 1960, The establishment of a cell strain (MAC-21) from a mucoid adenocarcinoma of human lung, *Cancer Res.* **20:**837–840.

Carr, K. E., 1971, Applications of scanning electron microscopy in biology, *Int. Rev. Cytol.* **30:**183–255.

Cavaliere, R., Ciocatto, E. C., Giovanella, B. P., Heidelberger, C., Johnson, R. O., Margottini, M., Mondovi, B., Moricca, G., and Rossi-Fanelli, A., 1967, Selective heat sensitivity of cancer cells, *Cancer* **20:**1351–1381.

Chandra, S., Moore, G. E., and Brandt, P. M., 1968, Similarity between leukocyte cultures from cancerous and noncancerous human subjects: An electron microscope study, *Cancer Res.* **28:**1982–1989.

Chopra, H. C., and Mason, M. M., 1970, A new virus in a spontaneous mammary tumor of a rhesus monkey, *Cancer Res.* **30:**2081–2086.

Clarke, J. K., Samuels, J., Dermott, E., and Gay, F. W., 1970, Carrier cultures of simian foamy virus, *J. Virol.* **5:**624–631.

Clarkson, B., 1967, Formal discussion: On the cellular origins and distinctive features of cultured cell lines derived from patients with leukemias and lymphomas, *Cancer Res.* **27:**2483–2488.

Clarkson, B., Strife, A., and DeHarven, E., 1967, Continuous culture of seven new cell lines (SKL-1 to 7) from patients with acute leukemia, *Cancer* **20:**926–947.

Clarkson, B. D., Thorbecke, J., DeHarven, E., and Miles, C., 1969, Immunoglobulin synthesis by human reticulum sarcoma cells *in vivo* and during long-term culture *in vitro*, *Cancer Res.* **29:**823–836.

Cooper, T. W., and Fisher, H. W., 1968*a*, Electron microscopic survey of the presence of microvilli in cultured mammalian cells, *J. Natl. Cancer Inst.* **41:**789–794.

Cooper, T. W., and Fisher, H. W., 1968*b*, Electron microscope observations on the attenuated attachment bridges of HeLa cells, *Exp. Cell Res.* **53:**663–665.

Costero, I., and Pomerat, C. M., 1951, Cultivation of neurons from adult human cerebral and cerebellar cortex, *Am. J. Anat.* **89:**405–467.

Dalton, A. J., and Haguenau, F., 1968, *Ultrastructure in Biological Systems*, Vol. III: *The Nucleus*, Academic Press, New York.

Dalton, A. J., and Stewart, S. E., 1972, Intracisternal A particles and C particles, *Science* **176:**319.

Dalton, A. J., and Zeve, V. H., 1967, A review of studies with the electron microscope on human leukemia and Burkitt's tumor, *Cancer Res.* **27:**2465–2470.

Dalton, A. J., Heine, U., Kondratick, J. M., Ablashi, D. V., and Blackham, E. A., 1973, Ultrastructural and complement-fixation studies on suspension cultures derived from human solid tumors, *J. Natl. Cancer Inst.* **50:**879–894.

Dawe, C. J., Banfield, W. G., Morgan, W. D., Slatick, M. S., and Curth, H. O., 1965, Growth in continuous culture and in hamsters of cells of a neoplasm associated with acanthosis nigricans, *J. Natl. Cancer Inst.* **33:**441–456.

De Harven, E., 1967, Human leukemic cells in tissue culture: An electron microscope survey, *Cancer Res.* **27:**2447–2464.

De Harven, E., Clarkson, B., and Strife, A., 1967, Electron microscopic study of human leukemic cells in tissue culture, *Cancer* **20:**911–925.

De The, G., Ambrosioni, J.-C., Ho, H. C., and Kwan, H. C., 1969, Lymphoblastoid transformation and presence of herpes-type viral particles in a Chinese nasopharyngeal tumor cultured *in vitro*, *Nature (Lond.)* **221:**770–771.

De The, G., Ho, H. C., Kwan, H. C., Desgrànges, C., and Favre, M. C., 1970, Nasopharyngeal carcinoma (NPC). I. Types of cultures derived from tumor biopsies and non-tumorous tissues of Chinese patients with special reference to lymphoblastoid transformation, *Int. J. Cancer* **6:**189–206.

Dingle, J. T., and Fell, H. B., 1969, *Lysosomes in Biology and Pathology*, Wiley, New York.

Djordjevic, B., and Tolmach, L. J., 1967, Responses of synchronous populations of HeLa cells to ultraviolet irradiation at selected stages of the generation cycle, *Radiat. Res.* **32:**327–346.

Dmochowski, L., 1960, Viruses and tumors in the light of electron microscope studies: A review, *Cancer Res.* **20:**977–1015.

Dmochowski, L., 1970, Comparison of leukemogenic and sarcomagenic viruses at the ultrastructural level, *Bibl. Haematol.* **36:**68–82.

Dmochowski, L., 1973, Unifying concepts of leukemia and related neoplasms in animals and man leading to the eventual control and prevention, *Bibl. Haematol.* **39:** in press.

Dmochowski, L., Taylor, H. G., Grey, C. E., Dreyer, D. A., Sykes, J. A., Langford, P. L., Rogers, T., Shullenberger, C. C., and Howe, C. D., 1965, Viruses and mycoplasma (PPLO) in human leukemia, *Cancer* **18:**1345–1368.

Dobrynin, Y. V., 1963, Establishment and characteristics of cell strains from some epithelial tumors of human origin, *J. Natl. Cancer Inst.* **31:**1173–1196.

Douglas, S. D., Borjeson, J., and Chessin, L. N., 1967, Studies on human lymphocytes *in vitro.* IV. Comparative fine structural features of the established Burkitt lymphoma cell lines AL-1, EB-2, and phytomitogen-transformed lymphocytes, *J. Immunol.* 340–346.

Dourmashkin, R. R., and Dougherty, R. M., 1961, Phagocytosis of crystalline particles by cells grown in tissue culture, *Exp. Cell Res.* **25:**480–484.

Eagle, H., 1955*a*, Propagation in a fluid medium of a human epidermoid carcinoma, strain KB *Proc. Soc. Exp. Biol. Med.* **89:**362–364.

Eagle, H., 1955*b*, Nutrition needs of mammalian cells in tissue culture, *Science* **122:**501–504.

Easterbrook, K. B., and Davern, C. I., 1963, The effect of 5-bromodeoxyuridine on the multiplication of vaccinia virus, *Virology* **19:**509–520.

Easty, D. M., 1967, Methods and applications of organ culture, in: *The Cancer Cell In Vitro* (E. J. Ambrose, D. M. Easty, and J. A. H. Wylie, eds.), pp. 50–62.

Easty, G. C., and Mercer, E. H., 1960, An electron microscope study of the surface of normal and malignant cells in culture, *Cancer Res.* **20:**1608–1613.

Edwards, G. A., and Fogh, J., 1960, Fine structure of pleuropneumonia-like organisms in pure culture and in infected tissue culture cells, *J. Bacteriol.* **79:**267–276.

Epstein, M. A., 1961, Some unusual features of fine structure observed in HeLa cells, *J. Biophys. Biochem. Cytol.* **10:**153–163.

Epstein, M. A., 1962, Observations on the mode of release of herpes virus from infected HeLa cells, *J. Cell Biol.* **12:**589–597.

Epstein, M. A., and Achong, B. G., 1965, Fine structural organization of human lymphoblasts of a tissue culture strain (EB-1) from Burkitt's lymphoma, *J. Natl. Cancer Inst.* **34:**241–253.

Epstein, M. A., and Barr, Y. M., 1964, Cultivation *in vitro* of human lymphoblasts from Burkitt's malignant lymphoma, *Lancet* **1:**252–253.

Epstein, M. A., Achong, B. G., and Barr, Y. M., 1964*a*, Virus particles in cultured lymphoblasts from Burkitt's lymphoma, *Lancet* **2:**702–703.

Epstein, M. A., Hummeler, K., and Berkaloff, A., 1964*b*, The entry and distribution of herpes virus and colloidal gold in HeLa cells after contact in suspension, *J. Exp. Med.* **119:**291–302.

Epstein, M. A., Barr, Y. M., and Achong, B. G., 1965, The behavior and morphology of a second tissue culture strain (EB-2) of lymphoblasts from Burkitt's lymphoma, *Brit. J. Cancer* **19:**108–115.

Erlandson, R. A., and De Harven, E., 1971, The ultrastructure of synchronized HeLa cells, *J. Cell Sci.* **8:**353–397.

Erlandson, R. A., Babcock, V. I., Southam, C. M., Bailey, R. B., and Shipkey, F. H., 1967, Semliki forest virus in HEp-2 cell cultures, *J. Virol.* **1:**996–1009.

Farquhar, M. G., and Palade, G. E., 1963, Junctional complexes in various epithelia, *J. Cell Biol.* **17:**375–412.

Fawcett, D. W., 1966, *The Cell: An Atlas of Fine Structure,* Saunders, Philadelphia.

Feller, W. F., Stewart, S. E., and Kantor, J., 1972, Primary tissue culture explants of human breast cancer, *J. Natl. Cancer Inst.* **48:**1117–1120.

Ferenczy, A., Fenoglio, J., and Richart, R. M., 1972, Observations on benign mesothelioma of the genital tract (adenomatoid tumor): A comparative ultrastructural study, *Cancer* **30:**244–260.

Finegold, I., Hirshaut, Y., and Fahey, J. L., 1968, Immunochemical and morphologic comparison of donor tissues with immunoglobulin-producing tissue culture lines from two patients with malignancies, *Cancer Res.* **28:**1538–1549.

Fisher, H. W., and Cooper, T. W., 1967, Electron microscope studies of the microvilli of HeLa cells, *J. Cell Biol.* **34:** 569–576.

Flaxman, B. A., 1972, Growth *in vitro* and induction of differentiation in cells of basal cell cancer, *Cancer Res.* **32:**462–469.

Flaxman, B. A., and Van Scott, E. J., 1968, Keratinization *in vitro* of cells from a basal cell carcinoma, *J. Natl. Cancer Inst.* **40:**411–422.

Flaxman, B. A., and Van Scott, E. J., 1972, Growth of normal human mammary gland epithelium *in vitro, Cancer Res.* **32:**2407–2412.

Flaxman, B., Revel, J. P., and Hay, E. D., 1969, Tight junctions between contact-inhibited cells *in vitro, Exp. Cell Res.* **58:**438–443.

Fogh, J., 1961, Filamentous organization of poliovirus particles, *Virology* **14:**495–497.

Fogh, J., and Hacker, C., 1960, Elimination of pleuropneumonia-like organisms from cell cultures, *Exp. Cell Res.* **21:**242–244.

Fogh, J., and Stuart, D. C., Jr., 1960, Intracellular crystals of poliovirus in HeLa cells, *Virology* **11:**308–311.

Fogh, J., Hahn, E., III, and Fogh, H., 1965, Effects of pleuropneumonia-like organisms on cultured human cells, *Exp. Cell Res.* **39:**554–566.

Foley, G. E., Lazarus, H., Farber, S., Uzman, B. G., Boone, B. A., and McCarthy, R. E., 1965, Continuous culture of human lymphoblasts from peripheral blood of a child with acute leukemia, *Cancer* **18:**522–529.

Fuse, Y., Price, Z., and Carpenter, C. M., 1963, A comparison of the fine structure of cultured MAC-21 and HeLa cells, *Cancer Res.* **23:**1658–1670.

Gazzolo, L., De The, G., Vuillaume, M., and Ho, H. C., 1972, Nasopharyngeal carcinoma. II. Ultrastructure of normal mucosa, tumor biopsies, and subsequent epithelial growth *in vitro, J. Natl. Cancer Inst.* **48:**73–86.

Gelderblom, H., Molling, K., and Watson, K. F., 1972, Detection of oncornaviruses of presumbably human origin, in: *Abstracts of the 7th Meeting of the European Tumour Virus Group,* p. 28, Sept. 25–27, Zierickzee, Netherlands.

Gelderblom, H., Bauer, H., Ogura, H., Wigand, R., and Fischer, A. B., 1974, Detection of oncornavirus-like particles in HeLa cells. I. Fine structure and comparative morphological classification, *Int. J. Cancer* **13:**246–253.

George, P., Journey, L. J., and Goldstein, M. N., 1965, Effect of vincristine on fine structure of HeLa cells during mitosis, *J. Natl. Cancer Inst.* **35:**355–375.

Gerber, P., and Monroe, J. H., 1968, Studies on leukocytes growing in continuous cultures derived from normal donors, *J. Natl. Cancer Inst.* **40:**855–856.

Gey, G. O., Coffman, W. D., and Kubicek, M. T., 1952, Tissue culture studies of the proliferative capacity of cervical carcinoma and normal epithelium, *Cancer Res.* **12:**264–265.

Glauert, A. M., Rogers, G. E., and Glauert, R. H., 1956, A new embedding medium for electron microscopy, *Nature (Lond.)* **178:**803.

Goldstein, M. N., 1971, Annulate lamellae in cultured neuroblastoma cells, *Cancer Res.* **31:**209–213.

Goldstein, M. N., Burdman, J. A., and Journey, L. J., 1964, Tissue culture of neuroblastomas. II. Morphologic evidence for differentiation and maturation, *J. Natl. Cancer Inst.* **32:**165–199.

Gori, G. B., and Lee, D. Y., 1964, A method for eradication of mycoplasma infections in cell cultures, *Proc. Soc. Exp. Biol. Med.* **117:**918–921.

Gregg, M., and Morgan, C., 1959, Reduplication in nuclear membranes in HeLa cells infected with adenoviruses, *J. Biophys. Biochem. Cytol.* **6:**539–540.

Grimley, P. M., and Moss, B., 1971, Similar effect of rifampin and other rifamycin derivatives on vaccinia virus morphogenesis, *J. Virol.* **8:**225–231.

Grimley, P. M., Rosenblum, E. N., Mims, S. J., and Moss, B., 1970, Interruption by rifampicin of an early stage in vaccinia virus morphogenesis: Accumulation of membranes which are precursors of viral envelopes, *J. Virol.* **6:**519–533.

Gyorkey, F., Min, K. W., Sinkovics, J. G., and Gyorkey, P., 1969, Systemic lupus erythematosus and myxovirus, *New Engl. J. Med.* **280:**333.

Hagmuller, K., and Leslie, I., 1962, The use of organ culture to study ^{131}I uptake and metabolism of thyroid tissue, *Exp. Cell Res.* **27:**396–400.

Hallauer, C., Kronauer, G., and Siegl, G., 1971, Parvoviruses as contaminants of permanent human cell lines. I. Virus isolations from 1960–1970, *Arch. Ges. Virusforsch.* **35:**80–90.

Harford, C. G., Hamlin, A., Parker, E., and Van Ravenswaay, T., 1956*a*, Electron microscopy of HeLa cells infected with adenoviruses, *J. Exp. Med.* **104:**443–454.

Harford, C. G., Hamlin, A., Parker, E., and Van Ravenswaay, T., 1956*b*, Globoid structures in the cytoplasm of rapidly growing HeLa cells, *J. Biophys. Biochem, Cytol.* **2:**347–350.

Harford, C. G., Hamlin, A., and Parker, E., 1957, Electron microscopy of HeLa cells after ingestion of colloidal gold, *J. Biophys. Biochem. Cytol.* **3:**749–756.

Harford, C. G., Hamlin, A., and Rieders, E., 1966, Electron microscopic autoradiography of DNA synthesis in cells infected with vaccinia virus, *Exp. Cell Res.* **42:**50–57.

Harris, H., Watkins, J. F., Ford, C. E., and Schoefl, G. E., 1966, Artificial heterokaryons of animal cells from different species, *J. Cell Sci.* **1:**1–30.

Hayflick, L., 1965, Tissue cultures and mycoplasmas, *Texas Rep. Biol. Med.* **23:**285–303 (Suppl.1).

Heine, U., 1969, Electron microscopic studies on HeLa cells exposed to the antibiotic toyocamycin, *Cancer Res.* **29:**1875–1880.

Hendee, W. R., Zebrun, W., and Bonte, F. J., 1963*a*, Anomalous structures in the cytoplasm of HeLa cells cultured in the presence of 5-bromodeoxyuridine, *J. Cell Biol.* **17:**675–680.

Hendee, W. R., Zebrun, W., and Bonte, F. J., 1963*b*, Effects of X-radiation on fine structure of HeLa cells, *Texas Rep. Biol. Med.* **21:**546–557.

Hinglais-Guillaud, N., 1960, L'ultrastructure de l'exocol normal de la femme, *Bull. Assoc. Fr. Cancer* **46:**212–252.

Hinuma, Y., and Grace, J. T., Jr., 1967, Cloning of immunoglobulin-producing human leukemic and lymphoma cells in long-term cultures, *Proc. Soc. Exp. Biol. Med.* **124:**107–111.

Hodge, L. D., Robbins, E., and Scharff, M. D., 1969, Persistence of messenger RNA through mitosis in HeLa cells, *J. Cell Biol.* **40:**497–507.

Hodges, G. M., 1970, A scanning electron microscope study of cell surface and cell contacts of "spontaneously" transformed cells *in vitro. Eur. J. Cancer* **6:**235–239.

Hooks, G., Gibbs, C. J., Chopra, H. C., Lewis, M., and Gajdusek, D. C., 1972, Spontaneous transformation of human brain cells grown *in vitro* and description of associated virus particles, *Science* **176:**1420–1422.

Hou-Jensen, K., Priori, E., and Dmochowski, L., 1972, Studies on ultrastructure of Ewing's sarcoma of bone, *Cancer* **29:**280–286.

Howatson, A. F., and Almeida, J. D., 1958, A method for the study of cultured cells by thin sectioning and electron microscopy, *J. Biophys. Biochem. Cytol.* **4:**115–118.

Humble, J. G., Jayne, W. H. W., and Pulvertaft, J. V., 1956, Biological interaction between lymphocytes and other cells, *Brit. J. Haematol.* **2:**283–294.

Iwakata, S., and Grace, J. T., Jr., 1964, Cultivation *in vitro* of myeloblasts from human leukemia, *N.Y. State J. Med.* **64:**2279–2282.

Jezequel, A. M., Shreeve, M. M., and Steiner, J. W., 1967, Segregation of nucleolar components in mycoplasma-infected cells, *Lab. Invest.* **16:**287–304.

Journey, L. J., and Goldstein, M. N., 1961, Electron microscope studies on HeLa cell lines sensitive and resistant to actinomycin D, *Cancer Res.* **21:**929–932.

Kallmann, F., Adams, J. M., Williams, R. C., and Imagawa, D. T., 1959, Fine structure of cellular inclusions in measle virus infections, *J. Biophys. Biochem. Cytol.* **6:**379–382.

Kelly, D. E., and Luft, J. H., 1966, Fine structure, development, and classification of desmosomes and related attachment mechanisms, in: *Congress of Electron Microscopy, Kyoto, Japan, 1966*, Vol. 2, pp. 401–402 Maruzen, Tokyo.

Kessel, R. G., 1968, Fine structure of annulate lamellae, *J. Cell Biol.* **36:**658–663.

Kim, J. H., and Perez, A. G., 1965, Ribonucleic acid synthesis in synchronously dividing populations of HeLa cells, *Nature (Lond.)* **207:**974–975.

Kim, J. H., and Stambuk, B. K., 1966, Synchronization of HeLa cells by vinblastine sulphate, *Exp. Cell Res.* **44**:631–634.

King, M. E., Godman, G. C., and King, D. W., 1972, Respiratory enzymes and mitochondrial morphology of HeLa and L cells treated with chloramphenicol and ethidium bromide, *J. Cell Biol.* **53**:127–142.

Klug, H., 1962, On the occurrence of lymphocytes in reticulum cells, *Experientia* **18**:317–318.

Kojima, K., and Kozuka, S., 1962, Structural changes in HeLa cells cultivated in serum-free medium, *J. Cell Biol.* **14**:141–144.

Krishan, A., and Hsu, D., 1971*a*, Binding of colchicine-3H to vinblastine and vincristine-induced crystals in mammalian tissue culture cells, *J. Cell Biol.* **48**:407–410.

Krishan, A., and Hsu, D., 1971*b*, Vinblastine-induced ribosomal complexes, *J. Cell Biol.* **49**:927–932.

Kuhn, N. O., and Harford, C. G., 1963, Electron microscopic examination of cytoplasmic inclusion bodies in cells infected with parainfluenza virus, type 2, *Virology* **21**:527–530.

Kumegawa, M., Cattoni, M., and Rose, G. G., 1967, Electron microscopy of oral cells *in vitro*. I. Annulate lamellae observed in strain KB cells, *J. Cell Biol.* **34**:897–901.

Kumegawa, M., Cattoni, M., and Rose, G. G., 1968, Electron microscopy of oral cells *in vitro*. II. Subsurface and intracytoplasmic confronting cisternae in strain KB cells, *J. Cell Biol.* **36**:443–452.

Lane, N. J., and Novikoff, A. B., 1965, Effects of arginine deprivation, ultraviolet radiation and X-ray radiation on cultured KB cells: A cytochemical and ultrastructural study, *J. Cell Biol.* **27**:603–620.

Lapis, K., and Bernhard, W., 1965, The effect of mitomycin C on the nucleolar fine structure of KB cells in cell culture, *Cancer Res.* **25**:628–645.

Lasfargues, E. Y., 1957, Cultivation and behaviour *in vitro* of the normal mammary eipithelium of the adult mouse. II. Observation of the secretory activity, *Exp. Cell Res.* **13**:553–562.

Lasfargues, E. Y., and Ozzello, L. J., 1958, Cultivation of human breast carcinomas, *J. Natl. Cancer Inst.* **21**:1131–1147.

Lenk, R., and Penman, S., 1971, Morphological studies of cells grown in the absence of mitochondrial-specific protein synthesis, *J. Cell Biol.* **49**:540–546.

Lentz, T. L., 1971, *Cell Fine Structure*, Saunders, Philadelphia.

Lettre, R., Siebs, W., and Paweletz, N., 1966, Morphological observations on the nucleolus of cells in tissue culture, with special regard to its composition, *Natl. Cancer Inst. Monogr.* **23**:107–123.

Lewin, P. K., and Moscarello, M. A., 1968, Nucleolar changes in HeLa cells grown in the presence of aminonucleoside, *Lab. Invest.* **19**:265–285.

Loni, M. C., 1971, Etude ultrastructurale de cellules KB infectees massivement par le virus de Newcastle. I. Developpement intracellulaire du virus et alterations cellulaires induites. II. Effet de la microirradiation ultraviolette sur les premiers stades de la multiplication du virus, *Arch Ges. Virusforsch.* **35**:269–289.

Loni, M. C., Burgers, M., and Hugon, J., 1967, Uptake of ferritin particles by ATP-stimulated HeLa cells, *Zellforschung* **76**:725–731.

Love, R., Soriano, R. Z., and Walsh, R. J., 1970, Effect of hyperthermia on normal and neoplastic cells *in vitro*, *Cancer Res.* **30**:1525–1533.

Lucas, L. S., Whang, J. J. K., Tjio, J. H., Manaker, R. A., and Zeve, V. H., 1966, Continuous cell culture from a patient with chronic myelogenous leukemia. I. Propagation and presence of Philadelphia chromosome, *J. Natl. Cancer Inst.* **37**:753–759.

Luibel, F. J., Sanders, E., and Ashworth, C. T., 1960, An electron microscopic study of carcinoma *in situ* and invasive carcinoma of the cervix uteri, *Cancer Res.* **20**:357–361.

Luft, J. H., 1961, Improvements in epoxy resin embedding methods, *J. Biophys. Biochem. Cytol.* **9**:409–414.

Luft, J. H., 1966, Fine structure of capillary and endocapillary layer as revealed by ruthenium red, *Fed. Proc.* **25**:1773–1783.

Macpherson, I., 1966, Mycoplasmas in tissue culture, *J. Cell Sci.* **1**:145–168.

Macpherson, I. A., and Allner, K., 1960, L-forms of bacteria as contaminants in tissue culture, *Nature (Lond.)* **186:**992.

Martinez-Palomo, A., LeBuis, J., and Bernhard, W., 1967, Electron microscopy of adenovirus 12 replication. I. Fine structural changes in the nucleus of infected KB cells, *J. Virol.* **1:**817–829.

Martinez-Palomo, A., Brailovsky, C., and Bernhard, W., 1969, Ultrastructural modification of the cell surface and intercellular contacts of some transformed cell strains, *Cancer Res.* **29:**925–937.

Martorelli, B., Jr., Parshley, M. S., and Moore, J. G., 1969, Effects of chemotherapeutic agents on two lines of human breast carcinomas in tissue culture, *Surg. Gynecol. Obstet.* **128:**1001–1006.

Mattern, C. F. T., and Daniel, W. A., 1965, Replication of poliovirus in HeLa cells: Electron microscopic study, *Virology* **26:**626–643.

Maul, G. G., and Brinkley, B. R., 1970, The Golgi apparatus during mitosis in human melanoma cells *in vitro, Cancer Res.* **30:**2326–2335.

Maul, G. G., and Romsdahl, M. M., 1970, Ultrastructural comparison of two human malignant melanoma cell lines, *Cancer Res.* **30:**2782–2790.

Mayor, H. D., Powell, B., and Trentin, J. J., 1964, Structure of the viral capsid of adenoviruses type 12 and 18, *Virology* **23:**614–616.

McCoy, T. A., and Neuman, R. E., 1956, The cultivation of Walker carcinosarcoma 256 *in vitro* from cell suspensions, *J. Natl. Cancer Inst.* **16:**1221–1229.

McDuffie, N. G., 1967, Nuclear blebs in human leukaemic cells, *Nature (Lond.)* **214:**1341–1342.

McGill, M., and Brinkley, B. R., 1972, Mitosis in human leukemic leukocytes during colcemid inhibition and recovery, *Cancer Res.* **32:**746–755.

McIntosh, J. R., and Landis, S. C., 1971, Distribution of spindle microtubules during mitosis in cultured human cells, *J. Cell Biol.* **49:**468–497.

Millong, G., 1961, Advantage of a phosphate buffer for OsO_4 solution in fixation, in: *Proceedings of the 18th Annual Meeting of the Electron Microscopy Society of America,* pp. 15–16 (abst.).

Miyamoto, K., 1971, Mechanism of intranuclear crystal formation of herpes simplex virus as revealed by the negative staining of thin sections, *J. Virol.* **8:**534–550.

Mollenhauer, H. H., 1964, Plastic embedding mixtures for use in electron microscopy, *Stain Technol.* **39:**111–114.

Mollo, F., and Stramignoni, A., 1967, Nuclear projections in blood and lymph node cells of human leukemias and Hodgkin's disease and in lymphocytes cultured with phytohaemagglutinin, *Brit. J. Cancer* **21:**519–503.

Monneron, A., and Bernhard, W., 1969, Fine structural organization of the interphase nucleus in some mammalian cells, *J. Ultrastruct. Res.* **27:**266–288.

Moore, G. E., Mount, D., Tara, G., and Schwartz, N., 1963, Growth of human tumor cells in suspension cultures, *Cancer Res.* **23:**1735–1741.

Moore, G. E., Kitamura, H., and Toshima, S., 1968, Morphology of cultured hematopoietic cells, *Cancer* **22:**245–267.

Moreno, G., 1971, Effects of ultraviolet micro-irradiation on different parts of the cell. II. Cytological observations and unscheduled DNA synthesis after partial nuclear irradiation, *Exp. Cell Res.* **65:**129–139.

Moreno, G., and Vinzens, F., 1969, Effets de la micro-irradiation ultra-violette sur differentes parties de la cellule. I. Etude en microscopie electronique sur coupes en serie transversales et sagittales, *Exp. Cell. Res.* **56:**75–83.

Moreno, G., Lutz, M., and Bessis, M., 1969, Partial cell irradiation by ultraviolet and visible light: Conventional and laser sources, *Int. Rev. Exp. Pathol.* **7:**99–137.

Morgan, C., Howe, C., and Rose, H. M., 1959*a*, Intracellular crystals of Coxsackie virus viewed in the electron microscope, *Virology* **9:**145–149.

Morgan, C., Rose, H. M., Holden, M., and Jones, E. P., 1959*b*, Electron microscopic observations on the development of herpes simplex virus, *J. Exp. Med.* **110:**643–656.

Morgan, C., Godman, G. C., Breitenfeld, P. M., and Rose, H. M., 1960, A correlative study by electron and light microscopy of the development of type 5 adenovirus, *J. Exp. Med.* **112:**373–382.

Morgan, C., Rifkind, R. A., Hsu, K. C., Holden, M., Seegal, B. C., and Rose, H. M., 1961, Electron microscopic localization of intracellular viral antigens by the use of ferritin-conjugated antibody, *Virology* **14:**292–296.

Morgan, C., Rose, H. M., and Mednis, B., 1968, Electron microscopy of herpes simplex virus. I. Entry, *J. Virol.* **2:**507–516.

Morgan, H. R., 1968, Ultrastructure of the surfaces of cells infected with avian leukosis-sarcoma viruses, *J. Virol.* **2:**1133–1146.

Morowitz, H. J., Tourtellotte, M. E., and Pollock, M. E., 1963, Use of porous cellulose ester membranes in the primary isolation and size determination of pleuropneumonia-like organisms, *J. Bacteriol.* **85:**134–136.

Morton, D. L., Hall, W. T., and Malmgren, R. A., 1969, Human liposarcomas: Tissue culture containing foci of transformed cells with viral particles, *Science* **165:**813–816.

Mouriquand, C., Mouriquand, J., and Arnaud, C., 1968, Etude cytologique de 42 cultures de tissus hematopoietiques humains et murins: Considerations sur quelques comportements cellulaires, *Pathol. Biol.* **16:**383–395.

Movat, H. Z., and Fernando, N. V. P., 1962, The fine structure of connective tissue. I. The fibroblast, *Exp. Mol. Pathol.* **1:**509–534.

Mussgay, M., and Weibel, Jr., 1962, Electron microscopical and biological studies on the growth of Venezuelan equine encephalitis virus in KB cells, *Virology* **16:**52–62.

Mustakallio, E., and Gronroos, J., 1957, Complement-fixation tests for antisera prepared against strain HeLa cell and 5 cell strains derived from human breast carcinoma, *Ann. Med. Exp. Fenn.* **35:** Suppl. 12.

Nadkarni, J. S., Nadkarni, J. J., Clifford, P., Manolov, G., Fenyo, E. M., and Klein, E., 1969, Characteristics of new cell lines derived from Burkitt lymphoma, *Cancer* **23:**64–79.

Nagayama, A., and Dales, S., 1970, Rapid purification and the immunological specificity of mammalian microtubular paracrystals possessing ATPase activity, *Proc. Natl. Acad. Sci.* **66:**464–471.

Nardone, R. M., Todd, J., Gonzalez, P., and Gaffney, E. V., 1965, Nucleoside incorporation into strain L cells: Inhibition by pleuropneumonia-like organisms, *Science* **149:**1100–1102.

Nass, M. K., and Nass, S., 1963, Intramitochondrial fibers with DNA characteristics, *J. Cell Biol.* **19:**593–611.

Nielsen, G., and Peters, D., 1962, Elektronmikroskopische Untersuchungen über die initialstadien der vaccine-virusinfektion von HeLa-Zellen, *Arch. Ges. Virusforsch.* **12:**493–513.

Nii, S., Morgan, C., Rose, H. M., and Hsu, K. C., 1968, Electron microscopy of herpes simplex virus. IV. Studies with ferritin-conjugated antibodies, *J. Virol.* **2:**1172–1184.

Novikoff, A., Albala, A., and Biempica, L., 1968, Ultrastructural and cytochemical observations on B-16 and Harding–Passey mouse melanomas: The origin of premelanosomes and compound melanosomes, *J. Histochem. Cytochem.* **16:**299-319.

Oettgen, G, A., Aoki, T., Old, L. J., Boyse, E. A., DeHarven, E., and Mills, G. M., 1968, Suspension culture of a pigment-producing cell line from a human malignant melanoma, *J. Natl. Cancer Inst.* **41:**827–843.

Overton, J., 1968, The fate of desmosomes in trypsinized tissue, *J. Exp. Zool.* **168:**203–206.

Ozzello, L., 1972, Ultrastructure of human mammary carcinoma cells *in vivo* and *in vitro*, *J. Natl. Cancer Inst.* **48:**1043–1050.

Paintrand, M., and Rosenfeld, C., 1972, Etude ultrastructurale de la glycocalix des leucocytes humains normaux et leucemiques en culture permanente: Comparaison entre deux lignees d'origine normale et deux lignees d'origine leucemique, *Compt. Rend. Acad. Sci. Paris* **274:**415–417.

Palade, G. E., 1952, A study of fixation for electron microscopy, *J. Exp. Med.* **95:**285–298.

Paweletz, N., 1969, Desmosomen in der Gewebekultur von Tumorzellen, *Naturwissenschaften* **56:**517–518.

Pfeiffer, S. E., and Tolmach, L. J., 1967*a*, Selecting synchronous populations of mammalian cells, *Nature (Lond.)* **213:**139–142.

Pfeiffer, S. E., and Tolmach, L. J., 1967*b*, Inhibition of DNA synthesis in HeLa cells by hydroxyurea, *Cancer Res.* **27:**124–129.

Phillips, D. M., and Phillips, S. G., 1971, Distinctive characteristics of two established cell lines, *J. Cell Biol.* **49:**803–815.

Pinkerton, H., Ghagat, B., Rana, M. W., and Holtwick, S., 1971, Histology and ultrastructure of cultured human tumor cells exposed to antisera to the nerve growth factor, *Cancer Res.* **31:**1483–1487.

Plata, E. J., Aoki, T., Robertson, D. D., Chu, E. W., and Gerwin, B. I., 1973, An established cultured cell line (HBT-39) from human breast carcinoma, *J. Natl. Cancer Inst.* **50:**849–862.

Porter, K. R., and Kallman, F., 1953, The properties and effects of osmium tetroxide as a tissue fixative with special reference to its use for electron microscopy, *Exp. Cell Res.* **4:**127–141.

Price, Z. H., 1967, The micromorphology of zeiotic blebs in cultured human epithelial (HEp) cells, *Exp. Cell Res.* **48:**82–92.

Priori, E., Dmochowski, L., Myers, B., and Wilbur, J. R., 1971, Constant production of type C virus particles in a continuous tissue culture derived from pleural effusion cells of a lymphoma patient, *Nature New Biol.* **232:**61–62.

Privat, A., Mandon, P., and Drian, M. J., 1972, Contribution de la microscopie electronique a balayage pour l'etude du tissu nerveux en culture organisee, *Exp. Cell Res.* **71:**232–238.

Puck, T. T., Marcus, P. I., and Ciecura, S. J., 1956, Clonal growth of mammalian cells *in vitro*, *J. Exp. Med.* **103:**273–284.

Pulvertaft, R. J. V., 1964, Cytology of Burkitt's tumour, *Lancet* **1:**238–240.

Pulvertaft, R. J. V., 1965, A study of malignant tumors in Nigeria by short-term tissue culture, *J. Clin. Pathol.* **18:**261–273.

Pulvertaft, R. J. V., and Humble, J. G., 1962, Intracellular phase of existence of lymphocytes during remission of acute lymphatic leukemia, *Nature (Lond.)* **194:**194–195.

Rabin, E. R., Benyesh-Melnick, M., and Brunschwig, J. P., 1967, Studies on acute leukemia and infectious mononucleosis of childhood. II. Ultrastructure of cultured lymphoblastoid cells, *Exp. Mol. Pathol.* **7:**196–207.

Rabson, A. S., O'Conor, G. T., Baron, S., Whang, J. J., and Legallais, F. Y., 1966, Morphologic, cytogenetic and virologic studies *in vitro* of a malignant lymphoma in an African child, *Int. J. Cancer* **1:**89–106.

Rasmussen, R. E., and Painter, R. B., 1966, Radiation-stimulated DNA synthesis in cultured mammalian cells, *J. Cell Biol.* **29:**11–19.

Recher, L., Parry, N. T., Briggs, L. G., and Whitescarver, J., 1971*b*, Difference in effects of proflavine and actinomycin D, *Cancer Res.* **31:**1915–1922.

Recher, L., Briggs, L. G., and Parry, N. T., 1971*a*, A re-evaluation of nuclear and nucleolar changes induced *in vitro* by actinomycin D, *Cancer Res.* **31:**140–151.

Recher, L., Sinkovics, J. G., Sykes, J. A., and Whitescarver, J., 1969, Electron microscopic studies of suspension cultures derived from human leukemic and nonleukemic sources, *Cancer Res.* **29:**271–285.

Recher, L., Chan, H., Briggs, L., and Parry, N., 1972, Ultrastructural changes inducible with the plant alkaloid camptothecin, *Cancer Res.* **32:**2495–2501.

Reed, M. V., and Gey, G. O., 1962, Cultivation of normal and malignant human lung tissue. I. The establishment of the adenocarcinoma cell strains, *Lab. Invest.* **11:**638–652.

Reith, A., and Oftebro, R., 1971, Structure of HeLa cells after treatment with glycerol as revealed by freeze-etching and electron microscopic methods, *Exp. Cell Res.* **66:**385–395.

Reynolds, E. W., 1963, The use of lead citrate at high pH as an electron-opaque stain in electron microscopy. *J. Cell Biol.* **17:**208–212.

Reynolds, R. C., Montgomery, P. O'B., and Karney, D. H., 1963, Nucleolar "caps," a morphologic entity produced by the carcinogen 4-nitro-quinoline-N-oxide, *Cancer Res.* **23:**535–538.

Reynolds, R. C., Montomery, P. O'B., and Hughes, B., 1964, Nucleolar "caps" produced by actinomycin D, *Cancer Res.* **24:**1269–1278.

Robbins, E., and Gonatas, N. K., 1964*a*, Histochemical and ultrastructural studies on HeLa cell cultures exposed to spindle inhibitors with special reference to the interphase cell, *J. Histochem. Cytochem.* **12**:704–711.

Robbins, E., and Gonatas, N. K., 1964*b*, Ultrastructure of a mammalian cell during the mitotic cycle, *J. Cell Biol.* **21**:429–463.

Robbins, E., and Jentzsch, G., 1969, Ultrastructural changes in the mitotic apparatus at the metaphase-to-anaphase transition, *J. Cell Biol.* **40**:678–691.

Robbins, E., and Marcus, P. I., 1964, Mitotically synchromized mammalian cells: A simple method for obtaining large populations, *Science* **144**:1152–1153.

Robbins, E., and Scharff, M., 1966, Some macromolecular characteristics of synchronized HeLa cells, in: *Cell Synchrony—Studies in Biosynthetic Regulation* (I. L. Cameron and G. M. Padilla, eds.), pp. 353–374, Academic Press, New York and London.

Robbins, E., Marcus, P. I., and Gonatas, N. K., 1964, Dye induced ultrastructural changes in multivesicular bodies: Acridine orange particles, *J. Cell Biol.* **21**:49–62.

Robbins, E., Jentzsch, G., and Micali, A., 1968, The centriole cycle in synchronized HeLa cells, *J. Cell Biol.* **36**:329–339.

Robbins, E., Pederson, T., and Klein, P., 1970, Comparison of mitotic phenomena and effects induced by hypertonic solutions in HeLa cells, *J. Cell Biol.* **44**:400–416.

Romsdahl, M. M., and Hsu, T. C., 1967, Establishment and biologic properties of human malignant melanoma cell lines grown *in vitro, Surg. Forum* **18**:78–79.

Rose, G. G., 1966, Cytopathophysiology of tissue cultures growing under cellophane membranes, *Int. Rev. Exp. Pathol.* **5**:111–178.

Rose, G. G., 1970, *Atlas of Vertebrate Cells in Tissue Culture*, Academic Press, New York and London.

Rose, G. G., Cattoni, M., and Pomerat, C. M., 1963, Observations on oral tumors *in vitro*. I. Zeiosis versus the nucleus and endoplasmic reticulum in strain KB, *J. Dent. Res.* **42**:38–53.

Rose, G. G., Cattoni, M., and Pomerat, C. M., 1964, Observations on oral tumors *in vitro*. II. Karyobiosis in strain KB cells, *J. Dent. Res.* **43**:580–605.

Rothblat, G. H., 1960, PPLO contamination in tissue cultures, *Ann N.Y. Acad. Sci.* **79**:430–432.

Rovin, S., 1962, The influence of carbon dioxide on the cultivation of human neoplastic explants *in vitro, Cancer Res.* **22**:384–387.

Sabatini, D. D., Bensch, K., and Barnett, R. J., 1963, Cytochemistry and electron microscopy: The preservation of cellular ultrastructure and enzymatic activity by aldehyde fixation, *J. Cell Biol.* **17**:19–58.

Salazar, H., Kanbour, A., and Burgess, F., 1972, Ultrastructure and observations on the histogenesis of mesotheliomas: "Adenomatoid tumors" of the female genital tract, *Cancer* **29**:141–152.

Sandborn, E. B., 1970, *Cells and Tissues by Light and Electron Microscopy*, 2 vols., Academic Press, New York and London.

Sanford, K., 1965, Malignant transformation of cells *in vitro, Int. Rev. Cytol.* **18**:249–303.

Saturno, A., 1963, The morphology of Mayaro virus, *Virology* **21**:131–133.

Scharff, M. S., and Robbins, E., 1966, Polyribosome disaggregation during metaphase, *Science* **151**:992–995.

Schneeberger, E. E., and Harris H., 1966, An ultrastructural study of interspecific cell fusion induced by inactivated Sendai virus, *J. Cell Sci.* **1**:401–406.

Schwartz, J., and Roizman, B., 1969, Similarities and differences in the development of laboratory strain and freshly isolated strains of herpes simplex virus in HEp-2 cells: Electron microscopy, *J. Virol.* **4**:879–889.

Seman, G., Gallager, H. S., Lukeman, J. M., and Dmochowski, L., 1971, Studies on the presence of particles resembling RNA virus particles in human breast tumors, pleural effusions, their tissue cultures and milk, *Cancer* **28**:1431–1442.

Shelton, E., and Dalton, A. J., 1959, Electron microscopy of emperipolesis, *J. Biophys, Biochem. Cytol.* **6**:513–514.

Shigematsu, T., and Dmochowski, L., 1973, Studies on the acid mucopolysaccharide coat of viruses and transformed cells, *Cancer* **31**:165–174.

Siegl, G., Hallauer, C., Novak, A., and Kronauer, G., 1971, Parvoviruses as contaminants of permanent human cell lines. II. Physicochemical properties of the isolated viruses, *Arch. Ges. Virusforsch.* **35**:91–103.

Siegl, G., Hallauer, C., and Novak, A., 1972, Parvoviruses as contaminants of permanent human cell lines, *Arch. Ges. Virusforsch.* **36**:351–362.

Silverstein, S. C., and Marcus, P. I., 1964, Early stages of Newcastle disease virus–HeLa cell interaction: An electron microscope study, *Virology* **23**:370–380.

Simard, R., 1970, The nucleus: Action of chemical and physical agents, *Int. Rev. Cytol.* **28**:169–211.

Simard, R., and Bernhard, W., 1966, Le phenomene de la segregation nucleolaire: Specificite d'action de certains antimetabolites, *Int. J. Cancer* **1**:463–479.

Simard, R., and Bernhard, W., 1967, A heat-sensitive cellular function located in the nucleolus, *J. Cell Biol.* **34**:61–76.

Simard, R., Amalyric, F., and Zalta, J. P., 1969, Effet de la temperature supraoptimale sur les ribonucleoproteines et le RNA nucleolaire. I. Etude ultrastructurale, *Exp. Cell Res.* **55**:359–369.

Sirtori, C., and Bosisio-Bestetti, M., 1967, Nucleolar changes in KB tumor cells infected with herpes simplex virus, *Cancer Res.* **27**:367–376.

Smith, G. F., and O'Hara, P. T., 1968, Structure of nuclear pockets in human leukocytes, *J. Ultrastruct. Res.* **21**:415–423.

Smith, U., Smith, D. S., and Yunis, A. A., 1970, Chloramphenicol-related changes in mitochondrial ultrastructure, *J. Cell Sci.* **7**:501–521.

Steel, C. M., 1972, Human lymphoblastoid cell lines. III. Co-cultivation technique for establishment of new lines. *J. Natl. Cancer Inst.* **48**:623–628.

Steel, C. M., and Edmond, M., 1971, Human lymphoblastoid cell lines. I. Culture methods and examination for Epstein–Barr virus, *J. Natl. Cancer Inst.* **47**:1193–1201.

Stewart, S. E., Lovelace, E., Whang, J. J., and Ngu, V. A., 1965, Burkitt tumor tissue culture, cytogenetic and virus studies, *J. Natl. Cancer Inst.* **34**:319–327.

Stewart, S. E., Kasnic, G., Jr., Draycott, C., and Ben, T., 1972, Activation of viruses in human tumors by 5-iododeoxyuridine and dimethylsulfoxide, *Science* **175**:198–199.

Stoebner, P., Miech, G., Sengel, A., and Witz, J. P., 1970, Notions d'ultrastructure pleurale. I. L'hyperplasie mesotheliale, *Presse Med.* **78**:1179–1184.

Stoker, M. G. P., Smith, K. M., and Ross, R. W., 1958, Electron microscopic studies of HeLa cells infected with herpes virus, *J. Gen. Microbiol.* **19**:244–249.

Storb, R., Amy, R. L., Wertz, R. K., Fauconnier, B., and Bessis, M., 1966, An electron microscope study of vitally stained single cells irradiated with a ruby laser microbeam, *J. Cell Biol.* **31**:11–29.

Strauli, P., Lindenman, R., and Haemmerli, G., 1971, Mikrokinematographische and elektronenmikroskopische Beobachtungen an Zelloberflachen und Zellkontakten der menschlichen Carcinom-Zellkulturlinie HEp 2, *Virchows Arch. Abt. B Zellpathol.* **8**:143–161.

Sykes, J. A., Recher, L., Jernstrom, P. H., and Whitescarver, J., 1968, Morphological investigation of human breast cancer, *J. Natl. Cancer Inst.* **40**:195–223.

Tawara, J. T., Goodman, J. R., Imagawa, D. T., and Adams, J. M., 1961, Fine structure of cellular inclusions in experimental measles, *Virology* **14**:410–416.

Tawara, S., 1966, A morphological study on the nucleus of HeLa cells infected with adenovirus type 12, in: *Electron Microscopy 1966*, Vol. 2 (Uyeda, ed.), pp. 187–188, Maruzen, Tokyo.

Tolmach, L. J., and Marcus, P. I., 1960, Development of X-ray induced giant HeLa cells, *Exp. Cell Res.* **20**:350–360.

Toner, P. G., and Carr, K. E., 1971, *Cell Structure: An Introduction to Biological Electron Microscopy*, Williams and Wilkins, Baltimore.

Toolan, H. W., 1954, Transplantable human neoplasms maintained in cortisone treated laboratory animals: H.S. No. 1; H. Ep No. 1; H. Ep No. 2; H. Ep No. 3; and H. Emb. No. 1, *Cancer Res.* **14:**660–666.

Toshima, S., Takagi, N., Minowada, J., Moore, G. E., and Sandberg, A. A., 1967, Electron microscopic and cytogenetic studies of cells derived from Burkitt's lymphoma, *Cancer Res.* **27:**753–759.

Toshima, S., Moore, G. E., and Sandberg, A. A., 1968, Ultrastructure of human melanoma in cell culture, *Cancer* **21:**202–216.

Tousimis, A. J., and Hilleman, M. R., 1957, Electron microscopy of type 4 adenovirus strain RI-67, *Virology* **4:**499–508.

Trujillo, J. M., Butler, J., Ahearn, M. J., Schullenberger, L. C., List-Young, B., Gott, C., Anstall, H. B., and Shively, S. A., 1967, Long-term culture of a lymph node tissue from a patient with lymphocytic lymphoma, *Cancer* **20:**215–224.

Tumilowicz, J. J., Nichols, W. W., Cholon, J. J., and Greene, A. E., 1970, Definition of a continuous human cell line derived from neuroblastoma, *Cancer Res.* **30:**2110–2118.

Uzman, B. G., Foley, G. E., Farber, S., and Lazarus, M., 1966, Morphologic variations in human leukemic lymphoblasts (CCRF-CEM cells) after long-term culture and exposure to chemotherapic agents, *Cancer* **19:**1725–1742.

Uzman, B. G., Saito, H., and Kasac, M., 1971, Tubular arrays in the endoplasmic reticulum in human tumor cells, *Lab. Invest.* **24:**492–498.

Venable, J. H., and Cogeshall, R., 1965, A simplified lead citrate stain for use in electron microscopy, *J. Cell Biol.* **25:**407.

Warocquier, R., and Scherrer, K., 1969, RNA metabolism in mammalian cells at elevated temperature, *Eur. J. Biochem.* **10:**362–370.

Watson, M. L., 1958, Staining of tissue sections for electron microscopy with heavy metals, *J. Biophys. Biochem. Cytol.* **4:**475–478.

Wheeler, C. P., Bowdon, E. J., Adamson, B. J., and Vail, M. H., 1971, Effects of certain nitrogen mustards upon the progression of cultured H.Ep. No. 2 cells through the cell cycle, *Cancer Res.* **30:**100–111.

Whitmore, G. D., 1971, Natural and induced synchronous cultures, *In Vitro* **6:**276–285.

Whitmore, G. F., and Gulyas, S., 1966, Synchronization of mammalian cells with tritiated thymidine, *Science* **151:**691–694.

Willoch, M., 1967, Changes in HeLa cell ultrastructure under conditions of reduced glucose supply, *Acta Pathol. Microbiol. Scand.* **71:**35–45.

Wischnitzer, S., 1970, The annulate lamellae, *Int. Rev. Cytol.* **27:**65–97.

Wolff, E., and Wolff, E., 1966, Culture organotypique de longue duree de deux tumeurs humaines du tube digestif, *Eur. J. Cancer* **2:**93–103.

Xeros, N., 1962, Deoxyriboside control and synchronization of mitosis, *Nature (Lond.)* **194:**682–683.

Yasuzumi, Y., and Sugihara, R., 1965, The fine structure of nuclei as revealed by electron microscopy, *Exp. Cell Res.* **40:**45–55.

Zajac, B., and Hummeler, K., 1970, Morphogenesis of the nucleoprotein of vesicular stomatitis virus, *J. Virol.* **6:**243–252.

Zeve, V. H., Lucas, L. S., and Manaker, R. A., 1966, Continuous cell culture from a patient with chronic myelogenous leukemia. II. Detection of a herpes-like virus by electron microscopy, *J. Natl. Cancer Inst.* **37:**761–773.

Zhdanov, V. M., Soloviev, V. D., Bektemirov, T. A., Ilyin, K. V., Bykovsky, A. F., Mazurenko, N. P., Irlin, I. S., and Yershov, F. I., 1973, Isolation of oncornaviruses from continuous human cell cultures, *Intervirology* **1:**19–26.

The Strategy of a Search for Viral Involvement in Human Cancer 15

F. KINGSLEY SANDERS

1. Introduction

The first suggestions that viruses could be concerned in the causation of neoplasia in birds were made over 60 years ago (Ellermann and Bang, 1908; Rous, 1911), to be followed, 20–30 years later, by compelling evidence (Bittner, 1942; Shope and Hurst, 1933; Gross, 1951) that viruses could similarly cause tumors in mammals. However, it is only recently that serious consideration has been given to the possibility that such a situation could also obtain in man. In principle, this has been because morphological, immunological, and biochemical, as well as biological, studies of animal model systems have established an association between viruses and neoplasms, particularly leukemias and sarcomas, in a whole range of mammalian species, extending from mice to primates (Dameshek and Dutcher, 1970), but similar studies have not so far led to the isolation and characterization of an authentic human cancer virus. This chapter represents an attempt to discover why this should be so, to decide what kind of evidence might be needed in the future to indicate viral involvement in the genesis of any one human tumor, and to see how current studies measure up to the criteria adopted.

F. KINGSLEY SANDERS Walker Laboratory, Sloan-Kettering Institute for Cancer Research, Rye, New York

Any search for viruses directly causative of human cancer divides itself naturally into three phases:

1. Guessing which of the wide spectrum of human tumors are most likely to have a viral etiology.
2. Deciding what experimental methods to adopt in order to obtain evidence of viral infection in human tumor material.
3. Deciding how to establish whether the infections observed play any part in the genesis of the tumors with which they have been associated.

2. *Selection of Human Tumor Material*

Since it has been established that many infectious agents can be vertically rather than horizontally transmitted (Gross, 1970)—i.e., that the chain of infection can pass from parent to offspring *in utero* or even via the germ cells (Bittner, 1952) rather than from individual to individual within a group of already separate organisms—it may be best to begin the selection of human tumors suitable for virological study by eliminating those with an obvious non-viral environmental cause (this leaves open the question of whether such nonviral causes may also operate by "activating" a virus latent within the cells of susceptible individuals, Huebner and Todaro, 1970; Kaplan, 1967). So excluded would be lung carcinoma in view of its strong correlation with cigarette smoking (Doll and Hill, 1952; Hammond, 1968), bladder carcinoma caused by β-naphthylamine (Boyland, 1963), gastric cancer with its obvious dietary association (Higginson, 1967), and, of course, cancer of the scrotum in chimney sweeps (Pott, 1775).

The next step is to select neoplasms where there is at least some evidence of transmissibility. African Burkitt's lymphoma, where the geographic distribution of cases has been strongly held to suggest a viral cause (Burkitt, 1962), is the first human tumor for which such a probability has been generally accepted (Epstein and Achong, 1973). Kaposi's sarcoma, another geographically restricted tumor, has also been associated with herpes virus infection (Giraldo *et al.*, 1972). Carcinoma of the cervix has many of the characteristics of a transmissible venereal disease. It has a higher incidence among low socioeconomic groups, among women having intercourse with uncircumcised males and among women who begin regular intercourse at an early age. It has a predictably low incidence among Jewish women other than prostitutes and is virtually unknown among virgins and nuns (Nahmias, 1969; Nahmias *et al.*, 1971). Herpes simplex virus type II infection has been strongly correlated with this condition on seroepidemiological grounds (Rotkin, 1973). This virus has, moreover, been recently isolated from male genital secretions (Centifanto *et al.*, 1972) and its genome detected in cells of a cervical carcinoma (Frenkel *et al.*, 1972).

There is also suggestive epidemiological evidence—although the association remains to be proven statistically—that Hodgkin's disease may be communicable. Vianna *et al.* (1971, 1972), on the basis of a careful investigation of past cases (confirmed by histopathology) and those of their close associates (established by personal interview), showed that more than 30 cases of Hodgkin's disease occurring since 1954 could be linked—either directly or through a symptomless carrier—with a group of four students with active Hodgkin's disease in an Albany high school at that time, the incubation period being up to 3 yr. A similarly linked chain of cases has been found in Mount Kisco, N.Y. (Vianna *et al.*, 1972), as well as suggestions that a similar mode of transfer may have been operating in the recent past in high schools in Nassau County, Long Island (Vianna and Polan, 1973). Cell cultures from patients with Hodgkin's disease have provided evidence of the presence of a herpes virus (Eisinger *et al.*, 1971), although its relationship to the etiology of this disease remains obscure.

Other human tumors which have less direct evidence to support their candidacy for a viral origin, since this at present rests mainly on an analogy with animal tumors of known viral cause, are breast cancer (Moore *et al.*, 1971) and one or more of the acute leukemias (Allen *et al.*, 1973). Tumors in cultures from patients with Hodgkin's disease have provided evidence of the presence of a herpes virus (Eisinger *et al.*, 1971), although its relationship to the etiology of this disease remains obscure.

In the case of animal tumor viruses, ultimately convincing evidence of oncogenicity is obtained when it can be shown that virus, injected by a suitable route into the species from which it was originally isolated, is capable of causing a tumor. It is noteworthy that evidence of transmissibility in nature (with the notable exception of Marek's disease, Biggs, 1968) is often lacking. Indeed, inoculation of tumor extracts into hosts identical, or at least closely related genetically, to the original donor seems necessary to establish transmissibility. For example, Gross leukemia was first isolated from an inbred line of mice (AKR) that had been selected for their high incidence of "spontaneous" leukemia (Gross, 1951). The first isolates of Rous sarcoma virus (RSV) were obtained by inoculation of chickens genetically related to the original donor (Rous, 1911). Feline leukemia virus (FeLV) (Jarrett *et al.*, 1964) is an example of the way oncogenic viruses can be found by using recipient individuals with at least a degree of immunological immaturity. All the above suggests that whether a cell responds to viral infection by becoming a tumor cell is determined not only by the nature of the infectious agent but also by whether the cell itself is transformable; this susceptibility can be genetically, and perhaps also environmentally, determined. Work on the genetics of mice (Boyse *et al.*, 1972) and poultry (Payne *et al.*, 1971) has shown that genes governing susceptibility to cellular transformation, expressed within the cells of individuals showing viral oncogenesis, are relevant to their positive response. Since (1) injection of material obtained from tumors into any human being is unthinkable on ethical grounds and (2) human beings, even siblings, are genetically heterogeneous (except in the case of identical twins), it is hardly surprising that infectious human leukemias and sarcomas directly mimicking the situation in mice and fowls have not so far been found. In this instance, it is of interest that the presence of Gross virus infection has been established in wild mice but that it has never been an obvious cause of leukemia in the wild; were it not for the attention focused on this agent by studies using highly inbred susceptible populations its presence in the wild might never have been suspected. Even bovine lymphosarcoma, prevalent in many herds of cattle with some evidence of transmissibility (Olson *et al.*, 1972) as well as strong evidence of viral involvement (Van der Maaten and Boothe, 1971; Miller and Olson, 1972), is unlikely to have its human counterpart, since the individuals of such herds are likely to have many genes in common.

In most virally induced tumors of animals, the virus itself was first isolated from the tumor tissue (Gross, 1970), and it would seem logical that this would be the first place to begin to look for a human tumor virus. But, with a noninbred population, it is not at all clear that this choice is correct. Marek's disease in chickens is caused by a highly infectious herpes virus that multiplies in feather follicles, is spread from individual to individual by feather dander, and is so highly resistant to the destructive effects of the environment that buildings that have housed chickens with Marek's disease remain a source of infection for a long time (Witter, 1972). Nevertheless, it is extremely difficult to recover virus from the tumors themselves (Churchill and Biggs, 1967). Related viruses infecting other species (Eidson *et al.*, 1972) do not appear to cause tumors in their natural hosts and, moreover, can be used to protect chickens against the tumors caused by Marek's disease virus.

However, if a virus is to be involved in human oncogenesis it must at some stage act on at least one cell to convert it to a tumor cell. Many tumors constitute clones, by definition derived ultimately from single cells. Evidence to support this is that many tissue culture lines of cells derived from Burkitt tumors are monoclonal IgM producers (Klein *et al.*, 1972); every human wart constitutes a single clone of cells (Murray *et al.*, 1971). If most virally induced tumors do consist of clones of cells, the key oncogenic event may take place during transient infection of a single cell that becomes "transformed," subsequently generating a clone of similarly altered progeny.

Thus unless we assume that genetic information from the virus is involved in transformation, becomes "integrated" in some way, and can be detected in later generations of the clone by appropriate methods, we may as well abandon the search for evidence of tumor viruses within the tumor cells themselves. Nevertheless, tumor cells are still the best places to begin looking for evidence of viral transformation, at least until we become convinced that such efforts must fail because all trace of the virus disappears from the clone once transformation has occurred.

So the starting material for any search for human oncogenic viruses is likely to be samples of human tissue that ought to consist predominantly of malignant cells of the tumor under investigation. In practice, the samples are likely to be tissue cultures derived from specimens of tumor removed surgically at operation or as part of the diagnostic process. Unfortunately, tumor biopsies consist of a mixture of cells, some normal, some malignant, and the cells of tissue cultures derived from such biopsies are similarly heterogeneous. The problem of identification of tumor cells in such cultures has been dealt with by other authors in this volume and will not be considered further here. It need only be stated that the condition posed—namely, that the cultures in which traces of viral infection will be sought should consist mainly of tumor cells—has rarely been met in the past. Cultures of human tissue, especially following one or more transfers *in vitro*—and prolonged cultivation may often be necessary to allow even partial expression of a cryptic viral genome (Sabin, 1965)—often consist mainly of fibroblasts, whatever their tissue of origin; fibroblasts appear to enjoy a selective advantage in the media and manipulations to which most tissue cultures are usually subjected. Fortunately, techniques are now available for the separation of tumor cells from contaminating fibroblasts and are described in Chapter 1. In combination with media that select positively for tumor cells (see Chapters 2, 3 and 4), such methods might lead to greater success in the production of "pure" cultures of human tumor cells. With many mouse tumors that have been difficult to establish in culture owing to overgrowth of contaminating fibroblasts, considerable success has been achieved by the technique of alternating passage between mice and tissue culture (Buonassisi *et al.*, 1962). Although fibroblasts have a slight advantage in tissue culture, they are overgrown by tumor cells *in vivo* and are soon eliminated. In the case of human tumors, alternate passage between tissue culture and athymic (*Nu/Nu*) (Pantelouris, 1971; Pantelouris and Hair, 1970) or immunosuppressed (Castro and Hamilton, 1972) mice might be considered as a means of selecting a tissue culture population consisting mainly of human tumor cells.

Quite apart from the fact that the culture conditions chosen may accidentally select against tumor cells, some tumor tissues may be difficult to establish in culture because short-lived elements in the original mixed population of cells from the tumor may interfere with the establishment of long-term cultures. This may have been true in the past with reference to attempts to establish long-term cultures of biopsied lymph nodes from patients with Hodgkin's disease (Grand, 1947; Rottino, 1949*a,b*). This difficulty has now been overcome by subjecting tissue fragments to a preliminary phase of organ culture on stainless steel grids (Eisinger, 1973; Pontén, 1967; Nilsson, 1971). During this phase, differentiated elements within the fragments fall out and are lost, rendering subsequent cultivation of the residual cell population possible by conventional methods. Using this technique, lymph node biopsies in virtually all positively diagnosed cases of Hodgkin's disease give rise eventually to long-term cultures of distinctive, large, irregularly oriented, thinly spread, pleomorphic cells, often with many lysosomes, and sometimes with eosinophilic inclusions (Eisinger *et al.*, 1971). It is not known whether these cells correspond to the neoplastic elements of Hodgkin's disease, since pathologists are not in fact agreed on what cells constitute the malignant component, although the majority opinion inclines to some form of malignant histiocyte; which would not rule out the cells described above. What is more important is that cells of this kind emerge as the predominant type in cultures derived in this way from biopsy specimens of all four histological types of the disease (Lukes and Butler, 1965). With other tumors where pathologists can identify the malignant cells with greater certainty, comparison of the morphology, karyology, and biochemistry of the cultured cells with those of the original biopsy specimen needs to be carried out and the identity of the cultured cells established beyond reasonable doubt.

3. *Methods for the Detection of Viruses in Human Tumor Cell Cultures*

Assuming that cultures believed to consist predominantly of tumor cells have been obtained, what are the means by which viruses can be sought in them? It is well known that the explantation of tissues into culture results many times in the emergence of viruses, carried into the culture along with the tissue of origin (Hsiung, 1968). Sanders (1973) has classified such viruses into three kinds:

1. *Passenger viruses* are carried into the culture in the form of complete, extracellular virions or lytically infected cells; they appear in culture because the tissue from which the culture was derived was infected *in vivo*, not because they are playing an etiological role.

2. *Indigenous viruses* are those that are frankly pathogenic in the appropriate circumstances (Epstein–Barr virus, EBV, has been identified as the cause of infectious mononucleosis, Henle *et al.*, 1968; Hirshaut *et al.*, 1968; herpes virus B is latent in the rhesus monkey but causes fatal disease in man, Andrews, 1967; Hull, 1974) but are normally introduced into tissue culture within latently infected cells, only to be induced to proliferate later by stimuli at present unknown.
3. *Cryptic viruses*, on the other hand, remain integrated within their host cells throughout their life in culture; they do not cause a cytopathic effect and do not often become induced or activated under the normal conditions of culture.

Classes (2) and (3) differ in degree rather than in kind, and all kinds of intermediate grades may exist, even with the same virus. Cell lines carrying Epstein–Barr virus can vary from those (Jijoye: Pulvertaft, 1967) in which a proportion of the cells can give rise to virus capable of infecting other cells (Miller *et al.*, 1972) to those (Raji: Pulvertaft, 1965) in which the presence of virus can only be demonstrated by nucleic acid hybridization (Zur Hausen and Schulte-Holthausen, 1970) or the "Epstein–Barr nuclear antigen" (EBNA) immunofluorescence test (Reedman and Klein, 1973). Such a virus can be either indigenous or cryptic. What follows is a listing of methods that can be used to detect viruses of these three classes in cells in culture, so that their appropriateness to the search for human tumor viruses can be assessed.

3.1. Inoculation of Tumor and/or Cultured Cell Extracts into Suitable Animal Hosts

Tumor and/or cultured cell extracts can be inoculated into suitable animal hosts. Suitability here can reside not only in species (e.g., mice), route of inoculation (e.g., intracerebral), or genetic constitution within a species (e.g., the use of genetically susceptible mice for arbovirus isolation) but also in pretreatment, possibly with immunosuppressive agents. By use of such methods, many viruses have been recovered from humans, not only from cancers but from nonneoplastic tissues as well. Gross (1970) gives a detailed account of much of this work. All such experiments, however, suffer from three major defects: (1) they fail to discriminate between potentially oncogenic and normally pathogenic agents; (2) viruses notoriously exert different effects in different host species (Andrewes, 1967), so that if an agent can be extracted from a human tumor that causes a tumor following animal inoculation, this does not mean that it was the agent that caused the tumor in man; (3) most common laboratory animals carry a veritable library of "silent" viral infections that may express themselves in frank symptoms following the inoculation of alien material (National Cancer Institute, 1966). It is thus incumbent on the investigator to show that any "human" agent, putatively isolated by animal inoculation, does not in fact come from the species inoculated; this has not always been appreciated in the recent past (Officer *et al.*, 1973).

3.2. Inoculation of Extracts into Tissue Cultures of "Indicator" Cells

The above objections apply less to virus isolations attempted by the inoculation of extracts into tissue cultures of suitable indicator cells. The latter can be controlled for the presence of latent viruses; and cellular alterations can be looked for that have at least some correlation with tumorigenesis (e.g., morphological transformation, Stoker and Abel, 1962; growth in soft agar, Macpherson and Montagnier, 1964). Moreover, cells from the same species, the same individual, or even the same tissue can be used as indicators. Cells from human individuals with genetic defects known to be associated with a heightened incidence of particular tumors (e.g., Down's syndrome, Todaro and Martin, 1967; xeroderma pigmentosum, Cleaver, 1969) can also be used in an attempt to find cells with a heightened susceptibility to any agent that may be present. But the inoculation of cell cultures with tumor extracts or tissue culture supernatants assumes that these will contain mature, extracellular, infectious virions of the agent sought able to invade the indicator cells used, and is thus by its nature weighted in favor of the isolation of passenger viruses. It is not surprising, therefore, that widespread use of this technique has not so far resulted in the isolation of an authentic human oncogenic virus.

3.3. Direct Search for Objects Resembling Virions

Objects resembling virions can be sought both in thin sections of cells and in material pelleted from tissue culture supernatants. Direct visualization, with the electron microscope, of appropriately prepared human material has resulted in many claimed demonstrations of viruses in human tumors, these being objects that have a morphology similar to that of known viral agents (Dmochowski *et al.*, 1969). Although it has been possible in many instances (e.g., herpes viruses) to find well-defined structures permitting the identification of particular viruses (e.g., EBV, Epstein *et al.*, 1964), with RNA tumor viruses, whose structure is less well established, electron microscopic observations on their own can be highly subjective (Stewart *et al.*, 1972). Where conclusions regarding the nature of a particle are based on its appearance alone, but not, for example, its frequency of occurrence as well as the demonstration of phenomena such as "budding" from the cell surface (Andervont, 1966; De Harven, 1968), the claim that such objects are viruses must be open to question. Even with such well-authenticated entities as "intracisternal type A" particles (Andervont, 1960), it is doubtful whether these should be called viruses since they have never been shown to be infective (Kuff *et al.*, 1968; Wivell, 1973).

3.4. *Search for Particles with the General Biophysical Properties of Viruses*

Particles with the general biophysical properties of viruses can be sought by labeling cultured cells with radioactive nucleosides, following by screening of the cultures for entities with the expected properties. Such entities should contain DNA or RNA, not both, packaged in a way to render the contained nucleic acid resistant to the action of relevant nucleases. Isopycnic density in sucrose, as well as sedimentation velocity and buoyant density of nucleic acid extracted from material so concentrated, can give clues to whether a "virus" has been obtained, as well as to its nature. For example, RNA-containing material banding at an isopycnic density of 1.14–1.16 can be suspected to be a mammalian oncornavirus (Nowinski *et al.*, 1970), and extracted DNA that has a buoyant density in CsCl of 1.71–1.73 may be thought to be derived from a herpes virus (Roizman and Spear, 1970).

Such tests, however, are not without their own hazards, as can be illustrated from the work of Eisinger *et al.* (1971). Human cell cultures derived from lymph node biopsies of patients with Hodgkin's disease were labeled with 5-^{3}H-uridine, and the tissue culture fluid was collected, passed through a 22-nm filter, pelleted, and centrifuged isopycnically on a sucrose gradient. A typical result is khown in Fig. 1. A marked peak of radioactivity banded at a sucrose concentration corresponding to a density of 1.20–1.22. Control cells from five other human cell lines and one hamster cell line were similarly labeled and treated as controls. Cells from (1) a human neuroblastoma (SK-N-SH), (2) a breast carcinoma (SK-BR-3), (3) a continuous cell line (SK-LN) from a normal lymph node, (4) strain WI-38 embryonic lung fibroblasts, and (5) the FL continuous line of human amnion cells all failed to show a similar uridine-labeled peak; (6) B34 hamster cells, a suspended-cell culture line that continuously sheds hamster sarcoma virus (HaSV) (Nowinski *et al.*, 1971), served as a positive control, since, when labeled in this way, they gave a peak banding at a density of 1.14–1.15. No peak was found

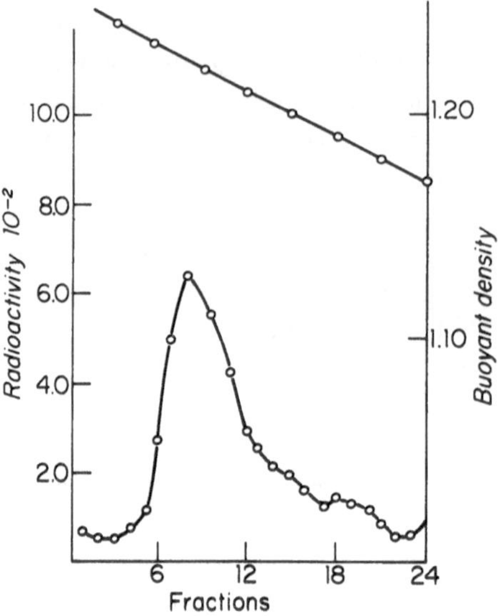

FIG. 1. Equilibrium density centrifugation of ^{3}H-uridine-labeled material excreted by attached cell line derived from a Hodgkin's disease lymph node.

following labeling with ^{3}H-thymidine. At first, it was considered that the presence of a ^{3}H-uridine peak in the Hodgkin's cell culture fluids was due to mycoplasma contamination (Todaro *et al.*, 1971). However, the following suggested that this was not so: (1) A mycoplasma species isolated from the culture line itself, grown up in broth and concentrated by centrifugation, banded in sucrose, not at 1.20–1.22, but at 1.24–1.26. (2) Cultures of FL amnion cells and WI-38 fibroblasts were deliberately infected with this same mycoplasma and labeled with ^{3}H-uridine in the manner described, and the tissue culture fluids were processed as before. No labeled peak was seen. Nevertheless, these experiments did not entirely rule out the possibility that mycoplasma contamination was in fact responsible for the ^{3}H-uridine band. Lemcke (1971) had examined the ability of mycoplasma to pass 22-nm filters, like those used in the preparation of the material studied here. Mycoplasma preparations passed through such filters lost infectivity by a factor approximately 5 $\log_{10}$, as judged by colony counts in agar. However, electron microscope examination of pelleted filtrates showed structures typical of mycoplasma. It should be pointed out that electron microscopy of thin sections, while allowing unequivocal identification of the presence of mycoplasma, may not distinguish between mycoplasma fragments and whole organisms. Fragmentation of mycoplasma following passage through a 22-nm filter might produce many pieces consisting of membrane-enveloped portions of mycoplasma cytoplasm. If they lack the organism's DNA, such pieces might band at a lower density than 1.24–1.26. The ^{3}H-uridine peak observed by Eisinger *et al.* (1971) may thus be due to the presence of mycoplasma fragments rather than whole organisms. Further evidence that this interpretation might be correct was found when RNA from the ^{3}H-uridine band sedimenting at 1.20–1.22 was extracted and cosedimented in a sucrose velocity gradient with ribosomal RNA markers derived from rat liver ribosomes. The result is shown in Fig. 2. Three peaks of labeled macromolecular RNA were seen, none of which coincided with 28S and 18S bands of the marker or with that expected for any known viral RNA. Two had sedimentation velocities intermediate between those of 18S and 28S, and the remainder, the largest, a somewhat slower velocity. All peaks were due to RNA, since treatment of the material with RNase eliminated them, all radioactivity now remaining at the top of the gradient. The labeled RNA was clearly not derived from human cells, but its position on the gradient is not inconsistent with a partial origin from mycoplasma (Markov *et al.*, 1969).

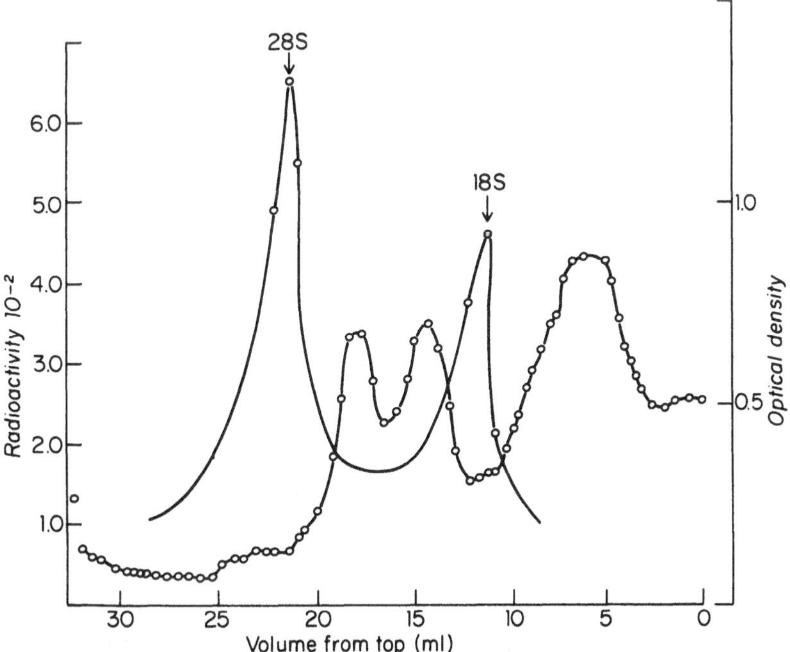

FIG. 2. Velocity sedimentation of ^{3}H-RNA extracted from ^{3}H-uridine-labeled material like that shown in Fig. 1. 18S and 28S RNA from rat liver ribosomes were added as a marker.

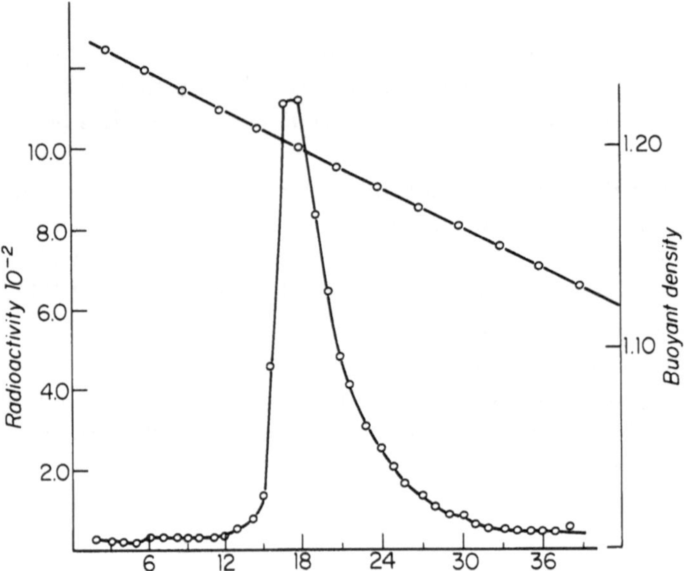

FIG. 3. Equilibrium density centrifugation of ^{3}H-thymidine-labeled material excreted by a "transferred" suspended cell culture derived from Hodgkin's disease.

However, certain of the Hodgkin's lymph node cultures observed by Eisinger *et al.* (1971) underwent a process of "lymphoblastoid" transformation, and came eventually to consist of floating cells. Labeling (Fig. 3), this time with tritiated thymidine, showed that these cells now excreted into the supernatant DNA-containing material, also banding at an isopycnic density of 1.20–1.22. This new peak did not seem due to mycoplasma contamination. Electron microscopy of sections of pelleted supernatants showed occasional double-enveloped virions resembling those of the herpes virus group. The sedimentation behavior of the peak, however, resembled that of herpes virus nucleocapsids rather than complete virions, and additional evidence from immunodiffusion showed tentatively that there was material present reacting with sera containing antibody against the group-specific nucleocapsid antigen of the herpes group.

Studies on EB virus-carrying cell lines have given similar results. DNA-containing material appears in tissue cultures of cells labeled with ^{3}H-TdR (Becker and Weinberg, 1972). Whether this is excreted into the medium, or comes from cells which die and disintegrate during the period of labeling is not yet certain; however, DNA extracted from this material has a buoyant density in CsCl of approximately 1.718, in the range typical for herpes viruses in general, and EB virus in particular.

3.5. Search for Immunological Evidence of Viral Infection

Immunological evidence of viral infection can be sought by appropriate serological methods, e.g., immunodiffusion (ID), immunofluorescence (IF), and complement fixation (CF). Such tests can be used in two different ways. The first is to look for evidence of infection by testing tumor cells and/or extracts against antisera that are either specific for individual viruses or else contain antibody against group-specific internal antigens associated with different families of viruses (e.g., herpes viruses). While such tests are of great value, the limits of how much antigen they can detect are uncertain, although they can be ranked in order of sensitivity (IF > CF > ID) Nevertheless, a negative result in any of these tests with tumor cell material does not imply that all trace of viral infection is absent. Moreover, all of these tests are plagued by nonspecific reactions, which must be very carefully controlled if their results are to be relied on. IF tests in particular are difficult to interpret, as their reading calls for experience as well as subjective judgment on the part of the observer.

Second, immunological reactions have been used to look for evidence of viral infection, and thus of disease relatedness, in sera from cancer patients, using antigens prepared either from tissue cultures of animal or human cells infected in the laboratory with known viruses (Sabin and Tarro, 1973; Hollinshead and Tarro, 1973) or from human cell lines carrying viruses suspected of an association with human cancer. Many of the antigen preparations used are themselves complex, and the multiplicity of antibodies present in most human sera makes the possibility of spurious cross-reactions a real one. An excellent example of such difficulties is given by the many studies made in an attempt to identify Epstein–Barr virus as the cause of at least one human cancer. Antibodies to this agent have a high prevalence in a variety of human conditions, both malignant and nonmalignant whether detected by IF or ID. Table 1 illustrates the wide spectrum of antibodies to EBV based on ID measurements and use of antigens prepared from a cell line in which there is a high level of expression of the EBV genome (Old *et al.*, 1968). By use of human cell lines which differ in the extent to which they express their contained EBV genome, a panel of suitable human sera, and the IF test, it has been possible to detect at least four different EBV-specified antigens: (1) viral capsid antigen (VCA) (Henle and Henle, 1966), (2) "early" antigen (EA) (Henle *et al.*, 1971), (3) "membrane" antigen (MA) (Klein, 1972), and (4) "EB virus nuclear" antigen (EBNA) (Reedman and Klein, 1973). Different cell lines express these antigens to varying degrees, hence the antibody status of each serum varies with the cell line used to assess it. The EBNA test at present seems to be the most promising since virtually all the cells of those lines which carry the EBV

TABLE 1

Precipitating Antibody to EBV Antigen in Human Sera[a]

Diagnosis	Number of sera tested	Percent positive
Burkitt's lymphoma	53	59
Nasopharyngeal carcinoma	63	86
Lymphosarcoma	30	53
Chronic lymphocytic leukemia	31	45
Hodgkin's disease	32	28
Acute leukemia	104	24
Other malignant disease		
Melanoma	12	17
Head and neck	141	13
Breast	38	11
Lung	22	5
Miscellaneous	34	12
Nonmalignant disease	157	9
Healthy subjects	127	8

[a]Data from Old *et al.* (1968).

genome also express the EBNA antigen (Reedman and Klein, 1973). In metaphase cells, moreover, the antigen appears to have a chromosomal location. EBV is the only virus at present detectable by this kind of test. However, it is likely that similar tests will be developed in the near future for detecting infection by other viruses, at least those whose genetic information becomes at least partially integrated into the cellular genome. At present, such tests have exciting possibilities for assessing the importance of DNA viruses in relation to human cancer. Their value with respect to possible RNA virus infection is less certain at the moment.

3.6. Cocultivation and/or Fusion

With the possible exception of the EBNA test, all the techniques discussed so far are more suitable for the recovery of passenger or indigenous than of cryptic viruses. The detection of the last may require more subtle approaches, such as cocultivation and/or fusion with cell types from various animal and human sources. The object of such techniques is to recover viruses that are difficult to isolate from tissue culture supernatants by conventional means. This may be because the material in the supernatants is

(1) unstable or (2) not in the form of fully infectious extracellular virus, but somehow able to pass from one cell to another when they are in contact. Cocultivation with normal peripheral blood (Henle *et al.*, 1967) and umbilical cord (Gerber *et al.*, 1969; Miller and Lipmann, 1973) leukocytes has been successful in demonstrating the presence of EBV in cells from which it cannot be otherwise recovered in infectious form, a positive result being recorded when the added lymphocytes themselves become "transformed" and give rise to a continuous cell line that can be shown to carry EBV (Nilsson *et al.*, 1972). Artificial cell fusion using inactivated Sendai virus (Koprowski *et al.*, 1967) can be of use in transmitting many viruses that are unable to travel from donor to recipient cells even when they are in contact. Both cocultivation and fusion studies will be aided when there is a means of distinguishing the two types of cells in the mixed cultures. This can be done when the donor and recipient cells are of opposite sex (Henle *et al.*, 1967), or by the use of indicator cells with special isozymes or chromosome markers, e.g., cells from Negroes with G6PD isoenzyme variant A (Boyer *et al.*, 1962) or patients with Klinefelter's syndrome (Stewart and Ferguson-Smith, 1958). Indicator cells which may have a special susceptibility to the agent in question (see Section 3.2) are an obvious choice for both cocultivation and fusion experiments.

3.7. Exposure to a Putative "Helper" Virus

Many instances are now known of animal "helper" systems where expression of a cryptic oncogenic virus in the form of extracellular virus requires the assistance of a second virus, able to provide the necessary envelope. Certain helper viruses, notably feline leukemia virus (FeLV), are able to replicate in cells from more than one species, including man (Jarrett *et al.*, 1969). This virus is also able to "rescue" the murine sarcoma virus (MSV) genome from mouse cells cryptically infected by this agent and then to infect cat cells, which release a hybrid feline sarcoma virus (FeSV) that is able to cause tumors in cats. FeLV is an obvious choice for an attempt to recover "sarcoma" information from human sarcomas.

3.8. Prolonged Cultivation

Prolonged cultivation has already been mentioned as a way of enhancing the expression of viral genomes in cultured human cells (Section 2) (Sabin, 1965). For example, EBV was first recovered from cells of the African Burkitt's lymphoma following prolonged cultivation *in vitro* (Epstein *et al.*, 1964). It could not be found in the original tumor. Similarly, the herpes virus nucleocapsid material found by Eisinger *et al.* (1971) in cultured Hodgkin's disease lymph nodes was not detected until the cells had been in culture for a considerable time and had undergone lymphoblastoid transformation. It is not understood at present why this should be so. Perhaps the process of adaptation to continuous growth in tissue culture brings about an alteration in the expressions of the cellular DNA that also allows expression of otherwise cryptic viral genetic information.

Another way to "induce" expression of otherwise dormant integrated viral genes may be transplantation to either an immunologically privileged site in a heterologous host or a nonprivileged site in a host treated by immunosuppression. Hirsch *et al.* (1972) have shown that activation of RNA tumor viruses in rodents can occur during the graft vs. host reaction and in mixed leukocyte culture, its presumed equivalent *in vitro*; the relevance of these observations to the apparently enhanced incidence of tumors or leukemia in human recipients of kidney (Hirsch *et al.*, 1971) and bone marrow (Fialkow *et al.*, 1971) transplants would appear obvious.

3.9. Attempted "Activation" of Cryptic Viruses

Suspect cells can be chemically treated in the attempt to "activate" cryptic viruses to complete their cycle of multiplication. Certain nucleoside analogues (bromo- or iododeoxyuridine) can be used to treat cultured cells and cause the activation of apparently cryptic viral genomes. Not only can DNA virus genomes (Gerber, 1972) be so activated but also RNA viruses, the products in the latter case ranging from the production of particular antigens considered to be virally specified (Weiss *et al.*, 1971) and consequently detectable by immunological methods up to complete infective type C viral particles (Lowy *et al.*, 1971; Aaronson *et al.*, 1971). Chemical treatment of 3T3 mouse fibroblasts cryptically carrying the genome of SV40 (a DNA virus) and then fusion of these cells with permissive African green monkey cells has the effect of causing many more 3T3 cells to become capable of making virus on fusion with permissive cells than when they are not treated chemically (Watkins, 1970). Chemical treatment, followed by cocultivation and/or Sendai-virus-induced fusion with suitable indicator cells, might thus be a sensitive way to detect cryptic viral infection of human tumor cells. Chemical activation by agents other than nucleoside analogues, perhaps water-soluble mutagens and carcinogens (Sanders, 1971; Igel *et al.*, 1969), X-rays (Gerber, 1964), mytomycin C combined with irradiation (Fogel and Sachs, 1970) and cell fusion (Burns and Black, 1968), and cancer "promoters" such as phorbol esters (Sivak and van Duuren, 1967) might also prove useful in this respect.

3.10. Search for Unusual Nucleic Acids or Enzyme Activities

A search can be conducted in cultivated tumor cells for unusual nucleic acids or enzyme activities similar to those known to be associated with viruses that are oncogenic in species other than man. Following the discovery of reverse transcriptase (Baltimore, 1970; Temin and Mizutani, 1970), the main thrust in recent years in this area has been to use molecular biological methods to detect cryptic viral genes in human material. These studies have been reviewed in detail (Temin and Baltimore, 1972), and it is not my intention to summarize them further here, but rather to classify those methods that have been used and to discuss their relevance to the human situation. Nucleic acid hybridization (Bolton and McCarthy, 1962; Gillespie and Spiegelman, 1965) has been widely used to look for viral "footprints" in human cells in the shape of unusual nucleic acids (Spiegelmann *et al.*, 1972*b*). This has been done in different ways, as illustrated in the following sections.

3.10.1. DNA Viruses: DNA/DNA Hybridization

The DNA/DNA hybridization method is to extract the DNA from virus labeled with radioactive tracers, denature it, and hybridize it with DNA from cells supposedly infected by this or a related virus. Except with SV40 virus (Gelb *et al.*, 1971), and presumably owing to the difficulty of obtaining virus with a sufficiently high specific radioactivity that remains viable, this method has not been widely used.

An alternative has been to use a DNA-dependent RNA polymerase *in vitro* to make a strongly labeled RNA probe, using the viral DNA as a template. This type of method has been used extensively to estimate the status of viral DNA in animal cells cryptically infected by polyoma and SV40 viruses (Westphal and Dulbecco, 1968; Sambrook *et al.*, 1968; Tai and O'Brien, 1969; Westphal and Kiehn, 1970; Levine *et al.*, 1970; Hirai and Defendi, 1971) and has indicated that multiple equivalents of the genome are present in such cells. Recent work suggests, however, that such a technique systematically overestimates the number of genomes present, which may be as much as fivefold less than the number suggested (Tooze, 1973, p. 370). RNA probes made *in vitro* have also been used to detect EBV DNA in human cells in which viral antigens (other than EBNA) cannot be detected by serological means (Zur Hausen and Schulte-Holthausen, 1970).

3.10.2. RNA Viruses: RNA/DNA Hybridization

In the RNA/DNA hybridization method, RNA extracted from radioactively labeled virions is used to detect DNA in the host cells that will hybridize with viral RNA. This method was originally used by Temin (1964) to find the supposed virally specified nuclear DNA in RSV-infected cells and was later refined considerably by Baluda (1972). The method suffers from two disadvantages: insensitivity due to a failure to obtain viruses with sufficiently high specific radioactivity, and an appreciable level of hybridization with DNA from control untransformed cells, perhaps because "normal" chicken cells may also have genes for many antigens present in the virus (Weiss *et al.*, 1971). Since a human oncornavirus has not yet been obtained, this method has not been used to look for its presence in human cells and cannot be considered sensitive enough to look for DNA capable of cross-reacting with animal oncornavirus RNA.

3.10.3. RNA Viruses: DNA/RNA Hybridization

The basis of the DNA/RNA hybridization method is to use virion reverse transcriptase and a viral RNA template to synthesize a highly radioactive DNA probe *in vitro*, to search for viral RNA in cells by hybridization of the probe with extracted cellular RNA, and then to recover the double-stranded hybrid using filters, hydroxyapatite columns, or sucrose, CsCl, or Cs_2SO_4 density gradient centrifugation. With known RNA tumor viruses, an effective way to produce such DNA probes is to employ the so-called endogenous reaction (Schlom and Spiegelman, 1971). Concentrated virion preparations, following treatment with the nonionic detergent NP-40, contain both reverse transcriptase and virion template RNA, and require the addition of the four nucleoside triphosphates to achieve synthesis *in vitro* of a DNA capable of hybridizing with viral RNA (Baltimore, 1970).

An application of this technique has been to use the endogenous reaction of known RNA-containing murine viruses (e.g., Rauscher leukemia, RLV; mammary tumor virus, MMTV) to prepare highly radioactive single-stranded DNA fragments, which are then tested for their ability to hybridize with RNA from human tumor cells. Since most oncornaviruses appear to contain a unique species of RNA with a sedimentation value of 70S, hybridization of the virally specified DNA with material having the biophysical properties of such an RNA in human cells can suggest that human tumor cells contain RNAs related to and perhaps having a similar origin as those of the murine tumor viruses. Experiments of this kind conducted with human tumor material have given remarkable results. DNA probes made using MMTV react only with RNA from patients with human breast cancer (Spiegelman *et al.*, 1972*a*)—not with normal breast tissue, and not with RNAs from lymphomas and leukemias (Spiegelman *et al.*, 1972*b*). In contrast, when the reaction endogenous to a murine leukemia virus is used to prepare DNA, the product fails to hybridize with breast cancer material, although it does so with nucleic acids from sarcomas (Kufe *et al.*, 1972), with RNA from human leukemias (Hehlmann *et al.*, 1972*a*), and with cells taken from patients with Burkitt's lymphoma, nasopharyngeal carcinoma (Kufe *et al.*, 1973), Hodgkin's disease (Hehlmann *et al.*, 1972*b*), and other lymphomas.

However, with Burkitt's lymphoma and nasopharyngeal carcinoma there is already strong evidence of association with herpes viruses (International Agency for Research in Cancer, 1972, pp. 261–396). Are two viruses possibly involved in these conditions, or is it necessary to consider that molecular probes of the kind outlined above may, on occasion, give false positive results? Recent studies on Marek's disease have shown that the fulminant epidemic form of the disease, characterized by high mortality and incidence of visceral tumors, occurs when chickens are exposed to simultaneous infection by Marek's disease herpes virus (MDHV) and a chicken leukosis virus (ALV). On the other hand, eukaryotic cellular DNAs from a wide range of vertebrate species have been shown to contain common sequences, there being more cross-reaction the more closely related the species concerned (Hoyer *et al.*, 1964). Human and murine DNAs contain many such common sequences. It is thus imperative that preparations of murine viruses used to synthesize specific radioactive DNA probes of complementary RNA in human cells be free from contaminants derived from mouse cells. On the other hand, type C viruses themselves have been associated with vertebrate species for a considerable evolutionary period, so it would not be unreasonable to suspect that the viruses themselves may have common nucleotide sequences; the existence of "interspecies" antigens, common to mouse, hamster, cat, and primate oncornaviruses (Geering *et al.*, 1970), can be cited as evidence of this. However, different strains of the murine leukemia and sarcoma viruses themselves show little homology (Stephenson and Aaronson, 1971), so it is difficult to understand why human tumor cells, if they contain nucleic acids associated with the presence of oncornaviruses, should react positively with molecular probes templated by murine virus RNAs, or why, should a human RNA tumor virus exist, the nucleic acid should cross-react to any significant degree. Moreover, the amount of RNA/DNA hybridization detected by Spiegelman and his colleagues was very small indeed, and even though it should be established that these RNAs in human cells are of viral origin, it remains to be shown that such RNAs are disease-related or, indeed, that they are present exclusively in tumor cells. As already pointed out, material obtained from human patients often contains much in addition to tumor cells (Section 2). "Normal" control tissue samples are similarly heterogeneous, their different constituent cell types not necessarily being there in the same proportions as in tumor tissue. A difference in reactivity with a given molecular probe between "tumor" and "control" cannot necessarily be ascribed only to the presence of tumor cells in the one specimen and not in the other.

Success has also attended a search made using human leukemic cells for intracellular enzyme activities (reverse transcriptase) like those of animal oncornavirus, the resemblance being asserted on the basis of a number of common properties:

1. When purified, the enzyme, found in about 30% of cases of acute granulocytic leukemia (Gallo *et al.*, 1970; Sarngadhavan *et al.*, 1972), has biochemical properties very similar to those of viral reverse transcriptase, including "preference" for the same synthetic and natural template–primer ribopolynucleotides.
2. The purified enzyme is immunologically related to reverse transcriptases from primate and, to a lesser extent, murine viruses (Todaro and Gallo, 1973).
3. Enzyme activity is recovered in a cytoplasmic particle with a discrete biochemical integrity and an isopycnic density of 1.16–1.17 (Sarin *et al.*, 1973).
4. The enzyme utilizes RNA as both template and primer for "endogenous" DNA synthesis (Gallo *et al.*, 1973).
5. This "endogenous" reaction produces a "simultaneous detection complex," suggesting that reverse transcriptase activity is tightly coupled *in vivo* to its 70S template RNA (Gallo *et al.*, 1973).

Biochemical fractionation methods have been used to recover entities with the expected properties (isopycnic density, reverse transcriptase activity, content of 70S RNA) from human breast cancer (Axel *et al.*, 1973; Feldman *et al.*, 1973) and, once more, Burkitt's lymphoma (Kufe *et al.*, 1973). If we accept such properties as unique to RNA tumor viruses, there still remain several puzzling features. With the virions of mammalian and avian oncornaviruses, an isopycnic density of 1.14–1.16 is associated with morphologically typical, *extracellular* type C particles, which do *not* occur intracellularly and arise by budding from the cell surface. Detergent treatment of such virions (necessary to reveal "endogenous" enzyme activity) gives rise to material that bands at a new density of $\geqslant$1.20 (Temin and Baltimore, 1972). Unequivocal, extracellular type C particles have not been found in human material, at any rate in the abundance necessary to demonstrate the endogenous reaction. Were they present, NP-40 detergent treatment should generate particulate material with enzyme activity but banding at a higher density; such material has recently been claimed by Feldman *et al.* (1973) to be recoverable from human milk.

To sum up, biochemical data of the type discussed in this section provide suggestive evidence of the presence of unusual nucleic acids and enzyme activities in material obtained from human tumor patients. Determination of whether their relationship to viral infection is indigenous or cryptic, and whether such viral infections are causally related to the tumors concerned, remains for further study.

4. Criteria for the Assertion That a Chosen Human Cancer Is Caused by a Specific Virus

The last phase of the establishment of a viral etiology for human cancer cannot begin until a well-qualified candidate virus has been isolated. Since its causal role cannot be established by direct inoculation into human beings, any involvements of a given isolated virus in the induction of human tumors must be indirectly based, requiring evidence of the following kinds:

1. *Multiple isolations of the same agent from different patients with the same disease should be obtained.* These would serve to rule out the possibility that the virus concerned was a passenger, and correlation of the facility of virus isolation with the stage of disease might give clues as to *how* the virus might be expressing its oncogenic potential. In this connection, it is of paramount importance to show that although human individuals without cancers might harbor the agent concerned, in frank cases infection by the virus must always precede the development of cancer. This criterion is of particular urgency since common, latent, human infections such as the herpes viruses are now suspected as a possible cause of cancer, whether alone or in association with such agents as radiation, chemical carcinogens, or other viruses.
2. As already stated, *the epidemiological rules followed by the agent in question in human populations should also be obeyed by the cancers it is alleged to cause* (e.g., herpes virus type II and cervical cancer; see Section 2).
3. *The virus should have the ability to "transform" human cells in culture by in vitro criteria, and such transformed cells should have the ability to grow into tumors when inoculated into suitably treated heterologous hosts* (see Section 2). It should be reiterated that successful induction of tumors by inoculation of the virus *by itself* into a heterologous host will not provide evidence of oncogenicity in man. Many viruses are known by now that appear not to be oncogenic in their natural hosts, although

they become so when they cross a species barrier. Thus herpes virus saimiri, a latent virus in the squirrel monkey, can induce lymphomas in the marmoset (Melendez *et al.*, 1972). Transformation of heterologous cells *in vitro* (judged equivalent to oncogenic conversion by accepted laboratory criteria) similarly does not imply oncogenic potential in the natural host. The finding that herpes simplex viruses types I and II, partially inactivated by ultraviolet light (Duff and Rapp, 1971) or photodynamically (Rapp *et al.*, 1973), are capable of transforming hamster cells *in vitro* demonstrates unequivocally that the genomes of these normally cytolytic DNA viruses contain integratable sarcomagenic information, but does not thereby implicate these viruses as a cause of tumors in man, although later success in the transformation of *human* cells (Rapp *et al.*, 1973), coupled with seroepidemiological evidence (Nahmias *et al.*, 1971), strongly suggests that this may indeed be the case. A further reminder that caution is needed when generalizing from tumor induction in animals to man is afforded by simian virus 40. Cytolytic in African green monkey kidney cells, it can transform human and mouse cells (Butel *et al.*, 1972). Nevertheless, at least two human isolates of viruses closely related to SV40 are known (Padgett *et al.*, 1971; Weiner *et al.*, 1972); neither has been implicated as a cause of tumors in man. Evidence that EBV virus, already implicated in human oncogenesis on serological and molecular biological grounds (International Agency for Research in Cancer, 1972, p. 2*ff*), is capable of causing tumors in the marmoset (Shope *et al.*, 1973) supports, but does not prove, a similar role in man.

4. *Antisera prepared against the virus should have the ability to neutralize its transforming ability and oncogenic potential, as defined under (3).*
5. *It should be demonstrated that virus-specific products (nucleic acids, antigens, enzymes, etc.) continue to be made by the tumor cells.* This criterion, and the possibility that it may not be an absolute requirement, has already been discussed (Section 2).
6. Finally, *there should be seroepidemiological evidence of an association between human infection and the incidence of tumors.* Although the occurrence of infection without tumor induction may be expected to be the rule rather than the exception, if all tumor patients do not give evidence of infection by *some criteria* then either (a) the tests employed are insufficiently sensitive or (b) the agent observed is not the only, or even the primary, cause of the tumor investigated.

There is as yet no one virus known that fulfills all these criteria as a *bona fide* human tumor virus. There do, however, appear to be two main groups of candidate viruses: (1) The RNA oncogenic viruses (see Tooze, 1973), well authenticated as the cause of many tumors in chickens and mammals, even primates (Theilen *et al.*, 1971), have not so far been implicated in human oncogenesis, although at least one contender (AT124) has not yet been entirely eliminated (Benveniste and Todaro, 1973). (2) DNA viruses of the herpes group have already been suggested as a cause of tumors in frogs (Lucké carcinoma), birds (Marek's disease), and mammals (tumors of cottontail rabbits and various monkey species), and there is much circumstantial evidence to involve them also in man (Burkitt's lymphoma, cervical carcinoma, Hodgkin's disease). If the definition of a tumor is expanded to include benign as well as malignant neoplasms, there are further candidates, such as papova viruses (human warts) and even pox viruses; the latter are known to cause benign tumors in Old World monkeys (Yaba virus, Niven *et al.*, 1961). The condition of molluscum contagiosum in man, known to be caused by a pox virus, has been inexplicably neglected. What such agents might do to a human individual whose immune system is impaired, whether by heredity or treatment, has yet to be imagined.

References

Aaronson, S. A., Todaro, G. J., and Scolnick, E. M., 1971, Induction of murine C-type viruses from clonal lines of virus-free BALB/3T3 cells, *Science* **174:**157.

Allen, P. T., Newton, W. A., Jr., Georgiades, J., Maruyama, K., East, J. L., Bowen, J. M., and Dmochowski, L., 1973, Studies on transforming activities from human solid tumor cells following co-cultivation with human leukemic bone marrow cells, in: *Proceedings of the Sixth Miles International Symposium on Molecular Biology*, Baltimore.

Andervont, H. P., (ed.), 1966, Suggestions for the classification of oncogenic RNA viruses, *J. Natl. Cancer Inst.* **37:**395.

Andrewes, C. H., 1967, *The Natural History of Viruses*, Weidenfeld and Nicolson, London.

Axel, R., Gulati, N., and Spiegelman, S., 1973, Particles containing RIDP and virus-related RNA in human breast cancers, *Proc. Natl. Acad. Sci.* **69:**3133.

Baltimore, D., 1970, Viral RNA-dependent DNA polymerase, *Nature (Lond.)* **226:**1209.

Baluda, M. A., 1972, Widespread presence in chickens of DNA complementary to the RNA genome of avian leukosis viruses, *Proc. Natl. Acad. Sci.* **69:**576.

Becker, Y., and Weinberg, A., 1972, Molecular events in the biosynthesis of Epstein–Barr virus in Burkitt lymphoblasts, in: *Oncogenesis and Herpesviruses*, p. 326, International Agency for Research in Cancer, Lyon.

Benveniste, R. E., and Todarok, G. J., 1973, Homology between type C-viruses of various species as determined by molecular hybridization, *Proc. Natl. Acad. Sci.* **70:**3316.

Biggs, P. M., 1968, Marek's disease: Current state of knowledge, *Curr. Topics Microbiol. Immunol.* **43:**93.

Bittner, J. J., 1942, Hormones, susceptibility, and milk influence in cancer, *Cancer Res.* **2:**710.

Bittner, J. J., 1952, Transfer of the agent for mammary cancer in mice by the male, *Cancer Res.* **12:**387.

Bolton, E. T., and McCarthy, B. J., 1962, A general method for the isolation of RNA complementary to DNA, *Proc. Natl. Acad. Sci.* **48:**1390.

Boyer, S., Porter, I. and Weilbacher, R., 1962, Electrophoretic heterogeneity of glucose-6-phosphate dehydrogenase and its relationship to enzyme deficiency in man, *Proc. Natl. Acad. Sci.* **48:**1868.

Boyland, E., 1963, *The Biochemistry of Bladder Cancer*, Charles C Thomas, Springfield, Ill.

Boyse, E. A., Old, L. J., and Stockert, E., 1972, The relation of linkage group IX to leukemogenesis in the mouse, in: *RNA Viruses and Host Genome in Oncogenesis* (P. Emmelot and P. Bentvelsen, eds.), p. 171, North-Holland, Amsterdam.

Buonassisi, F., Sato, G., and Cohen, H. T., 1962, Hormone producing cultures of adrenal and pituitary tumor origin, *Proc. Natl. Acad. Sci.* **48:**1184.

Burkitt, D. C., 1962, Determining the climatic limitations of a children's cancer common in Africa, *Brit. Med. J.* **27:**1019.

Burns, W., and Black, P., 1968, Analysis of simian virus 40—induced transformation of hamster kidney clones *in vitro*. V. Variability of virus recovery from cell clones inducible with mitomycin C and cell fusion, *J. Virol.* **2:**606.

Butel, J. S., Tevethia, S. S., and Melnick, J. L., 1972, Oncogenesis and cell transformation by papova virus SV40: The role of the viral genome, *Advan. Cancer Res.* **15:**1.

Castro, J. E., and Hamilton, D. N., 1972, Human tumour xenografts, *Brit. J. Surg.* **59:**312.

Centifanto, Y. M., Drylie, D. M., and Deardourff, S. L., 1972, Herpes-virus type 2 in the male genitourinary tract, *Science* **178:**318.

Churchill, A. E., and Biggs, P. M., 1967, Agent of Marek's disease in tissue culture, *Nature (Lond.)* **215:**528.

Cleaver, J. E., 1969, Xeroderma pigmentosum: A human disease in which an initial stage of DNA repair is defective, *Proc. Natl. Acad. Sci.* **63:**428.

Dameshek, W., and Dutcher, R. M., 1970, *Proceedings of the Fourth International Symposium on Comparative Leukemia Research*, Cherry Hill, N.Y., 1969, Karger, Basel and New York.

Darai, G., and Munk, K., 1973, Human embryonic lung cells abortively infected with herpesvirus hominis type 2 show some properties of cell transformation, *Nature (Lond.)* **241:**268.

De Harven, E., 1968, Morphology of murine leukemic viruses, in: *Experimental Leukemias* (M. Rich, ed.), p. 97, Appleton Cross, New York.

Dmochowski, L., Seman, G., and Gallagher, H. S., 1969, Viruses as possible etiologic factors in human breast cancer, *Cancer* **24:**1241.

Doll, R., and Hill, A. B., 1952, A study of the aetiology of carcinoma of the lung, *Brit. Med. J.* **2:**1271.

Duff, R., and Rapp, F., 1971, Oncogenic transformation of hamster cells after exposure to herpes simplex virus type 2, *Nature (Lond.)* **233:**48.

Eidson, C. S., Klever, S. H., and Anderson, D. P., 1972, Vaccination against Marek's disease, in: *Oncogenesis and Herpesviruses*, p. 147, International Agency for Research in Cancer, Lyon.

Eisinger, M., 1973, Human lymph nodes, in: *Tissue Culture Methods and Applications* (P. F. Kruse and M. D. Patterson, eds.), p. 65, Academic Press, New York and London.

Eisinger, M., Fox, S. M., De Harven, E., Biedler, J. L., and Sanders, F. K., 1971, Virus-like agents from patients with Hodgkin's disease, *Nature (Lond.)* **233:**104.

Ellermann, V., and Bang, O., 1908, Experimentelle Leukemia bei Huhnern, *Zentralbl. Bakteriol. Abt. I (Orig.)* **46:**595.

Epstein, M. A., and Achong, B. C., 1973, The EB virus, *Am. Rev. Microbio.* **27:**1624.

Epstein, M. A., Achong, B. G., and Barr, Y. M., 1964, Virus particles in cultured lymphoblasts from Burkitt's malignant lymphoma, *Lancet* **1:**702.

Feldman, S. P., Schlom, J., and Spiegelman, S., 1973, Further evidence for oncornaviruses in human milk: The production of cores, *Proc. Natl. Acad. Sci.* **70:**1976.

Fialkow, P. J., Thomas, E. D., Bryant, J. I., and Neumann, P. E., 1971, Leukemic transformation of engrafted human bone marrow cells *in vivo*, *Lancet* **1:**251.

Fogel, M., and Sachs, L., 1970, Induction of virus synthesis in polyoma tranformed cells by ultraviolet light and mitomycin C, *Virology* **40:**174.

Frenkel, N., Roizmann, B., Cassai, Z., and Nahmias, A., 1972, A DNA fragment of herpes simplex 2 and its transcription in human cervical cancer tissue, *Proc. Natl. Acad. Sci.* **69:**3784.

Gallo, R. C., Yang, S. S., and Ting, R. C., 1970, RNA dependent DNA polymerase of human acute leukemia cells, *Nature (Lond.)* **228:**927.

Gallo, R. C., Miller, N. R., Saxinger, W. C., and Gillespie, D., 1973, Primate RNA tumor virus-like DNA synthesized endogenously by RNA-dependent DNA polymerase in virus-like particles from fresh human acute leukemic blood cells, *Proc. Natl. Acad. Sci.* **70:**3219.

Geering, G., Aoki, T., and Old, L. J., 1970, Shared viral antigen of mammalian leukemia viruses, *Nature (Lond.)* **226:**265.

Gelb, L. D., Kohne, D. E., and Martin, M. A., 1971, Quantitation of SV40 sequences in African green monkey, mouse and virus-transformed cell genomes, *J. Mol. Biol.* **57:**129.

Gerber, P., Virogenic hamster tumor cells: Induction of virus synthesis, *Science* **145:**833.

Gerber, P., 1972, Activation of Epstein–Barr virus by 5-bromodeoxyuridine in "virus-free" human cells,*Proc. Natl. Acad. Sci.* **69:**83.

Gerber, P., Whang-Peng, J., and Monroe, J. H., 1969, Transformation and chromosome changes induced by Epstein–Barr virus in normal human leucocyte cultures, *Proc. Natl. Acad. Sci.* **63:**740.

Gillespie, D., and Spiegelman, S., 1965, A quantitative assay for DNA-RNA hybrids with DNA immobilized on a membrane, *J. Mol. Biol.* **12:**829.

Giraldo, G., Bethe, E., Coeur, P., Vogel, C. L., and Dhru, P. S., 1972, Kaposis sarcoma: A new model in the search for viruses associated with human malignancies, *J. Natl. Cancer. Inst.* **49:**1495

Grand, C. G., 1947, Tissue culture studies of lymph nodes of Hodgkin's disease, *Cancer Res.* **7:**49.

Gross, L., 1951, "Spontaneous" leukemia developing in C3H mice following inoculation, in infancy, with A-K leukemic extracts, or AK embryos, *Proc. Soc. Exp. Biol. Med.* **103:**509.

Gross, L., 1970, *Oncogenic Viruses,* 2nd ed., Pergamon Press, New York and London.

Hammond, E. C., 1968, Quantitative relation between cigarette smoking and death rates, *Natl. Cancer Inst. Monogr.* **28:**3.

Hehlmann, R., Kufe, D., and Spiegelman, S., 1972*a*, RNA in human leukemic cells related to the RNA of a mouse leukemia virus, *Proc. Natl. Acad. Sci.* **69:**435.

Hehlmann, R., Kufe, D., and Spiegelman, S., 1972*b*, Viral related RNA in Hodgkin's disease and other human lymphomas, *Proc. Natl. Acad. Sci.* **69:**1727.

Henle, G., and Henle, W., 1966, Immunofluorescence in cells derived from Burkitt's lymphoma, *J. Bacteriol.* **91:**1248

Henle, W., Diehl, V., Kohn, G., Zur Hausen, H., and Henle, G., 1967, Herpes-type virus and chromosome marker in normal leukocytes after growth with irradiated Burkitt cells, *Science* **157:**1064.

Henle, G., Henle, W., and Diehl, V., 1968, Relation of Burkitt's tumor-associated herpes-type virus to infectious mononucleosis, *Proc. Natl. Acad. Sci.* **59:**94.

Henle, G., Henle, W., Klein, G., Gunvèn, P., Clifford, P., Morrow, R. H., and Ziegler, J. L., 1971, Antibodies to early Epstein–Barr virus-induced antigens in Burkitt's lymphoma, *J. Natl. Cancer Inst.* **46:**861.

Higginson, J., 1967, Etiological factors in gastrointestinal cancer in man, in: Proceedings of the 9th International Cancer Congress, Tokyo, 1966, *VICC Monogr.* **10:**30.

Hirai, K., and Defendi, V., 1971, Homology between SV40 DNA and DNA of normal and SV-40 transformed Chinese hamster cells, *Biochem. Biophys. Res. Commun.* **42:**714.

Hirsch, M. S., Black, P. H., and Proffit, M. R., 1971, Immunosuppression and oncogenic virus infections, *Fed. Proc.* **30:**1852.

Hirsch, M. S., Phillips, S. M., Solnik, C., Black, P. H., Schwartz, R. S., and Carpenter, C. B., 1972, Activation of leukemic viruses by graft-versus-host and mixed lymphocytic *in vitro, Proc. Natl. Acad. Sci.* **69:**1069.

Hirshaut, Y., Glade, P., Moses, H., Manaker, R., and Chesin, L., 1968, Association of herpes-like virus infection with infectious mononucleosis, *Am. J. Med.* **47:**520.

Hollinshead, A. C., and Tarro, G., 1973. Soluble membrane antigens of lip and cervical carcinomas: Reactivity with antibody for herpesvirus non-virion antigens, *Science* **179:**698.

Hoyer, B. H., McCarthy, B. J., and Bolton, E. T., 1964, A molecular approach in the systematics of higher organisms, *Science* **144:**959.

Hsiung, G. D., 1968, Latent virus infections in primate tissues with special reference to simian viruses, *Bacteriol. Rev.* **32:**185.

Huebner, R. J., and Todaro, G. J., 1970, Oncogenesis of RNA tumor viruses as determinants of cancer, *Proc. Natl. Acad. Sci.* **64:** 1087.

Hull, R. N., 1964, in: *The Herpesvirus* (A. S. Kaplan, ed.), p. 390, Academic Press, New York and London.

Igel, H., Huebner, R., Turner, H., Kotin, P., and Falk, H., 1969, Mouse leukemia virus activation by chemical carcinogens, *Science* **160:**1624. International Agency for Research in Cancer, 1972, *Oncogenesis and Herpesviruses*, Lyon.

Jarrett, O., Laird, H., and Hay, D., 1969, Growth of feline leukemia virus in human cells, *Nature (Lond.)* **224:**1208.

Jarrett, W. F. H., Martin, W. B., Crichton, G. W., Dalton, R. G., and Stewart, M. F., 1964, Leukemia in the cat: Transmission experiments with leukemia (lymphosarcoma), *Nature (Lond.)* **202:**566.

Kaplan, H. S., 1967, On the natural history of the murine leukemias (presidential address), *Cancer Res.* **27:**1325.

Klein, G., 1972, EBV-associated membrane antigens, in: *Oncogenesis and Herpesviruses*, p. 295, International Agency for Research in Cancer, Lyon.

Klein, E., van Furth, R., Johansson, B., Ernberg, I., and Clifford, P., 1972, Immunoglobulin synthesis as cellular marker of malignant lymphoid cells, in: *Oncogenesis and Herpesviruses*, p. 253, International Agency for Research in Cancer, Lyon.

Koprowski, H., Jensen, F., and Steplewski, Z., 1967, Activation of production of infectious tumor virus SV40 in heterokaryon cultures, *Proc. Natl. Acad. Sci.* **61:**42.

Kufe, D., Hehlman, R., and Spiegelman, S., 1972, Human sarcomas contain RNA related to the RNA of a mouse leukemia virus, *Science* **175:**182.

Kufe, D., Magrath, V., Ziegler, V., and Spiegelman, S., 1973, Burkitt's tumors contain particles encapsulating RIDP and high molecular weight virus-related RNA, *Proc. Natl. Acad. Sci.* **70:**737.

Kuff, E. L., Wivel, N. H., and Lueders, K. K., 1968, The extraction of intracisternal A-particles from a mouse plasma-cell tumor, *Cancer Res.* **28:**2137.

Lemcke, R. M., 1971, Sizing small organisms, *Nature (Lond.)* **229:**492.

Levine, A. S., Oxman, M. N., Henry, P. H., Levin, M. J., Diamondopoulos, G. T., and Enders, J. F., 1970, Virus-specific deoxyribonucleic acid in simian virus 40–exposed hamster cells: Correlation with S and T antigens, *J. Virol.* **6:**199.

Lowy, D. R., Rowe, W. P., Teich, N., and Hartley, J. W., 1971, Murine leukemia virus: High-frequency activation *in vitro* by 5-iodo-deoxyuridine and 5-bromo-deoxyuridine, *Science* **174:**155.

Lukes, R. F., and Butler, J. J., 1965, The pathology and nomenclature of Hodgkin's disease, *Cancer Res.* **26:**1063.

Macpherson, I., and Montagnier, L., 1964, Agar suspension culture for the selective assay of cells transformed by polyoma virus, *Virology* **23:**29.

Markov, G. G., Bradrarova, I., Mintchera, A., Petrov, P., Shushkov, N., and Taner, R. G., 1969, Mycoplasma contamination of cell cultures: Interference with ^{32}P labeling pattern of RNA, *Exp. Cell. Res.* **57:**374.

Melendez, L. V., Hunt, R. D., Daniel, M. D., Fraser, C. E. O., Barahana, H. H., Garcia, F. G., and King, N. W., 1972, Lymphoma viruses of monkeys; herpesvirus saimiri and herpesvirus ateles, the first oncogenic herpesviruses of primates—A review, in: *Oncogenesis and Herpesvirus*, p. 451, International Agency for Research in Cancer, Lyon.

Miller, G., and Lipmann, M., 1973, Release of infectious Epstein–Barr virus by transformed marmoset leukocytes, *Proc. Natl. Acad. Sci.* **70:**190.

Miller, G., Shope, T., Lisco, H., Stitt, D., and Lipmann, M., 1972, Epstein–Barr virus: Transformation, cytopathic changes, and viral antigens in squirrel monkey and marmoset leukocytes, *Proc. Natl. Acad. Sci.* **69:**383.

Miller, J. M., and Olson, C., 1972, Precipitating antibody to an internal antigen of the C-type virus associated with bovine lymphosarcoma, *J. Natl. Cancer Inst.* **49:**1459.

Moore, D. H., Charney, J., Kramarsky, B., Lasfargues, E. Y., Sarkar, N. H., Brennan, M. J., Burrows, J. H., Surat, S. M., Paymaster, J. C., and Vaidya, A. B., 1971, Search for a human breast cancer virus, *Nature (Lond.)* **229:**611.

Morton, D. L., and Malmgren, R. A., 1968, Human osteosarcomas: Immunological evidence suggesting an associated infectious agent, *Science* **162:**-279.

Murray, R. F., Hubbs, J., and Payne, B., 1971, Possible clonal origin of common warts (verruca vulgaria), *Nature (Lond.)* **232:**50.

Nahmias, A. J., 1969, Association of genital herpesvirus with cervical cancer, *Int. Virol.* **1:**187.

Nahmias, A. J., Naib, Z. M., and Josey, W. E., 1971, Herpesvirus hominis type 2 infection: Association with cervical cancer, and perinatal disease, *Perspect. Virol.* **7:**73.

National Cancer Institute, 1966, Viruses of laboratory rodents, *Natl. Cancer Inst. Monogr.*, No. 20.

Nilsson, K., 1971, High frequency establishment of human immunoglobulin producing lymphoblastoid lines from normal and malignant lymphoid tissue and peripheral blood, *Int. J. Cancer* **8:**432.

Nilsson, K., Klein, G., Henle, G., and Henle, W., 1972, The rôle of EBV in the establishment of lymphoblastoid cell lines from adult and foetal lymphoid tissue, in: *Oncogenesis and Herpesviruses*, p. 285, International Agency for Research in Cancer, Lyon.

Niven, J. S. F., Armstrong, J. A., Andrewes, C. H., Pereira, H. G., and Valentine, R. C., 1961, Subcutaneous "growths" in monkeys produced by a pox virus, *J. Pathol. Bacteriol.* **81:**1.

Nowinski, R. C., Old, L. J., Sarkar, N. H., and Moore, D. H., 1970, Common properties of the oncogenic RNA viruses (oncornaviruses), *Virology* **42:**1152.

Nowinski, R. C., Old, L. J., O'Donnell, P. V., and Sanders, F. K., 1971, Serological identification of hamster oncornaviruses, *Nature New Biol.* **230:**282.

Officer, J. E., Telson, N., Estes, J. D., Fontanilla, E., Rongey, R. W., and Gardner, M. B., 1973, Isolation of a neurotropic type C virus, *Science* **181:**945.

Old, L. J., Boyse, E. A., Geering, G., and Oettgen, H. F., 1968, Serologic approaches to the study of cancer in animals and in man, *Cancer Res.* **28:**1288.

Olson, C., Miller, L. D., Miller, J. M., and Hoss, H. E., 1972, Transmission of lymphosarcoma from cattle to sheep, *J. Natl. Cancer Inst.* **49:**1463.

Padgett, B. L., Walker, D. L., Zu Rhein, G. M., Eckroade, R. J., and Dessel, B. H., 1971, Cultivation of papova-like virus from human brain with progressive multifocal leukoencephalopathy, *Lancet* **1:**1257.

Pantelouris, E. M., 1971, Observations in the immunobiology of "nude" mice, *Immunology* **20:**247.

Pantelouris, E. M., and Hair, J., 1970, Thymus dysgenesis in nude (*nu/nu*) mice, *J. Embryol. Exp. Morphol.* **24:**615.

Payne, L. N., Pani, P. H., and Weiss, R., 1971, A dominant epistatic gene which inhibits cellular susceptibility to RSV (*RAV-o*), *J. Gen. Virol.* **13:**455.

Pontén, J., 1967, Spontaneous lymphoblastoid transformation of long-term cell cultures from human malignant lymphoma, *Int. J. Cancer* **2:**311.

Pott, P., 1775, *Chirurgical Observations*, London.

Pulvertaft, R. J., 1965, A study of malignant tumors in Nigeria by short-term tissue culture, *J. Clin. Pathol.* **18:**261.

Pulvertaft, R. J., 1967, Unpublished data quoted by Zur Hausen, H., Henle, W., Hummeler, K., Diehl, V., and Henle, G., Comparative study of cultured Burkitt tumor cells by immunofluorescence, autoradiography and electronmicroscopy, *J. Virol.* **1:**830.

Rapp, F., Jui-Lies, H. L., and Jerkovsky, M., 1973, Transformation of mammalian cells by DNA-containing viruses following photodynamic inactivation. *Virology* **55:**339.

Reedman, B. M., and Klein, G., 1973, Cellular localization of an Epstein–Barr virus (EBV)–associated complement-fixing antigen in producer and non-producer lymphoblastoid cell lines, *Int. J. Cancer* **11:**499.

Roizman, B., and Spear, P., 1970, Herpesviruses: Current information on the composition and structure, in: *Comparative Virology*, p. 186, Academic Press, New York.

Rotkin, I. D., 1973, A comparison review of key epidemiological studies in cervical cancer related to current search for transmissible agents, *Cancer Res.* **33:**1353.

Rottino, A., 1949*a*, *In vitro* studies of lymph nodes involved in Hodgkin's disease. I. Liquefaction of culture medium, *Arch. Pathol. (Chicago)* **47:**317.

Rottino, A., 1949*b*, *In vitro* studies of lymph nodes involved in Hodgkin's disease. II. Tissue culture studies; formation, behavior and significance of the multinucleated giant cell, *Arch. Pathol. (Chicago)* **47:**328.

Rous, P., 1911, A sarcoma of the fowl transmissible by an agent from the tumor cells, *J. Exp. Med.* **13:**397.

Sabin, A., 1965, Manifestations of latent viral genetic material in experimentally produced cancers and search for such manifestations in human cancers, *Israel J. Med. Sci.* **1:**93.

Sabin, A. B., and Tarro, G., 1973, Herpes simplex and herpes genitalis viruses in etiology of some human cancers, *Proc. Natl. Acad. Sci.* **70:**3225.

Sambrook, J., Westphal, H., Srinivasan, P. R., and Dulbecco, R., 1968, The integrated state of DNA in SV-40 transformed cells, *Proc. Natl. Acad. Sci.* **60:**1288.

Sanders, F. K., 1971, Problems in the study of oncogens *in vitro*, *Med. Clin. North Am.* **55:**653.

Sanders, F. K., 1973, The presence of viruses in uninoculated tissue cultures: Sources and methods of detection, in: *Contamination in Tissue Culture* (J. Fogh, ed.), p. 243, Academic Press, New York and London.

Sarin, P. S., Abnell, J., and Gallo, R. C., 1973, in: *International Symposium on Control of Transcription* (A. Hollander, ed.), Plenum Press, New York.

Sarngadhavan, M. G., Sarin, P. S., Reitz, M. S., and Gallo, R. C., 1972, Reverse transcriptase activity of human acute leukemic cells: Purification of the enzyme response to AMV 70S RNA and characterization of the DNA product, *Nature New Biol.*, **240:**67.

Schlom, J., and Spiegelman, S., 1971. Simultaneous detection of reverse transcriptase and high molecular weight RNA unique to oncogenic RNA viruses, *Science* **174:**840.

Shope, R. E., and Hurst, E. W., 1933, Infectious papillomatosis of rabbits, *J. Exp. Med.* **58:**607.

Shope, T., DeChairo, D., and Miller, G., 1973, Malignant lymphoma in cottontop marmosets after inoculation with Epstein–Barr virus, *Proc. Natl. Acad. Sci.* **70:**2487.

Sivak, A., and van Duuren, B., 1967, Phenotypic expression of transformation: Induction in cell culture by a phorbol ester, *Science* **157:**1443.

Spiegelman, S., Axel, R., and Schlom, J., 1972*a*, Virus-related RNA in human and mouse mammary tumors, *J. Natl. Cancer Inst.* **48:**1205.

Spiegelman, S., Schlom, J., Axel., R., and Kufe, D., 1972*b*, Molecular probing for a viral etiology of human cancer, University of Texas, M. D. Anderson Hospital and Tumor Institute, 25th Annual Symposium in Fundamental Cancer Research.

Stephenson, J. R., and Aaronson, S. A., 1971, Murine sarcoma and leukemia viruses: Genetic differences determined by RNA–DNA hybridization, *Virology* **46:**480.

Stewart, J., and Ferguson-Smith, M., 1958, Klinefelter's syndrome: Genetic studies, *Lancet* **2:**117.

Stewart, S. E., Kasmi, G., Jr., Draycott, C., and Ben, T., 1972, Activation of viruses in human tumors by 5-iododeoxyuridine and dimethyl sulfoxide, *Science* **175:**198.

Stoker, M., and Abel, P., 1962, Conditions affecting transformation by polyoma virus, *Cold Spring Harbor Symp. Quant. Biol.* **27:**375.

Tai, H. T., and O'Brien, R. L., 1969, Multiplicity of viral genomes in an SV-40 transformed hamster cell line, *Virology* **38:**698.

Temin, H., 1964, Homology between RNA from Rous sarcoma virus and DNA from Rous sarcoma virus-infected cells, *Proc. Natl. Acad. Sci.* **52:**323.

Temin, H. M., and Baltimore, D., 1972, RNA-directed DNA synthesis and RNA tumor viruses, *Advan. Virus Res.* **17:**129.

Temin, H. M., and Mizutani, S., 1970, RNA-dependent DNA polymerase in virions of Rous sarcoma virus, *Nature (Lond.)* **226:**1211.

Theilen, G. H., Gould, D., Fowler, M., and Durgwatt, P. L., 1971, C-type virus in tumor tissue of a woolly monkey *(Lagothrix* sp.) with fibrosarcoma, *J. Natl. Cancer Inst.* **47:**881.

Todaro, G. J., and Gallo, R. C., 1973, Immunological relationship of DNA polymerase primate and mouse leukemia virus reverse transcriptase, *Nature (Lond.)* **244:**206.

Todaro, G., and Martin, G., 1967, Increased susceptibility of Down's syndrome fibroblasts to transformation by SV40, *Proc. Soc. Exp. Biol. Med.* **124:**1232.

Todaro, G. J., Aaronson, S. A., and Rands, E., 1971, Rapid detection of mycoplasma-infected cultures, *Exp. Cell Res.* **65:**256.

Tooze, J., ed., 1973, *The Molecular Biology of Tumor Viruses*, Cold Spring Harbor Laboratory, Cold Spring Harbor, N.Y.

Van der Maaten, M. J., and Boothe, A. D., 1971, Isolation of a herpes-like virus from lymphosarcomatous cattle, *Arch. Ges. Virusforsch.* **37:**85.

Vianna, N. J., and Polan, A. K., 1973, Epidemiologic evidence for transmission of Hodgkin's Disease, *New Eng. J. Med.* **289:**499.

Vianna, N. J., Greenwald, P., and Davies, J. N., 1971, Extended epidemic of Hodgkin's disease in high school students, *Lancet* **1:**1209.

Vianna, N. J., Greenwald, P., Brady, J., and Davies, J. N., 1972, Hodgkin's disease: Cases with features of a community outbreak, *Ann. Int. Med.* **77:**169.

Watkins, J., 1970, The effects of some metabolic inhibitors on the ability of SV40 virus in transformed cells to be detected by cell fusion. *J. Cell Sci.* **6:**721.

Weiner, L. P., Herndon, R. M., Narayan, O., Johnson, R. T., Shah, K., Rubinstein, L. J., Presiosi, T. J., and Conley, F. K., 1972, Virus related to SV40 in patients with progressive multifocal leukoencephalopathy, *New Engl. J. Med.* **286:**385.

Weiss, R. A., Friis, R. R., Katz, E., and Vogt, P. K., 1971, Induction of avian tumor viruses in normal cells by physical and chemical carcinogens, *Virology* **46:**920.

Westphal, H., and Dulbecco, R., 1968, Viral DNA in polyoma and SV40 transformed cell lines, *Proc. Natl. Acad. Sci.* **59:**1158.

Westphal, H., and Kiehn, E. D., 1970, The *in vitro* product of SV40 DNA transcription and its specific hybridization with DNA of SV40 transformed cells, *Cold Spring Harbor Symp. Quant. Biol.* **35:**819.

Witter, R. L., 1972, Epidemiology of Marek's disease—A review, in: *Oncogenesis and Herpesviruses*, p. 111, International Agency for Research in Cancer, Lyon.

Wivel, N. A., Lueders, K. K., and Kuff, E. L., 1973, Structural organization of murine intracisternal particles, *J. Virol.* **11:**329.

Zur Hausen, H., and Schulte-Holthausen, H., 1970, Presence of EB virus nucleic acid in a "virus-free" line of Burkitt tumor cells, *Nature (Lond.)* **227:**245.

Helper Activity for the Defective Friend Leukemia Virus in Human Malignant Cell Cultures* 16

AUDREY FJELDE

1. Introduction

The search for a possible viral etiology for human malignancy is at the forefront of current cancer research. Faced with the difficulties present in human investigation, scientists have found it necessary to use indirect approaches. This area of cancer research is further complicated by the fact that the necessary information for malignancy may be present in a cell without demonstrable virus particles. The genetic constitution of the host is an important factor controlling the expression of malignancy, and it has been shown that an agent causing only a mild infection in human beings can cause a malignant lesion in other species (Trentin *et al.*, 1962). A genetic basis for leukemogenesis has been described (Lilly *et al.*, 1964; Odaka and Yamamoto, 1962).

The study presented in this chapter can be considered as another investigation of ways to cope with the kinds of problems mentioned. The use of cultures of human malignant tissue first demonstrated that human extracts had helper activity for the incomplete murine Friend leukemia virus

*Supported in part by Damon Runyon Grant 1192 and W. Walker Fund.

AUDREY FJELDE Roswell Park Memorial Institute, Buffalo, New York

SFFV (Steeves *et al.*, 1971*c*; Fjelde *et al.*, 1971). This effect (HHA), human helper activity, has been investigated via the General Clinical Research Center, Roswell Park Memorial Institute, during the past 3 yr. In addition to HHA, lymphomas have shown reverse transcriptase and 70S RNA homologous with Rauscher leukemia virus (RLV) (Speigelman *et al.*, 1973; Kufe *et al.*, 1974) and have also demonstrated heterophile antigen (Milgrom *et al.*, 1973). A pyrimidine analogue, 3 deazauridine, has been found to inhibit helper activity (Fjelde and Bloch, 1973).

Human malignant tissue has properties similar to those of murine malignant tissue and also shows evidence of the presence of antigens associated with infectious mononucleosis. Although a few electron microscopic pilot studies have not revealed virus particles in the culture fluid, a situation such as that existing in Marek's disease (Peters *et al.*, 1973), i.e., a cooperation of two virus types, may account for some of the difficulties inherent in attempting to demonstrate a cancer virus infectious for humans. Human peripheral blood cultures from both leukemic and normal donors, after establishment, demonstrate the presence of herpes-type virus (Moore *et al.*, 1969).

A modification of an assay for murine helper leukemia viruses made possible the detection of helper activity in extracts of human tissue from malignant sources. Normal tissue did not show this activity. The helper activity, first detected in spleen cell cultures from patients suffering from lymphoreticular disease, increased the spleen focus forming efficiency of the polycythemic murine Friend leukemia virus designated "spleen focus forming virus" (SFFV). The described activity of the human tissue extracts appears to share several important properties usually associated with leukemogenic viruses of animals. Among the extracts which can help the deficient Friend virus are those that contain murine leukemia viruses, feline leukemia virus, and Rous sarcoma virus.

The method we are using to study human material is briefly as follows: tissue is minced in tissue culture medium with fetal calf serum and the cells are centrifuged out immediately or cultured. The supernatant, used for the helper activity assay, is centrifuged at 75,000*g* for 2 h in the Spinco. The pellet is resuspended in phosphate-buffered saline (PBS) and injected intravenously with the SFFV virus into genetically suitable mice. In the pilot study, human spleen cell cultures from patients with chronic myelogenous leukemia (CML) were the best source of activity. Since hematopoietic cultures from CML patients show one of the few human karyotypic abnormalities associated with malignancies, the Philadelphia chromosome, an attempt was made to determine whether the abnormality was linked to the presence of helper activity. This chromosome tends to disappear during *in vitro* establishment of the cells; however, the "M" line, originated by J.

Pauly from CML peripheral blood, continued to show both the Philadelphia chromosome and helper activity. Electron microscopy revealed that the line was contaminated with mycoplasma and carried herpes-type virus particles. Subsequent studies have shown that the "helper activity" was "enhancement" and resembled the activity found in mice stimulated by endotoxin. A study of CML lines from 15 patients with and without the chromosomal abnormality showed no correlation with the presence of helper activity (Table 1).

Steeves *et al.* (1971*b*) have described human helper activity for the SFFV murine leukemia in an investigation reported at the Comparative Research Leukemia Symposium in Padua. Activity was detected in 20 of 31 spleens of patients having hematopoietic neoplasms, and no activity was seen in normal spleens (0/14) or in fetal spleen cultures (0/7). The human extracts showing helper activity had the same filtration patterns as murine helper through Diaflow membranes (Amicon Corp., Lexington, Mass.) of graded porosity.

2. *The Nature of Human Helper Activity*

The underlying principle of the human helper activity assay is based on the *Fv-1* allele in the murine host. In the B-type host, an indigenous helper

TABLE 1

Philadelphia Chromosome Studies[a]

Tissue	Diagnosis	Assay	Philadelphia chromosome	Line established
Spleen	CML	Positive	(+)	(+)
Spleen	CML	Positive	(+)	
Spleen	CML	Positive	(+)	
Spleen	CML	Negative	(+)	
Blood	CML	Negative	(−)	
Spleen	HD	Positive	(+) ?	
Spleen	CML	Positive	Not done	(+)
Bone marrow	CML	Positive	(+)	
Bone marrow	CML	Negative	(+)	
Bone marrow	CML	Negative	(+)	
Bone marrow	CML	Positive	Not done	(+)
Blood	CML	+/−	(+)	
Bone marrow, blood	CML	Negative	(+)	
Tumor cells	CML	Negative	(+)	(+)
Tumor cells	CML	Positive	(+)	(+)

[a]Shows the lack of correlation between the persistence of the Philadelphia chromosome and positive HHA. CML, Chronic myelogenous leukemia; HD, Hodgkin's disease.

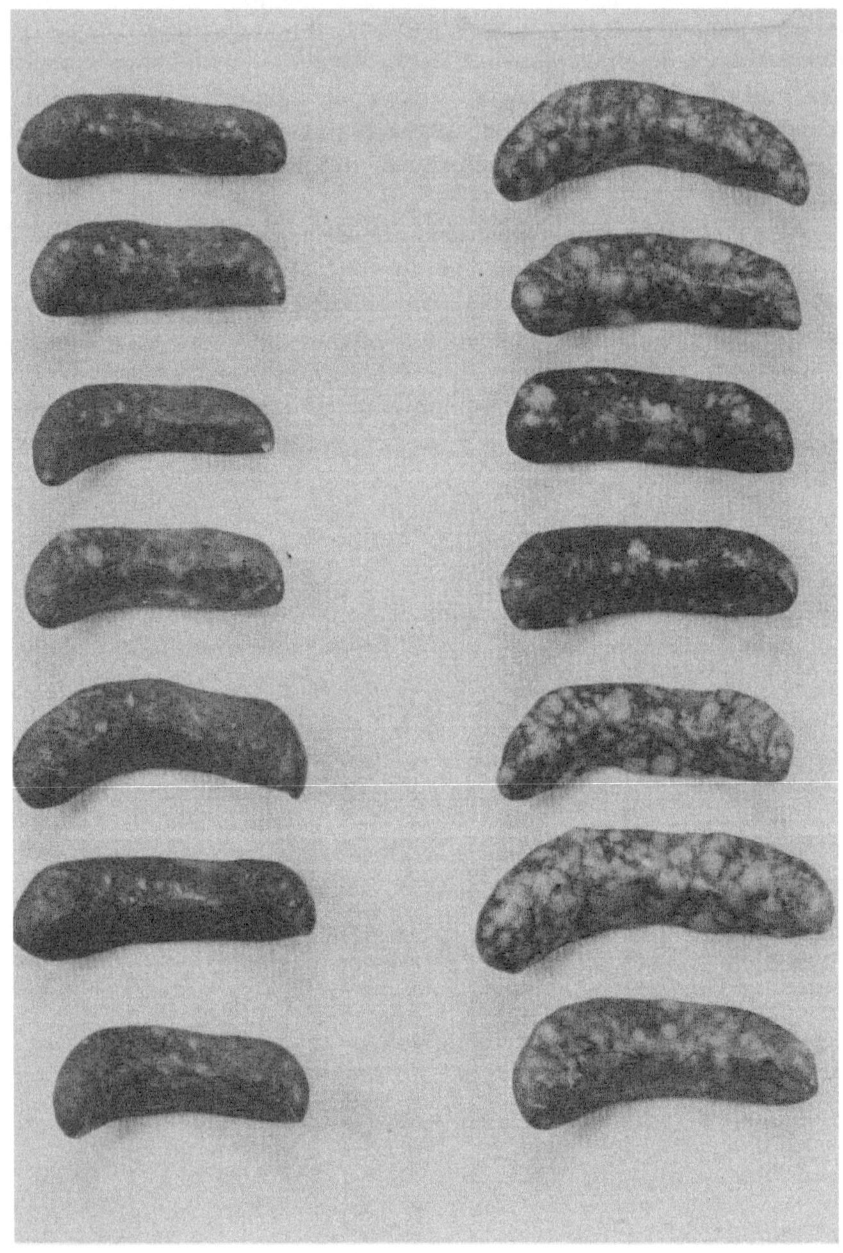

FIG. 1. Spleens from B-type mice injected with Friend virus SFFV(LLV) alone (left) and injected with SFFV(LLV) plus human helper extracts (right).

lymphatic leukemia virus (LLV) in the polycythemic Friend virus complex is repressed. When repression occurs, other RNA leukemia viruses can act as helpers. The helper effect is shown in Fig. 1. Spleens from mice injected with polycythemic Friend virus alone are shown on the left, and on the right are shown spleens from mice injected with Friend virus together with human helper extracts, having the typical foci of erythroblastic stem cells. Dr. Friend considers the target cell for Friend virus to be a primitive stem cell which would differentiate along the erythroid pathway.

The HHA assay is based on the cumulative findings of several scientists. The Friend virus was reported by Friend in 1957 (Friend, 1957), and in 1962 Mirand proposed that his Friend virus stocks might reasonably be considered a "Friend virus complex." He reported the presence of the indigenous helper LLV, which causes lymphatic leukemia in rats (Mirand and Grace, 1962). Dawson and Fieldsteel have also described a lymphatic leukemia virus (1969) and a chronic remittent type of Friend disease (1973). In 1964, Axelrad and Steeves reported an assay system for murine leukemia viruses; the virus complex used is designated SFFV(LLV). The LLV is expressed (foci on the ninth day in the spleen) in a genetically receptive mouse and inhibited in the nonreceptive mouse. When the indigenous LLV is repressed, other helper viruses can be substituted (Steeves *et al.*, 1971*a*). This helper assay method was modified and used to detect helper activity in supernatant media from cultured malignant human cells. the growth of hematopoietic cell types resembled that seen in peripheral blood cultures (Fjelde, 1969; Fjelde, 1972). Preliminary electron microscopic studies have not revealed viral particles in human material giving positive activity; however, evidence has been obtained showing that human malignant tissue demonstrating helper activity also contains DNA hybridizable with the RNA of RLV mouse leukemia virus.

The relationship between the deficient SFFV Friend virus and the indigenous LLV helper virus has been investigated in many studies, which have been summarized by Eckner (1973). It seems that the associated helper virus is functional late in the viral synthesis cycle and that the early stages are helper independent.

Studies (Pincus *et al.*, 1971; Rowe *et al.*, 1973) have demonstrated that the *Fv-1* locus controls susceptibility to murine leukemias; the *b* allele, dominant for resistance to N-tropic viruses is present in B-type mice. Lilly (1970) has also described a second gene, *Fv-2*, affecting the response to Friend virus.

3. *Pilot Studies and Methods*

In our studies, spleen cultures were routinely totally removed from flasks after incubation. Cells attached to the bottom of the flask were removed by scraping. The total culture was centrifuged at 9000g (International centrifuge HR-1) for 10 min in order to remove the cells, which were either stored or subcultured. The supernatant fluid was then centrifuged at 75,000g in the Spinco. The pellet was resuspended in PBS and stored in sealed ampules at −196°C or used immediately for the HHA assay in B-type mice with the $Fv\text{–}1^r$ gene, dominant for resistance to the indigenous LLV, thus permitting a second helper to function.

The concentrated human extract was injected intravenously into mice together with the SFFV, and the number of foci in the spleens of these mice was compared with the number found in the spleens of mice injected with SFFV alone. On the ninth day, grossly visible foci were present, and after fixation of the spleens in Bouin's fixative the foci larger than 0.5 mm in diameter were counted. The Δ value represented the value obtained after dilution factors and background SFFV activity were estimated. A ΔFFU value above 1500 was considered positive.

Since RNA viruses from several species had been shown to have a helper function for SFFV, it was of interest to devise an experiment for testing possible helper activity in human neoplasms. Spleens, bone marrow, and peripheral blood were used to demonstrate the presence of helper activity in cultures from patients with lymphoreticular diseases. Activity was also found in a bone marrow culture from a child with neuroblastoma. Subsequently, activity has been found in all neuroblastomas investigated (6/6). Routinely, tumors or spleens were prepared as cell suspensions in G-16 glass culture bottles with a nucleated cell population of approximately 5×10^6/ml.

In the first HHA assays reported, helper activity was recovered from cell cultures of spleens of patients suffering from chronic myelogenous leukemia, lymphosarcoma, and Hodgkin's disease, but not from cultures of normal human spleens. Surgical specimens were used in the studies and processed immediately after removal. The spleens were provided by the General Clinical Research Center at Roswell Park Memorial Institute and by nearby hospitals.

The overall research plan is shown in Fig. 2 and the method of processing in Fig. 3. Spleens were cut into convenient pieces, washed with PBS, and subsequently minced in small amounts of complete medium with serum. The cell suspension was removed and the mincing process repeated several times. Stationary 200- or 100-ml cultures with a nucleated cell population of 5×10^6 cells/ml were used as a unit source of HHA. In pilot experiments, a variety of tissue culture methods were tested. The best results were obtained using Eagle's medium (MEM) with 10% fetal calf serum (FET) and an incubation period of 48 h.

Time studies (Fjelde, 1973) of cultures showed that peaks of activity occurred at zero and 48 h. Cell suspensions obtained in PBS instead of

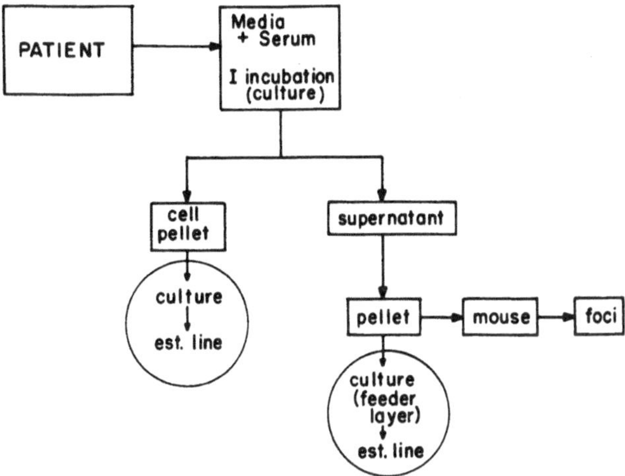

FIG. 2. Method of studying human helper activity (HHA). Cells and tissue from the patient are processed as shown and also investigated for the presence of heterophile antigen and virus–specific 70S RNA.

complete medium were usually low in activity. Cultures treated with phytohemagglutinin (PHA) were also low in activity, as were those in which trypsinized cells were used. PHA was used in an attempt to induce mitosis and possibly increase cell division, and perhaps in the process find out whether a mitogen or a mitogen-sensitive cell is important in the induction of spleen foci. In subsequent experiments, the use of a mitogen has not always brought about a decrease in helper activity. These studies are in progress at the present time, as are studies concerning the importance of

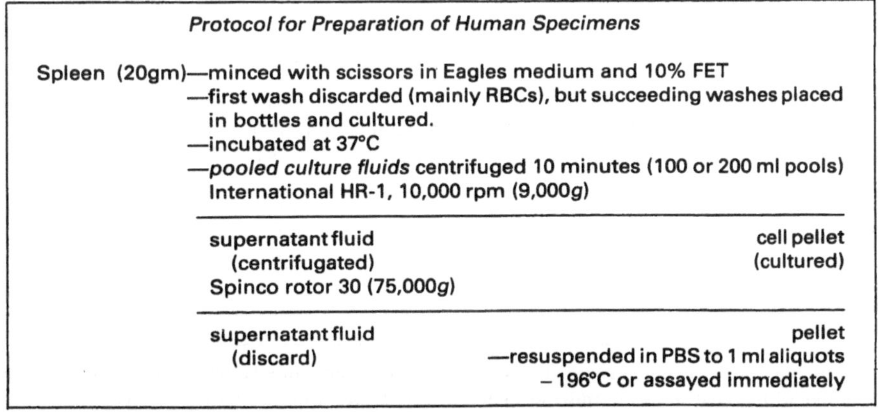
Protocol for Preparation of Human Specimens

Spleen (20gm)—minced with scissors in Eagles medium and 10% FET
—first wash discarded (mainly RBCs), but succeeding washes placed in bottles and cultured.
—incubated at 37°C
—*pooled culture fluids* centrifuged 10 minutes (100 or 200 ml pools) International HR-1, 10,000 rpm (9,000*g*)

supernatant fluid (centrifugated) Spinco rotor 30 (75,000*g*) | cell pellet (cultured)

supernatant fluid (discard) | pellet —resuspended in PBS to 1 ml aliquots −196°C or assayed immediately

FIG. 3. Method used in preparing human cell and tissue extract for the HHA assay.

TABLE 2

Time Study of HHA from a Human Spleen Culture from a Patient with Hodgkin's Disease[a]

	Foci	Average	FFU/ml	ΔFFU/ml
Pse	0,0,0,0,0,1,3	0.57	314	
Day 0	1,4,7,7,9,15,24	9.57	3828	3514
1	0,0,2,2,2,4,5	2.14	857	543
2	3,4,4,6,8,10,10	6.43	2571	2257
3	1,3,3,7,10,10,12	6.51	2628	2314
4	0,1,1,1,3,3,3	1.71	685	371
5	0,0,3,3,6,7,9	4.14	1657	1343
6	0,0,1,2,2,9	2.35	933	619
7	0,0,1,1,2,6,6	2.28	914	600
Pse	0,0,0,0,0,1,6	1.00	314	

[a]The helper activity is highest on days 0, 2, and 3. The top and bottom lines represent the intravenous injection of the Friend virus SFFV(LLV) alone into seven mice, and the other values represent the Friend virus together with the human extract on days 0 through 7 of cultivation.

arginine and asparagine. The untreated spleen specimens undergo microbiological investigation, and rare cultures which show contamination are not used. None of the human spleens examined to date for mycoplasma has shown contamination.

Table 2 shows the level of helper activity at different times of incubation. When spleens from leukemic mice were similarly cultured, no peak was seen (Table 3), and the helper activity or leukemogenicity could sometimes be

TABLE 3

Time Study of a Murine Helper[a]

	PBS	Indicator	Moloney helper	Mean number of foci	FFU/ ml	ΔFFU/ ml
	3.98	0.02		1.93	771	
MolLV, 1 h	2.98	0.02	1.0	2.57	1028	257
MolLV, 2 days	2.98	0.02	1.0	5.28	2114	1343
MolLV, 3 days	2.98	0.02	1.0	11.85	4743	3972
MolLV, 4 days	2.98	0.02	1.0	13.52	5428	4657

[a]The top line represents the Friend virus alone and the other values represent the Friend virus together with an extract from murine spleen infected with Moloney leukemia virus (MolLV). The helper activity, which increased during a 4-day period, represents an increase in virus titer during cultivation.

TABLE 4

Murine Spleens Infected with Friend Virus[a]

No.	Treat-ment	Culture	Route of inoculation	Number of dead Friend leukemia/ number inoculated	Latent period (days)	Percent dead
1	—	Day 5	i.p.	0/4	—	0
2	IUdR	Day 5	i.p.	4/4	113	100
3	—	Day 24	i.p.	0/4	—	0
4	IUdR	Day 24	i.p.	1/4	86	25
5	IUdR	Day 42	i.p.	1/4	61	25
6	IUdR	Day 42	i.v.	4/4	49	100

[a]Demonstrates a retention of leukomogenicity and focus-forming capacity of spleen cultures from Swiss mice infected with Friend virus and treated with IUdR.

demonstrated (Tables 4 and 5) irregularly for long periods of cultivation. Some of the neuroblastoma cultures showed "spotty" retention of helper activity. This activity was not related to mycoplasmal contamination.

An attempt was made to determine whether culture media of various compositions would influence the maintenance or growth of human tumor cells from cultured spleens. Two of the metabolites tested were arginine and asparagine. However, RPMI-1640, which contained both, was less effective

TABLE 5

Leukemogenicity of Murine Spleen Cultures[a]

	Control				IUdR			
	Cells (i.p.)		Supernatant (i.v.)		Cells (i.p.)		Supernatant (i.v.)	
	Number positive	Latent period (days)	Number positive	Latent period (days)	Number positive	Latent period (days)	Number positive	Latent period (days)
Day 0	3/10	51						
Day 2	1/5	44	3/5	44	1/5	23	4/5	46
Day 4	1/5	48	4/5	41	0/5	—	1/5	31
Day 7	0/5	—	1/5	46	0/5	—	1/5	52
Day 14	1/5	45	0/5	—	0/5	—	1/5	45
Day 21	0/5	—	1/5	25	0/5	—	0/5	—

[a]Demonstrates the leukemogenicity of spleen cultures from Swiss mice injected with Friend virus, tested after various periods of incubation. The routine method described for culturing human spleens was used; the cells from each culture were injected intraperitoneally and the supernatant was concentrated and injected intravenously.

for producing helper activity than Eagle's medium with only arginine. Complete medium with fetal calf serum was better than phosphate-buffered saline on day 0 for making the extract for this assay. PHA, which affects the lymphoblastoid stem cell and would presumably compete for cells the LLV needed, was added to cultures and reduced considerably the number of erythroblastic foci in the helper assay compared with the controls (Steeves *et al.*, 1971*c*; Fjelde *et al.*, 1971).

Perhaps the target cell for SFFV is a very primitive reticuloendothelial cell which could develop into either an erythroid or a lymphoid cell. Perhaps the human material (nucleic acid?) giving the helper effect was removed by the PHA and was therefore not present in the culture medium used for the assay. Trypsinized cultures used for helper assay yielded less helper activity than the nontrypsinized controls.

Hematopoietic cells are dependent on their environment for necessary metabolites, and amino acids such as asparagine and related enzymes are important. Anything in the environment that deprives the cell of the necessary substrate would affect the propagation of the cell type. Competing organisms making or using the metabolites would influence the growth of a cell (tumor) population (Simberkoff *et al.*, 1969). It has been pointed out that endotoxin (Thomson, 1969) has a stimulating effect on the focus formation, presumably increasing the numbers of target cells present in the spleen. This effect would be considered enhancement rather than helper activity. The two effects can be differentiated by the demonstration of one-hit or multiple-hit curves using dilution techniques.

4. *Characteristics of Human Neuroblastoma Cells and Other Cells in Culture*

When injected intravenously with the polycythemic Friend virus in mice which repress the indigenous helper virus (LLV), extracts from neuroblastomas functioned as a helper in producing spleen foci. Six neuroblastoma cell lines, which consist of two cell types and have a characteristic growth pattern, have remained diploid. One cell population consists of spindle-shaped or stellate cells which attach to the glass and form long interconnecting projections. The second population consists of small floating cells attached to each other. These cells can be seen forming masses on the cell layer. Passages are made from the floating masses, which then attach and form a new two-cell-type culture. In one study (Fjelde and Freeman, 1973), no viruses were found in cultures treated with 5′-iododeoxyuridine and other agents. In contrast to normal brain, neuroblastoma cultures have all

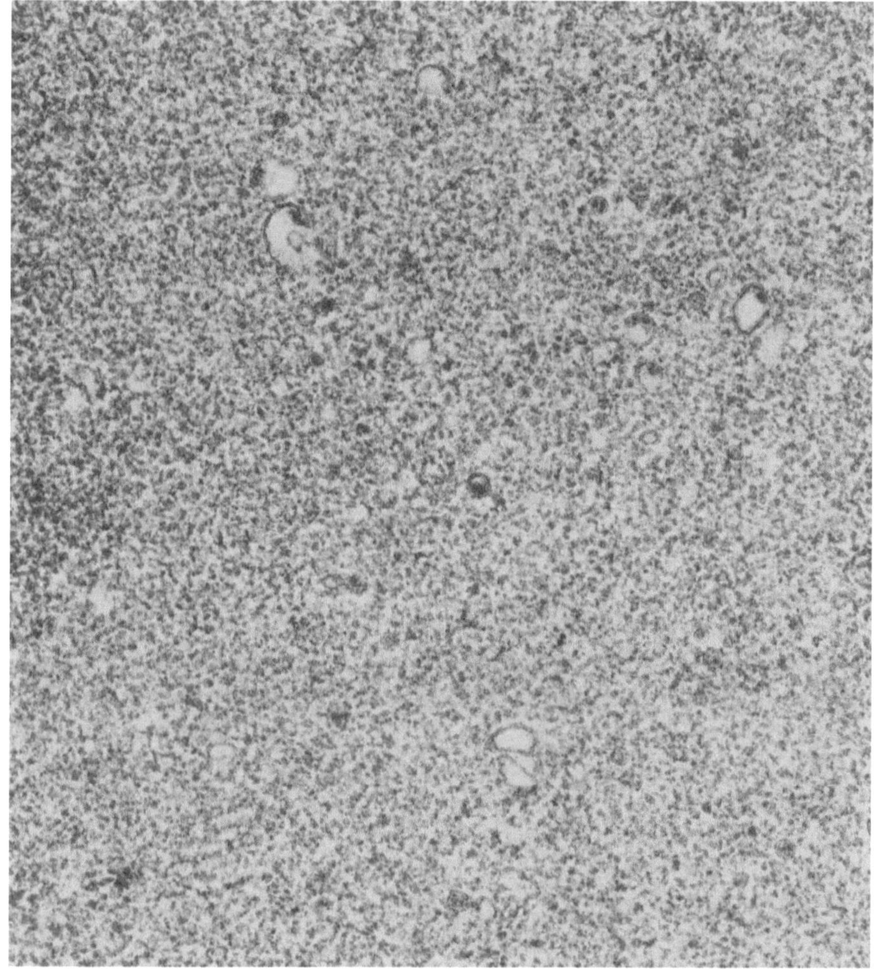

FIG. 4. Electron micrograph of a pellet used for the demonstration of human helper activity from a neuroblastoma.

shown helper activity (Fig. 4). In preliminary unpublished studies, lymphomatous spleens and neuroblastoma tumors showing helper activity have also shown RNA which is homologous to murine RLV-RNA. Later studies of the lymphomas have been published (Spiegelman *et al.*, 1973).

A number of cell lines have been derived directly from human tissue showing helper activity and from such tissue cocultivated with normal human embryo cells. Other cell lines from human embryo cells and other human lines have been treated with extracts showing helper activity and all grow rapidly.

TABLE 6

Neuroblastoma Cultures[a]

Source	ΔFFU/ml	Significance
Bone marrow	1800	Positive
Bone marrow	2914	Positive
Tumor	2400	Positive
Tumor	1593	Positive
Tumor	1477	(Positive)
Tumor	2023	Positive

[a]Shows some of the HHA values typical for neuroblastoma cultures. Values above 1500 were considered positive.

Some of these cultures, particularly those derived from neuroblastoma tumors, have been examined for the presence of virus particles. None has been found.

Although some of the established neuroblastoma lines have continued to show helper activity, no activity has been seen in other lines after establishment or in cell lines the author has established from various tumors and other tissue.

One subline of HS1-Fjelde established in 1952–53 at Sloan-Kettering Institute from a human sarcoma (Fjelde, 1955) has acquired mycoplasmal contamination and strongly enhances focus formation with the Friend virus (Eckner *et al.*, 1974*b*) but is not a true helper. Other lines, HEp-1 and HEp-2, also established by the author in 1952–1953, showed no enhancement or helper activity. A series of (unpublished) studies have been done with different malignant human cell lines and clones, established by the author and maintained in culture for a period of one to several years. The lines were derived from peripheral blood, bone marrow, spleen, skin, xeroderma pigmentosum tumors, sarcomas, and a colon tumor producing fetal antigen (CEA) (line Col-Fj-1). None of the routinely cultured lines has to date shown C-type particles in preliminary electron microscopic studies. The neuroblastomas (6/6) have shown initial positive HHA values (Table 6) in the murine spleen focus forming assay. The activity disappears during prolonged cultivation but has reappeared in some lines irregularly. These established lines and other freshly cultured malignant cells are considered to be likely candidates for testing the theory that human malignant cells contain repressed or unexpressed oncogenes which could be affected by a trigger mechanism during cultivation. Prolonged cultivation, cocultivation with other cells with DEAE-dextran, 5′-bromodeoxyuridine (BUdR), or 5′-

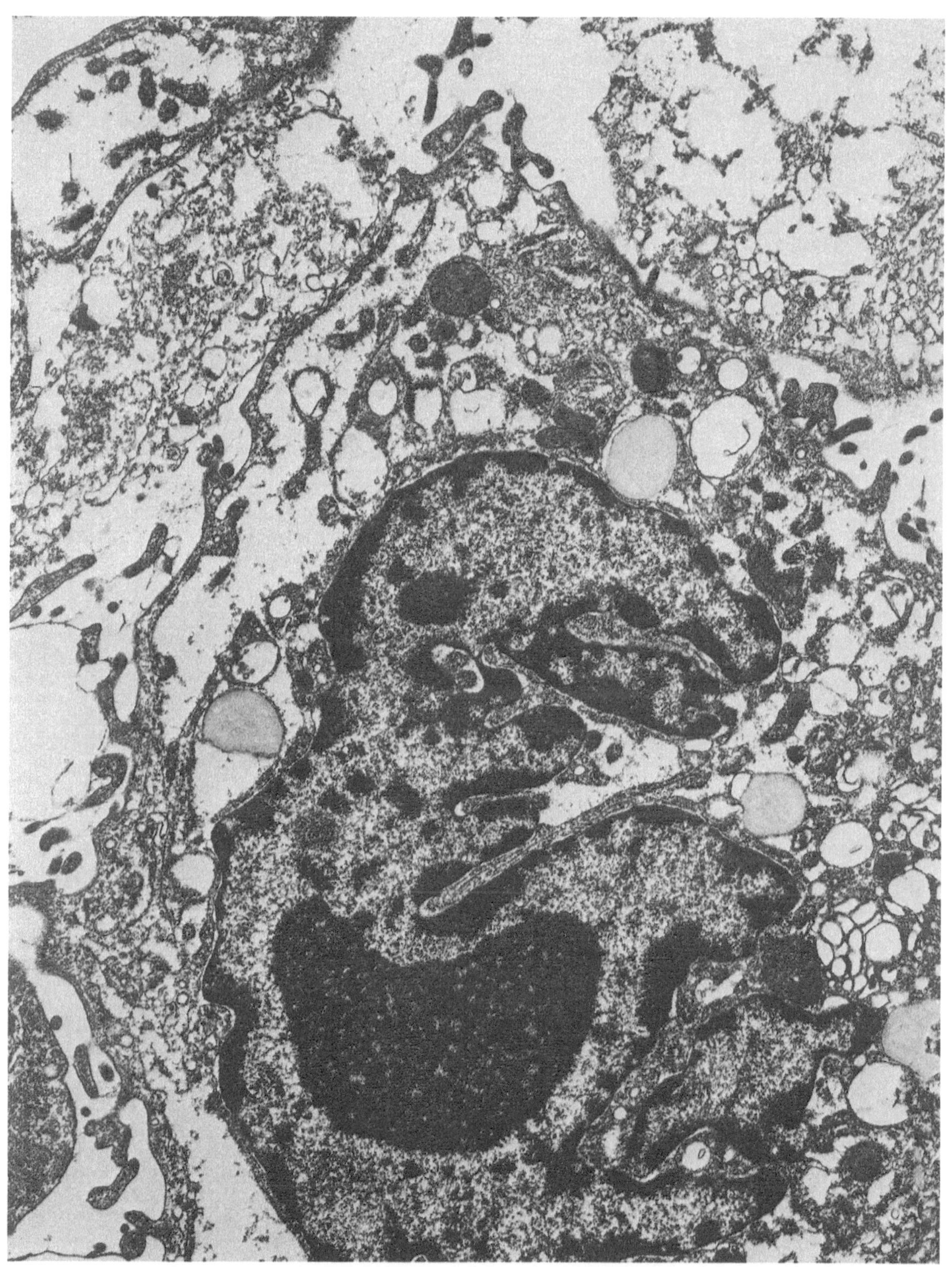

FIG. 5. Electron micrograph of a neuroblastoma large-type cell.

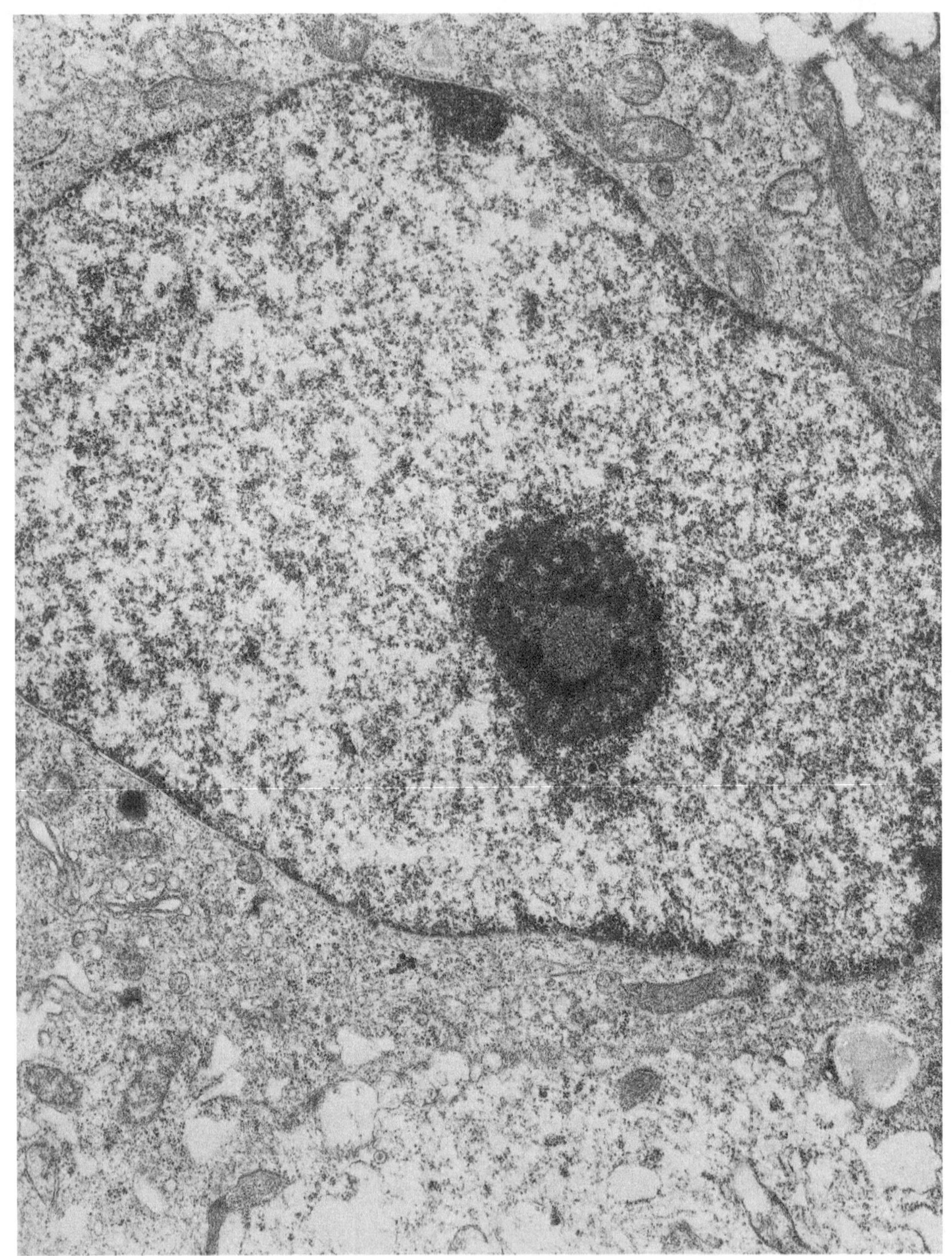

FIG. 6. Electron micrograph of a neuroblastoma small-type cell.

iododeoxyuridine (IUdR), and treatment of embryo cultures with pellets from centrifuged (70,000–80,000*g*) culture (malignant cell) supernatant are some of the methods in use in the attempt to induce evidence of viral activity. These established lines and treated monolayers have not been as yet examined for virus particles.

Neuroblastomas have been described as usually occurring in young children and metastasizing profusely to the liver and often to bones and other organs. They are composed of rather small, indifferent-looking cells, often with peculiar balls or rosettes. J. H. Wright recognized these as similar to cells peculiarly aranged among the fetal sympathetic formative cells and proposed the name "neuroblastoma," which has been widely accepted. Some of these neurological tumors are peculiar in being familial, many families having been described in which several members were affected in successive generations. Neuroblastomas can also spontaneously disappear.

The original culture pattern resembles that of the histological sections described in textbooks. The elaborate interconnecting processes seen are characteristic of brain cells in culture. Although no viruses have been seen in our studies, neuroblastoma cultures should be good candidates for a study of possible human tumor virus.

Since morphological observation of cells in the established neuroblastoma cultures suggested that small lymphocytes might be present, a careful study with the light microscope and the electron microscope was done. Figures 5 and 6 show that the two cell types seen probably represent stages in maturation. Small (floating) cells and large attached cells with typical elongated processes can be seen. Neither mycoplasmas nor viruses were seen in numerous electron microscopic preparations. In studying the development from day 0 to establishment, rosette formations are seen first and finally the two cell types. New attached large-cell cultures can be started from floating small cells.

5. *Attempts to Inhibit Helper Activity with Chemotherapeutic Agents*

Since experiments with human malignant tissue suggested the possible presence of a C-type viral agent, further experiments were designed to determine whether helper activity could be inhibited *in vivo* by a known antiviral agent, 3-deazauridine, an inhibitor of RNA viruses (Wang and Bloch, 1972).

In pilot experiments, 3-deazauridine inhibited the helper activity of human malignant tissue extracts for the defective Friend spleen focus forming virus complex, SFFV(LLV). This inhibition of helper activity was

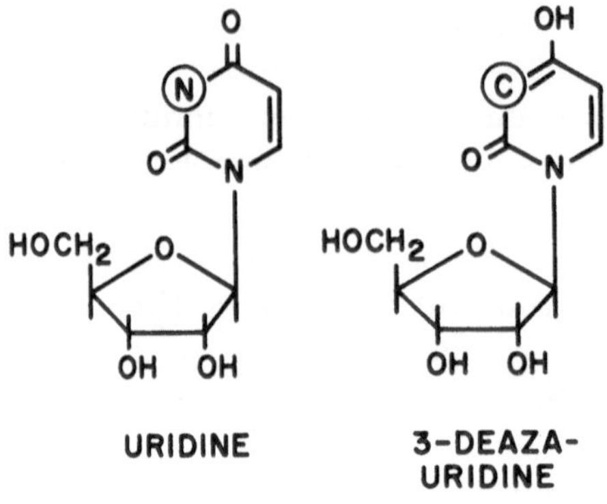

FIG. 7. Chemical structure of 3-deazauridine, an analogue of uridine.

demonstrated under conditions where the natural helper (LLV) was inhibited. These experiments were conducted in collaboration with Dr. A. Bloch at Roswell Park Memorial Institute. The inhibition of activity was demonstrated with tissues from a variety of human malignancies including neuroblastoma and several lymphomas, Hodgkin's disease, reticulum cell sarcoma, and lymphosarcoma (Fjelde and Bloch, 1973). The chemical structure of 3-deazauridine (3D), a pyrimidine analogue shown to be growth-inhibiting for microorganisms, tumor cell lines, and some tumors *in vivo*, is shown in Fig. 7. 3-Deazauridine undergoes phosphorylation, and its inhibiting activity is probably exerted at the nucleotide stage at which it accumulates in the cell.

Tissue from surgery was minced in complete medium and the cells were centrifuged out immediately or cultured. The supernatant, used for the helper assay, was centrifuged at 75,000*g* for 2 h in the Spinco. The pellet was resuspended in PBS and injected intravenously into mice, and the spleen was examined for foci 9 days after injection. The method of estimating the helper effect is shown in Table 7. The Friend virus is injected intravenously with and without the helper and the difference is estimated. Table 8 shows a representative human helper assay done routinely in our laboratory together with assays containing uridine or the analogue 3-deazauridine. The top and bottom values represent the Friend virus alone. NB in lines 2, 3, and 4 represents a neuroblastoma assay (highly positive) and HD represents a Hodgkin's disease extract, which unfortunately lost activity during storage after the preliminary screening.

The spleens of the mice treated with the neuroblastoma preparation and the Friend virus all showed the characteristic foci of Friend leukemia cells, the average being 2957 focus-forming units per milliliter per spleen. When

TABLE 7

Human Helper Activity (HHA) Assay[a]

	Helper	Spleen count	X	FFU/ml	ΔFFU/ml	Significance
FV	—	5,9,7,3,1,—,—	25/5	364		Control
FV	NB	1,28,60,15,13,42,48	207/7	2957	2593	Positive
FV	HD	2,1,1,3,2,3,2	14/7	200	0	Negative
FV	—	1,1,2,3,3,5,—	15/6	364		Control

[a]Illustrates the method of estimating the helper effect. The Friend virus (SFFV) is injected intravenously with and without the helper, and the difference is estimated. The study shows a representative HHA assay done routinely in our laboratory. The top and bottom values represent the Friend virus alone, (310)NB is a neuroblastoma assay (positive), and HD represents a (negative) Hodgkin's disease extract.

the background value, i.e., the FFU/ml value for Friend virus alone, was subtracted, the so-called Δ value was 2593. Uridine was used as a second control. The results on lines 2 and 3 are not significantly different. When 3D was substituted for uridine, many of the mice showed no spleen foci or small numbers of foci. We have found that we occasionally observe what appears to be a stimulation (79 value) in one or two mice in a series of completely negative animals. We have previously reported in other studies that a small

TABLE 8

Spleen Focus Forming Assay Demonstrating HHA Inhibition[a]

Inoculum	Chemical	Indi-cator	Helper	Spleen count		FFU/ml	ΔFFU/ml
						Average	
FV control	—	FV	—	5,9,7,3,1,—,—	25/5	364	////
FV + 310	—	FV	NB	1,28,60,15,13,42,48	207/7	2957	2593
FV + 310 + UR	UR	FV	NB	0,25,34,39,48,—,—	146/5	2920	2556
FV + 310 + 3D	3D	FV	NB	0,2,0,0,8,56,79	145/7	2071	1707
FV + 338	—	FV	HD	7,7,0,0,10,5,5	34/7	486	122
FV + 338 + 3D	3D	FV	HD	0,0,0,0,2,0,0	2/7	28.57	0
						Average	
FV control	—	FV	—	1,1,2,3,3,5,—	15/6	364	////

[a]HHa assay used to test inhibition in a B-type mouse using (1) Friend virus (FV), (2) FV plus human helper 310 (extract from a neuroblastoma, NB), (3) FV plus 310 plus uridine (UR), (4) FV plus 310 plus 3D (analogue), and (5) FV plus 338 (extract from a spleen from a patient with Hodgkin's disease (HD)), (6) FV plus 338 plus 3D.

amount of a cytotoxic drug appears to be stimulating. Only one of seven mice showed foci (two) when treated with 3D and an extract from a Hodgkin's spleen. The preparation in this case showed a higher value when tested in the preliminary screening procedures. In this study, it seems that the two compounds 3-deazauridine and uridine are decidedly different in their effect on the helper activity and that the uridine control mice do not show the inhibiting effect seen in the 3D-treated mice.

We have found activity in spleens of patients suffering from lymphoreticular diseases. The activity from these spleens is related to the degree of involvement—spleens showing greater numbers of pathological cells also show a higher degree of helper activity. Normal control spleens have not shown significant helper activity.

Table 9 shows a series of lymphoma spleens, most of which had lost activity during storage, but which had shown high activity in previous screening. The top line represents the average value (186) of the two controls (172 and 200) consisting of the Friend virus alone. With the exception of number 5, all of the lymphomas showed decreased focus formation when treated with 3D.

TABLE 9

3D-Treated Cultures[a]

Treatment	Patient No.	Indicator	Helper	FFU/ml	Δ FFU/ml
Combined controls	—	FV	—	186	—
Control 1	—	FV	—	172	—
	1	FV	RCS	2087	1901
	2	FV	L	2677	2491
	3	FV	L	2750	2564
3D	3	FV	L	1228	1042
	4	FV	HD	740	554
3D	4	FV	HD	150	0
	5	FV	L	329	143
3D	5	FV	L	813	627
	6	FV	LS	733	547
3D	6	FV	LS	266	80
	7	FV	HD	977	791
3D	7	FV	HD	416	230
	8	FV	HD	587	401
3D	8	FV	HD	300	114
Control 2	—	FV	—	200	—

[a]Shows decreased helper activity in 3D-treated human helper extracts assayed in B-type mice. RCS, Reticulum cell sarcoma; L, lymphoma; HD, Hodgkin's disease; LS, lymphosarcoma.

TABLE 10

Induction of Spleen Foci in B-type and N-type mice[a]

Treatment	Indicator	Helper	X	FFU/ml	ΔFFU/ml
			Balb/C		
				Average	
—	FV	—	31.71	4485	////
—	FV	LS	51.67	10,334	5849
3D i.v.	FV	LS	0	0	0
3D i.p.	FV	LS	51.43	10,286	5801
				Average	
—	FV	—	13.14	4485	////
			Swiss		
—	FV	—		Confluent	
3D i.v.	FV	LS		Confluent	
3D i.p.	FV	LS		Confluent	

[a]Shows results of the human helper assay (HHA) in Balb/C (B-type) mice, which repress the indigenous Friend leukemia helper. The same preparation was injected into Swiss mice (N-type), which permit the indigenous helper LLV to function, eliminating the effect of a B-tropic helper. LS, Human lymphosarcoma extract; FV, SFFV(LLV) indicator virus.

In Table 10, 3D was used in two ways: (1) injected intravenously together with the Friend virus in the usual method for expressing the helper systems and (2) separately by the intraperitoneal route. In Table 10, the top section represents results in mice which repress the indigenous helper permitting the human helper to function. Intraperitoneal injection exerted no effect on the assay; however, the simultaneous injection of the helper, the virus, and the 3D combined just prior to injection decreased the Δ value to 0. A value of 5801 Δ FFU/ml was seen with the FV and its human helper, and an inhibition with the 3D. In a pilot study when the same preparations were used in a receptive Swiss mouse in which the LLV (indigenous virus) was effective, the spleens in both treated and untreated were confluent, suggesting that at this dosage the 3D was effective on the human helper, but not on the complete complex when the indigenous helper was functioning. Taken together, these data suggest a possible viral nature of the helper from human malignant tissue, and represent further investigation of the nature of the helper activity.

3-Deazauridine, which inhibits a broad spectrum of nononcogenic viruses, has been shown by Shannon and Westbrook (1973) to interfere with

Gross leukemia virus replication *in vitro*. Gross virus can function as a helper for the deficient Friend virus in the assay. The analogue also inhibits RNA virus-induced cytopathic effects (Shannon *et al.*, 1972).

6. A Correlation of the Degree of Human Splenic Involvement with the Presence of 70S RNA, Heterophile Antigen, and Helper Activity for the Friend Leukemia Virus SFFV

Although the viral etiology of many animal malignancies is well established, it has been difficult to obtain proof of the existence of an oncogenic human counterpart. Recently attention has focused on RNA viruses and C-type particles. Investigators (Priori *et al.*, 1971) have reported a C-type particle in cultured human malignant tissue. Gilden and Oroszlan (1971) state that

> RNA viruses of the C-type appear at the present to be the most likely candidates for hypothetical human cancer viruses in spite of the current lack of a legitimate human isolate. The search for a human cancer virus may have to be modified to a search for a human oncogene or proteins homologous to those of known mammalian C-type viruses. The identification of a potential human oncogene might be possible by cross hybridization between the isolated provirus DNA of other mammalian C-type viruses and human tumor cell DNA.

It is possible that viruses as such might never be found: however, a method which induced viral replication in human cell cultures has been reported by Sarah Stewart (Stewart *et al.*, 1972). She describes the use of IUdR and DMSO as a method of activating a virus in a nonproducing established cell line from a human rhabdomyosarcoma. Others using a similar system (Lowry *et al.*, 1971) have reported the use of IUdR and BUdR in activating murine leukemia virus in a mouse tissue culture which grew as a virus-negative line.

Aronson *et al.* (1971) have reported similar studies with clonal lines of virus-free mouse cells. They feel that their studies provided strong evidence that genetic information can be passed from cell to progeny cell for many generations without being expressed, representing a mammalian system comparable to the lysogenized bacteria.

Such cells showed the reverse transcriptase which Schlom and Spiegelman (1971) have described as evidence for the presence of an oncornavirus. They present a method which permits detection of RNA tumor viruses. Temin (1964; Temin and Mizutani, 1970), Baltimore (1970), and Spiegelman *et al.* (1970) have described the enzyme capable of using the viral RNA template to produce a complementary DNA copy. DNA related to the RNA of mouse leukemia has been demonstrated (Kufe *et al.*, 1972) in human sarcoma. Similar studies with human and mouse mammary tumors have been reported.

Using a special culture system and a cloned cell line from Friend leukemic tissue, Friend has observed that a derepression of leukemic cells can take place, permitting maturation of erythroblastic cells to benzidine-positive normoblasts (Friend *et al.*, 1971). Cultures of Friend tumor cells can be obtained which show virus particles that are noninfective. She has used such cells to immunize mice against the Friend disease.

6.1. Studies Showing the Presence of Heterophile Antigen

Tissue from patients investigated in the human helper studies was also studied for the presence of heterophile antigen by means of absorption of infectious mononucleosis sera (Milgrom *et al.*, 1973). The titer of lysins for bovine red blood cells was significantly reduced by spleen preparations from patients having lymphoreticular diseases (Table 11). The value obtained

TABLE 11

Summary of Studies on Heterophile Antigen[a]

Spleen cells used for absorption		Pathology	Reduction
Lymphomas	HD14	2+	23
	HD28	3+	19
	HD13	4+	18
	HD29	3+	17
	HD19	2+	14
	HD7	+	13
	HD18	±	11
	HD14A	±	7
	HD23-1	±	7
	HD23-2	±	7
	LS11[b]	4+	22
	LS12	3+	17
	L15	±	16
	LS22	±	6
	LS26	+	4
	RCS17	±	12
Neuroblastoma 16		Tumor	7
Seven normal spleens		Normal tissues	1–5

[a]Shows the effect of absorption of infectious mononucleosis sera with spleen cells on lysis of bovine erythrocytes. Values above 10 were considered to be positive. HD, Hodgkin's disease; LS, lymphosarcoma; L, lymphoma; RCS, Reticulum cell sarcoma.

[b]Showed very high degree of focus formation (confluent) in HHA assay and also 70S RNA, identical with spleen 297 in Table 13.

correlated well with the degree of involvement of the spleen, more antigen being present when spleens showed nodules and tumor masses. Control normal human tissue showed no heterophile antigen. Neuroblastomas to date have shown no evidence for the presence of heterophile antigen, although human helper activity was consistently present in all tumors. Subsequent studies have shown that leukemic spleens also demonstrate heterophile antigen. The results seem to indicate that malignant transformation of human lymphocytes might be accompanied by the acquisition of the heterophile antigen. It has been proposed that the formation of antibodies by infectious mononucleosis patients is the result of the appearance of the heterophile antigen, and that the formation of these antibodies might account for the benign character of this disease, which closely resembles malignant hematopoietic diseases, or the malignant character of the human lymphomas, which in our study possess the antigen but not the antibodies. Others have demonstrated heterophile antigen on human lymphoid cells in culture. Most of these cells were infected with the Epstein–Barr virus. Results of our investigation are summarized in Table 11, in which the close correlation of spleen involvement with the heterophile antigen values can be seen. Spleens were studied from patients with Hodgkin's disease, lymphosarcoma, reticulum cell sarcoma, chronic lymphocytic leukemia, and chronic myelogenous leukemia. The most involved spleens also showed the highest HHA. In the spleens tested, LS11 gave highest HHA (confluent foci) and extremely high heterophile antigen values and 70S RNA and DNA homologous to RLV RNA. The spleen identified as LS11 is identified in Table 13 as 297. These pilot studies suggest that spleens from patients with Hodgkin's disease, lymphosarcoma, and reticulum cell sarcoma show evidence of heterophile antigen, while normal spleens and tumors from neuroblastoma patients do not. The findings demonstrated were obtained in collaboration with Drs. Milgrom and Kano. The significance of these studies in relation to helper activity is not known. However, the specimens showing the highest number of tumor cells also showed the highest activity. Some of the Hodgkin's disease spleen biopsies contained visible masses of characteristic cells. The degree of involvement was designated as follows: solid mass of cells, 4+; profuse nodules, 3+; many nodules, 2+; occasional nodule, +; rare or none, ±. Buffy coat cells and spleens from leukemia patients contained large numbers of leukemic cells.

The effects of absorption of infectious mononucleosis sera with pathological cells on lysis of bovine erythrocytes are shown in the right-hand column of Table 11. It has been proposed that formation of heterophile antibodies by patients suffering from infectious mononucleosis is a result of the appearance of a novel antigen, the heterophile antigen, in virus-infected tissues of the patients. Since infectious mononucleosis rather closely resembles malignant blood diseases, it is tempting to speculate that heterophile antibodies may play some role in its benign character.

It cannot be explained at present why patients with lymphoma fail to form heterophile antibodies. It is possible that the mechanism which prevents formation of heterophile antibodies by patients suffering from lymphoma, and possibly also from leukemia, may be of basic importance for the malignant character of these diseases.

6.2. *Attempts to Demonstrate Virus Particles*

Since the nature of the human helper activity was not clearly elucidated by the assay system or by electron microscopic studies, further investigations were undertaken in an attempt to determine whether viruses or virus-related material might be present. The original investigations were undertaken in order to determine whether human sources could contribute a helper function in the standard mouse assay for leukemia viruses (Fig. 8). When spleen cultures showed that this was possible, further studies were done for reverse transcriptase and RNA homologous to the DNA made from Rauscher leukemia virus. Preliminary findings had shown that human neuroblastomas and spleens from patients having lymphoreticular disease

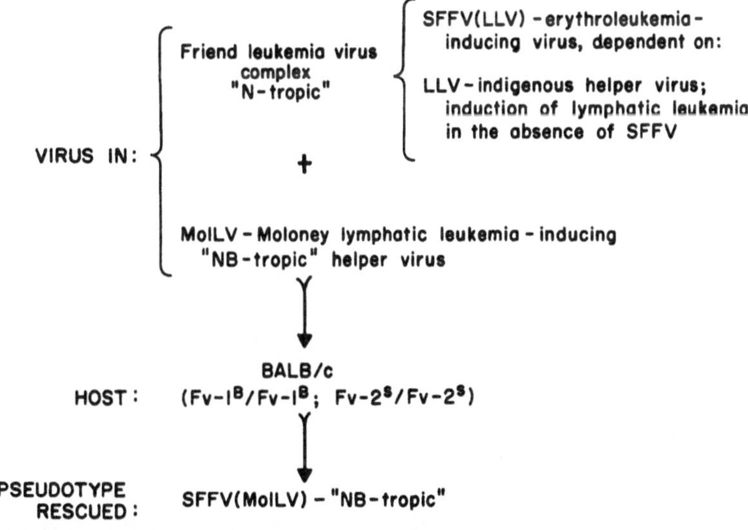

FIG. 8. Scheme for production of human pseudotypes (HuLH) in mice which restrict the indigenous helper LLV. From Eckner (1973).

TABLE 12

Summary of Studies on 70S RNA[a]

Diagnosis	Number	Number positive	Percent positive	Average cpm positive	Average cpm negative	RNase sensitive	Hybridization: With tumor RNA	Hybridization: With normal RNA
Lymphoma[b]	40	31	77.5	353	16	14/14	9/9	0/9
Controls	15	1	7	175	14	—	—	—

[a]Shows a summary of studies on the presence of viral-specific 70S RNA in human lymphomas. Hybridization was possible with tumor RNA, not with normal tissue RNA. Further details are given in Table 13.
[b]35 Hodgkin's disease, 4 lymphosarcoma, 1 lymphoreticular cell sarcoma.

had helper activity and also reverse transcriptase and viral-specific RNA homologous to RLV RNA. A summary of some data from the human lymphomatous spleens and one out of 15 control spleens showed positive values for reverse transcriptase. All of nine lymphomatous spleens positive for human helper activity also contained viral-specific RNA homologous to MLV in hybridization studies. Details of this study are shown in Table 12 and in Tables 13, 14, and 15 from Spiegelman *et al.* (1973).

7. *Characterization of HHA as Either Enhancing or True Helper in Function*

Cells and tissue from 375 different individuals, more than 500 different specimens, have been used for studies related to helper activity, viral-specific 70S RNA, and heterophile antigen and for determination of culture characteristics and establishment. Established lines, as well as the original cultures, and extracts from these sources have been frozen for future reference.

Established lines, in addition to lines from lymphomatous and leukemic spleens, include those derived from neuroblastoma (six lines), melanoma, xeroderma pigmentosum and other skin tumors, and a colon tumor producing fetal antigen (CEA).

A strain was established from adult Fallopian tubes from a pregnant patient treated for malignancy. Skin, lung, kidney, spleen, and thymus strains were established from the fetus. Various tissues from normal embryos were also established for cocultivation studies. All of these lines

TABLE 13

Summary of Studies Testing for Viral-Specific RNA in Human Malignant Spleens

Tumor	cpm 70S	Rxn[a]	RNase sensitivity
	Hodgkin's disease		
1. 249	133	+	+
2. 234	109	+	NT[b]
3. 211	344	+	+
4. Lo	1236	+	+
5. RP	601	+	NT
6. RP (lymph node)	49	+	NT
7. 263	159	+	+
8. 274	112	+	+
9. 218	9	−	
10. 223	474	+	NT
11. 241	92	+	+
12. 270	20	−	
13. 245	619	+	+
14. 252	71	+	NT
15. 227	12	−	
16. 269	622	+	+
17. 218	2956	+	+
18. SZ	221	+	NT
19. 253	42	+	NT
20. 259	42	+	NT
21. 229	48	+	NT
22. 248	125	+	+
23. 281	16	−	
24. 283	16	−	
25. 293	116	+	+
26. 286	59	+	NT
27. 284	13	−	
28. AK	109	+	NT
	Lymphosarcoma		
1. 228	295	+	+
2. 244	42	+	+
3. 297	1581	+	NT
4. 224	185	+	NT
5. 262	24	−	
6. 254	128	+	NT
	Reticulum cell sarcoma		
1. 24405	83	+	+
2. 268	112	+	+
	average = 302 cpm		

From Spiegelman *et al.* (1973).

[a]Twenty-nine of 36 positive (80.6%), 7 of 36 negative (19.4%); average of positives 371 cpm, average of negatives 16 cpm.

[b]Not tested.

TABLE 14

Control Spleens Showing Negative Values for 70S RNA and Reverse Transcriptase

Diagnosis	Specimen	cpm 70S	RXN
1. Glioblastoma	24409	14	–
2. Malignant melanoma	24408	4	–
3. Cancer of pancreas	24407	5	–
4. Multiple myeloma	24404	15	–
5. Cancer of lung	24406	22	–
6. Anemia	24412	19	–
7. Myocardial infarction	24413	4	–
8. Arteriosclerotic heart disease	24414	6	–
9. Hodgkin's disease (noninvolved spleen)	JG	11	–
10. Myocardial infarction	24435	29	–
11. Meningioma	24417	20	–
12. Myocardial infarction	24432	22	–
13. Carcinoma of breast	24415	1	–
14. Hodgkin's disease (noninvolved spleen)	250	25	–
		—	–
		average = 14 cpm	

From Spiegelman *et al.* (1973).

TABLE 15

Hybridization of Lymphoma DNA-^{3}H Product with Tumor pRNA and Normal Spleen pRNA, with RLV and AMV RNA, or with RD-114 and RSV TNA[a]

Lymphoma DNA-^{3}H	Tumor pRNA	Normal spleen pRNA	RLV RNA	AMV RNA
1. 234	+	–	+	–
2. 211	NT	NT	+	–
3. 241	+	–	NT	NT
4. 224	+	–	NT	NT
5. 229	+	–	NT	NT
6. 286	+	–	NT	NT
7. 228	+	–	+[b]	[c]

From Spiegelman *et al.* (1973).

[a]Summarizes the results obtained from annealing reactions of DNA-^{3}H synthesized in human lymphomas with cellular and viral RNAs. The data indicate that human lymphomas contain particles which encapsulate reverse transcriptase and a 70S RNA related to that of RLV and RD-114.

[b]RD-114 RNA.

[c]RSV RNA.

have a normal diploid karyotype. Positive helper extracts from 150 patients are under investigation. Some of these studies are aimed at differentiating between "helper" and "enhancement" effects in spleen focus formation and are being done in collaboration with R. Eckner and E. Mirand (Fjelde *et al.*, 1974*a,b*; Eckner *et al.*, 1974*a*), using human leukemia helper (HuLH).

To investigate the apparent ability of HuLH extracts to provide a virus-like helper function for defective SFFV (Fig. 9), we have used biologically active material prepared from lymphoid tumors and from the spleens of patients with chronic myelogenous leukemia and Hodgkin's disease. Titration of defective SFFV in the presence of excess HuLH material converted the multiple-hit dose–response curve to a one-hit (or near one-hit) pattern. HuLH material was also similar to murine leukemia virus helpers in that it was inactivated after exposure to ultraviolet light or incubation at 56°C for 60 min. In contrast, mycoplasmas and some leukemic tissue extracts which have been shown to enhance the estimated titer of SFFV did not provide a true helper function. Titration of SFFV in the presence of these preparations did not convert the observed multiple-hit dose–response curve to a one-hit pattern. Enhancing agents were not sensitive to ultraviolet inactivation and resisted heat inactivation when incubated at 90°C for 20 min. We conclude from these data and others that 20–30% of all human leukemic tissue extracts tested provide true "helper activity" for SFFV and that this activity is not due to mycoplasma or the presence of other known enhancing agents. Typical curves for helper activity are shown in Fig. 9. We have also investigated the BeWo human

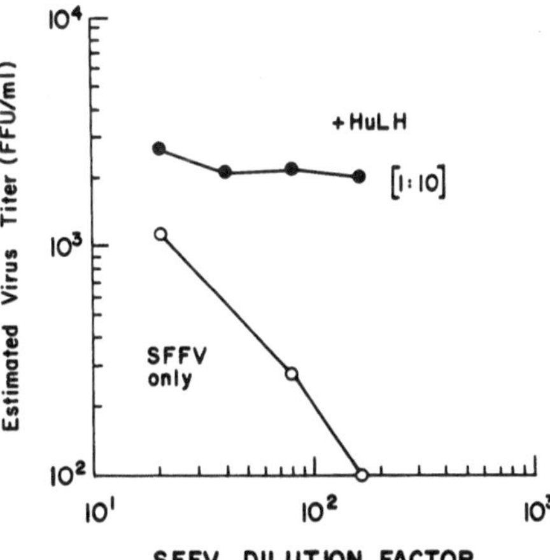

FIG. 9. Types of curves obtained in comparison of an enhancing agent with true helper activity in mice. O, SFFV alone; ●, SFFV with a true human helper, demonstrating a one-hit dose–response curve.

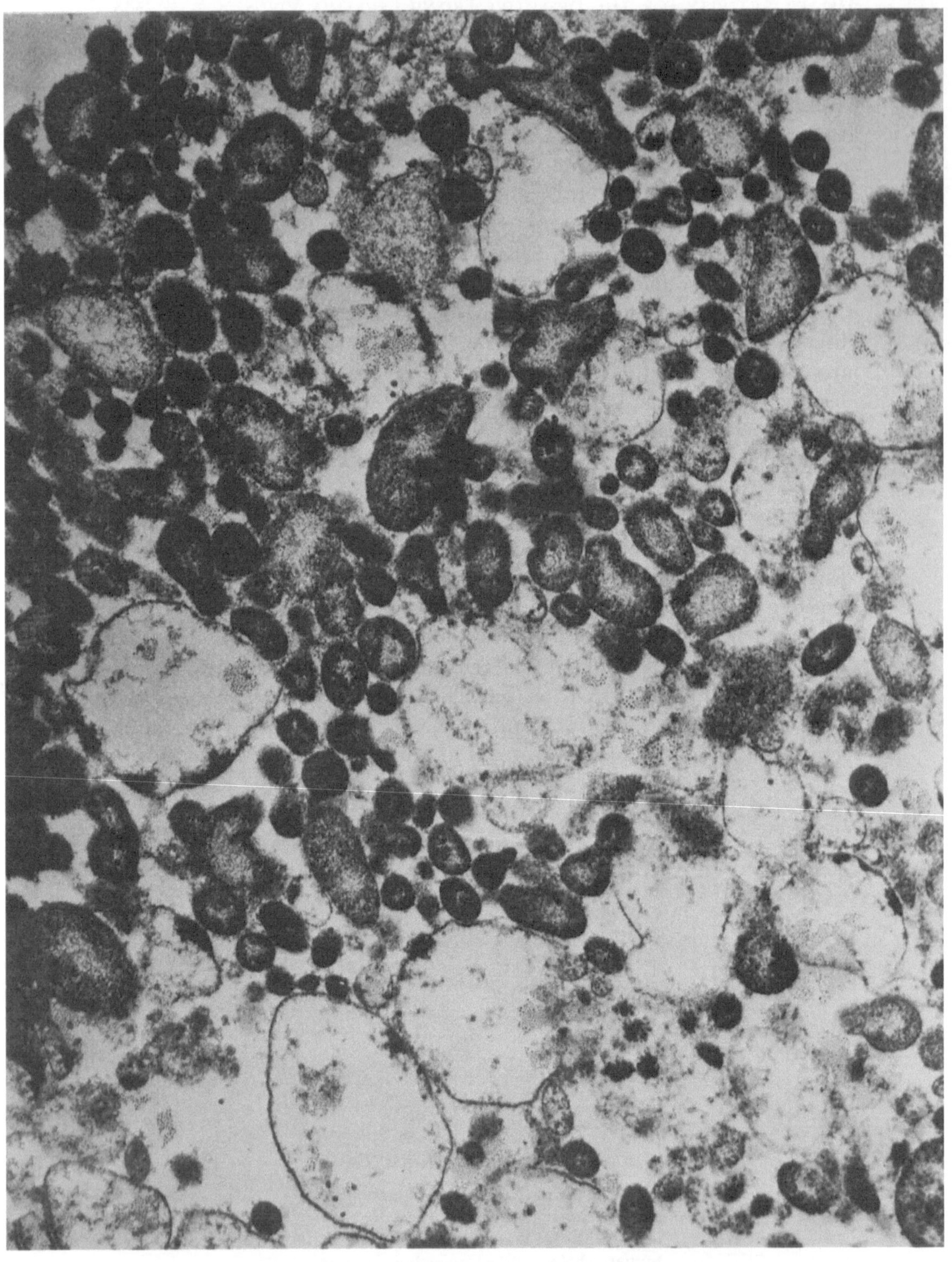

FIG. 10. Electron micrograph of mycoplasma from the BeWo line showing enhancement with the Friend virus.

trophoblast cell line (Patillo and Gey, 1968). Preliminary studies of BeWo showed that enhancing activity for SFFV was present in lines from two different sources. One line heavily contaminated with mycoplasma (Fig. 10) showed a high degree of enhancement with a typical multiple-hit curve. Mycoplasma has been implicated as a source of helper activity (Steeves and Minowada, 1973). The magnitude of the response of Friend virus was enhanced two to five times. A mycoplasma-free line has been tested at one dose and showed fourfold increase in activity; Friend virus alone showed a focus forming value (FFU) of 100 and together with BeWo culture concentrates showed a ΔFFU value of 1000. Impure gonadotropin made from the cultures was investigated and showed no enhancement *in vivo*, no suppression of B-cell function *in vivo* (Jerne technique), and no suppression of T-cell function *in vitro* using Balb/C thymocytes with phytohemagglutinin or concanavalin A. Commercial gonadotropin, however, did show T-cell suppression and some leukemogenic enhancing effect, which is different from the human helper activity described by us for SFFV. We tentatively conclude that an enhancing agent is associated with the trophoblast line which possibly mediates the enhancement effects via the T-cell population (Fjelde *et al.*, 1974).

Friend spleen focus forming virus (SFFV), always present with the indigenous lymphatic leukemia virus (LLV), penetrates the target cell, an erythroid stem cell, and produces the typical erythroblastic disease. Presumably the SFFV can infect the target cell in either a sensitive or a resistant mouse, but is unable to multiply in the (*Fv-1*^{s}) sensitive (N-type) mouse without the help of the N-tropic LLV and is unable to multiply in the (*Fv-1*^{r}) resistant (B-type) mouse without the help of a B- or NB-tropic helper virus. The helper viruses, lymphatic leukemia viruses, when acting alone can cause lymphatic leukemia, possibly infecting a different target cell, i.e., a lymphoblastoid type. Two different lines of hematopoietic cells may be involved, erythrogranulocytic and lymphoid, and two or three different viruses, SFFV, N-tropic helper LLV, and, in resistant mice, also the B-tropic helper virus. An immunodepression, presumably involving B-type lymphocytes, accompanies Friend leukemia (Bennett and Eckner, 1973). It is not known whether the reticuloendothelial cell population includes a common stem cell for both the erythroid and lymphocytic pathways; however, virus particles have been seen in plasma cell types in a morphological study (Koo *et al.*, 1971).

We conclude that a helper virus or helper infectious nucleic acid would increase the number of spleen foci produced by Friend virus in a repressive host and also depress the host's immune competence, and that erythroblastic target stem cells are necessary in order to induce foci. We have obtained evidence of helper effect from human malignant hematopoietic tissues, and

TABLE 16

RPMI 1 × Eagle's Medium Used for Human Helper Assay Studies[a]

L-Arginine (free base)	17.4	Folic acid	1.0
L-Cystine	6.0	*i*-Inositol	1.0
L-Glutamine	146.0	Nicotinic acid	1.0
L-Histidine (free base)	3.2	Pyridoxal HCl	1.4
L-Isoleucine (allo free)	26.2	Riboflavin	0.1
L-Leucine (methionine free)	13.1	Thiamine HCl	1.0
L-Lysine HCl	22.75	Calcium chloride	140.0
L-Methionine	7.5	Disodium phosphate · $7H_2O$	113.4
L-Phenylalanine	8.5	Glucose	2000.0
L-Threonine (allo free)	11.9	Magnesium chloride · $6H_2O$	100.0
L-Tryptophan	2.0	Magnesium sulfate · $7H_2O$	100.0
L-Tyrosine	18.0	Monopotassium phosphate	60.0
L-Valine	11.7	Phenol red	5.0
Biotin	1.0	Potassium chloride	400.0
Calcium pantothenate	1.092	Sodium bicarbonate	350.0
Choline chloride	1.0	Sodium chloride	8000.0

[a]Amounts are given in milligrams per liter.

from neuroblastomas. Virus particles have not been seen in electron microscopic studies; however, the human tissue, including neuroblastoma (unpublished), has shown "reverse transcriptase" and RNA homologous to RLV. Human tumors arising from hematopoietic cells have heterophile antigen, while neuroblastoma cells apparently do not. Apparently the formation of foci would be adversely affected in situations in which (1) virus or infectious nucleic acids were made ineffective, (2) the target cell was unavailable, and (3) the immunocompetence of the host was increased. It seems likely that enzymes, antigens, nutrients, and other cell types could influence the expression of helper activity in addition to the presence of infectious virus or infectious nucleic acids. Amino acids and related enzymes play an important role in both the animal assays for HHA and the tissue culture studies. Many reports and reviews concerning this area of study are available (Muller-Berat, 1969; Astaldi *et al.*, 1969; Sorkin, 1969; Hersh, 1971). Apparently the medium used for most of the HHA studies (Table 16) furnished a suitable environment for the helper activity, which as yet has not been clearly defined. The environment is a critical factor in cell survival. The HHA assay system is currently being used in experiments designed to elucidate the factors concerned in controlling the immunocompetence of the host as well as other factors concerned in the survival of the host. It seems that some of the "enhancing" agents can mimic some of the functions of the true helper system.

8. References

Aronson, S. A., Todaro, G., and Skolnick, E. D., 1971, Induction of murine C-type viruses from clones of virus-free Balb/3T3 cells, *Science* **174:**157.

Astaldi, G., Burgio, G. R., Kre, J., Genova, R., and Astaldi, A. A., Jr., 1969, L-Asparaginase and blastogenesis, *Lancet* **1:**423.

Axelrad, A. A., and Steeves, R. A., 1964, Assay for Friend leukemia virus: Rapid quantitative method based on enumeration of macroscopic spleen foci in mice, *Virology* **24:**513.

Baltimore, D., 1970, RNA-dependent DNA polymerase virions of RNA tumor viruses, *Nature (Lond.)* **226:**120.

Bennett, M., and Eckner, R. J., 1973, Immunobiology of Friend virus leukemia, in: *Virus Tumorigenesis and Immunogenesis* (W. S. Ceglowski and H. Friedman, eds.), pp. 387–414, Academic Press, New York.

Dawson, P. J., and Fieldsteel, A. H., 1969, Inhibition of Friend virus-induced splenomegaly by an associated lymphatic leukemia virus, *Proc. Soc. Exp. Biol. Med.* **132:**898.

Dawson, P. J., and Fieldsteel, A. H., 1973, Genetic factors in chronic remittent Friend disease, *Cancer Res.* **33:**2456.

Eckner, R. J., 1973, Helper-dependent properties of Friend spleen focus-forming virus: Effect of the *Fv-1* gene on the late stages in virus synthesis, *J. Virol.* **12:**523.

Eckner, R. J., Fjelde, A., and Mirand, E. A., 1974*a*, Antigenic alterations of defective Friend virus grown with human leukemic tissue extracts (in press).

Eckner, R. J., Han, T., and Zeigel, R., 1974*b*, Enhancement of friend virus-induced focus-formation by mycoplasmas: Distinction from viral-associated helper activity, in preparation.

Fjelde, A., 1955, Human tumor cells in tissue culture, *Cancer* **8:**845.

Fjelde, A., 1969, The establishment of mammalian cells in culture, in: *Axenic Neomammalian Cell Reactions* (G. Tritsch, ed.), pp. 1–24, Marcel Dekker, New York.

Fjelde, A., 1972, The establishment in culture of permanent lines of hematopoietic cells, and recent virus studies done with haematopoietic cells, in: Proceedings of the 1971 Meeting of the European Tissue Culture Association, *Symp. Biol. Hung.* **14:**37.

Fjelde, A., 1973, Prolonged leukemogenicity in long term cultures of leukemic mouse spleens, session in depth on carcinogenesis *in vitro*, in: Annual Meeting of the Tissue Culture Association, *In Vitro* **8:**432.

Fjelde, A., and Bloch, A., 1973, Inhibition by 3-deazauridine of helper activity provided by human malignant tissue extracts for the induction of leukemia in mice, in: *Abstracts of the Annual Meeting of the American Society for Microbiology* (May), p. 223 (in press).

Fjelde, A., and Freeman, A., 1973, Characteristics of human neuroblastoma, *Proc. Am. Assoc. Cancer Res.* **14:**108 (in press).

Fjelde, A., Steeves, R. A., and Mirand, E. A., 1971. Effect of culture conditions on recovery of helper activity from human leukemic cells, *In Vitro* **6:**376.

Fjelde, A., and Bourke, R., 1974*a*, The presence in the BeWo human trophoblast line of helper or enhancing activity for the Friend spleen focus-forming virus (SFFV), *Proc. Am. Assoc. Cancer Res.* **34:**103 (in press).

Fjelde, A., Eckner, R. J., and Mirand, E. A., 1974*b*, Characterization of helper extracts from human malignant tissue as different from agents able to enhance the expression of Friend spleen focus-forming virus (SFFV), in preparation.

Fjelde, A., Eckner, R. J., and Mirand, E. A., 1974*c*, Partial characterization of helper extracts from leukemic humans (HuLH): Distinction from agents able to enhance the expression of Friend spleen focus-forming virus (SFFV), *In Vitro* **9:**366.

Friend, C., 1957, Cell free transmission in adult Swiss mice of a disease having the characteristics of a leukemia, *J. Exp. Med.* **105:**307.

Friend, C., Scher, W., Holland, J. G., and Sato, T., 1971, Hemoglobin, synthesis in murine virus-induced leukemic cells *in vitro*: Stimulation of erythroid differentiation by dimethylsulfoxide, *Proc. Natl. Acad. Sci.* **68:**378.

Gilden, R. V., and Oroszlan, S., 1971, Structural and immunologic relationships among mammalian C-type viruses, *J. Am. Vet. Med. Assoc.* **158:**1099.

Hersh, E., 1971, Immunosuppression by L-Asparaginase and related enzymes, a review, *Transplantation* **12:**368.

Koo, G. C., Ceglowski, W. S., Higgins, M., and Friedman, H., 1971, Immunosuppression by leukemia viruses. V. Ultra-structural studies of antibody forming spleens of mice infected with Friend leukemia virus, *J. Immunol.* **106:**799.

Kufe, D., Hehlman, R., and Spiegelman, S., 1972, Human sarcomas contain RNA related to the RNA of a mouse leukemia virus, *Science* **175:**182.

Kufe, D., Hehlman, R., Peters, W., Fjelde, A., and Spiegelman, S., 1974, Particles encapsulating RNA-instructed DNA polymerase and high molecular weight virus related RNA in human lymphomas, in preparation.

Lilly, F., 1970, Identification and location of a second gene governing the spleen focus response to Friend leukemia in mice, *J. Natl. Cancer Inst.* **45:**163.

Lilly, F., Boyse, E. A., and Old, L. J., 1964, Genetic basis of susceptibility to viral leukemogenesis, *Lancet* **2:**1207.

Lowy, D. R., Rowe, W. P., Teich, N., and Hartley, J. W., 1971, Murine leukemia virus: High-frequency activation *in vitro* by 5-iododeoxyuridine and 5-bromodeoxyuridine, *Science* **174:**155.

Milgrom, F., Kano, K., and Fjelde, A., 1973. Studies on heterophile antigen in lymphoma and leukemia spleens by means of absorption of infectious mononucleosis sera, *Int. Arch. Allergy Appl. Immunol.* **45:**631.

Mirand, E. A., and Grace, J. T., Jr., 1962, Induction of leukemia in rats with Friend virus, *Virology* **17:**364.

Moore, G. E., Gerner, R. E., Kitamura, H., Minowada, J., and Fjelde, A., 1969, Lymphocytic cell lines derived from normal individuals, in: *Proceedings of the Third Annual Leucocyte Conference* (W. O. Rieke, ed.), pp. 177–198, Appleton-Century-Crofts, New York.

Muller-Berat, C. N., 1969, Immunosuppressive action of L-asparaginase studied by means of the localized haemolysis in gel assay (L.H.G.A.), *Acta Pathol. Microbiol Scand.* **77:**750.

Odaka, T., and Yamamoto, T., 1962, Inheritance of susceptibility to Friend mouse leukemia virus, *Japan J. Exp. Med.* **32:**405.

Patillo, R. A., and Gey, G. O., 1968, The establishment of a cell line of human hormone-synthesizing trophoblastic cells *in vitro, Cancer Res.* **28:**1231.

Peters, W. P., Kufe, D., Schlom, J., Frankel, J. W., Prickett, C. O., Groupé, V., and Spiegelman, S., 1973, Biological and biochemical evidence for an interaction between Marek's disease, herpesvirus and avian leukosis virus *in vivo, Proc. Natl. Acad. Sci.* **70:**3175.

Pincus, T., Hartley, J. W., and Rowe, W. P., 1971, A major genetic locus affecting resistance to infection with murine leukemia viruses. I. Tissue culture studies of naturally-occurring viruses, *J. Exp. Med.* **133:**1219.

Priori, E. S., Dmochowski, L., Myers, B., and Wilbur, J. B., 1971, Constant production of type C–virus particles in a continuous tissue culture derived from pleural effusion cells of a lymphoma patient, *Nature New Biol.* **232:**61.

Rowe, W. P., Humphrey, J. B., and Lilly, F., 1973, A major genetic locus affecting resistance to infection with murine leukemia viruses. III. Assignment of the *Fv-1* locus to linkage group VIII of the mouse, *J. Exp. Med.* **137:**850.

Schlom, J., and Spiegelman, S., 1971, Simultaneous detection of reverse transcriptase and high molecular weight RNA unique to oncogenic RNA viruses, *Science* **174:**840.

Shannon, W. M., and Westbrook, L., 1973, Inhibition of Gross leukemia virus replication by 3-deazauridine, *Proc. Am. Assoc. Cancer Res.* **14:**28.

Shannon, W. M., Arnett, G., and Schabel, F. M., 1972, 3-Deazauridine: Inhibition of ribonucleic acid virus-induced cytopathogenic effects *in vitro, Antimicrob. Agents Chemother.* **2:**159.

Simberkoff, M. S., Thorbecke, G. J., and Thomas, L., 1969, Studies of PPLO infection. V. Inhibition of lymphocyte mitosis and antibody formation by mycoplasma extracts, *J. Exp. Med.* **129:**1163.

Sorkin. E., 1969, *The Immune Response and Its Suppression*, S. Karger, Basel.

Spiegelman, S., Burny, A., Das, M. R., Keydar, J., Schlom, J., Travnicek, M., and Watson, K., 1970, DNA-directed DNA polymerase activity in oncogenic RNA viruses, *Nature (Lond.)* **227:**1029.

Spiegelman, S., Kufe, D., Hehlmann, R., and Peters, W. P., 1973, Evidence for RNA tumor viruses in human lymphomas including Burkitt's disease, *Cancer Res.* **33:**1515.

Steeves, R. A., and Minowada, J., 1973, Mycoplasmas provide helper activity for Friend spleen focus-forming virus in mice, *Proc. Am. Assoc. Cancer Res.* **14:**71.

Steeves, R. A., Fjelde, A., and Mirand, E. A., 1971*a*, Specificity of helper activity for Friend spleen focus-forming virus, *Proc. Am. Assoc. Cancer Res.* **12:**57.

Steeves, R. A., Fjelde, A., and Mirand E. A., 1971*b*, Demonstration of helper activity with human leukemic tissue extracts, in: *Comparative Research Leukemia Symposium*, Padua, Italy, September.

Steeves, R. A., Fjelde, A., and Mirand, E. A., 1971*c*, Helper activity of human leukemic tissue extracts for leukemia virus expression in mice, *Proc. Natl. Acad. Sci.* **68:**2391.

Stewart, S. E., Kasnia, G., Draycott, C., and Ben, T., 1972, Activation of viruses in human tumors by 5-iododeoxyuridine and dimethylsulfide, *Science* **175:**198.

Temin, H. M., 1964, Nature of the provirus of Rous sarcoma, *Natl. Cancer Inst. Monogr.* **7:**557.

Temin, H. M., and Mizutani, S., 1970, RNA-dependent DNA polymerase in virions of Rous sarcoma virus, *Nature (Lond.)* **226:**1211.

Thomson, S., 1969, An assay method for target cells of Friend spleen focus-forming virus, *Proc. Am. Assoc. Cancer Res.* **10:**93.

Trentin, J. J., Yabe, Y., and Taylor, G., 1962, The quest for human cancer viruses, *Science* **137:**835.

Wang, M. C., and Bloch, A., 1972, Studies on the mode of action of 3-deazapyrimidines. I. Metabolism of 3-deazauridine and 3-deazacytidine in microbial and tumor cells, *Biochem. Pharmacol.* **21:**1063.

Index